THE HEALTH HUMANITIES IN GERMAN STUDIES

THE HEALTH HUMANITIES IN GERMAN STUDIES

Edited by Stephanie M. Hilger

BLOOMSBURY ACADEMIC
LONDON • NEW YORK • OXFORD • NEW DELHI • SYDNEY

BLOOMSBURY ACADEMIC
Bloomsbury Publishing Plc
50 Bedford Square, London, WC1B 3DP, UK
1385 Broadway, New York, NY 10018, USA
29 Earlsfort Terrace, Dublin 2, Ireland

BLOOMSBURY, BLOOMSBURY ACADEMIC and the Diana logo
are trademarks of Bloomsbury Publishing Plc

First published in Great Britain 2024

Cover design: Rebecca Heselton
Cover image © andipantz / iStock

A catalog record for this book is available from the British Library.

Library of Congress Cataloging-in-Publication Data
Names: Hilger, Stephanie M. (Stephanie Mathilde), editor.
Title: The health humanities in German studies / edited by Stephanie Hilger, University of Illinois Urbana-Champaign, USA.
Description: London ; New York : Bloomsbury Academic, 2024. | Series: Bloomsbury handbooks | Includes bibliographical references and index.
Identifiers: LCCN 2023052673 (print) | LCCN 2023052674 (ebook) | ISBN 9781350296183 (hardback) | ISBN 9781350296190 (paperback) | ISBN 9781350296206 (pdf) | ISBN 9781350296213 (ebook)
Subjects: LCSH: Medicine and the humanities–Germany. | Literature and medicine–Germany. | Medicine–Germany–Philosophy.
Classification: LCC R702 .H434 2024 (print) | LCC R702 (ebook) | DDC 610.943–dc23/eng/20240124
LC record available at https://lccn.loc.gov/2023052673
LC ebook record available at https://lccn.loc.gov/2023052674

ISBN: HB: 978-1-3502-9618-3
ePDF: 978-1-3502-9620-6
eBook: 978-1-3502-9621-3

Typeset by Integra Software Services Pvt. Ltd.

To find out more about our authors and books visit www.bloomsbury.com and sign up for our newsletters.

CONTENTS

ILLUSTRATIONS

CONTRIBUTORS

Katharina Bahlmann is Research Associate at the Johannes Gutenberg University Mainz. She studied philosophy and art history, and received her PhD with a study on Arthur C. Danto and the end of art. She has taught philosophy of perception and art theory at several German art schools. At Mainz University, she is leading a research project on the development of rare disciplines in the German higher education system. Since 2016, Katharina Bahlmann has organized a number of workshops in the field of Medical Humanities, together with Anita Wohlmann, focusing on questions of perception and perspective.

Heike Bartel is Professor in German Studies and Health Humanities at the University of Nottingham. She leads interdisciplinary research projects at the interface of arts & humanities and health sciences, with particular focus on under-researched and marginal groups. She has worked extensively in the field of eating disorders, trauma, and gender-based violence. Her recent publications include the monograph *Men Writing Eating Disorders: Autobiographical Writing and Illness Experience in English and German Narratives* (2020) and the award-winning (*THE* 2021) arts-based training tool for healthcare professionals "Consider Eating Disorders in Men" accredited by the Royal College of General Practitioners. https://www.nottingham.ac.uk/research/groups/hungry-for-words.

Eleoma Bodammer is Reader in German at the University of Edinburgh. She has published on German writers 1750–1830, in particular on Goethe, Schiller, Hoffmann, and Stolberg, and in the fields of disability in German literature and Anglo-German cultural exchange. She is the co-editor of *Disability in German Literature, Film, and Theater* (2010).

Alec Cattell is Associate Director of the Teaching, Learning, and Professional Development Center and Director of the Ethics in Teaching & Learning Program at Texas Tech University. He holds a PhD in German from the University of Waterloo. He also teaches German language, literature, film, and cultures of the German-speaking world in the Department of Classical & Modern Languages & Literatures at Texas Tech. His scholarship includes publications on representations of disability, disability rhetorics, and disability aesthetics in German literature. He has also published on language pedagogy and curriculum design.

Necia Chronister is Professor of German at Kansas State University. Her research centers on contemporary literature, women writers, discourses of unification, and embodiment. She has published on Jenny Erpenbeck, Judith Hermann, Antje Rávik Strubel, and Juli Zeh, among other contemporary authors, in both academic venues and the literary magazine *World Literature Today*. Her monograph, *Domestic Disputes: Examining Discourses of Home and Property in the Former East Germany*, was published in 2021.

Benjamin R. Davis, Academic Specialist in the Department of Linguistics, Languages, and Cultures at Michigan State University, earned his PhD in German with graduate certification in Women, Gender, and Sexuality Studies from Washington University in St. Louis (2014). Prior to coming to Michigan State, he served as Visiting Assistant Professor of German at UNC-Greensboro. His research focuses on the representation of gendered resistance, “queer” subjectivities, and political possibilities in Early Modern German literature and culture. His broad teaching and service record includes Cultural Studies and German courses at all levels, academic advising, curriculum development, program direction, and supporting education abroad.

Stefani Engelstein is Professor of German Studies and of Gender, Sexuality, and Feminist Studies at Duke University. Her work addresses German and British literature and science, aesthetics, gender, political theory, and the history of knowledge. She is the author of *Sibling Action: The Genealogical Structure of Modernity* and of *Anxious Anatomy: The Conception of the Human Form in Literary and Naturalist Discourse*. Her current book project is entitled *The Opposite Sex*. She has been the recipient of Guggenheim, NEH, Humboldt, and Fulbright Fellowships and is a frequent Visiting Scholar at the Leibniz Center for Literary and Cultural Research, Berlin.

Katharina Fürholzer has been a postdoc in the department “Aging of Individuals and Society,” University of Rostock, since 2022. Prior to that, she worked, among others, at the Institute for the History, Philosophy and Ethics of Medicine, Ulm University, and spent three years as a postdoctoral visiting scholar at the Program of Comparative Literature & Literary Theory, University of Pennsylvania. Her research is grounded in the Medical Humanities, with a particular interest in correlations between medical and literary ethics. Current focuses include poetic approaches to aphasia as well as ethics and aesthetics in the context of postmortal dignity.

Mariacarla Gadebusch Bondio has led the Institute for the Medical Humanities at the University of Bonn since 2017. Following her studies in philosophy, history of science (University of Milan), history of medicine, and Romantic literature (Freie Universität

Berlin), she began her scientific career in history and ethics of medicine at the University of Greifswald. From 2011 to 2017, she headed the Institute for History and Ethics of Medicine at the Technical University of Munich. Her main research interests lie in the intersections between medicine and philosophy and include topics such as norm and deviance in medical discourses, medical fallibility, evidence practices, patient narratives, ethics and cancer, and ethical-cultural challenges of gender-sensitive issues in medicine.

Heidi Hausse is Assistant Professor of History at Auburn University. Her research examines the intersections of culture, medicine, and technology in the German-speaking lands of early modern Europe. Her book, *The Malleable Body: Surgeons, Artisans and Amputees in Early Modern Germany*, examines surgical treatises and prosthetic artifacts to uncover a transformation in the practices and attitudes surrounding surgical and artificial intervention in the body. Her work on surgery and prosthetic technology has appeared in *The Sixteenth Century Journal* and *Technology and Culture*. She is currently collaborating with a mechanical engineer to develop a 3D-printed prototype of a sixteenth-century mechanical hand.

Katja Herges is Assistant Professor at the Center for Interdisciplinary Research into Health and Illness at the University of Wrocław. Previously, she worked in medical ethics and clinical psychiatry. In addition to her medical degree, she has earned a PhD in German studies and feminist theory and research from the University of California, Davis. Her academic interests include German life writing and contemporary literature, visual cultures of illness, gender and illness, and mental health. Her edited volume *Contested Selves: Life Writing and German Culture* (together with Elisabeth Krimmer) was published in 2021.

Stephanie M. Hilger is Professor of Comparative Literature and German at the University of Illinois at Urbana-Champaign, where she also holds an appointment in the Carle Illinois College of Medicine. Her research puts the study of eighteenth-century European culture into dialogue with the Health Humanities. She is the author of *Women Write Back* (2009) and *Gender and Genre* (2014). She has also edited *New Directions in Literature and Medicine Studies* (2017) and co-edited *Bodies in Transition in the Health Humanities* (2019) and *The Early History of Embodied Cognition* (2015). She is currently completing a book manuscript, *Medicalizing Difference: The Eighteenth-Century Construction of the "Hermaphrodite"* Her new research explores the work of physician-poets in the context of increasing disciplinary specialization in the eighteenth century.

Davina Höll is Assistant Professor at the Obama Institute for Transnational American Studies at Mainz University. Her dissertation, *Das Gespenst der Pandemie,* dealt with the politics and poetics of cholera at the interface of literary studies and medical history. As a post-doctoral researcher in the EXC 2124 "Controlling Microbes to Fight Infections" at Tübingen University, she investigated microbiome research's historical, epistemological, ethical, and cultural implications. In her current work on More-Than-Human conceptualizations in the face of anthropocentric crisis, she focuses on connections between knowledge production and literature, art and science, and popular culture, especially at the intersection of Medical and Environmental Humanities.

Joela Jacobs is Assistant Professor of German Studies at the University of Arizona and the founder of the Literary and Cultural Plant Studies Network (see plants.arizona.edu). Her research and publications focus on nineteenth- to twenty-first-century German literature and film, Plant Studies, Animal Studies, Environmental Humanities, Jewish Studies, the History of Sexuality, and the History of Science. She is currently completing a monograph about the nonhuman and marginalized human figures in literary grotesques (*Grotesken*) from Panizza to Kafka. With Dr. Nike Thurn, she hosted a virtual event series on the centenary of Panizza's death (see panizza.arizona.edu).

Gabi Kathöfer is Associate Professor of German at the University of Denver. She analyzes German settler colonialism in Brazil at the intersection of medical, racial, and cultural definitions of (dis-)ability. Nineteenth-century Western understanding of abled-bodiedness centered on concepts of productivity, autonomy, and agency, offering a normative framework for Germans' self-definition as a country of work. However, it also led to the exclusion of presumed disabled and disposable bodies, in the German states as well as in the context of German settlements abroad. Focusing on German national identity construction as a "fit body" (body politic) in opposition to deviant "Others," Kathöfer examines German settlements as Indigenous spaces and places in which Indigenous lives and knowledges were deemed worthless. Moreover, Kathöfer calls for bridges not only between Western Sciences and Humanities Studies, but also between Western and Non-Western knowledges, especially Indigenous epistemologies, to build transdisciplinary relationships and relational frameworks for an ecology of knowledges and toward global cognitive justice.

Bastian Lasse received his BA in German Studies, with minors in History and Pedagogy (2015), and his MA in Literary Studies (2018) at Bielefeld University. He has been pursuing his PhD in Harvard's Department of Germanic Languages and Literatures since 2018. His publications on topics related to narratology and postcolonial and gender studies focus on texts from German realism, modernism, and late modernism in a postmodern world. His dissertation engages with narratives by Wilhelm Raabe, Theodor Fontane, as well as Alfred Döblin and W.G. Sebald in order to carve out a narratology of forgetting.

Priscilla Layne is Professor of German and Adjunct Associate Professor of African Diaspora Studies at the University of North Carolina at Chapel Hill. Her book, *White Rebels in Black: German Appropriation of Black Popular Culture*, was published in 2018. She has also published essays on Turkish German culture, translation, punk, and film. She recently translated Olivia Wenzel's debut novel, *1000 Coils of Fear*, from German into English. She is currently finishing a manuscript on Afro German Afrofuturism and a critical guide to Rainer Maria Fassbinder's film *The Marriage of Maria Braun*.

Heikki Lempa is Priscilla Payne Hurd Chair in the Arts and Humanities and Professor of Modern European and German History at Moravian University. He is the author of *Spaces of Honor: Making German Civil Society, 1700–1914* (2021), *Beyond the Gymnasium: Educating the Middle-Class Bodies in Classical Germany* (2007), and *Bildung der Triebe. Der deutsche*

Philanthropismus (1768–1788) (1993). He is also a co-editor of *Feelings Materialized* (2020) and *Staging Authority* (2022) and currently working on a book-length monograph on *The Bodies of the Others: German Sports, Medicine, and Dance in a Global Context, 1700–1914.*

Brian McInnis is Senior Lecturer in German at Christopher Newport University. His research focuses on sensibility and neurology in the eighteenth century and on memory. He studies the philosophy, medical function, and representation of emotion and sensibility in the eighteenth century and the role of memory in twentieth- and twenty-first-century literature. He is currently working on additional studies of Johann August Unzer's magazine *Der Arzt: Eine medicinische Wochenschrift.*

Madalina Meirosu is Assistant Professor of Romanian Studies in the School of International Letters and Cultures at Arizona State University in Tempe. Meirosu has presented her research on race, disability, gender, illness and the environment, and fictional representations of artificial intelligence at national and international conferences. Her published work includes contributions to the Romanian Academy's German-Romanian Dictionary, translations from German into Romanian and English, and articles on migration and race, gender, and illness. She has published in the *Journal for Narrative Inquiry in Bioethics* and has several new articles forthcoming, including an accepted submission to *Literature and Medicine.*

Elizabeth "Biz" Nijdam is Assistant Professor in the Department of Central, Eastern, and Northern European Studies at the University of British Columbia in Vancouver, Canada, where she lives and works on the traditional, ancestral, and unceded territories of Musqueam, Squamish, and Tsleil-Waututh Nations. She is currently completing her book manuscript *Graphic Historiography: Teaching History & Memory through Comics and Graphic Novels.* Biz's research and teaching interests include comics studies, migration and refugee studies, feminist methodologies in the graphic arts, and intersections between Indigenous studies and German and European studies. Biz also sits on the Executive Committee of the International Comic Arts Forum and the Executive Board of the Comics Studies Society.

Anke Pinkert is Associate Professor of German, Cinema & Media Studies, and Conrad Humanities Scholar in the College of Liberal Arts & Sciences at the University of Illinois Urbana-Champaign. She is the author of *Film and Memory in East Germany* (2008) and has published widely on postwar, Post-Holocaust memory, post-communist culture, and more recently on the bio-politics of mass incarceration. Her monograph, *Remembering 1989: Future Archives of Public Protest*, is forthcoming with University of Chicago Press.

Marina Rauchenbacher is a postdoctoral researcher in the Department of German Studies, University of Vienna. Together with Susanne Hochreiter and Katharina Serles, she has been working on their joint research project *Visualities of Gender in German-Language Comics* (funded by the Austrian Science Fund) since 2019. She is also associated with the Viennese historical-critical edition of Arthur Schnitzler's early works at the Austrian Academy of Sciences. Her research focuses on German-language literature, comics, visual culture studies, and gender theory. She has co-founded the Austrian Association for the Research and Promotion of Comics (OeGeC) and is board member of aka—Arbeitskeis Kulturanalyse. https://www.univie.ac.at/germanistik/marina-rauchenbacher/.

Julia Roos is Associate Professor of History at Indiana University, Bloomington. Her research focuses on twentieth-century Germany, gender, sexuality, and race. She is the author of *Weimar Through the Lens of Gender: Prostitution Reform, Woman's Emancipation, and German Democracy, 1919–1933* (2010), and of numerous articles and book chapters on the history of prostitution, propaganda, and biracial German "occupation children." She currently is completing a book manuscript entitled *(Re)Making Race in Germany: Biracial "Occupation Children," 1920–1960*. The study explores continuities and realignments in twentieth-century German racial discourse over Germans of color and the black "Other."

Allison Schmidt is a Lecturer in International Relations at the University of Pennsylvania. She has published articles in the *Journal of Migration History* and *Central European History*. She is currently working on her book manuscript, based on her dissertation, "Crossing Germany: Eastern European Transmigrants and Saxon State Surveillance, 1880–1924."

Amanda Sheffer directs the German and European Studies programs at the Catholic University of America in Washington, DC. She has chaired and serves on the American Association of Teachers of German (AATG) special interest group focusing on Austria, Switzerland, and Liechtenstein and received the national FL-A-CH award for her teaching contributions on Austria in 2017. Her research focuses on the literary doctor-patient relationship at 1900.

Nicole Thesz is Professor of German at Miami University in Oxford, Ohio. Her monograph *The Communicative Event in the Works of Günter Grass* appeared in 2018. She has written articles and book chapters on Grass, GDR literature, German film, fairy tale, ecocriticism, as well as on medicine and literature. Currently, she is writing a monograph on nature and the non-human in German folk and literary fairy tales.

Anne Waldschmidt is Professor of Sociology and Politics of Rehabilitation, Disability Studies, and Director of the International Research Unit in Disability Studies (iDiS) at the University of Cologne. She was a visiting professor at the universities of Leeds, Stockholm, and Vienna. From 2018 to 2023, she was a member of the Scientific Committee of the European Union Agency for Fundamental Rights. Her research focuses on political representation and participation of persons with disabilities, disability rights movements, personal autonomy and independent living, European disability policies, disability history, social theory of disability, sociology of knowledge, and discourse analysis.

Anita Wohlmann is Associate Professor in Contemporary Anglophone Literature at the University of Southern Denmark, Odense, where she is a member of the Center for Uses of Literature and the Center for American Studies. She has been involved in Narrative Medicine since 2015 and coordinates the German Network for Narrative Medicine as well as the teaching of Narrative Medicine in Odense (together with Cindie Aaen Maagaard). Anita's research focuses on metaphors, stereotypes, age and aging, illness narratives, and life writing. Her newest monograph is *Metaphor in Illness Writing: Battle and Fight Reused* (2022).

FOREWORD

Boundaries and Interdisciplines: Where Health Humanities Meets Literature & Science in German Studies

STEFANI ENGELSTEIN

It is part of the fecundity of interdisciplinary fields that they evade definition, and both the field of Health Humanities and of Literature and Science fit this expectation. If any one such interdisciplinary field is already indistinct in its outlines, the task of viewing it in the context of a contiguous, equally slippery field might appear a hopelessly unproductive endeavor. However, looking more closely at the ways in which interdisciplines come to define themselves in practice can prove productive far beyond the particular fields in question. In this case, each discipline offers a challenge to the other that, taken together, also push us to articulate more clearly the value of the humanities in general.

Calls for interdisciplinarity go back decades now, and yet we rarely pause to ask what we mean when we call a field interdisciplinary. Are we referring to a collaboration between scholars who each represent a traditional discipline? To an individual research program that crafts an approach incorporating elements of methods that traditionally belong to two distinct disciplines? To an investigation that sets syncretic goals, merging the generally divergent expected outcomes of two disciplines? Or rather to fields that use the methodology of one discipline to approach topics and questions associated with another? Is it the audience that is presumed to include multiple disciplines? While all of these undertakings may fit our understanding of interdisciplinarity, each leads to a fundamentally different kind of task and the answers to these questions may distinguish fields whose object of inquiry is quite proximate.

With this background in mind, my goal here is to explore the relationship between two vibrant fields that would seem necessarily to lie adjacent to each other or to intersect. If we take science to incorporate aspects of medicine, and literary studies to belong to the humanities, the juxtaposition of the two fields takes on the appearance of a strange chiasm, in which one leg of each is, at least in part, a subdivision of the corresponding half of a leg of the other. And indeed, there are as a result overlaps in the objects and topics explored by both fields. As we will see, however, they have been characterized by different approaches and in divergent relationships to the question of goals. Meanwhile, within German Studies, the two fields are less distinct from each other than elsewhere, demonstrating a porousness or promiscuity in questions, methods, and goals that might hold potential for thinking expansively about methods and goals across the humanities, indeed, may push us to think about the very relationship of the humanities to goals, to teleology.

The Medical Humanities as a named field had its simultaneous beginnings in humanities departments and in medical education in the US as early as the 1970s, arising from a concern that specialization and an emphasis on the scientific aspect of medicine were reducing the ability of new physicians to engage empathetically and with personal attention to their patients.[1] The "primal scene" of medical humanities, as Anne Whitehead and Angela Woods have noted, is therefore the "clinical encounter between the doctor and the patient" (2016, 2). The first journals of the field included not only the *Journal of Medical Humanities*, with its first issue published in 1980, but also *Literature and Medicine*, founded just two years later, reflecting the centrality of narratives of illness to the new field. As Stephanie Hilger notes, "the majority of these interdisciplinary ventures originated in literature departments" (2021, 301). The Medical Humanities were thus from the beginning in an unusual position, as the majority of its practitioners were trained in the humanities and based primarily in literature departments. Their audience, however, was diverse, as they programmatically engaged with students in medical schools or, with increasing frequency, with undergraduates with medical professional aspirations. Research was however often directed to other researchers within the medical humanities field. Moreover, faculty and administrators on both sides of the institutional divide generally understood the goals of the field as centered on improving the way that doctors interacted with their patients. While both ethics and art always had a place within Medical Humanities, its center of gravity was occupied by fiction, viewed as a force that could humanize readers through mechanisms of identification that were assumed to elicit empathy. Fiction about patients facing and managing illness and other medical conditions, navigating healthcare systems, and coming to terms with suffering therefore held center stage. Rita Charon's concept of "narrative medicine" has also shaped the field significantly by focusing on the way that narrativizing defines the patient for the doctor whether consciously or not. When broadened appropriately and intentionally, she argues, such narrative formation can both inculcate empathy in the physician and enable more effective treatment through a more wholistic understanding of the patient's situation and symptoms. While these methods lie within the humanities, they tend toward one particular form of affect studies, while the goals are atypical for the humanities, conforming more closely to the better health outcomes envisioned by the medical profession.

Recently, however, newer developments have enlarged the original scope of the Medical Humanities. Allied fields like the Health Humanities have arisen that extend the claims of benefits derived from humanities and arts practices to patients, while under the new designation of Critical Medical Humanities, scholars have moved beyond the interpersonal relationship of medical practitioner and patient. Their research agenda now includes investigating dynamics and practices in the laboratory, as well as analyzing health policy while posing ethical questions. In addition, the introduction of the new term marks a shift within the field of literature and medicine from a focus on narrative action or plot toward an inclusion of language, structure, and visual elements (Whitehead and Woods 2016, 3–5). Graphic medical fiction and the interaction of text and image it entails have received a great deal of recent attention. Anne Whitehead and Angela Woods, as well as Alan Bleakley, have recently interrogated the definition of empathy and questioned its standing as the most appropriate or most significant value to be sought in an engagement with the humanities. Bleakley has instead embraced and adapted Jacques Rancière's theory of aesthetics as an avenue to reshape the sensible through disruptive disjunctures that he calls dissensus, an idea to which we will return.

The tendencies of Health Humanities have therefore shifted in the recent past in a direction contrary to that of the literary fields in general; after a generation of turning away from such phenomenological responses, a newly named post-critical turn in literary studies has begun to welcome affect, particularly identification and empathy, as a recognized and significant part of the literary experience. Practitioners such as Rita Felski, most prominently, but also Martha Nussbaum and Elizabeth Anker have explored the relationship of such emotion not only to pleasure in the reading process, but also to political benefits for democratic sensibilities. This return to an affective approach has belatedly aligned certain currents within the broader field with some of the earlier tendencies of Medical Humanities, just at a moment when segments of Health Humanities have, in turn, embraced the critical tendencies away from which post-critical approaches have turned. In the process, one might argue, the Health Humanities has expanded the ways in which it claims interdisciplinarity, engaging with the methods, problems, and questions of multiple disciplines and beginning to examine the past as well as the present.[2] As a result, the trajectory of Health Humanities is bringing it closer to that of Literature and Science in methodology, as Literature and Science has remained largely committed to the critical approaches that marked its beginning. However, unlike Health Humanities, Literature and Science has remained circumspect about articulating goals beyond the specifics of any particular research findings.

Just as literary criticism that engages with disease within literary texts is much older than the named field of Medical Humanities, criticism that analyses the role of science within literature is older than the contemporary field of Literature and Science. While the field as currently practiced derives from the same period in which the Medical Humanities arose, namely the early to mid-1980s, the conjoined terms as an object of inquiry can be traced back at least to an MLA panel in 1938 that focused on science and literature of the early eighteenth century.[3] Early investigations of the relationship between science and literature had tended to envision literature as reacting to—and generally positioning itself against—scientific practices and methods. A new approach—which Steven Meyer goes so far as to call a new field under the same name (Meyer 2018, 4)—arose in the 1980s. The contemporary interdisciplinary field largely continues to follow principles summarized by George Levine in the preface to the volume by which he inaugurated the University of Wisconsin Press series Science & Literature in 1987. He claimed "that science and literature are two alternative but related expressions of a culture's values, assumptions, and intellectual frameworks; second, that understanding science in its relation to culture and literature requires some understanding not only of its own internal processes, but of the pressures upon it exercised by social, political, aesthetic, psychological, and biographical forces; third, that the idea of 'influence' of one upon the other must work both ways" (Levine 1987, vii). Levine thereby countered C.P. Snow's enduring concept of the two cultures with insistence on a single complex and interconnected culture. A decade later, Elinor Shaffer would instead speculate on the now-established field of Literature and Science as a Third Culture, a concept which Snow had evoked in a later edition of his work as a possible avenue to mediate between the sciences and humanities (Snow 1963; Shaffer 1998, 2). Shaffer adds to Levine's reciprocity the insight that literary critical methods of analysis and interpretation enable a direct critical engagement with scientific discourse, on the one hand, and also reveal a critique within works of literature that itself counters scientific claims to be the sole arbitrator of reality (1963, esp. 5, 11). The role of literature specifically in such studies is therefore at least twofold. First, it is perceived as a critical form in its own right that engages with social, psychological, ethical, and epistemological preconditions, assumptions, consequences, and contradictions. In addition, its techniques, i.e. its aesthetic form, afford ways of thinking, perceiving, and understanding that are multivalent and non-reductionist. While belied by the general term for this field, there was from the beginning an allied emphasis on visual studies alongside literature, both in the form of art criticism and through analyses of scientific illustrations.

While the interests of early Medical Humanities lay largely in the present, and have only recently begun to expand to other eras, early forays into Literature and Science frequently focused on the period around 1800 across Europe and the United States, and this period has remained a center of gravity within the field. In English departments, work on Darwin by Levine and Gillian Beer in the 1980s created an additional ongoing concentration of works in Literature and Science on the mid- to late-nineteenth-century. While the Health Humanities illuminates the human relationships designated by many physicians as the "softer" side of medical practice, Literature and Science looked from the beginning at the methods and practices by which truth claims were made, and did so while rendering visible the human interactions—in labs and in governments, in funding mechanisms, in scientific societies and in society in general—that were inextricable from the practices of building consensus for such truth claims, thus confounding the distinction of "hard" and "soft." While the Health Humanities remains focused on human experiences and practices, Literature and Science has also explored human investigations of the empirical world beyond humans, including animals and plants as well as geology and cosmology.

In spite of these distinctions, the two fields often wander through similar terrain. As mentioned above, Rita Charon, in *Narrative Medicine: Honoring the Stories of Illness* (2006), advocates for patients by striving to make doctors aware of the way their interactions with patients build narratives that affect the conclusions they draw. The more such narratives are attuned to details, the more humanizing the interaction, the more accurate the diagnosis, and the better medicine can serve to alleviate suffering and disease, she urges. In an equally foundational work of Literature and Science, *Sexual Visions: Images of Gender in Science and Medicine between the Eighteenth and Twentieth Centuries* (1989), Ludmilla Jordanova is similarly interested in the discursive practices of medicine. For Jordanova, medicine involves interpersonal interactions and therapeutics, but also an interest in experimental practice and the work of other naturalists and scientists investigating living organisms (1989, 17). The "images" of her title emerge not only visually, but also in "literature, political theory, art, natural history, medicine, law, social commentary and so on" (1989, 2). Jordanova's target here, the construction of sex and gender in culture, works through science and medicine as disciplines of growing institutional and cultural significance in the period she explores. Narrative for Jordanova is not limited to literature, however. In an article entitled "Writing Medical Identities 1780–1820" (1998), Jordanova analyzed the predilection of physicians to publish narrative histories of medicine that allowed them to advocate for certain practices through offering positive and negative critiques of past practitioners and by projecting a desired future of the profession. Both Charon and Jordanova thus view narrative practice among physicians as important sites for analysis. The former, however, is focused on contemporary interactions in the hope of making doctors conscious of their own behavior so that they can direct their methods toward grasping patients more fully, and thus treat them more comprehensively. The latter, on the other hand, reaches into the past and traces communal epistemological networks through which the doctor can develop new methodologies, influence future medical practice, establish authority among other practitioners, and legitimize medicine as an authority in the public realm. Both scholars thus pursue connections between community and epistemology, but in different arenas.

While the outline above provides a brief history of the two approaches, when we move to the field of German Studies, we must quickly acknowledge that the two fields become harder to distinguish. Within American German Studies, the Medical Humanities rose to visibility in the late 1980s and 1990s in the work of Sander Gilman, whose research on disease and representation defined his work during a period that including his term as President of the Modern Language Association of America (1995), bolstering the new field across the modern languages and literatures as well as in German Studies specifically. Whether focusing on German topics, as in his 1995 *Franz Kafka: The Jewish Patient*, or roaming widely across the globe, as in his transnational 1988 work, *Disease and Representation: Images of Illness from Madness to AIDS*, Gilman's approach to the Medical Humanities has had much in common with the field of Literature and Science. He combines text, image, and practice, in forms such as literature, art, and medical writing and is as interested in the physician's as in the patient's experience. He situates both within the context of larger social forces as they intersect with psychological forces that, for Gilman, are best approached through psychoanalysis. Temporally, Gilman's work often follows a long historical trajectory even while also illuminating the present. His goals are therefore critical ones directed both at society and at the aesthetic dimension of texts rather than at humanizing physicians.

Literature and Science in German Studies emerged as a field closer to the turn of the millennium. As in English, it focused first on the period around 1800, not least because of Goethe's pivotal position in both arenas, but it soon expanded to other periods as well. The national characteristics of intellectual life in Germany have also meant that Literature and Science in German Studies often draws heavily on the history of philosophy as well. In fact, the field encompasses diverse priorities in the disciplines under analysis. Helmut Müller-Sievers, in *Self-Generation: Biology, Philosophy, and Literature around 1800* (1997), for example, was focused primarily on the philosophical recoding of scientific terminology into new concepts, while Robert Richards in *The Romantic Conception of Life: Science and Philosophy in the Age of Goethe* (2002), excavated both science and philosophy in fine-tuned ways, while pursing literature through more distanced readings. Michel Chaouli in *The Laboratory of Poetry: Chemistry and Poetics in the Work of Friedrich Schlegel* (2002) explored Lavoisier's revolution in chemistry as a dominant strain of Schlegel's literary theory, while Simon Richter in *Missing the Breast: Gender, Fantasy, and the Body in the German Enlightenment* (2006) encompassed physiology and medicine within the wide cultural span of discourse analysis. With the appearance of Richter's work, my own *Anxious Anatomy: The Conception of the Human Form in Literary and Naturalist Discourse* (2008), and Jocelyn Holland's *German Romanticism and Science: The Procreative Poetics of Goethe, Novalis and Ritter* (2009), literature and science came to weigh equally as appropriate objects for close analysis within criticism that juxtaposed the two. Paradigmatically, Holland explored three figures who themselves straddled the line between science and literature in her nuanced explorations of Goethe's biological, Novalis/Hardenberg's mechanical and chemical, and Ritter's chemical, electrical, and magnetic interests alongside their literary work. Analyzing the tools and instruments of generation and self-generation, of narration, and of technological production in Romantic science and literature, Holland here rejected the common perception of a Romantic celebration of organicism in opposition to mechanistic views of pro/creativity. All of these diverse approaches as well as a newer emphasis on technology have continued to proliferate, as attested to by works by Christine Lehleiter (2014), Leif Weatherby (2016), and Sarah Pourciau (2017), as well as newer work by many of the scholars noted above; Müller-Sievers (2012), Engelstein (2017), and Holland (2019).

As I mentioned early in this essay, medicine and science are concepts that could be mapped into a Venn diagram with overlapping circles. Medicine as a discipline is practiced not only in the clinic or hospital, but also in the laboratory and on the dissecting table, wherever that may be located, as well as in the study where medical texts are written. Sciences under the names of natural history and later of biology traverse species boundaries between the human and the non-human. Medical science has always been in dialogue with those fields that investigated animal anatomy and physiology and even botany. Scholarship in German Studies has often delved into this nexus of science and medicine in critical work that dwells at the juncture of Literature and Science and Medical Humanities. One might think here of my own 2008 monograph, *Anxious Anatomy: The Conception of the Human Form in Literary and Naturalist Discourse*, mentioned above, which drew on obstetrics, surgery, physiology, and theories about race, as well as on theories of reproduction that cut across the human/animal/plant divide. Employing this scope allowed me to demonstrate how teleology, which played a central role in the epigenesis-preformationism debate and was theorized by Kant as a necessary constituent of the life sciences, also simultaneously came to serve as ideological legitimation for grounding social and political structures on the perceived constitution of the human body. One could locate works by scholars of later historical periods, such as Johannes Türk (2011) and Alys George (2020), in this same in-between space, interested in medicine as a discursive and experimental practice alongside other scientific fields in the context of literary experimentation and interrogation of the human—and sometimes non-human—body. For George, for example, the paradigmatic relationship of physician to the ill in modernism unfolds not in the examining room, but in the autopsy room. Both medicine and politics claim power over the vulnerable body, politics before death and medicine after it (106), leaving a trail of mutilated veterans and dissected corpses that mark the medicalized modern era in relation to its violence.

In the last two decades, as animal studies, environmental studies, and plant studies have emerged and also flourished in the humanities, these fields have shared methodologies with Literature and Science as a field and have often been categorized as subfields. The current volume demonstrates the productive fluidity of these boundaries with Medical Humanities as well, emphasizing the immediate relevance to human medical science of each of these surrounding and intersecting fields.

Returning to the questions mapped out at the beginning of this essay, we can now ask what the consideration of these two overlapping fields has revealed with respect to the stakes of interdisciplinarity. The Medical Humanities has experienced a shift, expanding both its methodologies and its goals. From an original focus on character and situational analysis in fiction as a resource for understanding human emotions in the service of improving outcomes for patients, the field has begun to incorporate literary and visual analysis with broader social and deeper aesthetic commitments. Literature and Science, like most fields in the humanities, frequently explicates its methodology and its immediate research goal, but as with much of the humanities outside the Medical Humanities, does not usually explicitly articulate a larger purpose for the knowledge it creates.

With these investments in mind, I would suggest that we could begin to see Literature and Science, under the productive pressure from the Medical Humanities to contemplate purposes, as an exemplary site to illuminate how the humanities paradigmatically embraces aesthetics without jettisoning all relation to teleology—an association, after all, which belongs to the genetic history of Literature and Science. It was Kant who, in the *Critique of Judgment*, established a partial analogy between organisms and aesthetic objects with respect to the role of teleology in judgements. Because no study of living organisms could advance without positing that organs and living processes have purposes, Kant granted teleology a place in the emerging discipline of biology as a regulative—rather than determinate—judgment. If organs were purposive with a hypothetical purpose, natural or artistic beauty was, however, purposive without purpose. The pleasure in beauty arose from the attunement of mind and orderliness, mind and structure, which initiated an infinite free play of the faculties in the face of such objects, ever seeking and probing and never able to settle. Classical aesthetics absorbed this lesson and carried it forward so consequentially that even now, after many revisions of the definition of the aesthetic, as well as periodic turns away from and then back to it, fields in the humanities remain supremely suspicious of purpose, of goal-setting.

At the same time, however, even classical aesthetics struggled to maintain the supposed autonomy of free play. In an immediate embrace and simultaneous rebuttal of Kant, Schiller both barred and granted a purpose to the experience of beauty, positing that only in the activation of such a play drive could the human be fully present in both its rationality and its sensuousness. This convergence displaced the aesthetic experience from pragmatic activity, but tendentiously posited it as preparatory for ethical social behavior and hence the foundation of a free, participatory state. Adorno poised aesthetics at the cusp of the purposeful, upholding the oscillation of autonomy and social critique as its paradigm. The appeal of Schiller's oscillation has lasted, particularly in a French context, and has most recently been taken up by Jacques Rancière in his definition of dissensus as a necessary driver of democracy and as itself a product of the aesthetic generation of new domains of the sensible. It is this theory that Bleakley has recently adapted to advocate for teaching the humanities as a way to deepen, on the one hand, "close noticing and diagnostic acumen" which he calls "sensibility" and equates with Rancière's modes of perception and, on the other hand, "ways of being affected, or openness to the conditions of others," which he calls "sensitivity" and equates with Rancière's regimes of emotion (2015, 3 and 4). Bleakley may here lean a bit more heavily into the instrumental than humanities scholars are comfortable with, but he does problematize the elements most frequently listed as medically productive borowings from the humanities, namely empathy (2015, 78–99) and creativity (2015, 100–131). If we were to accept that the withholding of closure constitutes a value, we might restate the pleasure of aesthetics as that of evocation and provocation, which entails an eliciting of thought and the affect that inevitably forms a part of thought, rather than a suspension of either, while barring arrival at any final conclusion about meaning.

The humanities, which study such aesthetic objects, absorb this allegiance to openness. And yet, it is not difficult to find many pragmatic benefits to the humanities, benefits we can all rattle off to administrators, from critical thinking to persuasive communication to logical argumentation to interpersonal skills. New knowledge is also a clear product of such studies. Bruno Latour, whose death during the writing of this foreword represents an immeasurable loss to both fields and their intersections, was always quick to point out the contribution of literary studies to the pursuit of science studies. By drawing on methodologies of close reading while recognizing the porousness of boundaries, literature and science as a field explicates the ways in which knowledge is formed through networks of exchange that implicate multiple branches of society, from policy to the imagination, from economics to experiments, and from the laboratory to the library—virtual or not.

The commitment to aesthetics in the humanities, however, moves scholarship a crucial step beyond both skills-based arguments and the revelations of complex truths. It cannot be fully captured in affective identification or in the expansive mode of creativity or in the power of critical interrogation. Rather, by incorporating attention to aesthetics, the humanities illuminate and exercise modes of forming, thinking, intervening, and creating that engage with both critique and affect while interrupting certainty and resisting closure. It is this oscillation toward and away from teleological thinking that characterizes humanistic inquiry. It is no betrayal of such openness, of such free play, to call this oscillation in itself valuable, to acknowledge that interrupting the striving for ends has deep worth. In a culture that increasingly accepts only marketability and health outcomes as frameworks for judging value, such a claim upholds the distinct perspectives, praxes, and intellectual work represented by the discipline. The creative potential of interdisciplinary fields does not arise from assimilating one to the other, but depends on working across boundaries while recognizing ongoing distinctions. Paradox or not, in an era in which practitioners of the humanities have been forced to defend their pursuits, it is important to articulate and acknowledge this value, the value of disrupting teleological goal-setting as a goal, first to ourselves.

NOTES

1. Cole, Carlin, Carson (2015, 4–6).
2. Institutional investment in the field in the form of certificates and minors for undergraduates tends to run a bit behind these developments, creating the potential for tension.
3. For the history of Literature and Science, see Steven Meyer's Introduction to the *Cambridge Companion to Literature and Science* and also Jay Labinger's *Connecting Literature and Science* (2022), here 24–25.

WORKS CITED

Beer, Gillian. 1983. *Darwin's Plots: Evolutionary Narrative in Darwin, George Eliot and Nineteenth-Century Fiction*. London: Routledge and Kegan Paul.

Bleakley, Alan. 2015. *Medical Humanities and Medical Education: How the Medical Humanities Can Shape Better Doctors*. London and New York: Routledge.

Chaouli, Michel. 2002. *The Laboratory of Poetry: Chemistry and Poetics in the Work of Friedrich Schlegel*. Baltimore and London: The Johns Hopkins University Press.

Charon, Rita. 2006. *Narrative Medicine: Honoring the Stories of Illness*. Oxford and New York: Oxford University Press

Cole, Thomas, Nathan Carlin, and Ronald Carson. 2015. *Medical Humanities: An Introduction*. New York: Cambridge University Press.

Engelstein, Stefani. 2017. *Sibling Action: The Genealogical Structure of Modernity*. New York: Columbia University Press.

Engelstein, Stefani. 2008. *Anxious Anatomy: The Conception of the Human Form in Literary and Naturalist Discourse*. Albany, NY: SUNY Press.

George, Alys. 2020. *The Naked Truth: Viennese Modernism and the Body*. Chicago: University of Chicago Press.

Gilman, Gilman. 1988. *Disease and Representation: Images of Illness from Madness to AIDS*. Ithaca and London: Cornell University Press.

Gilman, Sander. 1995. *Franz Kafka: The Jewish Patient*. New York and London: Routledge.

Hilger, Stephanie. 2021. "Medical Humanities and the Eighteenth Century." *Goethe Yearbook*. 28: 301–306.

Holland, Jocelyn. 2009. *German Romanticism and Science: The Procreative Poetics of Goethe, Novalis, and Ritter*. New York and London: Routledge.

Holland, Jocelyn. 2019. *The Lever as Instrument of Reason: Technological Constructions of Knowledge around 1800*. London: Bloomsbury Press.
Jordanova, Ludmilla. 1998. "Writing Medical Identities 1780–1820." In *The Third Culture: Literature and Science*, edited by Elinor S. Schaffer, 204–216. Berlin and New York: Walter de Gruyter.
Jordanova, Ludmilla. 1989. *Sexual Visions: Images of Gender in Science and Medicine between the Eighteenth and Twentieth Centuries*. Madison, WI: University of Wisconsin Press.
Kant, Immanuel. 1913. *Kritik der Urteilskraft. Gesammelte Schriften*. Ed. Königlich Preußischen Akademie der Wissenschaften. I.5: 167–485. Berlin: Georg Reimer.
Labinger, Jay. 2022. *Connecting Literature and Science*. New York and London: Routledge.
Lehleiter, Christine. 2014. *Romanticism, Origins, and the History of Heredity*. Lewisburg: Bucknell University Press.
Levine, George. 1987. "Introduction. One Culture: Science and Literature." In *One Culture: Essays in Science and Literature*, edited by George Levine, 3–32. Madison: The University of Wisconsin Press.
Meyer, Steven. 2018. "Introduction." In *Cambridge Companion to Literature and Science*, edited by Steven Meyer, 1–22. Cambridge and New York: Cambridge University Press.
Müller-Sievers, Helmut. 1997. *Self-Generation: Biology, Philosophy, and Literature around 1800*. Stanford: Stanford University Press.
Müller-Sievers, Helmut. 2012. *The Cylinder: Kinematics of the 19th Century*. Berkeley: University of California Press.
Pourciau, Sarah. 2017. *The Writing of Spirit: Soul, System, and the Roots of Language Science*. New York: Fordham University Press.
Richards, Robert J. 2002. *The Romantic Conception of Life: Science and Philosophy in the Age of Goethe*. Chicago and London: The University of Chicago Press.
Richter, Simon. 1992. *Laocoon's Body and the Aesthetics of Pain*. Detroit: Wayne State University Press.
Richter, Simon. 2006. *Missing the Breast: Gender, Fantasy, and the Body in the German Enlightenment*. Seattle: University of Washington Press.
Schiller, Friedrich. 1962. *Über die ästhetische Erziehung des Menschen in einer Reihe von Briefen. Werke*. Nationalausgabe. Ed. Benno von Wiese. Weimar: Böhlau Verlag. 20.1: 309–412.
Shaffer, Elinor. 1998. "Introduction: The Third Culture – Negotiating the 'Two Cultures.'" In *The Third Culture: Literature and Science*, edited by Elinor S. Schaffer, 1–14. Berlin and New York: Walter de Gruyter.
Snow, C. P. 1959. *The Two Cultures and the Scientific Revolution*. New York: Cambridge University Press.
Snow, C. P. 1963. *The Two Cultures: And a Second Look: An Expanded Version of The Two Cultures and the Scientific Revolution*. Cambridge/New York: Cambridge University Press.
Türk, Johannes. 2011. *Die Immunität der Literatur*. Frankfurt a/M: Fischer Verlag.
Weatherby, Leif. 2016. *Transplanting the Metaphysical Organ: German Romanticism between Leibniz and Marx*. New York: Fordham University Press.
Whitehead, Anne and Angela Woods. 2016. "Introduction." In *The Edinburgh Companion to the Critical Medical Humanities*, edited by Anne Whitehead and Angela Woods; Assoc. Ed. Sarah Atkinson, Jane MacNaughton, and Jennifer Richards, 1–31. Edinburgh: Edinburgh University Press.

ACKNOWLEDGMENTS

This edited volume has been many years in the making. The idea for it began to germinate in 2017, when my volume *New Directions in Literature and Medicine Studies* was published, and I realized that there was a need for a similar collection with a focus on German Studies. My research into questions of embodiment, however, first led me to co-edit a collection on *Bodies in Transition in the Health Humanities* (2019), before I was able to return to this project in 2020. 2020 was, of course, the year when the Covid pandemic hit and, while the pandemic created obstacles for a project that involved a great number of contributors, it also highlighted the need to engage deeply with questions of disease and health across time and space.

Given its long genesis, there are many people to thank, first and foremost the contributors without whose ground-breaking work at the intersection of the Health Humanities and German Studies this volume would not even exist. Their research shows us the excitement that emerges when new intellectual paths are forged and provides us with directions for future scholarship. Thank you also to my editor at Bloomsbury, Ben Doyle, and his assistant editor, Laura Cope, who have been enthusiastic about the volume from the moment that I first shared the idea with them.

I am grateful for my home institution, the University of Illinois at Urbana-Champaign, which, over the past decade, has supported my work with a number of grants that have made it possible for me, a scholar of literature, to venture into the field of medicine and health and eventually become a contributor to the field of the Health Humanities. Interdisciplinary research needs institutional investment and the path of those who do this type of work can be circuitous but it often leads to fortuitous discoveries that give rise to further opportunities. Over the past decade, the Humanities Research Institute at Illinois under the leadership of Antoinette Burton has provided a home for those interested in exploring these issues in the form of a research cluster. A special thank you goes to my co-PI, Justine Murison, and the core members of the research group, "The Art of Medicine," which was funded by the Presidential Initiative to Celebrate the Arts and the Humanities at the University of Illinois.

Our discussions on the intersection between the humanities and medicine culminated in a speaker series, community outreach events, and curricular development initiatives, which all fed into this collection in both direct and indirect ways.

A thank you also to the students in the classes that I developed with the support of my home institution. Teaching literature to medical students and discussing issues of health and medicine with graduate students in the humanities has had more benefits than I can enumerate here. Our conversations on the role of the humanities in identifying the social determinants of health and structural inequalities have, I believe, outlined a path for what it means to be self-aware healthcare practitioners and engaged scholar-teachers who acknowledge their own positionality and embeddedness in existing power structures. Our thoughts on these issues were deeply shaped by the Covid pandemic, which crystallized many topics that had been percolating in Health Humanities scholarship and teaching for years. The genesis of many of the articles in this volume also lies in the early days of the pandemic and is reflected in the authors' commitment to approach questions of health and wellness from the perspective of the humanities.

Last but definitely not least I am deeply appreciative of my husband and my daughter who were wonderful company during the pandemic, when the days were long but the working hours short. Thank you!

INTRODUCTION

Intersections: Health Humanities and German Studies

STEPHANIE M. HILGER

The idea for this volume has been percolating for many years. As a scholar of German (and more broadly European) literature and culture, my turn toward the Health Humanities began when I started researching the eighteenth-century representation of so-called "hermaphrodites" in popular broadsides and medical writing.[1] In my quest to understand nonbinary and nonconforming individuals, I attended a course on embryology taught in my university's medical college, hoping to get definitive answers to my many questions and to dispel the mythical explanations that eighteenth-century scientists, despite all assertions to the contrary, often still upheld. The course outlined the development, in utero, of all major organ systems. When I entered the lecture hall, I stepped into a world that was alien yet fascinating. Soon, my head was spinning, trying to process concepts like gastrulation, embryogenesis, gamete, and ectoderm. At the same time that this terminology from the realm of embryology was foreign to me, it was embedded in a narrative structure that was intimately familiar because it resembled many of the stories that I, as a professor of literature, taught and read regularly. Cells were anthropomorphized as the protagonists in a story that took many twists and turns alongside the way to a fully formed human at the end of a nine-month period. They were "motivated," I soon learned, and "migrated" along an arduous path, crossing "bridges," "aqueducts," and "canals." During the lecture on the urogenital system, which I had eagerly awaited in my quest to understand what was *really* going on with nonbinary individuals, phrases such as "appear to," "should be," and "not fully understood" emanated from the lectern. There was no undisputed truth to be culled from present-day medical literature with which I could simply and unequivocally contrast the mistakes of the past regarding "hermaphrodites." Many gaps and ambiguities remain in science's understanding of the different steps that transform an undifferentiated cell mass to a fully formed human. Science does not follow a teleological path; instead, it is marked by ruptures, revisions, and rethinking. At the time, I was not fully aware yet that, with my research on eighteenth-century "hermaphrodites", I had positioned myself in the uncomfortable yet productive space where different disciplines meet.

Gradually, I began to think more broadly about the work situated at the intersection of the two fields that my work most closely engaged, German Studies and the Health Humanities. Over the past several decades, this scholarly intersection has surfaced and become more visible because of developments in the respective disciplines. Each discipline emerged under specific conditions and has a complex history that has profoundly shaped the type of research done under its heading. The term "German Studies" appears self-evident at first in that it references the study of all things German. What these "things" are, however, is contested and can, depending on the scholar, range from literature, in the sense of *belles lettres*, to other types of cultural production, as well as history, politics, and economics. In turn, the term "German" poses multiple questions as it leaves open its exact referent, ranging from the national to the linguistic, the cultural, and the political. The term "studies" conversely does not specify the scholarly approach toward the topic of German, however defined. The statement that "German Studies" is the Anglo-American version of "Germanistik" is true, yet it at the same time constitutes an oversimplification and erases the specific contexts of historical and disciplinary developments.

The early stirrings of *Germanistik* emerged in the seventeenth century when German began to replace Latin as the language of learning. The study of German language and literature, rather than just French, was heavily promoted by "Sprachgesellschaften," language societies, that emerged during this time. These developments continued in the eighteenth and nineteenth centuries when *Germanistik* became an integral part of the humanities. As Christian Buhr posits, "um 1800 [setzte] ein Prozess der Disziplinbildung ein" ["a process of disciplinary formation began around 1800"] (Buhr et al. 2015, xiii). The first professorship in the field was given to Friedrich Heinrich von der Hagen in Berlin in 1810. This disciplinary development was in tune with the Romantic interest in medieval literature as an expression of national history and the desire to position German literature on the same footing as other European national traditions. As a result of this history, the two main branches of *Germanistik* were philology and literature (Buhr et al. 2015, x). Over the course of the centuries, *Germanistik* became a full-fledged discipline, as marked by its institutionalization in universities in German-speaking lands. The complex history of the discipline of *Germanistik* itself became a subject of study with the creation, in 1972, of the *Arbeitsstelle für die Erforschung der Geschichte der Germanistik* in Marbach. When *Germanistik* moved across the Atlantic and was incorporated into Anglo-American institutions of higher education, which, as Louis Menand et al. have pointed out, were themselves modeled on German universities, the focus remained on these branches. Due to large-scale immigration from German-speaking lands in the nineteenth century, German was the second most commonly spoken language and the most commonly taught foreign language in the US until the First World War.[2] German language learning and the study of the literary output by canonical authors such as Goethe and Schiller were the mainstay of German departments. German history was typically taught, often in the context of central European history, in history departments.

In the wake of the two world wars, especially the Second World War and the Holocaust, both *Germanistik* and so-called *Auslandsgermanistik* became politically laden and controversial fields. If, in Theodor Adorno's famous words, writing poetry after Auschwitz was barbaric, could studying literature, especially German literature, be any less so? In their contribution to the fortieth anniversary issue of the *German Studies Review*, one of the main journals of the discipline, Celia Applegate and Frank Trommler summarize the effects of the Second World War on the study of German literature and history in the US:

> The postwar result, however, saw German history strengthened as an academic subject within departments of history, but the once-influential German language and literature suffering the consequences of Nazi Germany's infamy. These latter subjects fell from grace and into increasing irrelevance in the eyes of American students. The study of modern German history, in contrast, flourished in the guise of a morality tale about how modern institutions and economies could develop into barbarism under antidemocratic, antiliberal leadership.
>
> (2016, 472)

In the postwar period, *Germanistik* in the sense of the study of German language and literature continued to exist, albeit in a less prominent position, alongside the study of German history, which was mainly taught as a "morality tale." This development, together with the broader cultural turn in the humanities, ushered in the gradual transformation of *Germanistik* and history into *German Studies* as the study of a broader concept of culture beyond canonical authors and traditional historiography.

A major step in the transformation of *(Auslands)germanistik* and German History into German Studies in the United States was the creation of a professional society. In 1976, Gerald Kleinfeld, professor of history at Arizona State University, founded the Western Association for German Studies (WGSA). Conceived of as a counterweight to the perceived elitism of East Coast institutions in general and the Conference Group for Central European History in particular, the WGSA presented itself not only as multidisciplinary but also as inclusive of younger scholars (Lennox and Weinberg 2016). In 1984, the WGSA was renamed the German Studies Association (GSA) and began to grow both nationally and internationally. This growth occurred in tandem with the presentation of German history as a "morality tale," which was reflected in the funding mechanisms for German Studies: "The proliferation of German Studies in North America was also the result of sizable investments by German foundations which were willing to support a nonaffirmative view of the country" (Jarausch 2016, 497). The *Deutsche Akademische Austauschdienst* (DAAD), the Alexander von Humboldt Foundation, the Max Kade Foundation, the Goethe Institute, and the German Marshall Fund were all instrumental in promoting the growth of a specific type of German Studies. As Ulrich Grothus observes, the creation of these "Deutschlandzentren" occurred first in the United States before the concept was exported to other countries.

On its website, the GSA describes itself as "the multi- and interdisciplinary association of scholars in German, Austrian, and Swiss history, literature, culture studies, political science, and economics. The GSA holds an annual conference and publishes a scholarly journal, the *German Studies Review*. Members are generally professors and advanced students at universities and colleges in North America, although there are several hundred members in Europe and Asia. Membership is open to anyone. Member of the American Council of Learned Societies (ACLS)" (German Studies Association website). The GSA defines "German Studies" by the types of fields (ranging from literature to economics), geographical reach (not exclusive to the German nation), and disciplinary approach (multi- and interdisciplinary).[3] Each element of this tripartite equation has evolved since the early days of the association. The issue of disciplinarity in particular is one that has generated intense debate, especially with respect to the question of establishing a dialogue between the two main branches represented in the GSA: German history, on the one hand, and German literature/language, on the other. Most of the authors included in the fortieth anniversary issue of the *German Studies Review* engage with the question of disciplinarity. Celia Applegate and Frank Trommler characterize the GSA as a "multidisciplinary enterprise bringing together history and German" (Applegate and Trommler 2016, 471) while Konrad Jarausch observes "more pluridisciplinarity [...] than interdisciplinarity" (Jarausch 2016, 495). Others use prefixes such as "multi," trans," and "cross" to characterize the relation between these two fields. The basis for this debate is the underlying feeling that, what the German Studies Association set out to achieve, namely the integration of history and literature/language (and thereby the renewed valuation of the more traditional *Germanistik* as the study of language and literature), never happened (or never did so completely) and that the study of history and the study of literature continue to occur on parallel rather than intersecting tracks, as witnessed in the sessions at the annual meeting of the GSA.

In order to counteract this disciplinary bifurcation and to encourage truly interdisciplinary rather than just multidisciplinary work, in 2008, the GSA began with the creation of networks with the goal of "bridging temporal epochs (avoiding a presentist approach); bringing in more disciplines (especially beyond history and literature); and constituting panels in which scholars from different disciplines talk to each other (and attract an audience that crosses disciplinary boundaries)" (Ward 2016, 518). The number and variety of GSA networks speaks to the diversity of research that is being conducted in various segments of academe. A listing of current networks shows that this research goes beyond the association's rather narrow mission statement as "German, Austrian, and Swiss history, literature, culture studies, political science, and economics:" Asian German Studies, Black Diaspora Studies, Digital Humanities, Emotion Studies, Environmental Studies, Comics Studies, Body Studies, Teaching, Family and Kinship, GDR Studies and German Socialisms, Law and Legal Cultures, Medieval and Early Modern German Studies, Music and Sound Studies, Queer and Trans Studies, Swiss Studies, Visual Culture, War and Violence (German Studies Association Website). As Janet Ward, one of the driving forces behind the actualization of the GSA's interdisciplinary aspirations, observes, there is "multidirectional creative flow" (2016, 518) between these networks and the multi-day seminars at the annual conference meetings, which were themselves inaugurated more than a decade ago. In addition, these networks and seminars establish connections to related research clusters at European academic institutions, thereby pointing at the multilateral ways in which the concept of German Studies circulates back and forth across the Atlantic. German Studies has evolved beyond the concepts of *Auslandsgermanistik* and German history as a morality tale into a discipline that influences the way "(all) things German" are researched and taught not only in the US but throughout the world.[4]

The GSA's emphasis on the importance of interdisciplinary work can be framed with the ongoing debate on the role and position of the humanities in institutions of higher education. The "crisis in the humanities" has been a topic of intense discussion for the past three decades, as can be witnessed not only in high-profile academic publications such as the *Chronicle of Higher Education* and *Inside Higher Ed* but also in op-eds in the popular press. As a professor of German at the University of Illinois at Urbana-Champaign, a land-grant university in the American Midwest, the editor of the present volume will outline important touchstones in the debate in the US academic context, with references across the Atlantic, where appropriate. One of the earliest and most influential book-length publications in this context, Michael Bérubé and Cary Nelson's *Higher Education under Fire: Politics, Economics, and the Crisis of the Humanities* (1995) posited that higher education is "under fire from every ideological hiding place, from inside as well as outside the groves of academe" (1994, 3): "This conjunction of crises—political, fiscal, intellectual—has its roots in the late 1960s, when the transformation of American higher education coincided with legitimation crises in numerous American institutions; but its modern manifestation is a quite recent phenomenon, picking up steam only in the last few years" (1994, 6). While, in the 1990s, this crisis was not at the forefront of most humanities faculty members' awareness, it now permeates discussions at every level, especially at public universities. Shrinking budgets, dropping enrollments, ballooning administrative structures, and the deprofessionalization of academic labor loom large in departmental meetings and dominate the many strategic planning documents and state-of-the-discipline reports that departments have to produce on a regular basis. While the exact nature of the discussion depends on the field—English, History, and Foreign Languages and Literatures departments, among others, all have specific yet related concerns—it always centers on the need to justify, legitimize, and defend the humanities from inside and outside attacks regarding the usefulness of a humanities degree.

One of the most influential reports to be published in the past decade was the American Academy of Arts and Sciences' *The Heart of the Matter* (2013), whose goal was the promotion of the humanities and social sciences alongside STEM disciplines. As Michael Bérubé and Jennifer Ruth have observed in *The Humanities, Higher Education, and Academic Freedom* (2015), this report generated significant discussions, with contributors focusing not, as intended, on the importance of the arts and sciences in education but on their decline. Bérubé and Ruth urge a rethinking of the crisis discourse, not only by contextualizing the drop in humanities majors historically and demographically, but also by arguing that the perceived crisis in the humanities is mainly one of employment, with tenure-line positions becoming increasingly rare. They are not the only ones to critique the crisis discourse. Another influential publication, Gordon Hutner and Feisal Mohamed's *A New Deal for the Humanities* (2015), also takes the AAAS report, which mainly looked at elite private institutions, as its starting point and reframes it specifically for the public research university. Hutner and Mohamed argue against "the current retooling of our public universities as technical colleges" (2015, 12) and for "an administrative recommitment to the principle of the comprehensive public research university" (2015, 4) by providing stable sources of funding, a shift away from science-based models of evaluating departments, and a general recommitment to liberal arts education. At the same time, they argue for a rethinking of current models of academic departments and single-subject majors. In their assessment, interdisciplinary fields such as digital, environmental, and medical humanities are poised to play an increasingly important role in the reshaping of the humanities.

Discussing the medical humanities in specific, John McGowan, in his contribution to A *New Deal for the Humanities*, argues for a reevaluation of the "humanities sensibility" (2015, 139) beyond the current, oftentimes cynical reference to it. The "characteristic methods of the humanities—which include attention to context, questions of meaning and value, and a focus on intersubjective interactions and individual motivations—encourage us to attend to worldly factors that pertain to human wellbeing" (2015, 139). Medical Humanities—and its more inclusive incarnation, the Health Humanities, which acknowledges that medicine only constitutes a small fraction of an individual's sense of wellbeing and encompasses the full range of disciplines in the delivery of healthcare and the patients themselves—plays a role in a context where, as a result of time, cost constraints, and ever-increasing specialization, the human dimension of healthcare has been relegated to the background in both education and research. Conversely, the Health Humanities has also established itself in the humanities, where humanities scholars have become more outspoken about the fact that their work is not situated in the metaphorical ivory tower but engages broad social and political processes. Health Humanities is a true interdisciplinary field in the sense defined by Gerald Graff: "interdisciplinary work, whether humanistic or not, is a creatively natural, not an unnatural process. That which happens on the interstices of a field regularly determines the next knowledge breakthrough—and eventually influences the emergence of new disciplines, or at the very least new articulations and self-understandings of existing ones" (2015, 517). Medical Humanities emerged naturally in the late 1960s and early 1970s at the same time that the humanities first came under attack and the medical profession was looking for a space to reflect on the meaning of the momentous changes resulting from the transformation of medical schools into high-powered research centers and the emergence of new technologies such as in vitro fertilization and organ transplantation.

The natural convergence between the humanities and medicine was acknowledged in the 2020 report by the Association of American Medical Colleges (AAMC), *The Fundamental Role of the Arts and Humanities in Medical Education: Branches from the Same Tree*. Both the AAMC report and the AAAS report, published seven years earlier, invoke an organic metaphor—trees and the heart—to highlight the centrality of the arts and humanities in twenty-first-century (medical) education. The AAMC report strategically quotes Albert Einstein who famously posited that "[a]ll religions, arts, and sciences are branches of the same tree" (2020, 5). Over the past decade, Medical Colleges have worked on actualizing the interconnectedness of these two disciplines by integrating arts and humanities components into their curricula. As a result, at present, according to the AAMC report, more than 94 percent of medical schools report having required or elective courses in the Medical

Humanities (AAMC 2020, 7). While there is debate about how well integrated into the curriculum these components actually are, there is a manifest desire to transcend what is perceived as a dangerous trend toward hyper-specialization.[5] Not surprisingly, according to the AAMC, more humanities majors than biology majors were accepted into medical school because "[m]edical school admissions committees seek to admit well-rounded humanistic learners to the field of medicine" (2020, 7). Humanities majors do not face any hurdles to admission, quite on the contrary. Majors in humanities subjects do not, as tuition-paying parents sometimes fear, lead to unemployment and precarity for their children.[6]

Parallel to the developments in medical colleges, which are incorporating arts and humanities elements, humanities departments increasingly thematize issues related to healthcare through the creation first of postgraduate,[7] Master's programs and then of undergraduate curricula in the Medical/Health Humanities.[8] The affinity between medicine and the humanities lies in the fact that medicine is not a hard science; rather, it is an interpretive practice that combines scientific and humanities-based modes of knowledge. Therefore, medicine also experiences what Catherine Belling has called the "hermeneutic anxiety" (2006, 376) that informs humanities research; it is an interpretive practice that gathers multiple, sometimes conflicting, types of information to reach a conclusion and decide on a course of action.

The seeds for the Medical Humanities were planted more than a century ago. Medical training in the US has been profoundly shaped by the 1910 Flexner report, which, in response to the perceived haphazard and low-quality training of medical students, standardized American medical education by focusing on biomedicine to the detriment of fields that were not seen as contributing directly to scientific medical education.[9] Students first focused on the dissection of corpses before facing the manifestation of diseases in living patients. Critics of Flexner's pervasive reforms, such as prominent physician William Osler, lamented the exclusion of any form of humanities inquiry from this educational model. The seeds of the Health Humanities can be traced to the late 1960s/early 1970s, a time of momentous change in the medical profession. One of the key figures in those early days was Edmund Pellegrino, Director of the Kennedy Institute of Ethics at Georgetown University, who called upon medical educators to refocus their attention on the moral dimension of medicine. These discussions led to the creation of, in 1967, the first humanities department in a medical school at Penn State University and, in 1969, the Society for Health and Human Values. In 1981, the *Journal of Medical Humanities* was first published (under the title of *Bioethics Quarterly*) at the Center for Bioethics and Humanities at the University of Colorado.[10] In 2000, in the UK, the Institute of Medical Ethics and the *British Medical Journal* founded the journal *Medical Humanities,* highlighting not only the important role played by medical ethics in the early days of the Health Humanities but also the intellectual exchange between scholars on both sides of the Atlantic.

At the same time that Pellegrino focused on medical ethics, Joanne Trautmann Banks, who was the first professor of literature at a medical school when she was appointed to Penn State University in 1972, highlighted the necessity of "read[ing], in the fullest sense" in order to increase medical practitioners' "tolerance for ambiguity" (1981, 36).[11] From her call gradually emerged the field of Literature and Medicine, which posited that training medical practitioners to read fully would provide them with interpretive skills that could improve patient care and might increase their empathy. With the establishment of the journal *Literature and Medicine* in 1982, these interdisciplinary scholarly endeavors found a home. The name of the journal reflected the reality that the majority of these interdisciplinary ventures originated in literature departments. Literature, in the sense of *belles lettres*, is perhaps the most "humanistic" of all humanities disciplines because it is often considered a production of art for art's sake. However, the contributors to the first issues of the journal demonstrated the exact opposite of this notion. In fact, another pioneer, Rita Charon, vehemently argued against instrumentalizing literature only to provide medical doctors with "a civilizing veneer" (2006, 226) by pointing out that writing a poem or quoting a philosopher does not necessarily make a better doctor. Similarly, Anne Hudson Jones, founding editor of *Literature and Medicine*, cautioned against the simplifying claim that engaging the humanities necessarily makes physicians more humane.

Many of the pioneers of the literature and medicine field focused on the textual features not only of literature but also of other types of discourse, including medical texts. Kathryn Montgomery Hunter's *Doctor's Stories: The Narrative Structure of Medical Knowledge* (1991) highlighted the role played by narrative in the doctor-patient encounter. In 2000, Ann Hunsaker Hawkins and Marilyn Chandler McEntyre edited the influential *Teaching Literature and Medicine* volume, which focused on practical pedagogical aspects in this new field. The best-known incarnation of the scholarly and pedagogical focus on narrative is Rita Charon's concept of "narrative medicine," which puts medical practitioners face to face with the textuality of their patients' experiences as well as their own.[12] Ronald Schleifer and Jerry Vannatta's *The Chief Concern of Medicine* pursues a similar aim, namely the integration of narrative knowledge into medical practice. These close reading practices were geared at simultaneously uncovering the textual dimension of medical discourse and demonstrating that literature does not constitute a self-referential aesthetic discourse but a powerful vehicle for social commentary.[13]

Literature and Medicine and medical ethics are two of the main strands—along with the history of medicine—that laid the foundation for the field of the Medical Humanities, which continues to expand in reach and aspirations. Most recently, as Paul Crawford observes, "medical humanities" has been replaced by "health humanities" to encompass not only the full range of disciplines involved in the delivery of healthcare (including fields such as dentistry, nursing, pharmacy, etc.) but also the patients themselves. In addition, this renaming "underscores the crucial distinction between medicine and health. As epidemiological evidence shows, medicine is only a minor determinant of health in human populations alongside other factors such as class, education, occupation, environment, race, and stigma" (Jones et al. 2017, 932).[14] The focus on these intersectional elements highlights the development of the field into a more inclusive one both in terms of content and form (graphic novels, blogs, and online discussion forums in addition to the more typical novels, short stories, and poetry). As Alan Bleakley has shown, the development of the Health Humanities in the United States was paralleled by developments in the United Kingdom, funded by such high-profile institutions as the Nuffield Trust and the Wellcome Trust. Bleakley, however, argues that the "arts and humanities [...] have merely nuanced medical practice, rather than offering fundamental critique and resistance" (2013, 23). He therefore posits the need for a "critical medical humanities" that "affords skepticism towards utilitarian models of health and well-being" (2013, 24) by confronting medical students with narratives that present challenging plots that force them to face political realities, also in the delivery of healthcare.[15] Catherine Belling argues that the role of the humanities in healthcare can best be understood as triangulating science and art. Excluding the humanities "deprives medical researchers, practitioners, and educators of a position from which they might understand their work as an historically, socially, and culturally contingent activity" (2017, 20): "the products of science and of the creative arts [...] all require the disciplines of the humanities in order to make sense, to be ethically enacted, to be rewarded or discouraged—to be understood as massively complex products of human knowledge of, response to, and action in the natural world" (2017, 23). This "making sense" is the point where the Health Humanities as practiced in Medical Schools intersects with the Health Humanities as an intellectual practice within the humanities itself.

Health Humanities has become a discipline, with journal publications, a professional organization (the Health Humanities Consortium), conferences, and textbook publications (sourcebooks, readers, etc.).[16] One of the challenges faced by the Health Humanities is the danger of being instrumentalized in the service of what Bleakley calls utilitarian models of health and well-being. The earlier mentioned debate about whether the humanities will necessarily make a doctor more humane crystallizes this concern. Terms such as "humane," "humanistic," "humanizing," and sometimes even "humanitarian" permeate discussions about the role of the Health Humanities in medicine and point at the danger of transforming the interdisciplinarity of the Health Humanities into a translational science. A particularly forceful critique of this utilitarian view of the humanities as a "handmaiden" to the sciences has been articulated by Martin Willis in the British context. Instrumentalizing the humanities for science, and the Health Humanities for medicine, runs the danger of shaping the humanities along the same model as the hard sciences, with expectations of outside funding, contributions to policy changes, similar investigative methods, etc. As Janet Ward forcefully posits, "[o]nly some parts of humanities research can follow the 'cure-for-cancer/save the planet' grid of expectations. What humanists write is often immediately relevant but that does not mean it can be immediately useful" (Ward 2016, 523). In the context of the increasing corporatization of higher education and its oftentimes disingenuous praise of the efficiency of the sciences versus the inefficiency of the humanities, an interdisciplinary field such as the Health Humanities becomes a testing ground for the limits and opportunities of interdisciplinarity. Lutz Koepnick's warning against falling into the trap of the "myths of the prefix" (2016, 501) in the context of an inter-, trans-, or cross-disciplinary field such as German Studies should therefore also be heeded by those working in the Health Humanities.

As a humanities discipline, German Studies intersects with the Health Humanities in various ways. If we think of the Health Humanities as a way to rectify the biomedical focus in healthcare, Germany plays an important role as the Flexnerian biomedical model of education had its roots in Abraham Flexner's travels to Germany: "[Donald] Barr (2011) argues that US doctors in the 1870s, who had visited Germany particularly to study laboratory sciences, started a long revolution in medical education that was brought to a head by the Flexner report (1910)" (Bleakley 2013, 18).[17] Fictionalized in Sinclair Lewis's 1925 Pulitzer Prize-winning novel *Arrowsmith*, this process is represented by the German scientist Max Gottlieb, who teaches the eponymous protagonist science-based medicine that eventually leads him to become a bacteriologist and develop a cure for the plague. Flexner's adaptation of German biomedicine can be contextualized with the broader influence that nineteenth-century German universities had on American higher education. Reflecting on these transatlantic connections in the development of Western biomedicine becomes especially productive when considering that the Medical/Health Humanities as a discipline has been imported into German, and more broadly European, academia as an intellectual platform from which to critique medicine's scientific and biomedical focus. In an acknowledgment of the field's Anglo-American roots, the field typically is called "Medical Humanities," as can be seen in the affiliations of some of the European contributors to this volume. Medicine and medical humanities circulate back and forth across the Atlantic in a multidirectional process of cross-fertilization. In this context, it is important to note that—due to the editor's academic home and training—this volume is firmly grounded in the Anglo-American, and more specifically US, tradition of the Medical/Health Humanities. The contributors to this volume, however, come from a variety of academic contexts—the US, UK, Austria, Denmark, Germany, and Poland—and they all, in one way or another, engage this tradition. They thereby invite us to reflect on the incarnation of the Health Humanities in different academic and cultural contexts—also beyond the German-language realm—and the ensuing productive transformations that the Health Humanities undergoes when it moves abroad, becomes institutionalized, and takes on different terminologies and incarnations.

In recent years, both the Health Humanities and German Studies have undergone a process of critically reflecting on their goals, methodologies, and practices. Alan Bleakley's call for a critical Medical Humanities can be situated in the context of these efforts: "Such an approach is political and practical, as well as aesthetic and ethical, where it provides a potential democratizing force for medical culture" (2013, 24). This critical, political, and democratizing stance forces medical practitioners, scholars, and pedagogues to acknowledge and critically engage with the social determinants of health and structural health inequities, which Covid-19 has highlighted, perhaps more visibly than ever before. In tandem with this critique of the conservative strain in the Health Humanities that merely nuances rather than rethinks and resists existing power asymmetries has emerged an awareness of the field's Eurocentric and Western focus. Claire Hooker and Estelle Noonan argue that the "discipline must continue to expand its scholarly and critical engagements with processes of Othering in biomedicine" (2011, 79). These calls for a critical rethinking of the Health Humanities can be framed with the broader effort to decenter and decolonize disciplines that has gathered steam over the past several years. As Ijeoma Opara has argued in the context of global health, there must be a "greater awareness about the lasting damages of colonialism, and the power asymmetries that are pervasive in global health:" "twirling in and out of social justice conversations and dancing on the edges of diversity, equity, inclusion (DEI) discourse is the maintenance of a power hierarchy in global health that is still predominantly white, cis-gendered, heterosexual, male, and European/American" (2021, n.p.). Central to the effort of uncovering and ultimately dismantling these power hierarchies is the concept of intersectionality, "because a critical analysis of colonialism is fundamentally intersectional and must locate its construction, and thus, deconstruction, at the intersection of white supremacy, global anti-Blackness, patriarchy, capitalism, ableism, classism, homo/transphobia, fatphobia, and xenophobia" (2021, n.p). Highlighting and exploring these intersections in the Health Humanities is a crucial step on the path toward realizing the discipline's full potential.

Returning to one of the earliest incarnations of the Health Humanities, narrative medicine, we can see how the concept of "narrative humility," as described by Sayantani DasGupta, can be mobilized for an engaged Health Humanities that consciously reflects on the intersectionality of identities:

> Taking a position of narrative humility means understanding that stories are relationships we can approach and engage with while simultaneously remaining open to their ambiguity and contradiction and while engaging in constant self-evaluation and self-critique about issues such as our own role in the story as listeners, our expectations of the story, our responsibilities to the story, and our ownership of the story [...] It simultaneously reminds us that there are larger sociopolitical power structures that marginalize certain sorts of stories and privilege others. Narrative humility suggests an inward orientation, requiring not only that we learn about others, but that we begin by learning about ourselves—how our past cadre of life stories has built our prejudices and preferences, and how by the very act of listening, we ourselves are always changed into different kinds of listeners.
>
> (2004, 7)

Acknowledging our positionality and embeddedness in existing power structures through narrative humility lays the foundation for a Health Humanities that is critical and political, both for those working in medicine and for those situated in the humanities. It circumvents the danger of merely providing doctors with what Rita Charon called "a civilizing veneer" (2006, 226) and a notion of "cultural competence" that all too often reifies those stereotypes that it sets out to dismantle. At the same time, a self-aware scholarly practice of the Health Humanities protects the discipline from being instrumentalized for medicine and instead positions itself in a way that critically engages and questions biomedicine's deepest foundations.

The goals of a critical Health Humanities intersect with those of German Studies, which has undergone similar efforts to decolonize and decenter its practices, most visibly represented by the scholarly collective Diversity, Decolonization, and the German Curriculum (DDGC), founded in 2016, and the publication of the related volume, *Diversity and Decolonization in German Studies* in 2020. DasGupta's notion of self-critique can be juxtaposed with German Studies' self-evaluation of its disciplinary practices and prejudices. As Gizem Arslan points out, current debates in German Studies focus on "its imbrication in ethnonationalism, the disciplinary extrusion of non-white populations, a limited and monolingual way of teaching language, as well as the universalization of white, male, and heterosexual experience in research and teaching" (2021, 421). German Studies scholars and pedagogues are increasingly interrogating the "constitutive role whiteness plays for German Studies" (2021, 422). The effort to decolonize German Studies by critically engaging the history of German settlers in North America and Germany's colonial history in Africa and Asia has broadened the effort to decenter the field.[18] As is the case in the Health

Humanities, the exploration of intersectional identities has led German Studies to enter into dialogue with fields such as critical race, gender studies, Black (European) Studies, and indigenous studies, among others. Like the Health Humanities, German Studies has been deeply changed by these approaches, both in scholarship and pedagogy, as these efforts at decentering and decolonizing have opened up pathways for "articulat[ing] the relevance of German Studies to diverse groups of students" (Criser and Malakaj 2020, 14) at a time when enrollments across the humanities—including the study of foreign languages and cultures—have been dropping. At the same time, "[d]ecolonizing foreign language education then means—among other things—resisting market pressures and corporate thinking that limit language study to its applicability in the workforce" (Criser and Malakaj 2020, 7). A critical rethinking of German Studies occurs in tandem with the broader effort to reframe the humanities in the twenty-first century.

Humanities disciplines' engagement with the intersectional identities of sex, gender, race, and ability has led to a renewed interest in the human body, theories of embodiment, and the related focus on what constitutes the human. In this context, Mererid Puw Davies and Sonu Shamdasani's edited volume *Medical Humanity and Inhumanity in the German-Speaking World* (2020) constitutes an important milestone in the exploration of the "the grey areas where discourses and practices of medicine designate and create both the human and the inhuman, both the humane and the inhumane [...] in German-speaking lands" (2020, xi). Even though Davis and Shamdasani's volume does not foreground the intersection of German Studies with the Health Humanities, the contributors' exploration of the human—and the related question of the humane, a focus of the Health Humanities—provides a bridge to this disciplinary interface and therefore to the present volume.

There is currently no book-length publication that explores the intersection between German Studies and the Health Humanities in its own right. The present volume seeks to fill this gap by presenting the work of scholars working in different disciplines (literature, history, disability studies, medical/health humanities), at institutions on both sides of the Atlantic (Austria, Denmark, Germany, Poland, the UK, and the US), and at different stages of their career (from junior researchers to senior scholars who have been pioneers in the field of German Health Humanities) who all apply a Health Humanities lens to subjects typically investigated under the rubric of German Studies. The conception of this volume as "state-of-the-art" means that, after surveying the field of German studies, the editor solicited contributions from scholars doing innovative and thought-provoking work. It is important to note that the contributors are all situated in a Western context—the United States, the United Kingdom, and Europe. This is both an acknowledgment of the institutional and intellectual intersection of the Health Humanities with German Studies and a call to broaden this exploration to other spaces, geographical, institutional, and intellectual. Also, the contributors are positioned in humanities disciplines, which reflects the institutional framework that promotes this type of interdisciplinary inquiry. Although there are physicians who, by training and interest, are humanists, rare are the instances of a physician who has the institutional space and time to produce this kind of work. In this sense, the scholarship presented here is, in Janet Ward's words, "relevant" for the medical field, even though it is not directly "useful" in the sense of being translational and immediately applicable to medical practice. The articles in the present volume provide a powerful critique and resistance to biomedicine. They constitute a critical German Health Humanities that is not bound by the utilitarian logic that has framed discussions of the usefulness of humanities research and teaching, which—as Stefani Engelstein powerfully argues in her preface to this volume—can limit what the humanities can actually achieve.

The volume is divided into seven sections, each of which represents a major research strand in the space where the Health Humanities and German Studies meet. The first section, "Medical Readings/Reading Medicine," presents scholarship that reads literary texts—novels, poems, and hybrid genres—that feature medical topics and medical conditions such as eating disorders, aphasia, and Covid-19. The authors use a lens that, in many ways, has been shaped by one of the earliest manifestations of the Health Humanities, narrative medicine; their analyses present a counterpoint to biomedicine by focusing on the issue of intersubjectivity. The next section, "Graphic Medicine," explores the particular subgenre of the graphic novel, which positions itself as a response to medical discourse. The authors in this section highlight the issue of embodiment by exploring the interplay between text and image and by recovering subaltern voices, especially those of patients. They thereby expand the goals of narrative medicine, which initially only focused on purely textual forms. The following five sections explore the cross-fertilization between the Health Humanities and other fields of inquiry that have come to the forefront in the effort to decenter and decolonize disciplinary discourses: disability studies, critical race studies, gender studies, trauma studies, and animal/environmental studies. The articles in the section on disability (section 3) discuss the representation of bodies that do not fit the norm by engaging with the medical and the social model of disability and its manifestation in different historical and cultural contexts. Similarly to the section on disability, the articles discussing race (section 4) trace the process by which bodies that are perceived as different become medicalized, pathologized, and eventually excluded from the body politic as the inscrutable and ultimately threatening Other. The question of alterity also undergirds the contributions to the section on gender (section 5), which explore the representation and exclusion of bodies that complicate binary notions of sex and gender. The effect of the exclusion of nonbinary identities is also traced in the section on trauma (section 6), an important area of inquiry in German Studies, especially in the context of the Second World War and the Holocaust. This section broadens the reach of trauma studies by including scholarship exploring trauma in pre-1945 texts, reaching back to the eighteenth century. Bodies that are marked as nonconforming are often presented as situated on the border between the human and the non-human. Animal and environmental studies, thematized in the last section (section 7), therefore constitute a productive space for the German Health Humanities. The articles here explore the representation of humans whose bodies and actions approximate those of animals and thereby highlight the interconnectedness between animals, humans, plants, and the broader environment. In light of the Covid-19 pandemic and the resurging interest in zoonotic diseases, the renewed focus on these multidirectional influences has been gaining momentum over the course of the past years.[19]

As this brief overview already shows, the transitions between the various sections are fluid, both because of the intersectional nature of identities and the fields that study them. For instance, the graphic medicine section ends with an article discussing a graphic novel that thematizes disability; it thereby provides a transition to the next section, on disability studies. Similarly, the section on race that follows disability studies begins with an article exploring the construction of racial others as disabled in colonial discourse. The section on race concludes with an article on the early modern period and thereby establishes a link to the subsequent section on gender, which starts with an article on early modern medical knowledge about female genitalia. In addition to these explicit transitions, the reader will be able to establish a dialogue between articles both within and across sections. For example, the article on intersex identities in the late nineteenth century can be read alongside the article on transgressive fifteenth-century bodies in the same section. Similarly, that same intersex article can be put into conversation with a number of essays in the section on disability because studies of intersex identities often question ableist perceptions of human bodies. The present volume can be used in different ways to explore various directions and developments in the field and explore connections between race and trauma, gender and the environment, and textual and graphic representations of disease. In this way, multiple thematic and methodological threads can be followed in this volume. The volume presents surveys, reflective writing, and pedagogical essays, alongside studies of specific texts and representations, allowing readers to create their own intersectional spaces within which they can situate their research.

The goal of *The Health Humanities in German Studies* is to present a diversity of approaches to the study of the intersection between German Studies and the Health Humanities, yet it does not claim or even aspire to be comprehensive. The connection between these two realms is constantly changing, contributing to its productivity and dynamic nature. In this sense, this volume presents examples of what is possible when we think beyond established boundaries and thereby imagine new paths for our research, teaching, and outreach efforts. This volume is an example of what Paul Jay calls an "*engaged* humanities" (2014, 152) that consists of "forms of engagement and outreach that connect a humanities education—and the competencies it teaches—to the public sphere and a host of vocations that sorely needs them" (2014, 153). The connection of the humanities to the public sphere is, of course, the core mission of the Public Humanities. Therefore, the present volume's exploration of the intersection between German Studies and the Health Humanities intersects with yet another emerging and gradually consolidating field of inquiry. Reframing the role of the humanities and the arts in academia and society at large as a public, in the sense of engaged, venture allows for a way to make these disciplines matter in concrete ways beyond their mere utilitarian instrumentalization by the sciences.

It is important to remember that the crisis discourse regarding the state and future of the humanities is not new, even though at times it might appear to be. More than fifty years ago, Max Horkheimer already observed: "In recent periods of contemporary society, the so-called human studies (*Geisteswissenschaften*) have had but a fluctuating market value and must try to imitate the more prosperous natural sciences whose practical value is beyond question" (1972, 191). Horkheimer not only cautions against thinking about intellectual inquiry in corporate terms but also warns of the separation between different disciplines and fields: "The isolated consideration of particular activities and branches of activity [...] requires for its validity an accompanying concrete awareness of its limitations. A conception is needed which overcomes the one-sidedness that necessarily arises when limited intellectual processes are detached from their matrix in the total activity of society" (1972, 199). Horkheimer's comments about the dangers of isolating inquiries from what he calls "their matrix in the total activity of society" echo those of Friedrich Schiller who, two hundred and fifty years earlier, had already expressed similar concerns. In his inaugural lecture as a professor of history at the University of Jena in 1789, "Was heißt und zu welchem Ende studiert man Universalgeschichte?" ("What Is and to What End Do We Study Universal History?"), Schiller contrasts the "Brotgelehrte" (the scholar who works for his bread) with the "philosophische Kopf" (1789, 5; philosophical head).[20] Schiller argues that the scholar who works primarily to earn an income is invested in separating his discipline from all others so as to protect his academic territory and carefully circumscribe his tasks. By contrast, the philosophical head incarnates the Enlightenment ideal of the universal scholar whose goal is to connect his studies to different disciplines in an effort to insert them into the "große Ganze der Welt" (1789, 7; the wholeness of the world). While Schiller specifically addresses his fellow historians, his lecture highlights the inadequacy of any type of epistemological endeavor that does not strive to understand the "Zusammenhang der Dinge" (1789, 7; connection between things) by failing to embed discipline-specific knowledge within a broader context.

Horkheimer's "matrix" and Schiller's "wholeness" both highlight the need to think beyond and across disciplines, to establish connections, and to build bridges between different approaches to the same topic. In this context, it behooves us to remember that, while the divide between the sciences and the humanities might appear as an immutable reality from a present-day perspective, it is actually a relatively recent phenomenon. A *de facto* interdisciplinarity reigned up to the Early Modern period, when the Cartesian mind-body dichotomy was gradually mapped onto the separation of the humanities and sciences, which were eventually characterized as "soft" and "hard." The eighteenth century was a transitional period when debates regarding disciplinary specialization came to the foreground, as Schiller's lecture demonstrates. Only in the nineteenth century was the separation of the sciences and the humanities institutionalized in the European system of higher education. From there, it was eventually disseminated globally by way of Anglo-American research universities in the twentieth century. While a majority of the work done in German Studies and the Health Humanities focuses on the present day or the recent past, this volume's inclusion of historical perspectives enables a rethinking of the debate about disciplinary specialization and the crisis discourse regarding the arts and humanities in the context of broader historical developments. This historical vantage point ultimately questions the binary division of knowledge into sciences and humanities and highlights medicine's epistemological status as an interpretive practice rather than a hard science. Exploring the intersection between the Health Humanities and German Studies allows for the creation of more fluid spaces of intellectual inquiry that, while harkening back to pre-nineteenth-century pursuits of knowledge, also point to the exciting future of interdisciplinary research.

NOTES

1. I encountered mentions of "hermaphrodites" while researching my second book, *Gender and Genre* (2015). My interest in the confluence of literary and medical discourses led to the publication of three (co)edited volumes: *The Early History of Embodied Cognition* (2015), *New Directions in Literature and Medicine Studies* (2017), *Bodies in Transition* (2019).
2. German immigration to North America accelerated in the early nineteenth century due to a number of factors such as the increasing violence of the Napoleonic Wars and the famine in German territories (see Hilger 2015, 144). For a discussion of eighteenth- and early nineteenth-century German immigration to North America, see Colin Calloway, Malathi Michelle Iyengar, Hartmut Lehmann, Liam Riordan, Lynne Tatlock, Mack Walker, Marianne Wokeck, and Susanne Zantop.
3. In tune with the GSA mission statement, the editorial statement of the *German Studies Review* defines itself as "the scholarly journal of the German Studies Association (GSA), the world's largest academic association devoted to the interdisciplinary study of the German-speaking countries [...] articles and book reviews on the history, literature, culture, and politics of the German-speaking areas of Europe encompassing primarily, but not exclusively, Germany, Austria, and Switzerland" (German Studies Association website). The most recent call-for-papers for the 2023 GSA convention defines German studies as follows: "The Program Committee cordially invites proposals on any aspect of DACHL (German, Austrian, Swiss, Liechtenstein) studies, including (but not limited to) history, Germanistik, film, art history, political science, anthropology, musicology, religious studies, sociology, and cultural studies" (German Studies Association website).
4. In this context, also see the creation of the "Food for Thought" forum at the GSA "with the aim of enhancing the visibility of the next generation of German studies scholars and to highlight new directions in scholarship" (Bahr and Gerstenberger 2023, 123).
5. Recognizing the structural and institutional challenges, the AAMC gives concrete examples for how to integrate humanities and arts into medical education in its fifty-four-page report.
6. See Phillip Bean for an insightful discussion of what it means to choose a "practical" major.
7. The first MA in Medical Humanities was created by the Institute of Medical Humanities, Texas Medical Branch, Galveston, in the 1970s. The first UK degree with such a designation was established at the University of Swansea in 1997.
8. For an overview of humanities baccalaureate programs in the United States and Canada, see https://case.edu/medicine/bioethics/education/health-humanities.
9. See Barr and Duffy for a contextualization of the Flexner report.
10. The *Bioethics Quarterly* was renamed *Journal of Bioethics* in 1982. It then became the *Journal of Medical Humanities and Bioethics* in 1985 before assuming its current title, *Journal of Medical Humanities* in 1989.
11. Among her many publications, Trautmann Banks' *Healing Arts in Dialogue* (1981) and *The Art of the Case History* (with Anne Hunsaker Hawkins, 1992) have been the most influential.
12. In Charon's expansive body of work on the topic of narrative medicine, see in particular *Narrative Medicine* (2006) and *Stories Matter* (with Martha Montello, 2002). For the German context, see Anita Wohlmann et al.'s *Narrative Medizin* (2022).
13. For a more detailed history of the field, see Hudson Jones, "Why Teach Literature and Medicine?" Also see Carson et al., Cole et al., Evans et al., and Jones et al.
14. With their article, Jones et al. (2017) responded to Rafael Campo's article, "The Medical Humanities, for Lack of a Better Term," written more than a decade earlier.

15. Another critique of the Medical Humanities can be found in Johanna Shapiro et al. (2009).
16. For the most prominent textbooks, see Evans and Finlay, *Medical Humanities* (2001), Crawford et al., *Health Humanities* (2015), Cole et al., *Medical Humanities* (2015), Jones et al., *Health Humanities Reader* (2014), Jones and Pachuki, *The Medical/Health Humanities* (2022), Goyal and Hegele, *Culture and Medicine* (2022).
17. See Barr, "Revolution or Evolution" (2011).
18. See Manthripragada, Ashwin, and Emina Mušanović.
19. In this context, see the One Health Initiative, which seeks to unite human and veterinary medicine: https://onehealthinitiative.com.
20. All translations are my own.

WORKS CITED

American Academy of Arts and Sciences (AAAS). 2013. *The Heart of the Matter*.

Applegate, Celia and Frank Trommler. 2016. "The Project of German Studies: Disciplinary Strategies and Intellectual Practices." *German Studies Review* 39, no. 3 (October): 471–492.

Arslan, Gizem. 2021. Review of Regine Criser and Ervin Malakaj, *Diversity and Decolonization in German Studies*. *German Quarterly* 94, no. 3 (Summer): 421–423.

Association of American Medical Colleges (AAMC). 2020. *The Fundamental Role of the Arts and Humanities in Medical Education: Branches from the Same Tree*.

Bahr, Katrin and Katharina Gerstenberger. 2023. "'Food for Thought': New Visions for the GSA." *German Studies Review* 46, no. 1: 123–143.

Barr, Donald. 2011. "Revolution or Evolution: Putting the Flexner Report in Context." *Medical Education* 45: 17–22.

Bean, Phillip. 2013. "Choosing a Practical Major." *New York Times* April 16.

Belling, Catherine. 2006. "Hypochondriac Hermeneutics: Medicine and the Anxiety of Interpretation." *Literature and Medicine* 25, no. 2 (Fall): 376–401.

Belling, Catherine. 2017. "Arts, Sciences, Humanities: Triangulating the Two Cultures." *Journal of Literature and Science* 10, no. 2: 19–25.

Bérubé, Michael and Cary Nelson, eds. 1994. *Higher Education Under Fire: Politics, Economics, and the Crisis of the Humanities*. London: Routledge.

Bérubé, Michael and Jennifer Ruth. 2015. *The Humanities, Higher Education, and Academic Freedom: Three Necessary Arguments*. London: Palgrave Macmillan.

Bleakley, Alan. 2013. "Towards a 'Critical Medical Humanities.'" In *Medicine, Health, and the Arts: Approaches to the Medical Humanities*, edited by Victoria Bates et al., 17–26. London: Routledge.

Buhr, Christian et al. 2015. "Einleitung." In *Ulrich Wyss: Geschichte der Germanistik-Gesammelte Aufsätze*, edited by Christian Buhr et al., vii–xv. Heidelberg: Winter.

Calloway, Colin G., Gerd Gemünden, and Susanne Zantop, eds. 2002. *Germans and Indians: Fantasies, Encounters, Projections*. Lincoln and London: University of Nebraska Press.

Campo, Rafael. 2005. "The Medical Humanities, for Lack of a Better Term." *JAMA* 294: 1009–1011.

Carson, Ronald, Chester Burns, and Thomas Cole, eds. 2003. *Practicing the Medical Humanities: Engaging Physicians and Patients*. Hagerstown: University Publishing Group.

Charon, Rita. 2006. *Narrative Medicine: Honoring the Stories of Illness*. Oxford: Oxford University Press.

Charon, Rita and Martha Montello. 2002. *Stories Matter: The Role of Narrative in Medical Ethics*. New York: Routledge.

Cole, Thomas et al. 2015. *Medical Humanities: An Introduction*. Cambridge: Cambridge University Press.

Crawford, Paul et al. 2015. *Health Humanities*. London: Palgrave Macmillan.
Crawford, Paul et al. 2010. "Health Humanities: The Future of Medical Humanities?" *Mental Health Review Journal* 15: 4–10.
Criser, Regine and Edvin Malakaj, eds. 2020. *Diversity and Decolonization in German Studies*. London: Palgrave Macmillan.
DasGupta, Sayantani. 2004. "Narrative Medicine, Narrative Humility: Listening to the Streams of Stories." *Creative Nonfiction* 52: 6–7.
Davies, Mererid Puw and Sonu Shamdasani. 2020. *Medical Humanity and Inhumanity in the German-Speaking World*. London: UCL Press.
Duffy, Thomas P. 2011. "The Flexner Report: 100 Years Later." *Yale Journal of Biology and Medicine* 84, no. 3 (September): 269–276.
Evans, Marilyn and Ilora G Finlay, eds. 2001. *Medical Humanities*. London: British Medical Journal Books.
Flexner, Abraham. 1910. *Medical Education in the United States and Canada: A Report to the Carnegie Foundation for the Advancement of Teaching*. New York: Carnegie Foundation.
German Studies Association Website. www.thegsa.org
Goyal, Rishi and Arden Hegele. 2022. *Culture and Medicine: Critical Readings in the Health and Medical Humanities*. London: Bloomsbury.
Graff, Harvey. 2015. *Undisciplining Knowledge: Interdisciplinarity in the Twentieth Century*. Baltimore: Johns Hopkins University Press.
Grothus, Ulrich. 2016. "German Studies in Nordamerika: Eine Außensicht." *German Studies Review* 39, no. 3: 645–654.
Hawkins, Ann Hunsaker and Marilyn Chandler McEntyre, eds. 2000. *Teaching Literature and Medicine*. New York: Modern Language Association.
Hilger, Stephanie. 2015. *Gender and Genre: German Women Write the French Revolution*. Newark: University of Delaware Press.
Hilger, Stephanie, ed. 2017. *New Directions in Literature and Medicine Studies*. London: Palgrave Macmillan.
Hilger, Stephanie and Lisa DeTora, eds. 2019. *Bodies in Transition in the Health Humanities: Intelligible States of Corporeality*. London and New York: Routledge.
Hilger, Stephanie and John McCarthy, Nicholas Saul, and Heather Sullivan, eds. 2015. *The Early History of Embodied Cognition from 1740 to 1920: The "Lebenskraft" Debate and Radical Reality in German Science, Music, and Literature*. Amsterdam and New York: Rodopi.
Hooker, Claire and Estelle Noonan. 2011. "Medical Humanities as Expressive of Western Culture." *Medical Humanities* 37: 79–84.
Horkheimer, Max. 1972. *Critical Theory: Selected Essays*. Trans. Matthew J. Connell et al. New York: Continuum.
Hudson, Anne Jones. 2017. "Why Teach Literature and Medicine? Answers from Three Decades." *New Directions in Literature and Medicine Studies*, edited by Stephanie Hilger, 31–48. London: Palgrave Macmillan.
Hunter, Kathryn Montgomery. 1991. *Doctor's Stories: The Narrative Structure of Medical Knowledge*. Princeton: Princeton University Press.
Hutner, Gordon and Feisal Mohamed. 2015. "Introduction." In *A New Deal for the Humanities: Liberal Arts and the Future of Public Higher Education*, edited by Gordon Hutner and Feisal Mohamed, 1–17. New Brunswick: Rutgers University Press.
Iyengar, Malathi Michelle. 2014. "Not Mere Abstractions: Language Policies and Language Ideologies in U.S. Settler Colonialism." *Decolonization: Indigeneity, Education & Society* 3, no. 2: 33–59.
Jarausch, Konrad H. 2016. "From National to Transnational German Studies: Some Historical Reflections, 1977–2017." *German Studies Review* 39, no. 3 (October): 493–503.
Jay, Paul. 2014. *The Humanities "Crisis" and the Future of Literary Studies*. London: Palgrave Macmillan.

Jones, Therese et al. 2014. *Health Humanities Reader*. New Brunswick: Rutgers University Press.
Jones, Therese, M. Blackie, R. Garden and D. Wear. 2017. "The Almost Right Word: The Move from Medical to Health Humanities." *Academic Medicine* 92, no. 7 (July): 932–935.
Jones, Therese and Kathleen Pachuki, eds. 2022. *The Medical/Health Humanities: Politics, Programs, and Pedagogies*. New York: Springer.
Koepnick, Lutz. 2016. "Critical Theory and the German Studies Association." *German Studies Review* 39, no. 3 (October): 553–563.
Lehmann, Hartmut, Hermann Wellenreuther, and Renate Wilson, eds. 2000. *In Search of Peace and Prosperity: New German Settlements in Eighteenth-Century Europe and America*. University Park: Pennsylvania State University Press.
Lennox, Sara and Gerhard L. Weinberg. 2016."Forty Years of the GSA, 1976–2016." *German Studies Review* 39, no. 3: 449–469.
Lewis, Sinclair. 1925. *Arrowsmith*. New York: Harcourt Brace.
Manthripragada, Ashwin and Emina Mušanović. 2020. "Accounting for Our Settler Colonialism: Toward an Unsettled German Studies in the United States." In *Diversity and Decolonization in German Studies*, edited by Regine Criser and Ervin Malakaj, 23–40. London: Palgrave Macmillan.
McGowan, John. 2015. "Can the Humanities Save Medicine, and Vice Versa?" In *A New Deal for the Humanities: Liberal Arts and the Future of Public Higher Education*, edited by Gordon Hutner and Feisal Mohamed, 131–144. New Brunswick: Rutgers University Press.
Menand, Louis, Paul Reitter, and Chad Wellmon. 2017. *The Rise of the Research University: A Sourcebook*. Chicago: University of Chicago Press.
Opara, Ijeoma. 2021. "It's Time to Decolonize the Decolonization Movement." https://speakingofmedicine.plos.org/2021/07/29/its-time-to-decolonize-the-decolonization-movement/
Riordan, Liam. 2002. "'The Complexion of My Country': The German as 'Other' in Colonial Pennsylvania." In *Germans and Indians: Fantasies, Encounters, Projections*, edited by Colin G. Calloway, Gerd Gemünden, and Susanne Zantop, 97–119. Lincoln and London: University of Nebraska Press.
Schiller, Friedrich. 1789. *Was heißt und zu welchem Ende studiert man Universalgeschichte? Eine akademische Antrittsrede*. Jena: In der akademischen Buchhandlung.
Schleifer, Ronald and Jerry B. Vannatta. 2013. *The Chief Concern of Medicine: The Integration of the Medical Humanities and Narrative Knowledge into Medical Practices*. Ann Arbor: University of Michigan Press.
Schleifer, Ronald and Jerry B. Vannatta. 2019. *Literature and Medicine: A Practical and Pedagogical Guide*. London: Palgrave Macmillan.
Shapiro, Johanna et al. 2009. "Medical Humanities and their Discontents: Definitions, Critiques, and Implications." *Academic Medicine* 84, no. 2 (February): 192–198.
Tatlock, Lynne and Matt Erlin. 2005. *German Culture in Nineteenth-Century America: Reception, Adaptation, Transformation*. Rochester: Camden House.
Trautmann Banks, Joanne. 1981. *Healing Arts in Dialogue: Medicine and Literature*. Carbondale: Southern Illinois University Press.
Trautmann Banks, Joanne and Anne Hunsaker Hawkins. 1992. *The Art of the Case History*. Baltimore: Johns Hopkins University Press.
Trommler, Frank. 2007. "Is Literature Still Central to German Studies?" *The German Quarterly* 80, no. 1: 97–105.
Walker, Mack. 1965. *Germany and the Emigration, 1816–1885*. Cambridge: Harvard University Press.
Ward, Janet. 2016. "Interdisciplinarity, German Studies, and the Humanities." *German Studies Review* 39, no. 3 (October): 517–527.
Willis, Martin, Waddington K. and J. Castell. 2017. "ScienceHumanities: Theory, Politics, Practice." *Journal of Literature and Science* 10, no. 2: 6–18.

Wohlmann, Anita, Daniel Teufel, and Pascal O. Berberat. 2022. *Narrative Medizin: Praxisbeispiele aus dem deutschsprachigen Raum*. Köln: Böhlau.

Wokeck, Marianne S. 2000. "German Settlement in the British North American Colonies: A Patchwork of Cultural Assimilation and Persistence." In *In Search of Peace and Prosperity: New German Settlements in Eighteenth-Century Europe and America*, edited by Hartmut Lehmann, Hermann Wellenreuther, and Renate Wilson, 192–216. University Park: Pennsylvania State University Press.

Zantop, Susanne. 1997. "The Beautiful, the Ugly, and the German: Race, Gender, and Nationality in Eighteenth-Century Anthropological Discourse." In *Gender and Germanness: Cultural Productions of Nation*, edited by Patricia Herminghouse and Magda Mueller, 21–35. Providence and Oxford: Berghahn Books.

Zantop, Susanne. 1997. *Colonial Fantasies: Conquest, Family, and Nation in Precolonial Germany, 1770–1870*. Durham: Duke University Press.

PART I

Medical Readings/Reading Medicine

CHAPTER ONE

"Verschlungen sitze ich/ neben der Sprache": Aphasic Poetry between Medicine and Metaphor

KATHARINA FÜRHOLZER

PRELIMINARY REMARKS

In a metaphorical sense, the phenomenon of aphasia (Greek: *ἀφασία*/*aphasía* = "speechlessness;" derived from *ἀ-*/*a-* = "without" + *φάσις*/*phásis* = "speech") seems firmly anchored in the history of literature: The loss and limits of language have captivated writers for thousands of years, the omnipresent topoi of silence and the unspeakable being only two examples for this ancient fascination. In its clinical form, this severe language impairment can be diametrically opposed to the mastery of both the spoken and the written word; one might just think of French poet Charles Baudelaire, who could only express the single phrase "Cré nom!" ["Damn!"] after suffering from stroke-related aphasia, which also signified the end of his literary career (Dieguez and Bogousslavsky 2007; Meißner 2019, 13–16). However, there is also a number of authors such as Samuel Beckett, Tomas Tranströmer, and Paul West who continued to write poetry and prose despite being aphasic. Next to that, the work of non-aphasic writers can display striking analogies to the aphasic breaking off and out of linguistic norms and conventions. In all these (con)texts, aphasia cannot only take on the role of a literary motif but also the effect as an aesthetic device that allows exploring the limits of language while at the same time enforcing and enabling new ways of expression. The potential correlations between aphasic and aesthetic forms of language crisis have hardly caught the eye of literary studies or the Medical Humanities.[1] This comes as a surprise, as aphasia inevitably leads us to the borders of language and questions familiar ways of saying and seeing the world, which is why its study promises enthralling insights not only for life sciences but also for literary studies. Against this backdrop, this article will look at poetry in which aphasia comes into play in either a medical or a metaphorical sense of the word, with the aim to gain a deeper understanding of the creative potential of linguistic destruction.

WORDS OF APHASIA

So, what is aphasia? In its clinical definition, this term comprises several forms of language disorders caused by brain lesions after completed speech acquisition (e.g., adults who suffered a stroke or craniocerebral injury). Impairments can occur in all language modalities (speech production, reception, reading, writing) and at all linguistic levels (phonology, morphology, semantics, syntax, pragmatics), making communication at times almost impossible.[2] Aphasias are usually distinguished in fluent forms (such as Broca's aphasia) and non-fluent forms (such as Wernicke's aphasia). They are characterized by the following symptoms:

Table 1.1 Standard forms of aphasia

NON-FLUENT FORMS	• heavily shortened style of speech; syntactically strongly reduced one to two-word sentences; missing inflected forms and functional words such as prepositions or declensions (agrammatism; telegraphic style) • phonetically distorted or semantically incorrect words (phonemic or semantic paraphasias) • impairment of speech or speech disorder (dysarthria) • difficulty finding words (anomia); speaking takes strong effort • relatively intact language comprehension • marked awareness of the disorder
FLUENT FORMS	• long, entangled, duplicated sentences; defective forms of inflection (paragrammatism) • phonetic or semantic neologisms • phonetically distorted or semantically incorrect words (phonemic or semantic paraphasias), up to exclusive use of neologisms (jargon) • excessive flow of speech (logorrhea) • heavily impaired language comprehension, up to word deafness (auditory verbal agnosia) • hardly any awareness of the disorder

For a more detailed overview of standard symptoms of aphasia, see Drummond (2006, 94–95, 146–152); Code (2010); Huber, Poeck, and Springer (2013, 41–50); Schneider, Wehmeyer, and Grötzbach (2014, 18–21); Hufschmidt, Lücking, and Rauer (2022).

In light of these symptoms, it may come as no surprise that people with aphasia may encounter severe difficulties when trying to make themselves understood in the world. In his autobiography, Wolfgang Niedecken, lead singer and founding member of the German rock group *BAP*, who suffered from stroke-related aphasia himself, once described this impuissance with a poem by Swedish writer Tomas Tranströmer:

> Ich konnte nicht lesen, weil die Buchstaben nach allen Richtungen davonstoben. Und wenn ich mich bemerkbar machen wollte, verstand man mich nicht, denn auch die Wörter, die ich selbst produzieren wollte, waren vor mir auf der Flucht, und meistens hechelte ich ihnen vergeblich hinterher. Der schwedische Lyriker Tomas Tranströmer, dem Ähnliches widerfahren war, fasste die Wortfindungsstörungen eines Schlaganfallpatienten einmal in die bezwingenden Verse: "Was ich sagen will,/glänzt außer Reichweite/wie das Silber/beim Pfandleiher." Ich wusste, was er meinte. Genau so war es. (Niedecken 2013, 86–87).[3]

> [I could not read because the letters dashed off in all directions. And when I tried to call attention to myself, I was not understood, because even the words I wanted to produce myself were on the run from me, and most of the time I was chasing them in vain. Swedish poet Tomas Tranströmer, who experienced a similar fate, once put a stroke patient's amnesic search for words into these compelling verses: "The only thing I want to say/ glitters out of reach/like the silver/in a pawnbroker's." I knew what he meant. That's exactly how it was.][4]

The loss of language control can deeply impair our self-perception, sometimes to such an extent that they might experience what Barbara Shadden calls "identity theft" (2005, 219). The impact that aphasia and the reactions of (non-aphasic) others may have in this regard is already noticeable in one of the most famous texts of aphasiology, namely the case study by Paul Broca. Broca was a French neurologist who contributed significantly to the foundations of modern aphasiology in the mid-nineteenth century, when he described his first encounter with his patient Louis Victor Leborgne, in medical history better known as "Monsieur Tan:"

> On April 11, 1861, a fifty-one-year old man, named Leborgne, [...] was brought to the general infirmary of Bicêtre [...] When he arrived at Bicêtre he had already been without speech for two or three months. He was in perfect health and intelligent and showed no difference from a healthy person except for the loss of speech. He came and went about the hospital, where he was known by the name of *Tan*. He understood everything that was said to him; he even had very fine hearing; but whatever question was posed to him, he always answered *tan*, *tan*, accompanied by very diverse gestures, by means of which he managed to express most of his thoughts. When the people who questioned him did not understand his miming, he easily became outraged and added a rude swearword to his vocabulary [...].
>
> (Broca 1994, 46–47; original emphasis)

Leborgne's reaction shows the frustration that other people's lack of understanding may cause in people with aphasia. At the same time, Broca's case study implicitly reveals a process over the course of which the patient becomes displaced by his impairment and thus affected in his former identity. After all, by being reduced to the nickname "Monsieur Tan," Leborgne's loss of language becomes accompanied by the loss of his name and thus of one of the core elements of personal identity. Due to their language impairments, people with aphasia may face severe difficulties to defend themselves against such kinds of encroachment, which may cause tremendous emotional distress, finding expression in reduced self-esteem, anger, depression, and suicidal tendencies (Code and Herrmann 2003; Parr 2007; Huber, Poeck, and Springer 2013, 136–142; Hilari and Cruice 2017; Hersh 2018).[5] Swiss writer Charles-Ferdinand Ramuz, who suffered a stroke and accompanying aphasia in 1943, described the emotional pain he experienced after his illness as "an extreme irritability with violent angers about nothing," an "extreme depression." He generally felt

> jeden Vergnügens beraubt: jener lebhaften Freude, die ich allem abgewann und die jedesmal ein inneres Erwachen veranlaßte, das seinerseits die Inspiration hervorrief,—nichts: eine Blume, eine Farbe an der Mauer, eine Musik, ein Vogelgesang. Und jetzt bin ich dagegen unempfindlich; eine bizarre Gleichgültigkeit gegenüber den Dingen und den Ereignissen. (Ramuz 1982, 413).[6]

> [deprived of any pleasure: the sharp moments of joy which came about anything, and which were always leading to an inner awakening, which itself led to inspiration; nothing, a flower, a colour, on the wall, music, a bird song: well, now, I am insensitive to this: some sort of odd indifference to things and events. (Bogousslavsky 2009, 141).]

The common public equation of language impairments with cognitive impairments can additionally contribute to the anguish of those affected by aphasia. This stigmatizing misconception has long been refuted—and a short anecdote about American poet and essayist Ralph Waldo Emerson, who became aphasic in old age, shows that the loss of language control can also lead to ingenious substitutions: "On a hot day, unable to articulate the word 'sun,' Emerson invited his companion into the shade with the phrase, 'Isn't there too much heaven on you there?'" (Paulsen 1981, 159).

BREAKING DISPLACEMENT: HANNE VAHLDICK'S "VERSCHLUNGEN SITZE ICH"

Despite (or maybe because of) its destructive nature, aphasia thus also has a creative potential. And notwithstanding its at times massive impact on a patient's language ability, aphasia does not necessarily mean the end of communication (e.g., Behrns, Ahlsén, and Wengelin 2010).[7] Depending on form and gravity, partial or total recovery may be possible, either spontaneously or with therapeutic help. In this regard, poetry may play a role in this process: Due to its focus on isolated single words and sounds and its use of a rhythm freed from potentially restricting norms of everyday language, poetry can offer a form of expression even when spontaneous language fails (Shafi and Carozza 2011). When approaching aphasia from a literary perspective, the recourse to poetry seems logical. After all, it is, as Ursula Rudnick once said, poetry, "which can best express the rupture of language and experience [...]. Unlike literary forms such as the novel and unlike philosophical analysis, poetry is not bound to a narrative structure. In its structure, poetry can mirror the fragmentation caused by destruction" (1997, 132).

In the poem "Verschlungen sitze ich" by Hanne Vahldick, a former teacher who was not even thirty years old when she had a stroke that resulted in hemiplegia and aphasia, poetic and aphasic forms such as the rupture and fragmentation of language permeate the lines. From its very first line, Vahldick's poem, which due to its biographical contextualization (Lutz 2013, 14, 224; Vahldick 2021) I will read as a direct reference to the poet's aphasia, confronts us with a world where familiarity has given way to confusion: "Verschlungen sitze ich/neben der Sprache." ["Entwined I sit/next to the language."] (Lutz 2013, 14).[8] The poem begins with "verschlungen" ["entwined"], a word that—highlighted by its prominent, incipient placement as well as an anaphoric echo in the synonymous "verworren" ["entangled"] only a few lines later—already alludes to a possible loss of order, orientation, and structure. The image is taken up by its form, as instead of a preposition such as "mit" ["with"], which one would expect in the context of this adverb, the sentence proceeds with a surprising "neben" ["next to"]. In their specific combination, the two verses thus create a notion of displacement that is mirrored in the poem's break with familiar rhetoric structures. This is further intensified by the last word of the sentence, as it is not a concrete human being or thing that is sitting next to the lyrical I, but "die Sprache" ["the language"], an objectified abstractum that is no longer understood as an integral part of the lyrical speaker but as an independent counterpart. The rhetorical image of this objectified language seems symbolic for the aphasic loss of control, as its dissociation repeals the hierarchical relationship between the I and the language—detached, language is no longer subject to the command and order of the lyrical speaker but has become self-contained, self-empowered. The lyrical I's dissociation from language as implicitly insinuated by the abstractum's objectification is strengthened not only through content (cf. the explicit proposition that the lyrical I remains "disjoint of the speaking" a few lines later) but also through form: After all, at no point are language and I joined in a single line. Continuing enjambments that create a separation between the lyrical speaker and terms related to language further exemplify this dissociation and reinforce the image of a self-empowered language that went astray.[9] Thus, the lyrical I's mouth remains, as it says in the poem, "mute" and even her smile is "entangled" (14), as if it had lost its original meaning and way, thus suggesting that aphasia has affected not only verbal but also nonverbal ways of expression. It is a bleak image with which the poem confronts the reader. This smile is not blithe but speaks of the confusion that preceded it and that it might cause, this way expressing doubt that the lyrical speaker's smile will be understood and returned by others.

As such, the lyrical I's confusingly confused mouth, her crooked smile, also alludes to the emotional pain this loss of language may cause. Accordingly, the lyrical I's world has turned into a "gruesome" (14) one, a world that consists of an eternal "battle" with words (14). Time and again, the attempt to (re)unite with language, to unify thoughts and words, fails, which is expressed in the verse's anomic breaking off into the white emptiness of the paper. Potential sentences become shattered in isolated fragments:

Aus dieser Sackgasse,
aus dieser Sprachstraße
verbissen kratze ich
mir das Gehirn. Ach, (Lutz 2013, 14)

[Out of this dead-end road,
out of this language route
clenched I scratch
my brain. Oh,]

Once familiar ways of communication have been rerouted into a cul-de-sac in which reciprocal conversations are no longer possible. Thus, the lyrical I's closed mouth no longer creates closeness, but is "verbissen:" It bites itself, jaws locked, a sharp-toothed fence that lets nothing in, nothing out, like a symbol for the aphasic disconnection of former paths of communications. And even when this dissociating mouth, or "gorge" (14), as the lyrical I at one point calls it, opens, it only decreases the confusion and thus distance to others (14). In this regard, an exclaimed "Ach" ["Oh"] at the end of the line of verse appears like a fainting wail of pain. Not even an exclamation point stresses this pain that is only separated by a tiny comma from the absorbing void that it adjoins—leaving the reader with a haunting feeling of the isolation that may mark a world lost to language.

Vahldick's "Verschlungen sitze ich" thus confronts the reader with a language that is segmented into small units, in verses mostly consisting only two to three words, at times broken off into isolated fragments, this way creating a confusion that gets further intensified by the lack of connecting components[10] and the distortion of familiar (syntactical, phonemic, semantical) structures.[11] As such, Vahldick's text mirrors the telegraphic, paraphasic language of non-fluent aphasia.[12] However, transferred into the aesthetic form of a poem, the distinction between symptom and style dissolves. The poem does not answer the question which breaches of norms are intended and which are not, which are due to the illness, and which correspond to a specific aesthetic decision. Oscillating between pathological destruction and poetic creation, Vahldick's aphasic poetry allows a glimpse into the abyss of aphasia and the shattering isolation that may follow its edge, while at the same time finding a language that can no longer be overheard.

THE POETIC MASTERY OF BROKEN LANGUAGE: RILKE'S *DUINO ELEGIES*

When taking a closer look at literary history, we can find a large number of poems concerned with the limits and loss of language that show, as I would argue, implicit analogies to the aphasic destruction of language we have seen in "Verschlungen sitze ich"—even though written by writers not suffering from any language impairments. Against this backdrop, I would like to approach the broken language of aphasia from an entirely different, no longer medical but purely metaphorical angle and contrast Vahldick's poem with the *Duineser Elegien* (*Duino Elegies*) by German poet Rainer Maria Rilke. The *Elegies* were written between 1912 and 1922 and hence during a time in Rilke's life that was marked by a devastating language crisis. But despite—or perhaps precisely because of—Rilke's distrust in language, the elegies are widely regarded as one of the most elaborate poetic stances toward language and the human condition. Rilke's work is distinguished by an unsurpassed artistry, an exceptional control over language, and a highly pronounced awareness for language's philosophical dimensions. That said, writer and work almost seem like the epitome of the anti-aphasic. I agree—and yet must object: it is precisely the poetic mastery of broken language which presents the *Duino Elegies*—not in a medical, but metaphorical sense—as a form of, as I call it, aphasic poetry—poetry that emphasizes the boundaries between what can and what cannot be said, eventually showing us the creative dimensions of the destruction of language. In the *Elegies*, we are confronted with these limits of language from the very beginning:

> Wer, wenn ich schriee, hörte mich denn aus der Engel
> Ordnungen? (Rilke 1923, 7)
>
> [And if I cried, who'd listen to me in those angelic
> orders? (Rilke 1977, 5)]

exclaims the lyrical speaker in the first elegy, brutally hurling the reader against the petrified walls that restrict and define the human condition. When reading further, one will notice that the *Elegies* are pervaded by terms such as "unspeakable," "silent," "mute," or "speechless," all of which evoke the oppressive premonition that being human means being cemented by language, no matter how vehemently one tries to make oneself understood, no matter to whom one turns for being heard, not even when transcending the human and invoking the angelic orders. This issue of orders frames the *Elegies* like alpha and omega. To quote one of the most poignant passages in this context:

> Und wir: Zuschauer, immer, überall,
> dem allen zugewandt und nie hinaus!
> Uns überfüllts. Wir ordnens. Es zerfällt.
> Wir ordnens wieder und zerfallen selbst. (Rilke 1923, 30)
>
> [And we: spectators, always, everywhere,
> looking *at* everything and never *from*!
> It floods us. We arrange it. It decays.
> We arrange it again, and we decay. (Rilke 1977, 59; original emphasis)]

This struggle to manage the physical and metaphysical orders of the world is mirrored in the *Elegies*' continuous disturbance of familiar orders of language and poetry. And this demolition is accomplished in the most elaborate way: Disordered rhythms and rhymes interrupt common patterns of speaking and hearing, poetic lines are chopped up in enigmatic enjambments, sentences are broken off by pauses and ellipses that—according to Romano Guardini—"ooze with the unspeakable" and are used whenever "Rilke wants to suggest something that cannot be said" (1961, 182, 217). All of this is rhetorically draped in ingenious inversions, nifty neologisms, and complex commoratios, to name just a few. Just as aphasia, these poetic destructions of familiar references and orders underline how little language is able to grasp the world. However, the paucity of *language* is not in the slightest equivalent to the paucity of *meaning*:

> Aber das Wehende höre,
> die ununterbrochene Nachricht, die aus Stille sich bildet. (Rilke 1923, 9)
>
> [But listen to the breathing,
> the endless news growing out of silence. (Rilke 1977, 9)]

Silence is filled with something that is beyond the human language but not the human condition; it is bulging with the inkling that the limits of our words are not the limits of our world.

This auspicious silence hidden behind the familiar orders of saying and seeing needs to be sought, found, explored—and the lyrical speaker does so in an aphasic-like breaking off and out of language. By breaking off familiar orders, the *Elegies* become a mirror of the shattering deficiency of language, of its harrowing confinedness to truly correspond to and with the complexities of human experiences. Once one has hit the apparently adamant wall of language, there usually appear to be only two options: to ignore it and continue to speak like nothing has changed, or to surrender and stop speaking at all. But like an aphasic patient, Rilke's lyrical speaker does not do either: He neither jumps to the one side nor the other but, instead, becomes an acrobat, a rope walker on the borders of language, balancing on the fine wall between the conventions of our familiar ways of speaking, and the inexpressible void that reputedly lies on the other side of the known. It is this vociferous protest against the restricting powers of both language and silence that distinguishes aphasic poetry such as Rilke's from other poetic destructions of language. As even though on the verge of being torn between the dualistic poles of the speakable and unspeakable, aphasic poetry dismantles the constraining, curtailing walls of language, thereby giving voice to both what can and what cannot be said, eventually creating a dialogue between the two, now united sides of the wall.

In Rilke's aphasic poetry, destruction and creation are thus inextricably intertwined. The loss of language is a radical experience that forces and, at the same time, allows us to rethink the physical and the metaphysical from an entirely new perspective, and in this way prevents linguistic inertia and intellectual stagnation. In loose reference to Martin Heidegger's postulate "Mit der gewöhnlichen Sprache [...] läßt sich die Wahrheit des Seins nicht sagen,"—"Ordinary language cannot express [...] the truth of being" (1989, 75)—I would therefore venture to say that not aphasia itself, but aphasic poetry can at times be seen as a potential form of the "ideal language" sought by language philosophy—a language freed from the constraining orders and deficient word-world-references of everyday language, thus paving the way for new paths in language and thought.

CONCLUSION: (UN)INTENDED IMPLICATIONS

It should go without saying that there is, of course, a vast difference between medical and metaphorical conceptions of aphasia. When approaching literature from a medical angle such as an aphasiological interpretation, one must be aware of the borders separating literature and medicine: What this paper explicitly did *not* want to do was to simply equate the literary with the medical, for example, to claim that every ellipsis must be understood as "aphasic," or, conversely, that an "aphasic" break in poetic language is always and compellingly expressed in the form of, for example, an enjambment. Rather, the juxtaposition of medical and metaphorical forms of aphasia aimed to make more recognizable and understandable certain analogies between different experiences of and confrontations with the limits of language. What is more, I also feel obliged to caution against "diagnostic" connotations that might accompany a "medical" approach toward literature, as they bear the risk that work and writer are associated with the disease or impairment highlighted by the reading, i.e., that the literary interpretation is (mis)conceived as a medical diagnosis. Such pathologizations must be counteracted in the most decisive manner. In this regard, the distinction between intentionality and non-intentionality cannot be emphasized enough: The disruptions and disturbances of clinical aphasia are not voluntary, but an expression of a physiological incapacity that can mean immense suffering for those affected. In contrast to that, in the poetry of a non-aphasic writer such as Rilke, the, as I have called it, aphasic-like breaking off and out of language is a sign of an absolute mastery of language. But while the results may be different, both an aphasic patient and a non-aphasic writer of broken poetry may nevertheless share a specific moment of unintentionality and suffering—which is the disturbing struggle for control caused by the collision with the limits of language. Nevertheless, I would argue that both the poetry of aphasic patients such as Vahldick's and the mastery of broken poetry such as Rilke's make us aware of what can and what cannot be said. What medical as well as metaphorical forms of aphasic poetry may thus evoke is an insight into what it means to approximate the verge of language as we know it, of what it means to feel like losing hold of language and, losing hold of oneself—however, by expressing the abyss, aphasic poetry at the same time may vanquish the void and thus oppose aphasic destruction with poetic creation.

NOTES

1. With a few notable exceptions; see in particular Jacyna (2000); Salisbury (2008); Salisbury (2010); Eagle (2014, 17–46); Plunka (2014); Salisbury and Code (2016); Salisbury (2022).
2. For an introduction to aphasia see, e.g., Drummond (2006); Wehmeyer and Grötzbach (2014); LaPointe and Stierwalt (2017); Papathanasiou, Coppens, and Potagas (2017); Raymer and Gonzalez-Rothi (2018); Grande and Hußmann (2018).

3. Torsten Rönnerstrand understands the poem's silver-metaphor as an inner, a mental speech that lives on in the patient despite his or her aphasia (Rönnerstrand 2006, n.p.). For a detailed analysis of Tranströmer's aphasic poetry, also with regard to the "aphasic" dimension of the poetic genre of haiku, see Fürholzer (2016); Fürholzer (2019, 189–210).
4. The English translation of Tranströmer's poem *April and Silence* is quoted from Tranströmer (2006, 199). Unless otherwise stated, all other translations are mine.
5. This is not least due to the widespread public association of aphasias with an intellectual disability, a misconception that has been proven wrong since the beginnings of aphasiology (Tesak 2005, 62; for a comprehensive English-speaking overview of the history of aphasiology, see Tesak and Code 2008).
6. Despite his impairment, Ramuz remained able to keep writing a diary, which thus represents an immediate and rather unfiltered aphasia document.
7. As aphasic poet Chris Ireland once said: "I have a language problem, not a communication problem" (Ireland and Black 1992, 355).
8. In 2021 Vahldick published her (illness) narrative *Harlekin: Erzählungen von Hanne* ("Harlequin: Narratives from Hanne"), in which this poem is included as well. All quotes of Vahldick's poem are taken from the original publication in Lutz (2013, 14).
9. Note the similarity between this image of an escaped language and Wolfgang Niedecken's flight metaphor when he says that the "Worte [...] waren vor mir auf der Flucht" ["words [...] were on the run from me"].
10. Cf., e.g., the missing verb in the line "Die Augen—aufmerksam" ["The eyes—attentive," 14].
11. Cf., e.g., the combination of—the figurative language of the—the idiom "sich das Gehirn zermartern/sich den Kopf zerbrechen" ["to rack one's brain"] and—the literal language of—"sich den Kopf kratzen" ["to scratch one's head"].
12. Cf. above cited symptoms of non-fluent aphasia.

WORKS CITED

Behrns, Ingrid, Elisabeth Ahlsén, and Åsa Wengelin. 2010. "Aphasia and Text Writing." *International Journal of Language Communication Disorders* 45, no. 2: 230–243.

Bogousslavsky, Julien. 2009. "'The Adventure': Charles-Ferdinand Ramuz's Extraordinary Stroke Diary." *European Neurology* 61, no. 3: 138–142.

Broca, Paul. 1994. "Notes on the Site of the Faculty of Articulated Language, Followed by an Observation of Aphemia; Translated from 'Remarques sur le siège de la faculté du langage articulé, suivies d'une observation d'aphémie (perte de la parole)', Bulletins de la Société Anatomique, 6: 330–357 (1861)." In *Reader in the History of Aphasia: From Franz Gall to Norman Geschwind*, edited and translated by Paul Eling, 41–49. Amsterdam: John Benjamins Publication.

Code, Chris and Manfred Herrmann. 2003. "The Relevance of Emotional and Psychosocial Factors in Aphasia to Rehabilitation." *Neuropsychological Rehabilitation* 13, no. 1–2: 109–132.

Code, Chris. 2010. "Aphasia." In *The Handbook of Language and Speech Disorders*, edited by Jack S. Damico, Nicole Müller, and Martin John Ball, 317–336. West Sussex: Wiley-Blackwell.

Dieguez, Sebastian and Julien Bogousslavsky. 2007. "Baudelaire's Aphasia: From Poetry to Cursing." In *Neurological Disorders in Famous Artists* 2, edited by Julien Bogousslavsky and Michael G. Hennerici, 121–149. Basel: Karger.

Drummond, Sakina S. 2006. *Neurogenic Communication Disorders: Aphasia and Cognitive-Communication Disorders*. Springfield: Charles C. Thomas.

Eagle, Chris. 2014. *Dysfluencies: On Speech Disorders in Modern Literature*. New York: Bloomsbury.

Fürholzer, Katharina. 2016. "Hinter der Agonie der Sprache der Geist: Zum aphasischen Bewusstsein in Tomas Tranströmers Lyrik." In *Geisteskultur zwischen Ästhetik und Poetik*, edited by Aneta Jachimowicz and Tomasz Żurawlew, 215–231. Würzburg: Königshausen & Neumann.

Fürholzer, Katharina. 2019. *Das Ethos des Pathographen: Literatur- und medizinethische Dimensionen von Krankenbiographien*. Heidelberg: Winter.

Grande, Marion and Katja Hußmann. 2016. *Einführung in die Aphasiologie*. Stuttgart: Thieme.

Guardini, Romano. 1961. *Rainer Maria Rilkes Deutung des Daseins: Eine Interpretation der Duineser Elegien*. München: Kösel.

Heidegger, Martin. 1989. *Gesamtausgabe* 65, edited by Friedrich-Wilhelm von Herrmann. Frankfurt am Main: Klostermann.

Hersh, Deborah. 2018. "From Individual to Global: Human Rights and Aphasia." *International Journal of Speech-Language Pathology* 20, no. 1: 39–43.

Hilari, Katerina and Madeline Cruice. 2017. "Quality-of-life Approach to Aphasia." In *Aphasia and Related Neurogenic Communication Disorders*, edited by Ilias Papathanasiou und Patrick Coppens, 287–310. Burlington: Jones & Bartlett.

Huber, Walter, Klaus Poeck, and Luise Springer. 2013. *Klinik und Rehabilitation der Aphasie: Eine Einführung für Therapeuten*. Stuttgart: Thieme.

Hufschmidt, Andreas, Carl Hermann Lücking, and Sebastian Rauer, eds. 2022. *Neurologie compact*. Stuttgart: Thieme.

Ireland, Chris and Maria Black. 1992. "Living with Aphasia: The Insight Story." *Working Papers in Linguistics* 4: 355–358.

Jacyna, L. S. 2000. *Lost Words: Narratives of Language and the Brain, 1825–1926*. Princeton: Princeton University Press.

LaPointe, Leonard L. and Julie Stierwalt, eds. 2017. *Aphasia and Related Neurogenic Language Disorders*. New York: Thieme.

Lutz, Luise. 2013. *Das Schweigen verstehen: Über Aphasie*. Berlin: Springer.

Meißner, Thomas. 2019. *Der prominente Patient: Krankheiten berühmter Persönlichkeiten*. Berlin: Springer.

Niedecken, Wolfgang. 2013. *Zugabe: Die Geschichte einer Rückkehr*. Hamburg: Hoffmann & Campe.

Papathanasiou, Ilias, Patrick Coppens, and Constantin Potagas, eds. 2017. *Aphasia and Related Neurogenic Communication Disorder*. Burlington: Jones & Bartlett.

Parr, Susie. 2007. "Living with Severe Aphasia: Tracking Social Exclusion." *Aphasiology* 21, no. 1: 98–123.

Paulsen, A. B. 1981. "Emerson and Aphasia." *Language and Style: An international journal* 14, no. 3: 155–171.

Plunka, Gene A. 2014. "Staging Aphasia: Jean-Claude Van Itallie's *The Traveller* and Arthur Kopit's *Wings*." In *Literature, Speech Disorders, and Disability: Talking Normal*, edited by Chris Eagle, 124–136. New York: Routledge.

Ramuz, Charles-Ferdinand. 1982. *Tagebuch 1896–1947*. Frauenfeld: Huber.

Raymer, Anastasia and Leslie Gonzalez-Rothi, eds. 2018. *The Oxford Handbook of Aphasia and Language Disorders*. Oxford: Oxford University Press.

Rilke, Rainer Maria. 1923. *Duineser Elegien*. Leipzig: Insel.

Rilke, Rainer Maria. 1977. *Duino Elegies and The Sonnets to Orpheus*. Translated by A. Poulin. Boston: Houghton Mifflin.

Rönnerstrand, Torsten. 2006. "Poesi ur afasi – ett tranströmerskt mirakel." *Tvärsnitt* 3, no. 4. https://web.archive.org/web/20111106023814/http://www.vr.se/huvudmeny/arkiv/2004/tvarsnittnr32004/poesiurafasietttranstromersktmirakel.4.64fbca2110dabf7901b80001106.html.

Rudnick, Ursula. 1997. "Reconstructing God-Language: The Poetry of Nelly Sachs." *European Judaism: A Journal for the New Europe* 30, no. 2: 131–150.

Salisbury, Laura and Chris Code. 2016. “Jackson’s Parrot: Samuel Beckett, Aphasic Speech Automatisms, and Psychosomatic Language.” *Journal of Medical Humanities* 37, no. 2: 205–222.
Salisbury, Laura. 2008. “‘What Is the Word’: Beckett’s Aphasic Modernism.” *Journal of Beckett Studies* 17, no. 1–2: 78–126.
Salisbury, Laura. 2010. “Sounds of Silence: Aphasiology and the Subject of Modernity.” In *Neurology and Modernity: A Cultural History of Nervous Systems, 1800–1950*, edited by Laura Salisbury and Andrew Shail, 204–230. New York: Palgrave Macmillan.
Salisbury, Laura. 2022. “Aphasic Modernism: Languages for Illness from a Confusion of Tongues.” In *The Edinburgh Companion to the Critical Medical Humanities*, edited by Anne Whitehead, Angela Woods, Sarah Atkinson, Jane Macnaughton, and Jennifer Richards, 444–462. Edinburgh: Edinburgh University Press.
Schneider, Barbara, Meike Wehmeyer, and Holger Grötzbach. 2014. *Aphasie: Wege aus dem Sprachdschungel*. Berlin: Springer.
Shadden, Barbara. 2005. “Aphasia as Identity Theft: Theory and Practice.” *Aphasiology* 19, no. 3–5: 211–223.
Shafi, Noel and Linda Carozza. 2011. “Poetry and Aphasia: A Clinical Outlook.” *Journal of Poetry Therapy* 24, no. 4: 255–259.
Tesak, Jürgen and Chris Code. 2008. *Milestones in the History of Aphasiology: Theories and Protagonists*. Hove: Psychology Press.
Tesak, Jürgen. 2005. *Geschichte der Aphasie*. Idstein: Schulz-Kirchner.
Tranströmer, Tomas. 2006. *The Great Enigma: New Collected Poems*. Translated by Robert Fulton. New York: New Directions Publishing.
Vahldick, Hanne. 2021. *Harlekin: Erzählungen von Hanne*. Egestorf: Buchverlag Andrea Schmitz.

CHAPTER TWO

The Totality Trap of Reading Illness: Unica Zürn's *The House of Illnesses*

ANITA WOHLMANN AND KATHARINA BAHLMANN

INTRODUCTION

This contribution examines the German writer and graphic artist Unica Zürn, her creative work and how it relates to her experiences of schizophrenia. Zürn's work does not easily fall into the popular genre of the illness narrative and pathography and thus "a form of autobiography or biography that describes personal experiences of illness, treatment, and sometimes death" (Hawkins 1993, 1). While illness is indeed the subject matter of several of Zürn's artistic works—among them *Das Haus der Krankheiten* (*The House of Illnesses*) (1958), *Dunkler Frühling* (*Dark Spring*) (1968), and *Der Mann im Jasmin* (*The Man of Jasmine*) (1971)—Esra Plumer has argued that Zürn uses illness primarily as a "consciously employed artistic methodology" and an intricate element of her process of production (2016, 6). In other words, as an artist, Zürn responds creatively to her experiences and appropriates them purposefully (Clements 2019, 202). Indeed, Zürn inventively plays with linear chronology and the fragmentary; she also muddies the boundaries between realist and non-realist aesthetics. In doing so, Zürn's work taps into some of the central concerns and controversies in the fields of Health Humanities and Narrative Medicine.

In Health Humanities, the role of narrative occupies a central role, especially in the subfield of Narrative Medicine. For one, scholars have emphasized the significant role of narrative in identity construction (Ricœur 1984; Bruner 1991; Eakin 2008) and as a therapeutic strategy when a person's life story is broken by illness and requires fixing through acts of restorying

(Brody 1994, 79; White 2001; Kenyon and Randall 1997). As "wounded storytellers" (Frank 1995), patients have increasingly used (semi-)autobiographical and fictional forms to come to terms with their experiences (Hawkins 1993) and, in doing so, they have employed some of the central functions of narrative: it invites us to articulate and make present what is otherwise latent, it helps explain experiences to ourselves and to others by creating a causal link between events, and, in the process, it promotes sense-making and a (deeper) understanding of what has happened. Interwoven with myths and metaphors, narratives thus give form, coherence, and meaning to what otherwise seems fragmented, arbitrary, and senseless.

However, other scholars have argued that the role of narrative has been grounded too firmly in limiting conceptualizations of the self to "a solid, unyielding core" and in imagining it as an ideal of "personal wholeness" (DeFalco 2009, 24). The emphasis on narrative and its affinity to "sequence, succession, causality, or closure" (Tammi 2006, 22) has been criticized for being too simplistic because these features may be restrictive or even harmful when they impose a false sense of unity or are idealized as normal and desirable (Woods 2011, 73–74). Anne Whitehead summarizes the debate by arguing that "mainstream medical humanities have reified narrative representation and defined it in limited and circumscribed ways; namely as *realist*, linear and working toward closure. Under the guise of interdisciplinarity, medicine has colonised a selective version of literature" (2017, 116; our emphasis). For this reason, Angela Woods (2013) and Sara Wasson (2018), for example, propose to also consider forms such as visual media and episodic, serial structures that value open-ended and fragmentary states and that invite meaninglessness and formlessness in, for example, non-realist aesthetics.

In juxtaposing handwritten diary entries with intricate drawings in an aesthetic context of surrealism and avant-garde art, Zürn's work *The House of Illnesses* (1958) negotiates core themes in health humanities and narrative medicine: there is a constant tension between fact and fiction as well as biographical detail and playful invention; the book explores power hierarchies between the dominant male Dr. Mortimer and an unnamed female patient and first person narrator, who is both complicit and resistant.[1] A diagnostic, medical gaze and the complexities of perception are thematized both *within* the text and on the level of the readers' *engagement with* the text; additionally, *The House of Illnesses* both invokes and simultaneously undermines a sense of coherence and unity, suggesting that any claim toward wholeness, closure, and semantic determinacy is ultimately a trap—a trap that Helga Lutz fittingly calls "Ganzheitsfalle," which we translate as "totality trap" (2003, 137).

In this article, we focus on the body images in *The House of Illnesses* and look more closely at Zürn's strategies of creation and fragmentation through both language and visualization. These strategies, we argue, self-reflexively invoke and destabilize any sense of semantic wholeness and totality. As we indicated above, Zürn's work is often approached in a dualistic, binary way: either Zürn's works on illness are understood as "direct products of [her] illness"—schizophrenia—or they are read as a form of appropriation, a conscious staging through "intentional artistic strategies that are intertwined with experiences of mental illness" and that aim at challenging our conventional patterns of perception and interpretation (Plumer 2016, 5; Lutz 2003, 169). Taking inspiration from Lutz' notion of the totality trap, we suggest that, in addition to these two important lenses, Zürn invites a broader perspective of non-binary approaches, juxtaposing diagnostic, medically informed readings, biographical approaches, historical contextualizations, a focus on the genre of the illness narrative and its affordances, as well as an exploration of her aesthetic strategies. This plurality of understanding the meaning(s) of Zürn's work can be usefully transferred to the pedagogical context of Narrative Medicine, which thematizes, among other things, the complexities of perception and the value of ambiguity in young doctors' professional identity formation.

After contextualizing the artist Unica Zürn and *The House of Illnesses*, we will focus on Zürn's use of body images and suggest several lenses through which the text can be read. At the end, we briefly describe how we have used excerpts from Zürn's text in a Narrative Medicine intervention at the Charité in Berlin that focused on the complexities of perception and the diagnostic gaze.

CONTEXT: UNICA ZÜRN

The work of Unica Zürn (Berlin, 1916—Paris, 1970) includes prose texts, anagram poems, drawings, and paintings, and is commonly situated in the context of (late) Surrealism (Henry, *DIE EINZIGE*, 47–48). On the one hand, this association can be explained by her long-standing relationship with the artist Hans Bellmer, whom she followed to Paris in 1953 and through whom she was introduced to a circle of renowned Surrealist artists such as Max Ernst and Hans Arp. On the other hand, aesthetic practices of Surrealism—the play with coincidence, change, and spontaneity—are also directly traceable in Zürn's works (Lutz 2003, 75; Brand-Claussen 2009, 109). In recent years, however, scholars have shifted toward a more differentiated classification of Zürn within art history. For one, they have highlighted the differences between Zürn's aesthetic and the works of Hans Bellmer and the classical Surrealists, for example, in the use of automatism (Lutz 2003, 75–84; Brand-Claussen 2009, 108; Plumer 2016, 121). For another, further artistic references within Zürn's works have been identified: avant-garde movements of the early twentieth century (Thüne 2011, 211), Berlin Surrealism (and especially the artists of the cabaret "Badewanne"), the works of Wols, Henri Michaux, and Antonin Artaud of the 1950s, in which the viewer's sensual receptivity is challenged by means of an abundance of small forms (Lutz 2003, 56–68, 84–93), as well as performance art more generally (Rupprecht 2006, 132–133).

Despite these multiple resonances and intersections, Zürn has not been adequately appreciated as an artist up until the turn of the millennium. This lack of recognition has been explained by the fact that Zürn was an autodidact (De Zanger 2015, 262). Moreover, her work plays with numerous biographical references which entailed that her works were primarily interpreted (and devalued) in light of her biography. Her romantic relationship to Hans Bellmer, for example, was viewed as an unequal master-pupil relationship, and Zürn's schizophrenia—which led to several stays in psychiatric clinics beginning in 1960, the break-up with Bellmer, and her suicide in 1970—suggested to scholars that she was a heartbroken, abandoned woman and a failed, wannabe artist (Lutz 2003, 21–28; Brand-Claussen 2009, 106).[2]

Since Zürn herself retrospectively dates the onset of her schizophrenia to 1957 (Brand-Claussen 2009, 110), it stands to reason that *The House of Illnesses*, written in 1958,[3] bears important traces of this experience. How then can we not interpret Zürn's text in light of her mental illness, especially when Zürn uses a first-person, female narrator who is in the thick of a mysterious, uncanny illness?

"AN ACE SHOT:" SUMMARY OF *THE HOUSE OF ILLNESSES*[4]

Zürn's narrator opens the diary with contradictory information that quickly unsettles a narrow biographical reading. The paratextual note "Die Geschichten und Bilder einer Gelbsucht" ["Stories and Pictures from a Bout of Jaundice"] introduces us to the manuscript. That jaundice is not the primary concern of the eponymous *House of Illnesses*—and maybe not even an issue after all—becomes clear in the first journal entry: Dr. Mortimer diagnoses an eye disease, describing it, oddly, as "Die beiden Herzen in Ihren Augen sind mitten durch die Brust geschossen" ["Both of the two hearts of your eyes have been shot right through the centre"] (Zürn, *House*, 10).[5] Dr. Mortimer's use of the phrase "Meisterschuss" ["ace shot"] (Zürn, *House*, 10) invites the reader to doubt the correctness of the diagnosis as well as Dr. Mortimer's medical authority. Moreover, in shifting from jaundice to an eye disease and, in the course of the text, to yet another, less specified illness (a mysterious attack of a "Todfeind" or "Mortal Enemy," Zürn, *House*, 25), we cannot help but doubt the reliability of the first-person narrator who remains vague and distant and oddly bodiless (Lutz 2003, 141). Presenting itself as a hand-written personal account that follows, in sequential order, the illness experiences of an unnamed woman, the ten, respectively eleven,[6] diary entries in *The House of Illnesses* are juxtaposed with seventeen drawings (ink and pencil on paper). The drawings not only visualize the events and experiences described in the text, in some cases they also contradict the text or contain other aspects such as subjective visualizations and fantasies (Thüne 2011, 213). In addition, the drawings themselves contain lines of text that temporally situate, describe, or comment on what is depicted (see Figures 2.1 and 2.2).

The story follows the narrator who recounts Dr. Mortimer's regular visits, her hallucinatory and delirious visions, as well her fantastic, dream-like walks through different, imagined rooms in the house of illnesses, such as "das Kabinett der Sonnengeflechte" ["the Cabinet of the Solar Plexuses"] (Zürn, *House*, 14), "das Zimmer der Augen" ["the Room of Eyes"] (49), "die Kammern der Hände" ["the Chambers of the Hands"] (37), and "[der] Raum der Herzen" ["the Suite of the Hearts"] (82) (Plumer 2016, 168). There are other figures or characters beside Dr. Mortimer: "der weißhaarige Herr, der [ihr] die Märchensuppe [ihrer] Kindheit Löffel für Löffel einflößte" [a "white-haired man [feeding her] the fairy-tale soups [of her] childhood"] (Zürn, *House*, 25), "der Fallensteller" ["trapper"] (38) who is both a dubious, untrustworthy creature but also protecting her from yet another character, the "Mortal Enemy," who is represented as a two-headed eagle (Zürn, *House*, 39; Plumer, 2016, 173). All characters appear to be Dr. Mortimer himself, or rather different versions or appearances of him. The narrator also mentions a "roter, lackierter Skorpion" ["red lacquer scorpion"], a "Buddhastatue aus Stein" ["small stone Buddha statue"], and a "Puppe aus Wachs" ["wax doll"] whose face is similar to the narrator's and whose body is pierced with black needles (Zürn, *House*, 86 (text), Zürn, *House*, 89 (drawing)). Like Dr. Mortimer, the narrator has a split self: a "bessere Hälfte" ["better half"]—described as "klug und weise" ["clever and wise"]—and a "schlechte Hälfte"

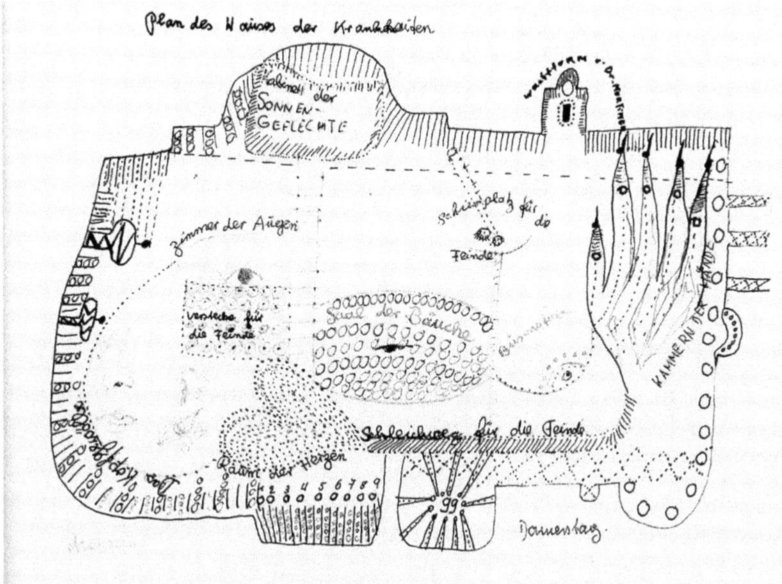

FIGURE 2.1: Unica Zürn, Haus der Krankheiten (1999). "Plan des Hauses der Krankheiten"—Berlin: Brinkmann und Bose. Copyright Herbach and Haase.

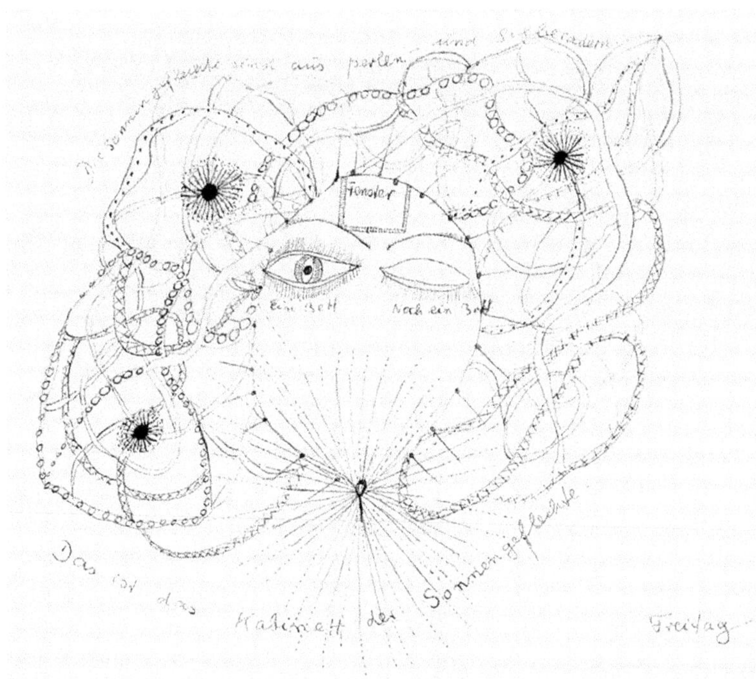

FIGURE 2.2: Unica Zürn, Haus der Krankheiten (1999). "Kabinett der Sonnengeflechte"—Berlin: Brinkmann und Bose. Copyright Herbach and Haase.

["bad half"] (Zürn, *House*, 70), both are in internal battle over what the illness means to her, which gains it affords her and how to deal with it. After an attempt to leave the house of illness, the narrator returns, finding the external world utterly bleak and depressing. At the end of the book, Dr. Mortimer gives her an ultimatum—either stay forever or leave—and she asks to be discharged and, at dawn, leaves the house, seemingly, for good.

But what (type of) house does she actually leave?

THE TOTALITY TRAP: ZÜRN'S BODY IMAGES

According to Helga Lutz, Zürn's house is a phantasmatic, hallucinatory entity that can be understood in different ways (2003, 137). For one, *Das Haus der Krankheiten* is a playful (although incomplete) inversion of the German word for hospital, "Krankenhaus" (Lutz 2003, 137), and thus the result of an aesthetic practice that is very germane to Zürn and her work with anagrams.[7] For another, the house also appears as a prison, a haunted house, and a ghost mansion with spooky characters and uncanny incidents (137). Most obviously, the house is also a metaphor for the human body and brings to mind Fritz Kahn's medical illustrations from the 1920s and 1930s.[8] Zürn's aesthetic, however, is entirely different from Kahn's, and her illustrations could not be more removed from Kahn's aspirations for science communication. As Figure 2.1 "Plan des Hauses der Krankheiten" ["Plan of the House of Illnesses"] (Zürn, *House*, 82) demonstrates, the topography of this phantasmatic, bodily entity is almost beyond recognition: body parts are spread across a two-dimensional map and labeled as rooms, such as the "Kabinett der SONNENGEFLECHTE" ["Cabinet of the SOLAR PLEXUSES"][9] or "Busenstube" ["The Bosom Parlour"]. As rooms, these organs can be entered and explored: the narrator mentions, for example, that she spent a sunny morning in the "Kammern der Hände" ["Chambers of the Hands"] (37)—her thumbnail more specifically—which she finds a quiet and festive place.

The house metaphor is interwoven with the prominent metaphor of illness as war or battle. As Figure 2.1 shows, the plan is reminiscent of the shape of a fortress, including palisades, a watchtower (which belongs to Dr. Mortimer), a secret path for enemies that extends across what looks like a courtyard, a shooting range and a hiding place for enemies. The map's aesthetic also suggests an innocent, child-like fantasy world known from fairytales. Once more, Zürn's strategies of wordplay take effect: the German word "Plan" signifies a map or blueprint, a proposition, and a game board ["Spielplan"] (Lutz 2003, 144). In a medical context, readers are often reminded of medical illustrations depicting cellular compartments in the context of cell biology; others identify the walls or boundaries of the house as a simplified illustration of the epidermis. In short, the drawings and the book as a whole provide a picture puzzle in which our perception is constantly shifting, and conflicting interpretations come to the fore (Lutz 2003, 143).

These shifting perspectives become particularly evident when we compare the plan or map[10] of the house of illnesses (Figure 2.1) with the drawing entitled "Kabinett der Sonnengeflechte" ["Cabinet of the Solar Plexuses"] (Zürn, *House*, 14; Figure 2.2). While the so-called plan (Figure 2.1) also features the cabinet in a miniature version, the cabinet in the plan has little in common with the full-page drawing in Figure 2.2. These dissimilar representations undermine the notion of a single body: the plural in "solar plexuses" already points to multiplicity; in addition, on the visual level, both the entire structure and the radiating circle at the bottom can be interpreted as a solar plexus (Thüne 2012, 135). In Zürn's artistic universe, the body is not a given, it is not a re-presentation, but a fleeting effect of writing and drawing, an assemblage of body fragments that are in the process of being rewritten, over and over again (Lutz 2003, 141). Accordingly, the great solar plexus is composed of other parts of the body, namely eyes and veins. The drawing also resembles a Medusa's head (Thüne 2012, 134) with one eye open and one eye closed, its hair made of "Perlen- und Silberadern" ["veins of pearl and silver"]. By labeling the eyes "Ein Bett" ["a bed"] and "Noch ein Bett" ["another bed"] and by placing a square "Fenster" ["window"] above them, the representation itself turns into a plan or map in which the nesting of space and body parts continues. Seen in this way, the illustration functions inversely to the plan of the house of illnesses: While the overall structure of the "Plan" (Figure 2.1) invokes an architecture that contains individual body parts, in Figure 2.2 the body part provides the overall structure in which architectural elements are inscribed. Such strategies of inversion, the use of word play, and the liberal juxtaposition of several body metaphors signal a constant shifting of meanings, a plurality of coexisting perspectives on illness and the body, and a confusingly vast texture of colliding ideas, images and voices, none of which lead to any closure or determinacy. The totality trap is constantly outwitted.

This openness and semantic indeterminacy of Zürn's text on level of content and aesthetic strategies lead us to hypothesize that the same sense of plurality is also required on the methodological level, asking us *how* we approach this representation of illness. After all, if Zürn's work circumvents semantic stability, it is unlikely that *one* approach will be able to offer any certainty—and thereby the satisfaction and gratification that comes with knowing what something "really" means. In fact, Zürn seems to mock such a detective's search for the truth and the "single story" when she makes subtle intertextual references to Sherlock Holmes in *The House of Illnesses*,[11] which, paradoxically, do not lead to a deeper understanding of the text (Lutz 2003, 150). Instead, such interspersed references, as Lutz argues, should be understood as a "bedeutungseröffnende Komponente" (150), an invitation to open up rather than close down the potential meanings of the text. Such semantic ambiguity compels, on the one hand, a plurality of approaches to Zürn's work; on the other, it also lies at the heart of interdisciplinary interventions, such as Narrative Medicine courses. To illustrate this claim, we offer a brief and necessarily incomplete overview of potential approaches to Zürn's text and its drawings and then illustrate how these approaches informed a Narrative Medicine course, in which we used an excerpt of Zürn's *The House of Illnesses*.

MULTIPLE ANGLES: APPROACHES TO *THE HOUSE OF ILLNESSES*

In our discussion so far, we have followed researchers like Helga Lutz, Esra Plumer, and Caroline Rupprecht in whose view Zürn is an artist who playfully and intentionally reconfigures her illness experience in order to explore its artistic potential. Rupprecht sees evidence for this artistic approach in the fact that Zürn's work appears too controlled and too carefully designed to have been created in a state of madness, or its immediate aftermath (2006, 133). This approach has many benefits because it counters a narrow understanding of illness as a deficit or abnormality, as a state of mere misery and stigmatization that requires treatment and overcoming. However, there are also (ethical) caveats to framing Zürn's text in this way. After all, it raises the question whether there are problematic gains to this creative "exploitation" of illness. Primary and secondary illness gains are well-known phenomena in medical psychology and describe a patient's personal benefits from being (and remaining) ill, such as attention, reduction of stress, inability to work, and access to drugs. In alignment with such practical gains, one can also wonder to what extent a use of illness for artistic reasons may involve a romanticization of the artist's condition: schizophrenia, from this perspective, is a "special" skill that grants Zürn a unique and exceptional access to the world and that functions as a crucial condition for her creativity and ingenuity as an artist.[12] Significantly, Zürn explicitly addresses such gains when her narrator openly admits that she welcomes her illness and wishes to prolong it. What remains open is the question if and to what extent Zürn—and by extension the narrator—indeed "exploits" her illness for professional gains as an artist.

This question invites biographical approaches that try to match facts about Zürn's life with her artistic work (see Henry 2010). While biographical readings do elucidate intriguing aspects—Henry explains, for example, that the highly ornamental aesthetic of Zürn's drawings is inspired by her exposure to oriental art in her childhood (38)—a focus on biography, like any other, singularly used approach, risks falling into a totality trap: one is easily lured into the detective work of gathering evidence in the hope that it will offer definitive explanations and allow closure to the hermeneutic endeavor. It risks overlooking or downplaying, however, how artworks are imaginative, drawing on exaggeration and therefore willfully distorting.

Joined with approaches from art history, a biographical lens opens up another perspective. As we outlined above, Zürn has been associated with surrealism, and this perspective collides in interesting ways with the diagnostic lens of, for example, a psychiatrist, who might see signs of delusions and hallucinations in the confused narrator. Following surrealist aesthetics, rationality and reason must be questioned. The experiences of the First World War upended grand conceptualizations about human logic and progress. According to Thomas Röske, surrealists "took the *fous* [the mentally ill; our translation] as an example and posited what they understood of their thinking, actions and creativity cogently against the traditional status quo—of which, to them, psychiatrists were excellent representatives" (2009, 10).[13] In the context of Surrealism, Unica Zürn was assigned a dual role: on the one hand, she was considered a surrealist artist, who used common surrealist procedures such as the fusion of figures in her drawings (Röske 2009, 16); on the other, she was deemed a personality who knew madness from within and created "outsider art"—an interpretation that was not always used to her benefit, as we discuss above (Brand-Claussen 2009, 106).

As a semi-autobiographical story about illness, *The House of Illnesses* also invites a discussion of the genre of the pathography, its affordances and complexities. Illness narratives are considered a genre of writing that gives intimate access to a subjective experience of illness—as opposed to a clinically defined disease—allowing (among others) healthcare professionals and relatives some insight into what it may feel like to be in "the kingdom of the sick" (Sontag 2002, 3). In the case of Zürn's *House of Illnesses*, 45 it is interesting, for example, to analyze the sensations with which the individual body parts or rooms are associated: Zürn refers to the cabinet of solar plexuses as "the noblest part" of her body while she attributes a "nasty feminine nature" to the heart. Another aspect would be the perception of interior and exterior space presented in the book, which repeatedly shifts and undermines the boundary between interior and exterior in the course of the illness experience.

A focus on the reader's experience (common in reader-response criticism) foregrounds the affective relationships between reader and text that Zürn's work solicits: Do its gaps confuse readers and create distance? Or do they activate a reader's imagination, thus leading to a deeper involvement with the text? Such questions tie in with the discourse about the role of illness narratives (and literature, more generally) in interdisciplinary contexts, such as medical education: To what extent may Zürn's text help cultivate empathy in readers by offering them a chance to change their perspective and better understand what it may feel like to live with a mental illness? If empathy cultivation is possible—a hypothesis that is still controversially discussed[14]—does it happen through identification with the narrator and her situation? Does the form of the text and its aesthetic strategies reproduce in readers the experience of confusion, uncertainty, delusion, and hallucination?

Finally, *The House of Illnesses* invites a diagnostic, medical gaze. Combined with insight about Zürn's medical biography, the experiences described in the text and drawings—"Visionen" ["visions"] (Zürn, *House*, 17), "seltsame Gedanken" ["strange thoughts"] (25), a "Fatamorgana" ["Fata Morgana"] (61)—can encourage trained healthcare professionals to go on a detective's search: Which symptoms can be identified? Which disease classification do they suggest? The role of the text is similar to the role of the patient (and her body or symptoms) in a doctor's office: both become the object of a medical gaze. Therefore, illness narratives—especially those that rely on explicit visualization, such as illustrations and films, thematize "how medicine *looks*" (Servitje 2019, 55). Such looking implies how medicine as an institution "*gazes* upon patients and populations;" the look also implies how medicine looks *like* to others, "how it *appears* in cultural productions" (55). In Zürn's text, medicine appears in a quite dubious way, and *The House of Illnesses* self-reflexively discusses the complications of a diagnostic gaze: it destabilizes, after all, any claim to diagnostic adequacy right from the start when the "story of jaundice" is followed by a questionable diagnosis of an eye disease. A diagnostic approach, like any other singular approach, fails to offer the determinacy and closure associated with it. Once more, we are left with a constant shifting of meanings, conflicting and even paradoxical interpretations.

There are, of course, more approaches to Zürn's text and many more issues that can be raised.[15] Our point here is that plurality and ambiguity—both *within* the text and in the encounter *with* the text—are invaluable assets. They encourage us to move beyond binary, dualistic approaches. Rather than asking "either/or" questions, we are challenged to adopt an "and/and" paradigm. For example, what happens if we understand Zürn's narrator as willfully unreliable *and* delusional against her better judgment *and* as self-reflexively staging her experiences? How is our understanding of illness and its artistic representation expanded if we move from a double consciousness to a consciousness of plurality and endless ambiguity? Which limitations and risks does such an expansion entail? How does each approach and the "evidence" it produces matter? For example, how does it affect our perception, feed into (professional) biases and impact the quality of our relation to the text/narrator? Are we distant, critical, suspicious, empathetic?

Clearly, Zürn's text is a thick fabric of conflicting ideas and voices that invites (and demands) endless possibilities of interpretative combinations (Lutz 2003, 149). In interdisciplinary pedagogical contexts such as Narrative Medicine, such a plurality is both a goal—in order to broaden perspectives and to encourage participants to think outside the box—and a controversial subject matter in its own right. After all, healthcare professionals and patients often desire coherence (as opposed to chaos), semantic clarity (as opposed to confusion), and closure (as opposed to interminable treatments and insecurity).

In our final chapter, we will illustrate briefly how our previous discussion translates into a pedagogical context at a medical university. Importantly, the premise of using a literary text or artwork like Zürn's in a medical context is based on plurality, too: we do not aim at bringing across a specific subject matter or predetermined learning goal. Instead, the text's semantic ambiguity, its interpretative openness, and the plurality of potential approaches carry a pedagogical value in its own right.

LEARNING TO SEE THE TRAP: ZÜRN IN A NARRATIVE MEDICINE CONTEXT

The interventions we describe are two smaller units within a three-week Narrative Medicine course that is taught by colleagues at the Charité university hospital in Berlin, Germany.[16] The elective is titled "Der diagnostische Blick" (The Diagnostic Gaze) and invites medical students to reflect on the complexities of perception, its sensory dimensions and limitations, as well as the professional biases it involves. The course draws on Narrative Medicine methodologies as established by Rita Charon and her colleagues at Columbia University (Charon et al. 2017). A unique feature of Charon's approach is the emphasis on theory and conceptual frameworks from, among others, literary theory, film studies, art philosophy, and performance theory, which Charon's program joins with central concerns in healthcare. Charon proposes a pedagogical model of close reading and reflective writing to improve medical students' narrative skills and to make them more attentive and more attuned care providers (Charon 2005). The learning goals are close attention to details in communication, a more holistic and complex understanding of illness and healthcare, a tolerance for ambiguity, as well as an awareness of one's own beliefs, values, and needs.[17] The discussion of artistic works is central to this concept and differs from the use of literary works in other areas where a literary text, for example, often *illustrates* a particular topic, serving as a departure point for a predetermined subject. Instead, in a Narrative Medicine-inspired context, the discussions focus on the text, bring out a text's aesthetic devices, and involve a constant returning to the text to test new hypotheses, observe how interpretations shift and, importantly, to allow participants to decide which topics and concerns they see in (or bring to) the text. Consequently, the conversation can go in any direction and the facilitator's role is to moderate the discussion, bring in clarifying terminology, and ensure that the group does not veer too far from the text.

In our segment of the Charité course, we introduce students to approaches to metaphors in healthcare and theories about human perception in art philosophy (Maurice Merleau-Ponty, Ludwig Wittgenstein, etc.), and we combine our theoretical inputs with practical exercises: students work with a metaphor and respond to a work of visual art through sketching or writing. In addition to other literary and visual artworks, we also hand out a copy of Zürn's "Plan of the House of Illnesses" (Figure 2.1) and ask students to describe what they notice. The question is deliberately broad, and students have learned by then that all responses are welcome and that they can comment on whatever strikes them, for example, or how the artwork affects them, thus combining both an attentive, close reading of the text and their own, subjective experiences. The responses we typically receive are very diverse and echo our previous discussion: students identify metaphors (house, fortress), they are reminded of classes in cell biology, they make detailed observations—for example, one student noticed that the drawing only references body parts of the upper body—and, when they have been introduced to Zürn's biography, some offer medically informed diagnoses. Others ask questions: Who does the canon in the shooting range belong to? And at what is it aimed—the enemy or the body itself? The plurality of observations and interpretations that the discussion brings to the fore may raise the expectation that we as teachers will eventually offer an explanation or a correct interpretation of Zürn's work. Predictably, this is not what we do. Our concern lies in clarifying how this plurality relates to medical practice and to healthcare more generally.

Multiperspectivity is central to medical education. Not only do students learn about human health and illness from multiple disciplinary angles—biology, chemistry, psychology, medical sociology—but they are also introduced to the biopsychosocial model of health and illness and use it in the form of a checklist when they take a patient's history. They also learn to attend to multiple sensory perceptions in the diagnostic process: they listen to a patient's words and her body's sounds (auscultation), they gather information by touch and visual perception. When we attend closely to Zürn's drawing, there is no checklist and, for the medical students' at least, there is no evident learned (and internalized) process of analysis. The students' observations are associative, creative, and open. What we foreground is the experience of the encounter, and we complement this experiential quality with self-reflection: How are our individual perceptions different from the others'? Why did *I* notice *this*? What do I bring into the encounter given my own biography? Which previous experiences, biases, interests form our individual perceptions? Such questions are related to exercises of self-experience in psychotherapeutic supervision and the processes of transference and countertransference in psychotherapy. They also speak to questions of professional identity formation: Which professional values, mindsets, and role models shape our perception? How does a healthcare professional balance the "culture of distance" that shapes the diagnostic, biomedical gaze and attitudes shaped by empathy and intersubjectivity that inform a more holistic theoretical frame (Ploeger 2022, 34–35)? These questions turn the topic of perception inward and involve a willingness to attend to (and become aware of) one's own's affects, which tend to be shifting, always contingent on multiple factors, and to which we do not always have complete access (Butler 2005).

Zürn's drawing "Plan of the House of Illnesses" also allows us to consider definitions of health and illness. Josie Billington argues that illness is not a clearly definable condition; it is on the spectrum of human existence, always fluctuating in how we evaluate it. Moreover, illness is not only bad. In the case of literary texts, Billington maintains that "books can help to find something in the person that is not merely 'ill', or something in the illness that is not simply 'bad'. So-called 'negative' experience ... can begin to be used as part of a continuum of existence, not just suffered" (2016, 11). This observation can be related to Zürn's work in many ways: illness probably crystallized her perception, efforts, and ways of being in the world.

The translatability and applicability of these ideas has limitations. At the end of our discussion, we typically do not hand out guidelines and checklists, and our course summaries are typically not condensed into pithy maxims and memorable anecdotes. The outcome for participants is therefore vaguer than they might expect and hope for, and this is a challenge that Narrative Medicine interventions often face. The issues we discuss directly inform clinical practice, but their relevance lies in shaping habits of mind, (self-)critical attitudes, and a sensibility toward phenomena that cannot be easily measured and categorized. There is much (justified) skepticism about the pedagogical impact of such interventions and while the literature reviews of Narrative Medicine programs show positive effects such as high participant satisfaction and positive outcomes across various competencies (e.g., Remein et al. 2019), many questions remain unanswered.[18] That students seem to be taking something important with them is reflected again and again in the course evaluations that we receive. Their answers, however, tend to be as diverse as the students, the facilitators, the pedagogical framings, and the course contexts more generally.

* * *

In the context of German medical education, Narrative Medicine interventions offer tools to respond to the national catalogue of learning goals for medicine (NKLM 2.0; https://nklm.de), such as compassion, self-awareness, and self-care. These competencies are difficult to convey, and medical educators often lack methodologies to do so. Narrative Medicine is one method that can be used. Although Zürn's *The House of Illnesses* can easily be replaced by other literary or artistic works, it offers an intriguing invitation to discuss core subjects in medical education. Moreover, it challenges some of the central assumptions and approaches in the field of Health Humanities. Most importantly, it reminds us that any approach, any interpretation, and any use in pedagogical contexts has to tackle the risk of falling into a totality trap, which offers the satisfaction of closure and the alleged certainty that comes with a single story and interpretation.

NOTES

1. Even though it is such a prominent element of *The House of Illnesses,* the doctor-patient relationship has not yet received much critical attention.
2. The image of the failed woman artist has also been associated with the failure of Zürn's marriage, which culminated in divorce four years before her relationship with Bellmer (1949) began and resulted in Zürn's separation from her two children.

3. The manuscript substantiates the link between author and narrator in the paratext where we learn that the text was written and sketched from April to early May 1958 in Ermenonville, a town north of Paris, where Zürn and Bellmer lived.
4. *Das Haus der Krankheiten* was first published as a facsimile in 1958 and with an added typescript version in 1969. The publishing house Brinkmann and Bose published a book version in 1986 and a second edition in 1999. In addition, a second typescript exists in German. The typescripts differ from each other as well as from the manuscript (Thüne 2011, 212). The English translation *The House of Illnesses* by Malcom Green was published in 1993 by Atlas Press, followed by a second edition in 2019.
5. There are no page numbers in Zürn's German text and for this reason, all German quotations appear without references. The English translation, by contrast, provides page numbers.
6. There are some differences between the manuscript and the typescript, see also footnote 4.
7. A similar playful strategy with words can be found with the name of Dr. Mortimer, which can be dissected into "mort" (death), "ort" (place), and "time" (Lutz 2003, 149).
8. Kahn is better known for his machine and factory metaphors, but there are other illustrations that compare the different areas of the brain, for example, to rooms in which "people" perform different tasks. A factory, of course, is also a type of house.
9. The cabinet represents the celiac (or solar) plexus, which is a system of nerves located in the abdomen behind the stomach.
10. The English translation of Zürn's book translates "der Plan" into "plan." For this reason, we continue to use "plan" here even though "map" might be the more accurate term.
11. Dr. Mortimer is also a character in Arthur Conan Doyle's "The Hound of the Baskervilles." Like Zürn's character, he is a doctor who is confronted with a mysterious illness (Lutz 2003, 150).
12. Such generalizations, and potential idealizations, of somatic and mental illnesses as well as neurodiverse conditions can be observed in representations of renowned artists, writers, and scientists. Vincent van Gogh's "madness" (which has been diagnosed as psychosis, epilepsy, depression, and schizophrenia; for an overview see Blumer 2002) and Temple Grandin's autism spectrum disorder are only two examples.
13. An important source for the Surrealists' examination of art of the mentally ill was Hans Prinzhorn's book *Bildnerei der Geisteskranken (Artistry of the Mentally Ill)* from 1922.
14. For a nuanced, critical discussion, see for example Suzanne Keen's *Empathy and the Novel* (2011) and Whitehead (2017).
15. Additional topics are, for example, the doctor-patient relationship, gender, and the therapeutic effects of writing. In addition, from a perspective of literary history, Zürn's work bears similarities with postmodern aesthetics and concepts. Zürn's intertextuality could be another concern for textual analysis, and a linguistic approach could focus on Zürn's use of word play.
16. We are grateful to Susanne Michl and Elise Siegert for inviting us to teach in their elective "Der diagnostische Blick" in February 2021 and July 2022 and to the students in both courses.
17. For a more comprehensive discussion of learning goals in Narrative Medicine and examples of how Narrative Medicine has been translated to medical education in German-speaking countries, see Wohlmann et al. (2022).
18. The long-term effects of these evaluations are still unclear, for example. Moreover, the studies also often rely on participants' self-evaluation and more objective measurements are often missing.

WORKS CITED

Billington, Josie. 2016. *Is Literature Healthy? The Literary Agenda*. Oxford: Oxford University Press.

Blumer, Dietrich. 2002. "The Illness of Vincent Van Gogh." *American Journal of Psychiatry* 159, no. 4: 519–526.

Brand-Claussen, Bettina. 2009. "Zu einigen Zeichnungen Unica Zürns/ On Several Drawings by Unica Zürn." In *Surrealismus und Wahnsinn/ Surrealism and* Madness, edited by Thomas Röske and Ingrid von Beyme, 105–112. Heidelberg: Verlag Das Wunderhorn.

Brody, Howard. 1994. "'My Story Is Broken: Can You Help Me Fix It?' Medical Ethics and the Joint Construction of Narrative." *Literature and Medicine* 13, no. 1: 79–92.

Bruner, Jerome. 1991. "The Narrative Construction of Reality." *Critical Inquiry* 18, no. 1: 1–21.

Butler, Judith. 2005. *Giving an Account of Oneself*. New York: Fordham University Press.

Clements, Charles. 2019. "A Fragmentary Illness: Review." *Journal of Modern Literature* 42, no. 1: 201–205.

Charon, Rita. 2005. "Narrative Medicine: Attention, Representation, Affiliation." *Narrative* 13, no. 3: 261–270.

Charon, Rita, Sayantani DasGupta, Nellie Hermann, Craig Irvine, Eric R. Marcus, Edgar Rivera Colón, Danielle Spencer, and Maura Spiegel. 2017. *The Principles and Practice of Narrative Medicine*. Oxford: Oxford University Press.

DeFalco, Amelia. 2009. *Uncanny Subjects: Aging in Contemporary Narrative*. Columbus: The Ohio State University Press.

De Zanger, Marion. 2015. "A Dreadful Lust for Forbidden Eyes. Unica Zürn and the Force of Imagination." In *Schmerz. Lust: Künstlerinnen und Autorinnen der deutschen Avantgarde*, edited by Lorella Bosco and Anke Gilleir, 251–270. Bielefeld: Aisthesis Verlag.

Eakin, Paul John. 2008. *Living Autobiographically: How We Create Identity in Narrative*. Ithaca: Cornell University Press.

Felski, Rita. 2008. *The Uses of Literature*. Oxford: Blackwell.

Frank, Arthur. 1995. *The Wounded Storyteller: Body, Illness and Ethics*. Chicago and London: University of Chicago Press.

Hawkins, Anne Hunsaker. 1993. *Reconstructing Illness: Studies in Pathography*. West Lafayette: Purdue University Press.

Henry, Ruth. 2010. *DIE EINZIGE: Begegnungen mit Unica Zürn*. Hamburg: Edition Nautilus.

Kenyon, Gary M. and William Lowell Randall. 1997. *Restorying our Lives: Personal Growth through Autobiographical Reflection*. Westport: Praeger.

Lutz, Helga. 2003. *Schriftbilder und Bilderschriften: Zum Verhältnis von Text, Zeichnung und Schrift bei Unica Zürn*. Stuttgart, Weimar: Verlag J.B. Metzler.

Ploeger, Cornelia. 2022. "Ärztliche Professionalität im Spannungsfeld von Einlassung und Distanz. Reflexionen am Beispiel des Spielfilms *Wit*." In *Narrative Medizin: Praxisbeispiele aus dem deutschsprachigen Raum*, edited by Anita Wohlmann, Daniel Teufel, and Pascal O. Berberat, 31–44. Köln: Böhlau.

Plumer, Esra. 2016. *Unica Zürn: Art, Writing and Postwar Surrealism*. London, New York: I.B. Tauris.

Prinzhorn, Hans. 1922. *Bildnerei der Geisteskranken. Ein Beitrag zur Psychologie und Psychopathologie der Gestaltung*. Berlin: Springer.

Remein, Christy Di, Frances Ellen Childs, John Carlo Pasco, Ludovic Trinquart, David B. Flynn, Sarah L. Wingerter, Robina M. Bhasin, Lindsay B. Demers, and Emelia J. Benjamin. 2019. "Content and Outcomes of Narrative Medicine Programmes: A Systematic Review of the Literature Through 2019." *BMC Open* 10.

Ricœur, Paul. 2004. *The Rule of Metaphor: The Creation of Meaning in Language*. Milton Park: Taylor & Francis.

Ricœur, Paul. 1984. *Time and Narrative*, vol. 1, translated by Kathleen McLaughlin and David Pellauer. Chicago. University of Chicago Press.

Röske, Thomas. 2009. "Inspiration und unerreichbares Vorbild – *L'art des fous* und Surrealismus/ Inspiration and Unreachable Paradigm – *L'art des fous* and Surrealism." In *Surrealismus und Wahnsinn/ Surrealism and Madness*, edited by Thomas Röske and Ingrid von Beyme, 9–19. Heidelberg: Verlag Das Wunderhorn.

Rupprecht, Caroline. 2006. *Subject to Delusions: Narcissism, Modernism, Gender*. Evanston: Northwestern University Press.

Servitje, Lorenzo. 2019. "Reading Film." In *Research Methods in Health Humanities,* edited by Craig M. Klugman and Erin Gentry Lamb, 55–77. Oxford: Oxford University Press.

Sontag, Susan. 2002. *Illness as Metaphor and AIDS and Its Metaphors*. London: Penguin Classics.

Tammi, Pekka. 2006. "Against Narrative ('A Boring Story')." *Partial Answers: Journal of Literature and the History of Ideas* 4, no. 2: 19–40.

Thüne, Eva-Maria. 2011. "Die neue Blickrichtung. Augenmetaphern und -zeichnungen in Unica Zürns 'Das Haus der Krankheiten.'" In *Sprache – Literatur – Literatursprache: Linguistische Beiträge*, edited by Anne Betten and Jürgen Schiewe, 211–227. Berlin: Erich Schmidt Verlag.

Thüne, Eva Maria. 2012. "Das Kabinett der Sonnengeflechte: Ein Beispiel von Text- und Bildbeziehung in Unica Zürns *Das Haus der Krankheiten*." In *Vielheit und Einheit der Germanistik weltweit*, edited by Franciszek Grucza, Vol. 4: *Sprache in der Literatur*, 133–138. Frankfurt am Main: Peter Lang.

Wasson, Sara. 2018. "Before Narrative: Episodic Reading and Representations of Chronic Pain." *Medical Humanities* 44, no. 2: 106–112.

White, Michael. 2001. "Narrative Practice and the Unpacking of Identity Conclusions." *Gecko: A Journal of Deconstruction and Narrative Ideas in Therapeutic Practice* 1: 28–55.

Whitehead, Anne. 2017. *Medicine and Empathy in Contemporary British Fiction: An Intervention in Medical Humanities*. Edinburgh: Edinburgh University Press.

Wohlmann, Anita, Daniel Teufel, and Pascal O. Berberat. 2022. *Narrative Medizin: Praxisbeispiele aus dem deutschsprachigen Raum*. Köln: Böhlau.

Woods, Angela. 2011. "The Limits of Narrative: Provocations for the Medical Humanities." *Medical Humanities* 37: 73–78.

Woods, Angela. 2013. "Beyond the Wounded Storyteller: Rethinking Narrativity, Illness and Embodied Self-Experience." In *Health, Illness and Disease: Philosophical Essays*, edited by Havi Carel and Rachel Cooper, 113–128. Stocksfield: Acumen.

Zürn, Unica. 1999. *Das Haus der Krankheiten*. 2nd ed. Berlin: Brinkmann und Bose.

Zürn, Unica. 2019. *The House of Illnesses: Stories and Pictures from a Case of Jaundice*. 2nd ed. London: Atlas Press.

CHAPTER THREE

Dr. Max Liebermann's Vienna: Diagnosis, Gender, and Criminality in Historical Crime Fiction

AMANDA SHEFFER

INTRODUCTION

Medicine and its intertwinement with a specific geographical location are at the center of the popular genre of historical crime fiction. While the broader crime fiction genre routinely takes place in medical and legal settings, historical crime fiction often explores constructed past settings for a modern audience's sensibilities based on detective fiction's traditions. Vienna around 1900, with its medical school and the central figure of Freud, is a site to examine the city's legacy, both historical and imagined, for contemporary audiences. This chapter explores one such popular series of novels, *The Liebermann Papers* (2005–18). These narratives were adapted into the television series *Vienna Blood* (2019–), which is a globally exported vision of medicine and crime in Vienna set in the years 1902–14.

During the nineteenth century, medical and scientific discourses become institutionalized in legal and criminal codes, which make these discourses central themes in detective and crime fiction. Bodies start to be categorized based on biological and pathological traits. Corporal differences according to the "social, racial, sexual, or moral" came to define notions of the "outsider" whom Alys George refers to as the "cultural Other" (George 2020, 3). The individual comes to embody larger societal debates, which attempt to use the supposed objectivity of science and medicine to justify prejudices, which are then enforced in the criminal code. The criminal code, in turn, labels individuals as “criminals.” In the context of medical discourse, the terms “disease,” “degenerate,” or “criminal” present the danger of reducing humans or groups to what Peter Shabad categorizes as “nonhuman monsters” (Shabad 2018, 83). Accordingly, what is labeled as crime “fluctuates with evolving cultural norms” (Levay 2019, 15).

Medicine diagnoses both the bodies of victim (cause of death) and perpetrator (cause of crime). In this way, medicine is reduced to the act of diagnosis to the detriment of other areas in the doctor-patient relationship such as aiding an individual’s “suffering” as Kathryn Montgomery Hunter phrases it (Hunter 1991, xvii–xviii). In this act of diagnosing, the doctor holds the power to label the body as healthy or sick in a way that can reinforce cultural and moral codes of the time. Since doctor-patient interactions reveal complex issues in society, detective and crime fictions have autopsied the [dead] body as a means of discussing broader historical, economic, social, racial, or political divisions. While these larger divisions represent complex social challenges, their embodiment in a character’s portrayal through diagnosis often serves as a simple explanation for the crime. Matthew Levay links this paradox to detective fiction and modernism: on the one hand it must show “the nuances of mental life” but these nuances make “it impossible for any narrative to deliver a comprehensive, unambiguous portrayal of character psychology” (Levay 2019, 26).

Twenty-first century medical crime narratives often dehumanize victims through brutal violence enacted on the body, often female and marginalized, for purposes of entertainment and marketability. Author Frank Tallis describes the genesis of *The Liebermann Papers* as an idea of his agent, who suggested both the detective and Victorian setting for a novel (franktallis.com 2018, paragraph 1). Tallis, who is a clinical psychologist and author, had just completed a book on Sigmund Freud and, after hearing a BBC broadcast on a Freud play, decided “Freud and Jung could no longer be regarded as ordinary mortals” (franktallis.com 2018, paragraph 1). Thus, Tallis “marr[ied] the Victorian murder mystery with the Freudian case study” (franktallis.com 2018, paragraph 1). This project offers interesting avenues for exploring medicine in Vienna at 1900 and for presenting case studies about *real* patients, most often young women who went to seek the help of a doctor at their most vulnerable.

This essay explores the construction of Vienna around 1900 in *The Liebermann Papers* as a simplified location of either high art or as a dark space leading toward National Socialism. In this context, I investigate the novel’s problematic conflation of the doctor’s diagnosis with detective work and the use of real patient files to create a crime fiction narrative that uses Freud’s Katharina case, which is well-known for its blaming of the victim. Finally, I will read the doctor/detective’s reveal scene in *Vienna Blood* (Book Two of the series) for its parallels with Conan Doyle’s Sherlock Holmes cases and the problem of making these reveals part of the doctor’s work. As Kathryn Montgomery Hunter suggests, medicine problematically regards itself as a science and in doing so forgets why the patient seeks out medical help—to receive relief from suffering (Hunter 1991, xvii–xviii). By exploring the approximation between the doctor’s work and the detective’s investigation, Hunter critiques medicine’s focus on technological diagnostic testing rather than care of the patient (Hunter 1991, xix).

This article challenges the metaphorical comparison of the doctor with the detective and this metaphor's extension to complex social issues equated with disease and illness.

THE LIEBERMANN PAPERS

The Liebermann Papers is a series of seven books, three of which have titles in the United States that are different from the UK originals (books one, four, and five). The series focuses on Dr. Max Liebermann, a "psychoanalyst and disciple of Sigmund Freud" according to the author, Frank Tallis (franktallis.com 2018, paragraph 5). Liebermann is a Jewish doctor in Vienna who shares strong similarities to the figure of Sherlock Holmes. Like Holmes, Liebermann has a partner, Oskar Rheinhardt, who is a police detective critical of police corruption and can work independently when needed to question authority. It should be noted that there are differences in the characters' backgrounds, the staging, as well as the narrative order of the books in the television adaptations. The focus of this chapter will be on the original books.

The series begins with *Mortal Mischief* (2005), or *A Death in Vienna* as it is known in the American market. The novels present Vienna at 1900 as an idealized version of Vienna juxtaposed with a dark (criminal) side. This idealized Vienna is described in Carl Schorske's foundational text, *Fin-de-Siècle Vienna: Politics and Culture* (1961), as the birthplace of modernism and as a "cultural temple of the aesthetic and psychological" (Beller 2001, 3). This approach to Vienna at 1900 has been critiqued by scholars like Steven Beller and Katherine Arens (Beller 2001, 2; Arens 2015, 15). In setting up an alternate representation of Vienna at 1900, Tallis's website outlines the Viennese political and intellectual models as comprising a "different set of thinkers" qualified as "German mystics, social Darwinists, and race theorists," which led to "Hitler's National Socialism" (franktallis.com 2018, paragraph 7). Tallis's bifurcated model operates in *Vienna Blood* (Book Two) when the discussion of the sewers, reminiscent of Graham Greene's *The Third Man*, suggests "It is a city beneath the city. Another Vienna that few, thankfully, ever see" (Tallis 2007, 401).

In the series, Tallis uses music, painting, and literature to help support a cultural form of tourism where English language readers will recognize names, places, and historical events. *The Liebermann Papers* assumes that readers already have a working knowledge of these Viennese forms, especially Freud. At key moments references seem to be missing, such as in book three, *Fatal Lies*, with its uncanny parallel to Musil's 1906 novel *die Verwirrungen des Zöglings Törleß* (*The Confusions of Young Törless*), which is set in an authoritarian male boarding school. The author, Robert Musil, or the protagonist, Törless, are not referenced in the novel until a "dossier," which is the author's postscript after the novel's completion, is presented (Tallis 2009, 434). This "dossier," which serves as a sort of reflective historical appendix to the novel, acknowledges the Austrian narrative tradition from which it takes its own crime narrative before the First World War, but also seeks to reconcile this moment at 1900 to forms of justice after the Second World War. For example, it links a discussion of the Eichmann trial and Arendt's "banality of evil" to themes in the crime novel that readers have just finished (Tallis 2009, 435). The books hereby provide a commentary on post-war forms of justice and accountability by linking past to present.

MEDICALIZING HISTORICAL CRIME FICTION

Before examining the gendered doctor-patient relationship and the doctor's diagnosis in historical crime fiction, it is important to review the close links between both medicine and crime fiction: the focus on the body as a central point. For this reason, there have been many stories linking detective work to that of the doctor's, most famously Dr. John Watson in the *Sherlock Holmes* novels by Arthur Conan Doyle. Historical crime fiction, like the larger crime fiction genre, seeks to uncover answers to challenges in a chaotic, modern mass society. Many of these stories provide commentary not only on the time period in which they are set but also on the time when they were written.

Crime fiction serves a need for justice and order. As Magdalena Waligórska defines it, "[crime] fiction provides entertainment by focusing on the darkest sides of reality, such as violence, murder, and injustice, and the genre is often seen as the escapist genre par excellence" (Waligórska 2014, 101). Thomas Knietsche argues that in historical crime fiction the crime in the story often is a metaphor for understanding [more complex] social and historical structures (Knietsche 2013, 117) embedded in a "commercial"/"lowbrow art" form (Levay 2019, 127). In this sense, historical crime fiction fills "the gaps historiography cannot fill" (Pezzotti 2016, 1). Historical crime fiction can therefore create and interpret collective memory and guilt—all while cautioning a modern, contemporary audience about parallels, imagined or authentic, to the present moment in the form of a cautionary tale. A recreated historical imaginary could be dangerous in its gap filling, yet Barbara Pezzotti notes this could be a form of "resistance" and "[generate] a new version of the past, a new outlook on the present, and a new group-shared expectations for the future" (Pezzotti 2016, 2). Scholars have recently turned their attention to the crime fiction genre for its complexity in glamorizing violence as entertainment, making "acceptable" the move to historical time periods where sexism, misogyny, and xenophobic practices were the norm, and dehumanizing the dead body of marginalized and vulnerable groups all the while having audiences recognize, contemplate, and challenge histories that have been presented in their education and cultural consciousness. This use of a past serves to suggest "a parallel between the paths of the investigation and the present of the reader and to comment upon contemporaneous events" (Pezzotti 2016, 4).

As scholars work on the historical and crime fiction genres, "there is an urgent need to think through the 'implications of the cultural fascination with crime'" (Levay 2019, p. 7). Drawing on Matthew Levay, I suggest there is a need to consider crime fiction in a global context as authors write about cultures of which they are not themselves a member and whose languages they do not speak.[1] These authors base their understanding of crime fiction on their own traditions, which may result in the creation of stereotypes, positive and negative. The Liebermann series is an example of writing outside of the national context, in this case about the Austrian context from a British perspective (franktallis.com 2018, paragraph 1). In these serial books, Vienna functions as a space of historical engagement in order to demonstrate a link between medical and criminal discourses and ideologies. For this purpose, the story invites a twenty-first century reflection on the Second World War and its crimes against humanity from a pre-First World War perspective.

MEDICINE & VIENNA AT 1900

Attempts at reconstructing Vienna at 1900, often referred to as "fin-de-siècle Vienna" after Carl Schorske's 1979 text of the same name, often result in an "idealized image," in Scott Spector's words (2001, 138). The neuroscientist Eric Kandel, who won the 2000 Nobel Prize for Physiology or Medicine, argues that the "idealized, romantic view of life in Austria" which he saw in art of the time "bears only the most tenuous relation to reality" that is "etched in my imagination" (Kandel 2012, xiv). Kandel's statement shows the historical city as a continual place of narrative reconstruction. According to Kandel, Maria Theresa and her son Joseph II "placed a premium on high-quality medicine because they viewed medical education and medical care as essential to the welfare of the state" (Kandel 2012, 22). In 1745, noted Dutch physician, Girard van Swieten, changed the school's approach to one of "a practice based on natural science" (Kandel 2012, 22). This focus on natural science was later expanded by Carl von Rokitansky when he took over the school in 1844 and "brought modernism to medicine by incorporating Darwin and a biological focus" (Kandel 2012, 23). It was Vienna at 1900 that opened up new discussions on the body and its relationship to the mind—both conscious and unconscious—that shaped medical thinking, both biological and psychological. I use the phrase "Vienna at 1900" to position my own approach, acknowledging the Schorskean tradition while allowing space for Alfred Pfabigan's "Vienna." Pfabigan's use of quotation marks around the term "Vienna" highlights Vienna as a construction and one of narrative production. He suggests that "'Vienna' was in a way a battleground for various ways of life and thought. Its character has to be sought less in particular traits than in the synthesizing power which this 'melting-pot-society' for a while possessed" (Pfabigan 2001, 155).

Vienna's historical status as a city of medical innovation is invoked to this day. The *Medizinische Universität Wien* (Medical University of Vienna) claims to be the largest medical school in the world citing three major reasons for this importance: "its history, its size and its excellent scientific performance" (Medical Programmes at the Medical University of Vienna 2022, paragraph 1). History is listed as a key element of the program's prestige. Some of its most prominent students include Sigmund Freud and Arthur Schnitzler. Another famous, yet also infamous, attendee was the criminologist Cesare Lombroso, whose name today is synonymous with practices of racial profiling and the "born criminal." Lombroso used biology and medicine to legitimize racist and xenophobic thinking, which made its way into police work. Matthew Levay describes the link between science and crime in Lombroso's approach:

> [Lombroso applies] the physiognomic indicators of degeneracy to the identification of potential criminals [...] Through his examination of their bodies and skeletal remains, Lombroso sought to classify criminals by their physical abnormalities, creating taxonomies of criminality to predict potential threats to a community [...] Lombroso advocated for his concept of the "born criminal," defined as an individual predisposed to crime due to a stunted family history.
>
> (Levay 2019, 9)

The work of detecting criminals became the scientist's and doctor's purview. They established the reasons why criminals acted, thereby attempting to create a sense of control in modern chaos through establishing pathological causality. This approach also impacted how "criminals" were sentenced. If a person could not be reformed because they were "born criminals" it would make no sense, it seemed, for society to attempt such a reform. This classification system based on perceived biological traits had significant implications for the coming decades: its ties to practices of eugenics and its attempted legitimization by privileging one ethnicity over another were inherent in the National Socialist legal code and mass genocide.

In the next section, I will examine the representation of medicine in Vienna at 1900 through an analysis of Frank Tallis' presentation of two examples of the doctor's work in *The Liebermann Papers*: one in a clinical setting with a female patient and one in the doctor's role as diagnosing detective. I will observe Freud's influence and appearance in the series as a fictionalized character through his Katharina case, which appears in book one *Mortal Mischief* (*A Death in Vienna*) as Dr. Liebermann desires a patient, Miss Lydgate. Next, I will look at the problematic and complex nature of conflating the moment of diagnosis with the detective's moment of reveal in the serial killer case in book two, *Vienna Blood*.

FREUD'S KATHARINA: MISS AMELIA LYDGATE & KATHERINE

Miss Amelia Lydgate is presented as a "hysterical" patient of Dr. Liebermann who experiences an attempted sexual assault by Herr Schelling.[2] It is clear to those familiar with Sigmund Freud and Josef Breuer's *Studies on Hysteria*, that there are strong similarities between Miss Lydgate and Freud's patient, Katharina. Ian Parker suggests that Katharina's case stands out because of its atypical situation: "The case of 'Katharina', which is actually only a brief conversation on a mountainside outside Vienna prompted by a young woman asking for help about her 'nerves', is unusual" (Parker 2006, 282). Katharina was a woman named Aurelia Kronisch and her conversation with Freud "took place in August 1893" (Parker 2006, 283). Freud's diagnosis stands out from his other cases and scholars have noted that he blames the victim (Parker 2006, 285). In his diagnosis, Freud attempts to save time due to his limited vacation contact, where he directly tells Katharina her diagnosis rather than allow for a talking cure where the patient gradually realizes her situation. Given these issues in the Katharina case, it stands out as a choice for a crime fiction narrative as it is not a typical representation of Freud's corpus and does not draw on more modern commentary of its handling of assault.

In *Mortal Mischief*, the fictionalized representation of Sigmund Freud holds Amelia responsible for her symptoms: "[p]erhaps her symptoms are not a defence as such against him, but a defence against her own powerful desire to reciprocate" (Tallis 2005, 284). The author thereby engages critiques of Freud's discourse of blaming the victim. While there is no explicit criticism of Freud in the novel, the audience is told that "Liebermann could not believe that Amelia Lydgate harboured a secret wish to be intimate with a man like Herr Schelling" (Tallis 2005, 284). In her attempt to confront an attempted sexual trauma, Amelia undergoes multiple therapy sessions while under a "hypnotised sleep" (Tallis 2005, 313), something which the real Freud later dismissed because not everyone was capable of being hypnotized. During these sessions Amelia describes how she attacked Herr Schelling with scissors to ward him off: ""He would have overpowered me—he would have—" her voice rose "—violated me"" and Liebermann replies: "An unconscionable, heinous crime" (Tallis 2005, 315). Dr. Liebermann qualifies the attempted assault on her as "unconscionable" and "heinous" (Tallis 2005, 315) and labels it a "crime" (Tallis 2005, 315). The remaining session is a conversation on criminality. At the same time that Liebermann acknowledges the criminality of the act, his assessment that "her actions appear to be explainable" also establishes that she is not a "threat to the social order" (O'Neill and Seal 2012, 43). Her "lack of agency serve[s] to reinforce sexist stereotypes of femininity" as Maggie O'Neill and Lizzie Seal describe in their analysis of the gendered approach to "deviance" (O'Neill and Seal 2012, 43).

Liebermann continues his judgement on the attempted assault as a form of reassurance that Amelia's desire to kill Herr Schelling is justified. He says, "'But you were being abused. His hands were on your body—you could smell his cologne. Remember the roughness of his face—grabbing, grabbing, grabbing ...'" (Tallis 2005, 316). Liebermann's repetition of "grabbing" returns her to the moment of the attempted assault. Experiencing it again does not heal but instead retraumatizes her. This repetition poses questions about the voyeurism permeating this scene, forcing the audience to "think through the 'implications of the cultural fascination with crime'" (Levay 2019, 7).

SHERLOCKIAN REVEAL AS DIAGNOSIS: *VIENNA BLOOD*

Seeing criminal detection as a medical diagnosis can oversimplify societal problems and dehumanize patients. In the second novel in the series, *Vienna Blood*,[3] the historical background of Vienna at 1900 and rising antisemitism are used for a serial killer case which is likened to that of Jack the Ripper—a criminal in England noted for his brutality against women by targeting their reproductive organs. The novel uses the plot of Mozart's *Die Zauberflöte* to depict a killing spree: the first victim, a snake in the zoo, is found under a statue of Mozart, the "Queen of the Night," her servants are depicted as murdered sex workers, the bird catcher "Papageno" is a victim, and the murdered Egyptian man is likened to Monostatos. Additionally, the story focuses on the freemasons, who also play a role in the Mozart opera. Serial killers, usually depicted as male, mark the "changing relations between self and society" (O'Neill and Seal 2012, 100). Serial killers often target "marginalized and culturally devalued social groups [which] can be perceived as reinforcing the dominant social order" (O'Neill and Seal 2012, 107). In *Vienna Blood*, a syphilitic painter, who has a similar biography as Adolf Hitler in his rejection from art school, kills people he deems morally unfit, for example: female sex workers and an Egyptian man living in Vienna in a homosexual relationship. This linking of psychology to criminology is further linked to the doctor's work through Liebermann's diagnosis and narrative's denouement. In an interview with the BBC, Tallis suggests a link between medicine and detective work:

> Psychoanalysis and crime investigation have much in common. Clues are like symptoms, and the detective is like a psychoanalyst, attempting to make connections in order to find an ultimate cause. A perpetrator is as elusive as a repressed, unconscious memory.
>
> (Frank Tallis 2019, paragraph 2)

With this link, Tallis seems to be following Freud in whose work the "dream analysis reads like a medical detective story. Freud attempts to decipher the psychic meanings of the figures, elements, and the events of his dream with the same investigative zeal he applied to the symptoms of his neurotic patients" (Kandel 2012, 67). Linking the moment of medical diagnosis to the moment of reveal, however, can be problematic and reductive. When labels of "illness" or "monstrosity" are applied to complex social issues, they become reduced and lack nuance, an inherent problem in all crime fiction. For example, Tallis calls National Socialism an "illness" which is an inadequate metaphor (Tallis 2007, 484) as it presents this ideology not as an active political choice but as a passive process. This reductivity in illness and criminality will be explored through the moment of "spot-diagnosis" in crime fiction. In his exploration of Sherlock Holmes and his criminal reveal, Wilbush describes the notion of "spot-diagnosis" as a practice in

> Oneupmanship [*sic*] [adding] interest to [the] subsequent explanation of the process by which it was putatively reached. Today, however, it is frowned upon probably not so much because not too rarely it proves inaccurate, but mostly because of a feeling that it does not satisfy scientific standards of diagnosis.
>
> (Wilbush 1992, 342)

"Spot-diagnosis" can present stereotypes, stigmas, and prejudices inherent in the deduction process. In crime fiction, the diagnosis is the moment the "criminal" is labeled and this is made legitimate through medical discourse for audiences. The conclusion of *Vienna Blood* seems to uphold Lombroso's suggestion that people are "born criminals" as the killer is *born with the illness* that the novel identifies as his reason for committing the crimes. Liebermann, the doctor, tells Rheinhardt, the police detective, how he "diagnosed" the painter Olbricht as the serial killer in a spot reading. Rheinhardt says: "He was born … syphilitic?" and Liebermann responds:

> "Indeed, and once I had established that fact, I immediately grasped the nature of his history. What kind of mother might have syphilis? A prostitute! Why might Olbricht despise other nationalities so much? Because they were her clientele: down-at-heel Hungarians, Poles, Czechs, and Jews, newly arrived in Vienna. These were the men who took her away from him. Why had *The Magic Flute* acquired such special significance for Olbricht? He had heard it being sung incessantly as a child—how could anyone forget these glorious melodies? And how might the son of a prostitute get to hear an opera? His mother must have rented a room next to a folk theater. The German nationalist doctrine of race hate provided the adult Olbricht with a rationale for many of his attacks."
>
> (Tallis 2007, 468)

In Liebermann's reasoning, being the child of a sex worker living next to a theater made Olbricht into a nationalist serial killer. Liebermann, the audience is told, "immediately" grasps this connection, which establishes the moment as a spot-diagnosis, pointing at his "genius."

Both the illnesses of the mother and son are morally coded through the act of sex work. While the murdered female sex workers from the novel's beginning are now forgotten for the analysis of the serial killer's body, his medical labeling also simplifies and obscures broader, more complex issues of nationalism, xenophobia, homophobia, and misogyny inherent in the serial attacks.

CONCLUSION

The Liebermann Papers, and its adaptation as a globally distributed television show, demonstrates that Vienna at 1900 remains a place of fascination for depicting fictional historical crimes in popular culture. The Austrian city of Vienna is depicted in a bifurcated manner, either as a city of art, music, literature, and architecture or as a city with hidden criminality and an exploration of taboos. Crime fiction's need for order and justice is at odds with the societal complexity that the genre also demands, especially in a historical setting. When the medical setting is combined with these larger challenges inherent to the genre, the need for the doctor-detective's clear-cut "spot-diagnoses," in the manner of Sherlock Holmes, competes with the responsibility to see the complexity of individuals and their living bodies. It is therefore imperative to explore more fully the treatment of the bodies of patients, victims, and perpetrators in the context of antisemitism, xenophobia, homophobia, and misogyny in Vienna at 1900.

NOTES

1. While cultural and artistic forms of Vienna at 1900 are depicted in the series, the limited use of German in the novel *Vienna Blood* does not follow conventions and has errors.
2. Miss Lydgate is not only the patient in this story but also the granddaughter of a noted hematologist; she continues his work as a sort of crime lab pathologist in later stories. In this context, the body can be read through the lens of gender and how this shapes the doctor-patient relationship as well as laws at 1900. In one way, male doctors used a biological, gendered discourse to prevent women from entering their profession and the university:

   > Male scientists and medical doctors regularly—and successfully—advanced essentialist claims that women were intellectually inferior, emotionally unequipped, and biologically unfit to become doctors, a profession that would purportedly distract women from their roles as mothers and wives. (George 2020, 77).

   At the same time, the women who wanted to study were labeled as *Mannweiber* (male women) because studying medicine seemed "undesirable" for their gender; men's own roles as fathers and husbands seemed not to be questioned. The legal code shaped how sex work regulated bodies (O'Neill and Seal 2012, 13). O'Neill and Seal note that this regulated "poor women involved through a combination of legal and medical discourses" (O'Neill and Seal 2012, 13).
3. *Vienna Blood* ("Wiener Blut") is a complex title suggesting more than murder and medicine. It also recalls Strauss's operetta of the same name, ties to the use of "blood" in National Socialist discourse, and, in modern times, the phrase "Vienna Blood" has been used in xenophobic advertisements by the Austrian far-right.

WORKS CITED

Arens, Katherine. 2015. *Vienna's Dreams of Europe: Culture and Identity Beyond the Nation-State*. New York: Bloomsbury Academic.

Beller, Steven. 2001. *Rethinking Vienna 1900*. New York: Berghahn Books.

Foucault, Michel. 1973. *The Birth of the Clinic: An Archaeology of Medical Perception*. 1st American ed. New York: Pantheon Books.

"Frank Tallis (Author of the Liebermann Novels)." 2019. *BBC* online. November 7, 2019. https://www.bbc.co.uk/mediacentre/mediapacks/vienna-blood/frank.

George, Alys X. 2020. *The Naked Truth: Viennese Modernism and the Body*. Chicago: The University of Chicago Press.

Hunter, Katherine M. 1991. *Doctors' Stories: The Narrative Structure of Medical Knowledge*. Princeton: Princeton University Press.

Kandel, Eric R. 2012. *The Age of Insight: The Quest to Understand the Unconscious in Art, Mind, and Brain: from Vienna 1900 to the Present*. New York: Random House.

Kniesche, Thomas W. 2013. "Weimar and Nazi Germany in Contemporary German Historical Crime Fiction." *Colloquia Germanica* 46, no. 2: 116–130.

Levay, Matthew. 2019. *Violent Minds: Modernism and the Criminal*. Cambridge: Cambridge University Press.

"Liebermann Papers 1 – Mortal Mischief." 2018. *Frank Tallis* online. Accessed January 8, 2018. https://www.franktallis.com/2018/01/08/the-liebermann-papers-1-mortal-mischief–2/.

Mazzarello, Paolo. 2011. "Cesare Lombroso: An Anthropologist Between Evolution and Degeneration." *Functional Neurology* 26, no. 2: 97–101.

McChesney, Anita and Jospeh W. Moser. 2013. "Introduction: Revolutionizing German-Language Crime Fiction." *Colloquia Germanica* 46, no. 2: 109–115.

"Medical Programmes at the Medical University of Vienna." Accessed 2022. *Medical University of Vienna*. https://www.meduniwien.ac.at/web/en/studies-further-education/study-programmes/.

O'Neill, Maggie and Lizzie Seal. 2012. *Transgressive Imaginations: Crime, Deviance and Culture*. Houndmills: Palgrave Macmillan.

Parker, Ian. 2006. "Katharina: Working Out Anxiety. Notes on Freud's Early Case." *Psychodynamic Practice* 12, no. 3: 281–291.

Pezzotti, Barbara. 2016. *Investigating Italy's Past through Historical Crime Fiction, Films, and TV Series: Murder in the Age of Chaos*. New York: Palgrave Macmillan.

Pfabigan, Alfred. 2001. "Freud's 'Vienna Middle.'" In *Rethinking Vienna 1900*, edited by Steven Beller, 154–170. New York: Berghahn Books.

Schorske, Carl E. 1981. *Fin-de-Siècle Vienna: Politics and Culture*. New York: Vintage Books.

Shabad, Peter. 2018. "Is Loyalty Really a Virtue? Shame and the Monstrous Other." In *Memories and Monsters: Psychology, Trauma, and Narrative*, edited by Eric R. Severson and David Goodman, 60–86. Abingdon, Oxon: Routledge.

Spector, Scott. 2001. "Marginalizations: Politics and Culture Beyond." In *Rethinking Vienna 1900*, edited by Steven Beller, 132–153. New York: Berghahn Books.

Tallis, Frank. 2005. *A Death in Vienna*. 1st American ed. New York: Grove Press.

Tallis, Frank. 2007. *Vienna Blood: A Novel*. 1st American ed. New York: Random House Trade Paperbacks.

Tallis, Frank. 2009. *Fatal Lies: A Novel*. 1st American ed. New York: Random House Trade Paperbacks.

Waligórska, Magdalena. 2014. "'Darkness at the Beginning': The Holocaust in Contemporary German Crime Fiction." In *Tatort Germany: the Curious Case of German-Language Crime Fiction*, edited by Todd Herzog and Lynn M. Kutch, 101–119. Rochester, New York: Camden House.

Wilbush, J. 1992. "The Sherlock-Holmes Paradigm – Detectives and Diagnosis." *Journal of the Royal Society of Medicine* 85, no. 6: 342–345.

CHAPTER FOUR

Teaching "Outbreak Narratives" during the Covid Pandemic

MADALINA MEIROSU

Every time I sat down to work on this essay, I found myself transported to that difficult semester in the fall of 2020 when I taught a course on pandemics during the Covid pandemic. As I considered the past, I found myself thinking of a line from *The Magic Mountain* (1924): "A strange, half-dreamy, half-scary sense of standing there and yet being tugged away at the same time, a kind of fluctuating permanence, that meant both a return to something and a dizzying, everlasting sameness" (22). I was pulled back into a time of mourning and despair, a time when friends or family were in the hospital, their lives in jeopardy; a time when I could not travel to be with my father, who was dying from cancer on another continent; a time that transported me back to a still earlier time in my life when, in my native Romania, store shelves were empty and a feeling of scarcity was in the air. During the fall of 2020, however, I lacked nothing: I had a roof over my head, a comfortable home, food, and a supportive spouse. And yet the possibility of not having food or heat in the near future awoke a deep-seated anxiety in me and intensified the insecurity I felt as I tried to navigate an uncertain world.

So each time I sat before a computer to work on this essay, I found myself recoiling from the past, in the grip of a need to curtain off that part of myself that is still in mourning. *I can't go on, I'll go on.* And in going on, I have decided to go against the grain and write in a more personal vein. In choosing this approach I am guided by one of the goals of the Medical Humanities, which is to explore the experience of illness, and this includes, according to Thomas Cole, Nathan Carlin, and Ronald Carson, understanding "how it feels to be a patient, a doctor, or a community affected by an epidemic" (13). You and I, dear reader, experienced this pandemic as members of the academic community, tasked with teaching under challenging circumstances, but in what follows I will speak on behalf of the smaller community of a classroom at Swarthmore College, where we sought to make the best of the first fully online semester during the Covid pandemic. I would like to say a few words, then, about the course I taught and the experience of teaching it.

WHY TEACH ABOUT PANDEMICS DURING A PANDEMIC? THE ORIGINS OF THE COURSE

This course on pandemics was a last-minute course proposal, after we learned that a number of students had chosen to take the Fall 2020 semester off in response to the College's decision to conduct all classes online. Consequently, we would not have our normal number of German-speaking students. More pertinent (and distressing) was that we would not have enough students for an advanced seminar in German. So at the eleventh hour I proposed a course on pandemics, featuring German literature in translation, that would introduce students from all disciplines to the political dynamics associated with infectious disease. I suggested this course in part because I was eager to teach a Medical Humanities course. Once the pandemic was upon us and the United States was mostly shut down, I found myself wanting to learn what other people had felt and experienced during earlier pandemics. As I was fairly familiar with the cholera pandemic of the nineteenth century, this was the infectious disease to which I turned first. The cholera pandemic had been a long, protracted affair; erupting toward the beginning of the century, with bouts of infection recurring over the next hundred or so years, its impact on the nineteenth century was considerable. And as I thought about Heinrich Heine's text on cholera, *Französische Zustände* (1833), which chronicled Parisians' reaction to an epidemic that was spreading rapidly and for which there was no cure, it struck me that many of the frightened reactions to a new disease exhibited by denizens of the nineteenth century were also on display in 2020. There were obvious parallels: xenophobia, the politicization of disease transmission and cure, and even conspiracy theories—for example, in the nineteenth century it was believed that poisoners were driving the cholera pandemic. In light of this belief, people who were discovered on the street with white powder on them were sometimes killed on the spot, even if the powders were intended as a cure for cholera. Jews (along with aristocrats in Revolutionary France) were often accused of poisoning as cholera rekindled old conflicts and served as a pretext for violence against those who were already ostracized or hated for political reasons.

I wanted to explore these parallels more closely, learning more about the reactions to pandemics, in the hope that this kind of study would afford both my students and myself an opportunity to think about what was happening at a remove, the stress of the immediate moment mediated by a more relaxed consideration of the past. And I was not alone in wanting to look to fictional representations of past pandemics. Newspapers, magazines, and blogs published reading lists of books about outbreaks. In departmental meetings conversations would swerve into a discussion of outbreak novels such as Albert Camus's *The Plague* and

Gabriel Garcia Marquez's *Love in the Time of Cholera*. It was as if people had suddenly discovered that pandemics are real, that they can afflict us in the present, and that they can bring the world to a standstill. And as a corollary to this, there was a new appreciation for how pandemics had afflicted people in the past, now that our vague knowledge of the bubonic plague and cholera had been concretized by this new pandemic sweeping the world. Camus put it best: "Everybody knows that pestilences have a way of recurring in the world, yet somehow we find it hard to believe in ones that crash down on our heads from a blue sky. There have been as many plagues as wars in history, yet always plagues and wars take people equally by surprise" (37).

Once I had settled on the general idea of teaching a course on the experience of pandemics, I proceeded to refine it. I decided that I wanted to teach a class in German studies that would employ a comparative approach. We would learn how German-speaking people dealt with pandemics, of course. But we would also look closer to home, particularly at how cholera, TB, and HIV/AIDS were received in New York and Philadelphia in the nineteenth and twentieth centuries. It was my hope that such a focus would give students who were learning remotely that semester an opportunity to feel connected to the Swarthmore area in some way as they inhabited the experience of New Yorkers and Philadelphians during earlier times of peril. I also hoped to show, by way of this comparative approach, cross-cultural patterns of response in the face of pandemics. For not only did Germans react in specific and sometimes troubling ways to large-scale infectious disease, Americans reacted in similar ways, often implementing the same measures found in the German response. To be sure, there was cross-continental communication and influence, both in the medical field, where doctors on both sides of the Atlantic engaged in a conversation about best practices when confronting epidemics, and in the political sphere, where governments paid close attention to the success and failure of measures on the other side of the Atlantic. Moreover, newspapers informed their reading public about measures taken against the crisis in other countries. Still, despite these interactions, it would seem that most human beings, no matter their location in time and place, exhibit the same basic range of responses to pandemics: denial, incredulity, despair, paranoia, xenophobia, and susceptibility to miracle cures and conspiracy theories.

SELECTING EPIDEMICS FOR STUDY

Why choose cholera, TB, and HIV/AIDS? To begin with, I thought it would be intriguing to juxtapose cholera with tuberculosis because the temporalities of these diseases are so different. Cholera spreads quickly and kills quickly, with patients sometimes dying within a few hours of infection. In the case of TB, patients sometimes lived decades with the disease, and even though the disease is contagious, the transmission rates are generally much less severe. I was attracted to this contrast, this slow/fast juxtaposition, and I thought it might provide a framework through which to look at cultural responses to the disease. In particular, if the disease progresses differently—for example, if it is much slower, as in the case of TB—is there still a strong tendency to resort to xenophobia and conspiracy theories in order to explain it?

As for HIV/AIDS, I originally intended to compare the public response to syphilis with the response to HIV/AIDS. Unfortunately, the Fall 2020 semester was shorter than usual (owing to the emergency addition of a January "term"), which would limit the thoroughness of the study of both diseases. And I was not able to find ideal German texts on syphilis that had been translated into English. But I was reluctant to jettison HIV/AIDS since I have vivid childhood memories of the way the disease was politicized. Those of us who lived behind the Iron Curtain in Eastern Europe were told that HIV/AIDS was a malady specific to the decadent West, a fitting consequence of imperialism. Of course, the disease was politicized in a different way in the US, where it was often regarded as a punishment for gay sex. Even the German attitude toward HIV/AIDS was bifurcated between an East German and West German attitude. In East Germany, people who contracted the disease were secreted out of sight as part of a general policy to associate the disease solely with the West. The result was that those who became ill in East Germany were isolated, as they suffered from a disease that was not officially acknowledged to exist in East Germany (Bochow 1993; Borneman 1987; Wasmuth 2002).

GOALS FOR THE CLASS

In addition to the goals listed on the syllabus, one of my hidden goals was to help students process their experience of the pandemic. I hoped to give them an opportunity, through non-traditional assignments involving creative engagement with the material, to work through the readings on multiple levels: these non-traditional assignments required students to engage the material both intellectually and emotionally, with heart as well as mind. The goal was an *embodied* response. The assignments forced them to acknowledge the emotional work that was required to do full justice to the materials they were given to read or watch.

One of my personal goals was to learn how to work with Scalar, a free, open-source publishing platform. Scalar allows students to create multimodal online projects; the project I had in mind was a Scalar book, with each student contributing a chapter. The students feel like they are writing a book, which excites them; it also inspires them to invest substantial time and energy so that their contribution to the collective project is worthy of it. Each student was responsible for a separate chapter in the book; they chose the specific theme of the chapter and supplied the content for the chapter. The various chapters would then be gathered together by an overarching introduction to the book, and the book would be published, ready to be read by whoever had the required link. The students could choose the scope of the audience for the book, whether it could be read by anyone who happened upon it online, or whether its readership was to be limited to those in the Swarthmore College community. So in addition to creating a syllabus on short notice, and while I scrambled to familiarize myself with the various technologies that were being put in place to teach remotely that semester, I began to learn Scalar as quickly as I could. It seemed a useful motivational tool for students, for I knew that motivation levels were trending downwards as students prepared for a full semester of online instruction. In fact, as I mentioned above, many students had chosen to take a semester off rather than engage in online learning. The best way to counteract the drudgery of online learning was to entice students with the prospect of an online book. This particular project took advantage of the fact that we were forced to meet online, while giving students the sense that there would be a finished product that they could show to anyone they chose. The project also equipped them with the tools required to work with Scalar in the future on other projects. And in the process of learning this technology, I also taught students how to compose a timeline in Timeline JS, another open-source tool that allows users to build interactive timelines.

COURSE ORGANIZATION AND THEMES

The Fall semester was only twelve weeks long and therefore shorter than usual. Having set aside the first week and the final week to introduce and sum up the course, I divided the remaining ten weeks among three major themes: cholera, TB, and HIV/AIDS. The first week introduced students to texts that provided a theoretical framework for the discussion of metaphors in literature and medicine. In addition to Priscilla Wald and Susan Sontag, we read Franz Kafka's *The Metamorphosis* (1915), which we interpreted from the perspective of living in isolation. Moreover, during our discussion two students who identify as queer spoke of how the story seemed to express their experience of coming out to a less than supportive family, and in particular the alienation they felt when they hunkered down with their family during the quarantine phase of the pandemic. As such, I was able to emphasize from the very beginning that the readings to come would do much more than simply teach students about German Literature.

The readings from the first section of the course devoted to cholera gave students a chance to read German literature in parallel with secondary texts that treated cholera from a global perspective. We finished this section with a viewing of F. W. Murnau's *Nosferatu* (1922) that, to my great surprise, was a class favorite and the topic of many analysis papers. We then made the transition from cholera to tuberculosis by spending a full week on vampires. We looked at how both cholera and tuberculosis were represented by vampires in fiction, as well as how these vampires express xenophobia and gender tensions. We began the second section of the course, on tuberculosis, by reading some texts on fever, including typhoid fever, and by watching the series *Charité* (2017–21), named after the Berlin hospital, which gave students a glimpse into the world of nineteenth century medicine. With this background in place, we spent the following three weeks reading Thomas Mann's *The Magic Mountain*, which allowed us to deepen our discussion of the relationship between time and illness. We also surveyed different types of cures for tuberculosis, as well as alternative medical treatments, that had originated in German-speaking spaces. We then read about tuberculosis in the United States, with a special focus on its impact in the Philadelphia area and Midwestern (South Dakota) Lakota communities. The third section of the course focused on HIV/AIDS; our readings brought us into the twenty-first century, thus setting the stage for the final week, when we considered what future pandemics might look like after asking how history influences the future.

CHALLENGES IN TEACHING THE COURSE DURING THE PANDEMIC

Let me begin with material challenges. I did not have access to a physical library, which significantly limited the materials I could use in the class. Many of the older texts I would have liked to work with, and which would normally have been held in reserve at the library for students, were not available in digital form. I was also unable to make copies of chapters to put on Moodle for my students. Another challenge lay in the fact that I could not be sure that students would have access to the specific version of all of the books I put on the syllabus. Under normal learning conditions, students could access the required version at the library, or take advantage of Swarthmore's book allowance program to purchase books from the Swarthmore bookstore. Neither of these options was available to students during the fall of 2020. I was also surprised to discover that so many relevant German texts were still untranslated. I had not expected many of the novels and short stories to be translated, of course, but I had expected more of Leopold von Sacher-Masoch's work, for example, to be available in English. I enlisted the help of librarians to help me track down translations, but their searches came to naught, as well. Consequently, I was forced to translate a number of the texts that I taught, producing original translations on the fly.

For all of these reasons, the preparatory work for the course took more time than I had originally anticipated. I had initially composed a syllabus that I thought would be interesting, but I had to rework it substantially owing to the dearth of English translations. Learning Scalar also took up much of my time, though I was extremely fortunate to be assisted by two librarians—Pamela Harris and Roberto Vargas—who not only provided guidance before the course began, but visited the class twice during the semester to assist the students as they worked with the program.

And then there were obstacles of a more personal nature. At the very beginning of the term I fractured my ankle, and so spent most of the semester in various splints. I was in a fair amount of pain at times, a pain that often became acute during the lengthy seminar. In order to minimize the discomfort, I taught while seated on the floor, my back against a bookshelf with my leg stretched out in front of me. But this only provided so much relief and I found myself needled with pain during the sessions and their immediate aftermath. I was thus in a situation of having to talk about pain and suffering in the very moment that I was in considerable pain, all the while doing my utmost to keep the pain from interfering with teaching the seminar and draining my energy. My teaching, too, was an *embodied* affair that semester. Furthermore, because my ankle and leg were not healing as expected, and because I did not have easy access to a doctor at that point in time, an additional layer of stress and worry came to the fore, which tapped into anxieties about Covid, interestingly. The feelings associated with my leg—that the discomfort is interminable and that it is not getting better—dovetailed with the dynamics of Covid itself, thereby intensifying my worried thoughts about Covid. For Covid, too, despite all the urgent efforts being made by research scientists, appeared to be never-ending, with no cure in view, no remedy to prop up our spirits. Isolation was our only remedy, and a taxing one, at that. At that point, being isolated for me was not only a matter of teaching from within the confinement of my home, but it also included my limited mobility, which exacerbated the sense of being trapped. Limited by a body that did not cooperate and confined to a house because of Covid left me feeling excruciatingly trapped at times. A final dimension of personal difficulty took the form of a father who was dying slowly, painfully, half a world away.

There were challenges of a technical nature, of course, of the kind familiar to most instructors of online courses. Swarthmore College worked hard to ensure that every student had access to a reliable computer, but once classes began it became clear that not every student had access to a reliable internet connection. The interruptions caused by dropped connections led to repeated summaries of what had been missed and generally degraded the quality of the discussion. The new Zoom setting also made it possible for students to absent themselves from the screen during my presentations and our general discussions; because it was Swarthmore's policy to allow students to switch off their cameras during class sessions, on one or two occasions I taught without any responsive human faces before me. These lectures left me feeling like I was talking to myself, as if I was doing one of the recordings for the mini-lectures that I would give them each week. The absence of live faces during our class was disconcerting and uncomfortable. I sometimes felt like Kafka's creature, an *Ungeziefer* that scared away the humans on the other side of the screen. In addition to this, each student had to cope with his or her unique living circumstances. Some of the students who were living with their families had a difficult time finding a quiet space in which to join the class. Distractions of all sorts—siblings shouting, parents cooking, TVs blaring—often interfered with their full participation. It was difficult to know what was going on with various students during the term, owing to the lack of in-person, face-to-face contact. Many of the students were markedly anxious, and it did not help that the Zoom set up was especially trying for students suffering from social anxiety. Sometimes they would write to me in advance of the class, explaining that they did not feel well and would prefer to participate without showing themselves. It was clear, though, that they were engaged to a point, for they still contributed to the chat and to class discussions, though it was difficult to gauge how "present" they actually were. I confess that I could relate to their occasional reluctance to expose themselves. I often did not feel like being in front of the computer, generating positive energy and smiling a smile I did not really feel. It was a chore to be "present." It is extraordinary difficult to teach in such a setting for someone who draws their energy from the classroom. When I teach in a classroom setting, it is not only the visual cues that let me know how deep I should delve into a particular issue or if my attempt to explain something has been successful. I am also attuned to the emotional atmosphere in the classroom; I can feel the undercurrents in the room and can therefore shunt to a different track, if needed. In an online environment, however, where half the students are hidden and the ones who are visible look stressed and mostly miserable, it is difficult to find the energy to be scintillating and inspiring, and it is difficult to discern if the students' faces lack energy because they do not understand what I am teaching them or because they are depressed.

Generally speaking, it was my impression that the students used the function of cutting the video as a kind of refuge. Still, I did my best to engage them. When a hidden student had been quiet for a while, I wrote them a private message in the chat or asked them a question. On the whole, I think it is fair to say that class discussions online during the pandemic were not as robust and spirited as they tend to be in the classroom. Many students were reticent to begin with, owing to the online environment and other unavoidable factors, such as showing up to class in one's bedroom, with one's bed and private space in the background, which meant that one's presence in class was fringed with embarrassment. Moreover, the class discussions in the Outbreak Narratives course were slightly more muted than discussions in my other online courses, though this was not because of a lack of interest on the part of the students. After all, the students who had enrolled in this course, which had been created at the eleventh hour, had either been so eager to take the course that they were willing to jettison one of the courses they had originally chosen for themselves, or they had stumbled upon this course as a more promising prospect than the course they had just dropped. The course satisfied no requirements for graduation; its only attraction for students was the subject matter.

One-on-one sessions were required in order to develop a rapport with each student that, had we convened on campus together, would have evolved more naturally. Like so many aspects of teaching that semester, this meant extra work. But the sessions were revealing. Sometimes students shared with me that they thought it would be difficult to think about infectious disease and pandemics when they were already engulfed in infectious disease and pandemic, but they found that immersion in these writings made it easier to endure the present crisis. It helped them to be reminded that these things happen, that the present crisis is not the only time that this has happened. And that every time that this had happened, even though people felt like the world was ending, the world did not end. What is required is to find the strength to endure by being together and talking about pandemics together. The students also said that the opportunity to be creative when contributing to the Scalar book gave them a way to work through some of the stresses brought on by the pandemic. The students were like little children when the book was completed; there was no containing their excitement.

FINDING WAYS TO KEEP STUDENTS ENGAGED

I went into the semester mindful of the challenges that quarantine and confinement would pose to students throughout the semester. Confinement by itself is inherently stressful; having to engage in serious intellectual work in this constricted environment would likely layer stress upon stress. I was especially worried that the standard demands placed on students at Swarthmore, which are notoriously challenging under normal circumstances, would be overwhelming for students in isolation. I was sensitive, too, to the fact that students' home environments were going to be part of the learning equation. Some students were quite alone and so had to contend with the debilitating effects of isolation. Other students shared a small space with large families. Some families did not appreciate how demanding intellectual work can be; other families were dysfunctional and consequently an additional source of agitation for students. All of these new challenges needed to be taken into account.

There was a general concern among Swarthmore faculty that students not feel overwhelmed by the amount of work required of them during this difficult semester. I thus found myself faced with a tricky question: will students be short-changed if I reduce the amount of work?

I began to deliberate about how to strike a balance between offering the kind of quality education that students expect and structuring the course in a less strenuous way in the hope that this would allow students to produce quality work. In the end I chose to assign a substantial amount of reading (for instance, we read the whole of *The Magic Mountain*). However, I did make an important concession. I reduced the length of our seminar from three hours to two hours, in order to reduce Zoom fatigue. I then supplemented our session with an hour's worth of recorded lectures that students listened to on their own time every week. I further divided these lectures into segments of manageable length (ten to fifteen minutes). This mirrored my practice in the classroom, where I try not to speak for long stretches. Instead, I look for ways to divide the lecture into shorter presentations, after which I put questions to the class in order to gauge understanding and encourage active learning. In the online course students were given multiple segments of the week's lecture along with questions to think about for each segment; when we gathered together for the seminar we compared our answers and related them to the readings.

I also offered the students reading guides that provided instructions for their readings. For example, when reading a novel as complex as *The Magic Mountain*, which can overwhelm the reader with its rich profusion of ideas, students often feel lost at sea if they are not given a specific orientation through the novel. I thus sought to provide a lodestar for students, asking them in advance to focus on the themes of time and illness as they read. I have found that reading without this intentional focus on one or two themes can produce "quiet" discussions in the classroom. The sheer size of *The Magic Mountain* proved a challenge and I was eventually forced to make a concession here as well. When students were given a lengthy reading assignment (say a 200-page section of the novel), in addition to having them focus their attention on specific themes, I would identify smaller page ranges that they were to read carefully, and even reread, so as to be able to contribute to the close reading of these passages during the class session.

I also sought to keep students engaged by asking them to be on the lookout for connections between our readings and current events. We discussed these parallels during every class session. At the beginning of the term students appeared doubtful that reading about nineteenth century cholera and other illnesses had much in common with current events. I could see the incredulity on their faces, which were front and center on the Zoom platform. And yet, starting with the second week, they began to share connections they were making between their readings and what was happening in their own historical moment. This unexpected applicability provided additional motivation for them and helped them stay engaged throughout the term. Even though none of these students were German majors, they discovered that through the reading of German literature they were acquiring knowledge that was relevant to them personally as they lived through a health crisis in the twenty-first century. Furthermore, over the course of the semester we had a number of discussions about how it is possible, whatever the subject of study, to acquire transferable knowledge and skills that will be relevant to one's career and later life, so long as one is mindful of what is taking place when one is learning. I thus tried to incentivize the students to invest themselves in the course by making it relevant to current events and by pointing out the value of all learning, even learning far afield from their majors.

I believe I was also able to help students stay connected to the course by being formally available to students for an hour a day, holding a virtual office hour during which students could "drop in" and discuss any concerns or questions they might have. Several students told me that just knowing that I was always available in this way helped to assuage some of their anxieties; this offer of daily access seemed to help students feel supported and even minimize their feelings of being overwhelmed. Furthermore, the consistency of my availability (11am EST every day) eliminated confusion, and the consistency also approximated the family-style feeling of support that students experience on the Swarthmore campus, where faculty tend to be available to students outside of formal office hours. Every other week I offered students anonymous surveys that enabled me to assess what was working and what was not working in the course. Their feedback helped me adjust my plans for the next two weeks. Also, based on their feedback I changed the structure of our in-class break. Students asked for smaller but more frequent breaks, which would allow them to move and stretch and fend off a Zoom-induced stupor.

During the semester we looked at art together. Because I wanted students to feel like they could contribute something new to the class, steering it in unexpected directions, I challenged them to find artists who were showcasing new art related to Covid. Knowing that they could always introduce a new find to the class, which we would discuss and consider in relation to our readings, encouraged personal investment and initiative. Throughout the term students shared images of paintings, samples of music, and even the occasional meme. Another effective motivational tool was the promise to familiarize students with the use of new digital platforms. Students were genuinely excited to learn how to create a timeline and a Scalar project. The idea of writing a book together, however, seemed daunting to some students, especially those students who associated a book with something created by "adults" (a word they often use to refer to faculty). Using information students had collected outside of class, we constructed the timeline during part of one of our sessions. There were the predictable hiccups that occur when using new technologies—some things worked, some things did not—but when the dust had finally settled we had produced the first item for the Scalar book. Once this first chapter of the book had been brought into being, the book began to feel real for the students.

It had been my hope that, during this seemingly never-ending dead time, the promise of a project that would come to fruition and achieve completion would communicate to students, perhaps at an unconscious level, that all things come to term and have an end, even pandemics. I was surprised to find students doubtful, for a long while, about their ability to pull off this project. One of the effects that isolation had on people was a festering negative energy and a lack of trust that "all will be well." Again, this was the first full semester that took place during the pandemic. During the first part of the semester students seemed to be wallowing in some sort of indeterminate misery that felt formless and interminable. And yet this murky indeterminacy, like the *tohu wa-bohu* of Genesis, or the formless interval of Plato's *khôra*, became the setting out of which something definite began to take form. The contrast was quite striking. Furthermore, there was something about seeing the project take shape, and in particular seeing their work gathered into a book, that helped to legitimize the work in their eyes, and led them to feel that they had produced quality work that did in fact deserve to be published. And so even though the semester was not taking place on campus, and even though there was a feeling in the air at times that the courses taking place this semester were not "real" courses (because, under normal circumstances, all courses at Swarthmore are in-person, students naturally assumed that their synchronous online courses would be *ersatz* and substandard), there was nevertheless a growing sense that this work was valuable.

Another choice I made in order to encourage engagement with the class—and this may be somewhat controversial in a German literature course—was to have students read a non-German novel that had just been published: Namwali Serpell's *The Old Drift* (2019). Serpell is an American-Zambian author whose work often focuses on postcolonial grief. *The Old Drift* explores how colonization plays a role in the transmission of disease. I chose to assign this book because I wanted students to experience something current, especially since it served as a palpable testimony that even though we are in the midst of a pandemic, and time seems to be standing still, creative work is still taking place and goals are being achieved. The choice of this text was meant to give students a sense, even a promise, of a better future. I also wanted to show students just how many of the things we had learned from our study of German literature were transferable to other literatures. Serpell's novel functioned as the payoff for all their hard work: it helped students appreciate how the meta-knowledge they had acquired during the course—how to do close readings, how to analyze metaphors of illness, how to situate a work within its cultural context, et cetera—could be applied to domains beyond German literature. Students would conclude the course mindful of the fact that they had not only learned about German literature, but they had also learned how to read literature in general, while also acquiring a special competence for literature that featured illness and medicine.

ASSIGNMENTS

As soon as students confessed to being worried that most of the final grade was based on writing assignments, I allowed students to rewrite their writing submissions. I added this safety net to another one that I had in place before the course began: a writing process consisting of multiple drafts with ample feedback from both myself and their colleagues in class. Curiously, not many students took advantage of the opportunity to rewrite. Students told me that knowing this opportunity for improvement was available to them reduced their stress considerably and led to better quality submissions. I introduced one other crucial safety net: I allowed for extensions, no questions asked. This seemed an obvious policy when teaching a course during a pandemic.

The amount of reading that I assigned per week naturally depended on the type of texts I was giving the students. The usual considerations were in play: how demanding the reading was, whether it is a primary or secondary, theoretical text, and so forth. I tried to anticipate points in the semester when attention spans would wane, or when students might feel overwhelmed by other kinds of tasks. I arranged the readings so that the lengthier and more difficult assignments took place during those periods in the semester when students were not under siege by other assignments. I used the reading guide to inform students about the degree of difficulty of the texts they were about to read. I also encouraged students to start reading more demanding texts early, in order to avoid being overwhelmed when the time came to have them prepared for class.

The creative final project caused a few students significant stress, as it forced them to produce something outside the parameters of normal academic work. One student admitted to some anxiety about having to work creatively, and so I gave her the option of writing an essay at the end in lieu of a creative project. This seemed to serve as a safety net for the student. With this fallback in place, she took a stab at the creative project and ended up submitting this as her final project. She later told me that the project gave her a sense of time redeemed, in that she was able to create something of value during this time of immobility. Once again, the enabling condition appeared to be the provision of a safety net, which allowed students to retreat to their comfort zone if needed. Simply knowing this option was available to them allowed students to challenge and invest themselves in creative projects that had cathartic value. The result was that they found themselves doing something new and exciting even as they may have felt trapped in their bedrooms.

The Scalar book was comprised of three different kinds of assignments. The third part consisted of the students' art projects and their accompanying artist statements. I will say more about these statements shortly. The first part of the book featured students' personal reflections about metaphors of illness in light of the texts they had read. For example, in response to their reading of Susan Sontag, students were asked to identify some of the ways that militaristic metaphors negatively influence lived illness—how they color the experience of chronic illness, for instance, or how they lead to shame when we feel that we are not strong enough to "fight" infection. One of the students concluded that new metaphors are needed if we are ever to be genuinely healthy: "Arundhati Roy's recent article 'The Pandemic is a Portal' describes Covid-19 (and illness at large) as an opportunity to give attention to, and challenge, the social tensions that disease so well exacerbates. Illness as journey instead of a battle and pandemic as a portal instead of a war allow me to look to the future with hope instead of despair."

This was followed by three response papers, which consisted of close readings of short texts chosen by the student. Throughout the semester I stressed that close reading was a transferable skill, that the art of listening deeply into a text, learning how to hear all it had to say to us, could also be directed to the students' daily experience of coping with the threat of illness while in isolation. Much was going on in the margins of our experience, if only we had ears to hear and appreciate it. We spoke of what was happening within us as we waited for a vaccine, a cure, an end that was at once a beginning. We considered how the posture of waiting for a sign in isolation placed us in a position similar to Hans Castorp's relationship with his thermometer in *The Magic Mountain*, as he waited day after day after day for it to show his temperature and reveal his fate—would he be able to leave or was it more of the same sanatorium for the (un)foreseeable future? Another student observed: "He is frantic, almost, to have an answer, to receive a verdict. But, like the other patients, he comes to terms with his condition. He is tired out after wasting away six of the seven minutes, and can do nothing but daydream, that activity which is most associated with time lost for naught. And there, finally, he loses his temporal sense."

ASSESSMENT

My concern to keep students motivated and engaged led me to give more weight to class participation in the final grade than I would under normal circumstances. Class participation included attendance, participation in class activities, along with evidence that they had listened to the pre-recorded lectures. The fact that 30 percent of the final grade was for class participation made it clear to students how vital class participation and investment was to the course. Naturally, this stimulated student participation. Of course, speaking in class can be a challenge for shy students, so I addressed this by allowing students to post in the chat window featured in Zoom. This reduced the anxiety of some of the more anxious students, especially those who are more comfortable typing than speaking aloud. Curiously, typing seems to be a “low stakes” mode of communication for many of my students.

The glaring differences in student working conditions gave me pause when it came to evaluating their work. Some students spent lockdown in luxurious homes, while other students spoke to me from the relative quiet of a closet. Given that students did not have the same level of access to basic staples of online learning such as high-quality internet, a private computer, and quiet time, it did not seem fair to expect the same quality of work from every student. Poor internet access, for example, would significantly hinder a student’s ability to do extensive research. So I was forced to resort to evaluating progress on a person-by-person basis. If a student demonstrated significant progress over the course of the semester, even if the overall quality did not rise to the level of a typical “A,” I awarded them a high grade. Desire and effort emerged as the key grading criteria, once I saw that students were not beginning from a level playing field. Some students availed themselves of the opportunity to rewrite papers, others did not, and I attribute the latter students’ failure to take advantage of this opportunity to their being frozen and generally “burned out.” This approach to grading was informed by disability studies, by trauma-informed pedagogy, and by universal design learning. These perspectives favor a flexible approach to grading that is able to do justice to different kinds of learners and different levels of ability. Moreover, my focus on students’ progress throughout the semester was consistent with the principles of universal design learning, as was my decision to allow students to produce an academic essay instead of a creative project if they felt more comfortable doing the former.

It is, of course, quite difficult to evaluate a creative project. What’s more, for those students who have chosen majors that do not value creative expression, the invitation to create an artistic project can be daunting, especially when it accounts for 35 percent of the final grade. Anticipating this, I divided the final project into two parts: the art project proper and an accompanying researched artist statement, in which students reflected on their work and made connections between it and material in class. The grade reflected the quality of the artistic statement. Still, this did not always assuage students’ anxiety, in part because many of them are overachievers, for whom it was important that the artistic component be excellent even though this had no bearing on their grade.

The final projects were impressive, even beautiful. They ranged from poetry to collages to cyanotypes, which are photographic prints that use sunlight and Prussian blue to produce an image. Our interest in the different temporalities associated with illness and isolation led one student to experiment with cyanotypes in their room, as there is something inherently compelling about a medium that depends so much on the time of exposure and that has the ability to reveal movement (or the lack of movement) in the space where the cyanotype undergoes development. The resulting hues of blue and the white, ghostly shadows cast by the objects and bodies in her room were in essence a visual representation of time unfolding during isolation. The student offered the following comment:

> My resulting cyanotypes are of an abstract quality which I feel speaks to the *rhythms* of light—in some regards, a visual sense of time determined by the ways in which the light is enabled to *move* within the space. Although my research into Helga Schmidt's work informed the formation of the project, after processing the prints I began to conduct research into ideas of rhythm as they relate to temporality. Theorist Paola Crespi likens rhythm to a ghost. She quotes Derrida: "Rhythm has always haunted our tradition, without ever reaching the center of its concerns" (4). She continues to explain that rhythm is a slippery concept to define—nothing seems to quite do it justice. It cannot be confined to the channels in which communication operates (3). Reflecting upon my project, I hope to sit with a similar sense of pertinent ambiguity. During my exaggerated confinement, temporality felt as if it dissolved into simply a rhythm. If rhythm sits at the core of temporal experience, perhaps experiencing illness involves a fundamental shift in internal rhythms—one which may at times be both generative and uncomfortable.

I found solace as I sat with the final projects and as I read the students' reflections. Despite the misery of Covid, quarantine and isolation, we had managed to create something of value. That these students, many of whom were new to serious literary analysis, and almost all of whom were riddled with anxiety during this period—anxious about creative projects, anxious about speaking about literature, anxious about doing close readings, and anxious about the state of the world—that they had trusted me, had given themselves over to a subject that was important to me, and had turned their immersion into outbreak narratives into something extraordinary, left me feeling like a gift had been given from them to me, from me to them, from the universe to all of us.

My final feeling, after the exhaustion finally lifted, was one of gratitude.

WORKS CITED

Bochow, Michael. 1993. "Einstellungen und Werthaltungen zu homosexuellen Männern in Ost-und Westdeutschland." In *Aids-eine Forschungsbilanz: Bericht über den Förderschwerpunkt "Sozialwissenschaftliche AIDS-Forschung" im Rahmen des Programms der Bundesregierung "Forschung und Entwicklung im Dienste der Gesundheit,"* edited by Cornelia Lange, 115–128. Berlin: Edition Sigma.

Borneman, John. 1987. "AIDS: Cultural Analysis/Cultural Activism." *October* 43 (Winter): 223–236.

Camus, Albert. 2012. *The Plague*. Translated by Stuart Gilbert. New York: Knopf Doubleday.

Cole, Thomas, Nathan Carlin, and Ronald Carson. 2015. *Medical Humanities*. New York: Cambridge University Press.

Crespi, Paola and Sunil Manghani. 2020. "Rhythm, Rhuthmos and Rhythmanalysis." In *Rhythm and Critique: Technics, Modalities, Practices*, edited by Paola Crespi and Sunil Manghani, 3–19. Edinburgh: University Press.

Heine, Heinrich. 1832. "Cholera in Paris." *Französiche Zustände*. Hamburg: Hoffmann und Kampe. projekt-gutenberg.org//heine/franzzus/franzus. Accessed 08.21.2020.

Mann, Thomas. 1996. *The Magic Mountain*. Translated by John E. Woods. New York: Vintage.

Schmidt, Helga. 2020. *Uchronia: Designing Time*. Basel: Birkhauser Architecture.

Wasmuth, Johannes. 2002. "Strafrechtliche Verfolgung Homosexueller in BRD und DDR." In *Nationalsozialistischer Terror gegen Homosexuelle. Verdrängt und ungesühnt*, edited by Burkhard Jellonnek and Rüdiger Lautmann, 173–186. München: Paderborn.

PART II

Graphic Medicine

CHAPTER FIVE

Comics from the German-Language Realm and Health Humanities: An Overview

MARINA RAUCHENBACHER

INTRODUCTION

Mental and physical illnesses, health, dis_ability,[1] and related socio-political issues are becoming increasingly significant in comics from the German-speaking world. As a result, for some years now, more attention has been paid to these topics in the—overall growing—comics research. In this context, *Graphic Medicine* and *Graphic Pathography* have become an important subfield in the Health Humanities.

The term *graphic medicine* was coined by the British physician and comic artist Ian Williams (Czerwiec et al. 2015, 4) and is to be understood as the "intersection of the medium of comics and the discourse of healthcare" (Czerwiec et al. 2015, 1). It often focuses on the educational role of comics (Green and Myers 2010, 1), diseases of various kinds, healthcare, people in the nursing professions, doctors, therapists, patient communication, treatment procedures, dis_ability, gender transition, pregnancy, menopause, aging, and so on.[2] The *Graphic Medicine Manifesto* (2015) sets out—as the title indicates—the field's principles and argues for the relevance of graphic works for medicine (Czerwiec et al. 2015).[3] Graphic medicine can be used to depict nonverbal processes, promote sensitivity among students toward patients, highlight social and political factors, and elaborate on the complexity of doctor-patient communication (Green 2015, 75). Furthermore, graphic medicine also allows for a rethinking of iconographies of illness and thus for addressing visual cultures linked to our notions of illness, or of what we understand by medicine (Williams 2015, 125).

Initially defined as a "sub-genre of graphic stories" (Green and Myers 2010, 1), Graphic Pathographies as "graphic illness and disability memoirs" are—in the light of "the memoir boom in general"—increasingly crucial in Health Humanities (Wegner 2020, 60; also, Schmidt 2020, 369).[4] The term references the original Freudian concept of *pathography*, which was functionalized by Anne Hunsaker Hawkins for Illness Studies to denote (auto) biographical works about "experiences of illness, treatment, and sometimes death" (Hawkins 1999, 1). These works contribute a wide variety of perspectives to medical discourse and allow for "retracing" and "materially reimagining" (Chute 2010, 2). Hillary Chute formulates this observation in reference to graphic memoirs by women dealing specifically with trauma, but it may apply also more generally to the (often painful) confrontation with illness. In response to a critique of the genre of autobiography (e.g., Schmidt 2020), Amelia DeFalco operates with the term *somatography*, which Thomas G. Couser defines as a memoir about "living with, loving, or knowing intimately someone with such a [physically or mentally suffering] body" (Couser 2009, 2). As DeFalco states, "autobiography typically reinforces the association of independence with identity, somatographies expose the dependency at the core of human relationships" (DeFalco 2016, 224). Comics thus contribute various perspectives to the discussion, be it with an (auto)biographical claim, in purely fictional form, or firmly pursuing an educational aspect. Research addresses these comics from a cultural theoretical perspective and focuses, for example, on narratological or aesthetic questions, on visual culture, and on discourse-analytical, sign-theoretical, and media-theoretical approaches.

The following analysis first briefly introduces the specific conditions of the comics medium and explores why comics, in particular, so prolifically and productively deal with health/illness ("Bodies and/in Comics"). Then, the central part of the essay aims to systematize relevant comics produced in the German-speaking world ("Topics: A Spotlight Overview").[5] However, it must be noted that comics are a hybrid medium that cannot be evaluated solely based on language; it is constituted by the very interaction between pictorial and textual elements. Comics research in the German-speaking world is heavily influenced by research in the Anglo-American world and cannot be thought of in isolation. In keeping with the publication at hand, however, this article highlights research that explicitly examines comics from the German-speaking world.

BODIES AND/IN COMICS

In comics, the repetitive pictorial representation of bodies is constitutive (i.a. Chute 2010; Frahm 2010; Klar 2011 and 2014; Rauchenbacher and Serles 2020; Szép 2020; Krüger-Fürhoff and Schmidt 2021).[6] Thus, those bodies are simultaneously *never* and yet *always* unique, as repetition inevitably entails difference.[7] Bodies must be drawn from different perspectives, and in different postures; they are fragmented and cropped, or cut off by the panel edge, and always multi-present—simultaneously in its repetitions (i.a. Frahm 2010; Klar 2011 and 2014; Rauchenbacher and Serles 2020). As a result of this repetitive structure, the comics medium is performative (Sina 2016, 13); bodies must continually be read and identified anew. For this reason alone, reading comics is a complex process that refers to one's perception, modes of reading, and classification strategies; it constantly challenges one to rethink one's knowledge.

In comics, bodies are thus given a specific significance and receive particular attention. As Elisabeth El Refaie points out, bodies can be represented in (autobiographical) comics "in ways that reflect their innermost sense of self, often by using a range of symbolic elements and rhetorical tropes to add further layers of meaning." She refers "to this process of engaging with one's own identity through multiple self-portraits as 'pictorial embodiment'" (El Refaie 2012, 51). Comics bodies are "material sites" (Donovan 2014, 239), which are used for processes of embodiment or—to put it differently—for the *graphic externalization* of emotions, thoughts, and mental or physical pain. In this context, El Refaie's functionalization of Drew Leder's concept of "dys-appearance" for Comics Studies proves instructive. Leder uses this term in a phenomenological discussion of illness and the body to describe a process of dissociation insofar as the body requires special attention when it is perceived as disturbing, different, or in opposition to the self (Leder 1990, 70). For comics analysis, this concept can be rethought insofar as the dissociative moment can be understood as the result of the repeated drawing of one's own body: "Every act of self-portraiture entails a form of dys-appearance, in the sense that one's body can no longer be taken for granted as an unconscious presence" (El Refaie 2012, 62). Comics experiment with attempts to manifest these dys-appearance processes and, in doing so, constantly have to choose new perspectives and new realizations for the body (Szép 2020, 92). Reading comic bodies is an "embodied process, which [...] makes it possible for readers to engage with the vulnerability of the Other articulated in the drawn lines" (Szép 2020, 24). Thus, comics are an effective medium for studying physical and mental illness and health precisely because the body is the graphic negotiating surface for the illness itself.

TOPICS: A SPOTLIGHT OVERVIEW

As already mentioned, in the German-speaking realm, graphic medicine is booming. Therefore, in the following section, I shall strive to offer an overview, grouped by topics that I identify as significant/frequent, with each chapter focusing on short individual analyses. This thematic clustering is intended neither as a diagnostic process nor as a pathologization of the comics, but instead follows the comics' content and accentuates the topics they address.

Due to the abundance of material, I will mainly concentrate on comics that emphasize topics explicitly relevant to the genre of graphic medicine. Beyond that, it must be stressed that medical discourses are often discussed in other types of comics as well (e.g., that deal with flight and war trauma or focus on trauma due to sexual abuse). Another limitation of this article regards the heterogeneous publication spectrum of comics, closely linked to the medium's history and its indie/alternative/DIY scene. In addition to publications by publishing houses, a wide variety of material is published in comic magazines, but also as self-publications, in book format or as zines. Additionally, webcomics and social media (above all Instagram) are becoming increasingly important. The following article attempts to cover as broad a spectrum as possible within the limits of its scope.

Eating Disorders

In particular, the topic of eating disorders offers a compelling insight into the spectrum between realistic-identificatory representations and abstraction/a deconstructive approach, which is fundamental for graphic medicine overall (Rauchenbacher 2024). While the former graphically quote ideal body concepts precisely because they must show the struggle with these ideals, the latter counteracts a graphically identificatory moment. In it, the claim of a didactic-pedagogical approach (designed especially for younger target groups) comes into conflict with a complex deconstructive, image-critical, and cultural-historical debate.

The thematization of eating disorders in comics is particularly productive because of the constitutive function of bodies in this medium. At the same time, the body, or rather its visual conception and perception, is a genuine component of the reflection on eating disorders. In this way, the social and socio-political classification (and stigmatization) of bodies—also centrally concerning gender—becomes subject to discussion (beauty ideals and gender coding). Furthermore, the body as a graphic area of negotiation for illness (see above) has particular relevance because eating disorders are about modifying bodies.

Four examples from German-speaking countries cover a wide range of (aesthetic) approaches. Ingrid Sabisch's *41,3 kg—Magersucht?* (2011) tells the story of a teenage girl who develops anorexia. A work that shares this comic's identificatory approach and has a similar overall plot is the educational comic *Ninette: Dünn ist nicht dünn genug* (2021) by the German Federal Centre for Health Education (BZgA). In contrast, Regina Hofer's *Blad* (2008/18) and Karin Krämer's *SIE* (2016) avoid realism, choosing instead to work with abstraction and a high degree of self-reflection when addressing the suffering bodies.

In Sabisch's *41,3 kg—Magersucht?*, young Jessica is confronted with her mother's aging and weight gain. Jessica starts fasting and develops an eating disorder, fuelled by online forums. Eventually, she receives treatment and then enters a clinic. However, it is only after she develops cardiac arrhythmia that she realizes the gravity of the situation and is eventually quasi-cured. From this summary, a straightforward, traceable plot already becomes evident, confirming a "positive 'narrative arc'" and a "happy ending," which must be considered a "rhetorical imperative" of many illness narratives (Couser 2016, 4). This comic is an apt example for the *paradoxical presence of the body*. Representations of the body seem unavoidable in order to allow a discussion of the topic. At the same time, however, the aesthetically unquestioned presence of the body can be criticized insofar as corporeality, and thus certain norms, are cited first and foremost, or, rather, the representation of the body, and thus the view of it, is only questioned to a limited extent or not at all. In its visual presence, the (sick) body continues to offer scope for identification, and, in fact, a particular visual-reading competence is required to classify the representations accordingly. This can be demonstrated by one figure in particular, who embodies an inner voice as well as the first-person narrator's ideal image: long hair, large eyes, and a narrow waist. Paradoxically, however, this very object of Jessica's addiction is presented unchallenged and unquestioned.

Regina Hofer's *Blad*[8] offers an autobiographical perspective on the subject and is far more complex in its storyline. The comic also does not focus on the idea of healing per se but remains open-ended. What is particularly striking about *Blad*—apart from the elaborate aesthetic realization—is that the comic body is not only the site where the illness is negotiated but is, rather, thematized as an artificial body itself, thus allowing questions of visual representability and perception to be discussed. Hofer works intensively with repetition; she constantly thematizes (self-)perception and focuses on the comic body's function as a site for the graphic negotiation of emotions, suffering, and thoughts (Rauchenbacher and Serles 2020). For example, the physical injury that the eating disorder causes to the body is matched by the extensive functionalization of the principal vulnerability of the comic body, which becomes evident, not least in the repeated use of split panels (Figure 5.1). At the same time,

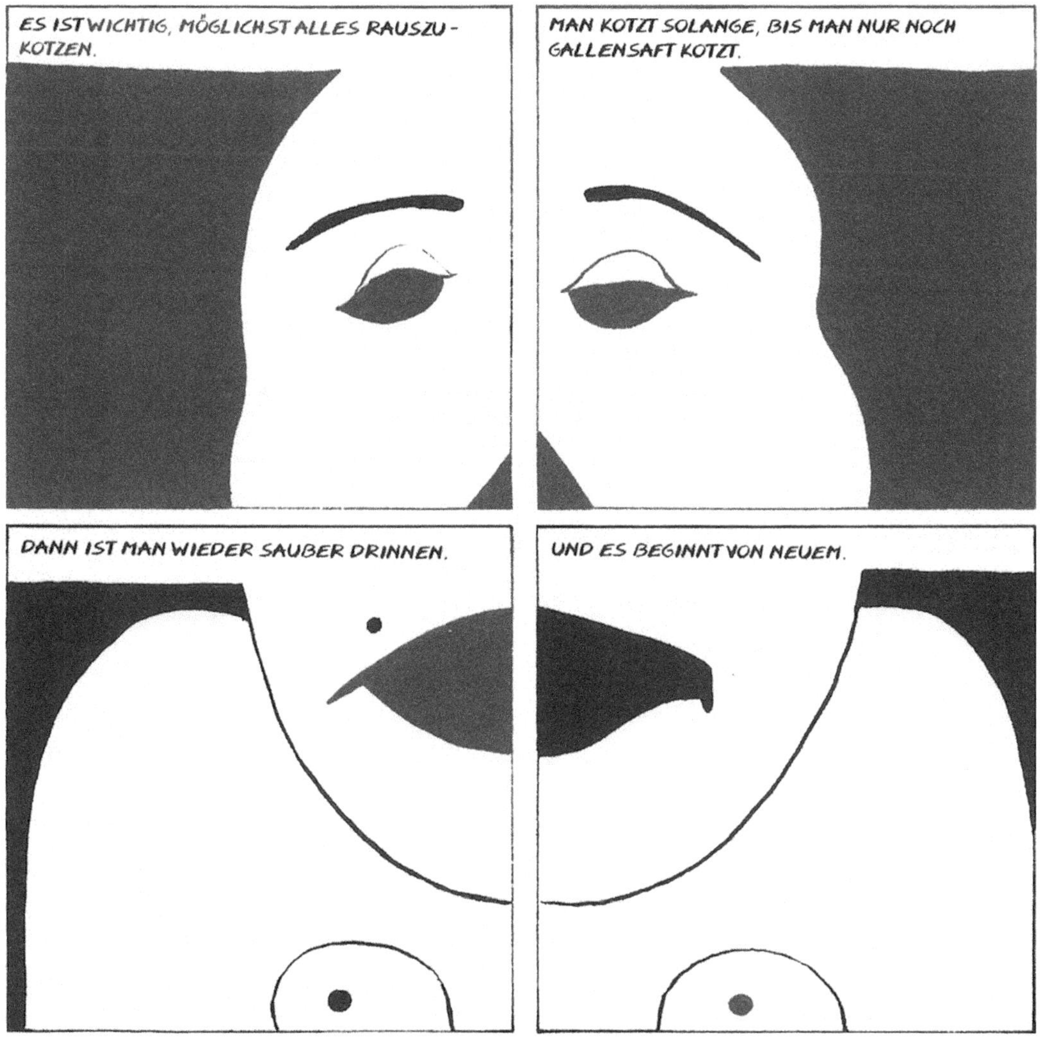

FIGURE 5.1: The (comic) body's vulnerability. Regina Hofer, *Blad* (2008/18). Wien: Luftschacht: 49. Copyright: Regina Hofer.

the incommensurability of the individual suffering depicted is made apparent by graphic representations that cannot always be deciphered at first glance, and text and images do not explicitly correspond to one another (Rauchenbacher 2022b).

Addictive Disorders and Drug Abuse

Discussing the impact of different addictive disorders and drug abuse is vital in comics in the German-speaking world and follows diverse (aesthetic) orientations and needs. Jürgen Wolsch's *Drogen* (2007) is an educational comic that introduces neurobiological processes and drug science. Elke Renate Steiner's *Risiken und Nebenwirkungen* (2010) creates seven characters that she uses to discuss prescription drug addiction (Schmidt 2020). In *Ton und Scherben* (2015), Jana Kreisl episodically portrays the effects that one man's alcoholism has on his wife and child. In *XES* (2020), Florian Winter autobiographically follows the still taboo subject of sex addiction.

Also of particular interest are the consequences of (one-time) drug abuse that takes place in coming-of-age comics. In *Filmriss* (2007), Kati Rickenbach thematizes a young woman's involuntary consumption of a drug, as well as the mental blackout that follows. Among the many subjects tackled in Lukas Jüliger's *Vakuum* (2013) is a teenager failing to come down from a drug trip (Lexe 2015). Sascha Hommer, Eric Wunder, and Hamed Eshrat adopt an autobiographical stance. Hommer recounts his drug abuse as a teenager in *Vier Augen* (2009); Wunder addresses his mother's heroin addiction in *Rauschgift* (2019). The "H" in Eshrat's *Coming of H* (2022) stands for "heroin," among other things, and thus for the drug abuse of the autobiographical avatar's best friend.

Rickenbach's *Filmriss* thematizes a central (anxiety-inducing) issue, especially for young women. Lela wakes up after a night of partying, has a hickey on her neck, and realizes that—as the comic's title suggests—she has had a mental blackout. Rickenbach shapes the search for memory criminologically and thematizes the threatening nature of the memory gap. The comic is consistently realized in eight-panel pages and contrasts different perspectives on the night's events.

Hommer's *Vier Augen* follows the story of the autobiographical avatar Sascha, who increasingly consumes drugs of various kinds. Hommer's black-and-white drawing style is characterized by clear structures, which he also uses to convey the protagonist's drug-induced delusions: People transform into monster-like figures or plant-like entities, until, finally, a permanent delusion remains, which Sascha experiences as a canine-esque mutating figure.

Aging

Of increasing importance is the examination of age/aging, its social stigmatization, and age-related changes and illnesses, geriatric care, and death (Krüger-Fürhoff 2021 and 2024; Lobnig 2021; Grünewald 2022; Klingenböck 2022; see also section "Death and Dying" in this essay). In 2015, the comic magazine *Strapazin* dedicated an issue to the topic, which offers diverse perspectives. In *Herbst in der Hose* (2017), Ralf König outlines—as already indicated by the title—a humorous approach to aging and andropause based on the couple Konrad and Paul (Krüger-Fürhoff 2021); humorous are also Peter Butschkow's cartoons in

Was geht'n im Alter so ab, Alter? (2018). In *Off the Blob: Gespräche mit Frauen über den Wechsel* (2019), Renate Mowlam draws on nine interviews to depict the physical, mental, and social effects of the menopause as well as coping mechanisms.

Additionally, dementia diseases have to be considered in connection with aging (Krüger-Fürhoff, Schmidt, and Vice 2022). Those are the subject of Flix's *Don Quijote* (2012), Thomas von Steinaecker and Barbara Yelin's *Der Sommer ihres Lebens* (2015/16/17) among other topics, (Klingenböck 2022), and Lika Nüssli's autobiographical comic *Vergiss dich nicht* (Krüger-Fürhoff 2021; Lobnig 2021). Steinaecker and Yelin's as well as Nüssli's works and Sheree Domingo's *Ferngespräch* (2019) are also particularly instructive concerning the elder care system (Krüger-Fürhoff 2021).

Cancer

While in the English-speaking world, Brian Fies' webcomic *Mom's Cancer* (2006) is one of the most discussed contributions to graphic medicine, comics on cancer have not yet been addressed to such an extent in the German-speaking world. In addition to Jutta Winkelmann's *Mein Leben ohne mich* (2016), Anna Faroqhi's *Krebs Kung Fu* (2017), and Sabine Dinkel's *Meine Arschbombe in die Untiefen des Lebens* (2018), two works by Ilse Kilic and Fritz Widhalm, *Ein kleiner Schnitt: Unser Krebsjahr* (2005) and *Kann ich solange zeichnen, bis alle Ängste verfliegen? Auf Nimmerwiedersehen, Krebs!* (2012), are noteworthy in particular. All of these comics are autobiographical, while Maki Shimizu's *Liebe Lust Prostata* (2018) is an adaptation of an autobiographical account by German journalist Friedrich W. Zimmermann. The children's comic *Trip mit Tropf* (2022) by Josephine Mark offers a humorous and sensitive approach to the subject.

Through the autobiographical avatars Ilse and Fritz in *Ein Kleiner Schnitt*, Kilic and Widhalm thematize Kilic's breast cancer, her treatment procedures, as well as the (social) impacts on everyday life. They work with sketchy drawings, contrast the complex medical terms with explanatory descriptions, functionalize humor, and, above all, mainly rely on the rhetorical element of understatement. The latter, in particular, draws attention to Kilic and Widhalm's meta-reflexive approach, which is already evident in the two covers, whose minimalistic graphic elements can be considered an understatement of the life-threatening processes they symbolize. The book cover of *Ein kleiner Schnitt* is light pink; beside the authors' names, the book's title, and the name of Kilic's independent publishing company, the cover only displays a discreet, irregular, vertical line, graphically symbolizing the comic's title. Even more subversive, the cover of *Kann ich solange zeichnen, bis alle Ängste verfliegen?* shows two red arches with small crosshatches and a small circle at the very bottom, symbolizing Ilse's sutures after her double mastectomy and her belly button.

In *Liebe Lust Prostata*, Maki Shimizu draws selected scenes from Friedrich W. Zimmermann's 2016 eponymous autobiographical account of his battle with prostate cancer. Shimizu's red, blue, and black drawings are both expressive and detailed; they underline the intense emotions evoked by the protagonist's cancer diagnosis and the consequences of prostate surgery (incontinence and impotence) as well as the (regained) sexual experience.

Shimizu's style is often sketchy, with different layers of drawing visible, which highlight individual scenes that stand on their own.

Covid-19

Throughout the Covid-19 crisis, graphic medicine has been given further impetus in the German-speaking world, with the number of comics and cartoons published online or on social media (such as Instagram) being innumerable. Also, cartoons are of particular interest as they allow the crisis and its social, political, physical, and psychological effects to be addressed pointedly (and humorously)—one such example being Ralf König's *Vervirte Zeiten* (2021)—and, to name just two of the numerous web publications, Kati Rickenbach's cartoons on Instagram and Renate Mowlam's series *Wir bleiben zuhause—Corona Comics* on her website. Both work with autobiographical avatars, as does Jutta Bauer's mostly cartoon-style work *Corona Diaries* (2021), Greta von Richthofen's graphic memoir *Das Gute am Ende des Tages* (2021), and Josep Rodes' *Corona Go Home: Tagebuch aus Varanasi* (2021). A didactic-educational approach is explored in Lilli L'Arronge's *Das geheime Tagebuch eines miesen Virus* (2021). In *Impfland* (2022), Federico Cacciapaglia frames the struggle with conspiracy theories and the search for a Covid-19 vaccine as a medieval quest.[9]

In *Corona Diaries*, Bauer draws and paints (ink and watercolor) in forty-one diary entries between March and July 2020, i.e., starting with the first lockdown in Germany, that offer everyday observations in a mixture of cartoons, sketches, and watercolor paintings. Additional statements or excerpts from emails accompany the predominantly single-sided entries. Bauer thus finds a specific graphic expression for each entry and, through this careful examination, also documents the focus on individual (seemingly irrelevant) experiences and the slowing down of (her) everyday life as a result of the lockdown.

L'Arronge's *Das geheime Tagebuch eines miesen Virus* was conceptualized specifically for children in cooperation with one of Germany's Youth Welfare Offices. The complex transmission processes, course of infection, immune defense, and hygiene measures are transferred into a vivid and colorful visual language and humorously told from the perspective of the titular "rotten" virus.

Death and Dying

Death and dying are much discussed in the genre of graphic medicine (see also section "Aging" in this essay). In the following, I shall therefore emphasize comics that specifically focus on this topic. An autobiographical approach is taken by Eva Müller in *Sterben ist echt das Letzte!* (2017), which examines the fascination with death and the fear it evokes, by Tina Brenneisen in *Das Licht, das Schatten leert* (2019), which tackles the subject of stillbirth, and by Markus Färber and Christine Färber in *Fürchtetal* (2021), which deals with the suicide of their father. Suicide is also the subject of Illi Anna Heger's *Minicomic 05: Laborlüftung* (2016) and Antonia Kühn's *Lichtung* (2018). In the latter, the mother's absence, a lack of understanding, and the voids left behind are reflected from the perspective of the child, Paul. Finally, in *Eremit* (2013), Marijpol explores a dystopian sci-fi world and the marketing of death, bringing a new, more social-critical perspective to the topic (Schmidt 2020).

In *Das Licht, das Schatten leert*, Brenneisen takes up the social taboo of stillbirth. Via two autobiographical avatars—the parents Tini and Fritzemann—Brenneisen discusses the suffering, the effects on the social environment, society's tabooing of the issue, and—through Tini's family—the inability to deal sensitively with the subject. Brenneisen works with expressive body and mimic depictions that emphasize the symbolic dimension of comic bodies as surfaces for the representation of suffering and mourning. This symbolic dimension is also made clear by the specific visualization of the dead child, Lasse. Metaphorically, the omnipresence of his absence is made clear by a romper suit, which is empty, i.e., graphically bodiless.

Färber and Färber's *Fürchtetal* is intriguing in terms of the interplay between the pictorial and textual layers. This autobiographical narration about suicide often dispenses—and this is unusual—with the depiction of the narrating or narrated characters. They are only represented schematically in varying degrees of abstraction or replaced by objects and abstract forms (Figure 5.2). *Fürchtetal* does not strive for a coherent narration that would follow a definite arc of suspense, but operates associatively, stringing tags of memories together.

Gender Transition and the Medical System

The increasing discussion of gender in German-language comics and the growing public and activist attention to intergender and, especially, transgender identities has also resulted in more engagement with gender transition and demands on society and the medical system. In *Hexenblut* (2014), Suskas Lötzerich reconstructs their story autobiographically, starting with their birth, when their sex could not be determined at the hospital (Hochreiter, Rauchenbacher, and Serles 2022). As the autobiographical avatar Suska—later Suskas—discovers, with the help of their mother, as a baby, they were operated on by a doctor—without their parents even being consulted. This medical brutality leads to a painful search for identity and a complicated, lengthy, and painful gender transition with several surgical procedures. The comic works with panels of different sizes, with the drawings repeatedly exceeding the frames, and with unframed depictions of varying sizes. This diverse page design expresses Suskas' restless search. In addition, *Hexenblut* is characterized by a constant focus on bodies and, above all, by en-face depictions, bringing the characters' emotions to the fore.

Gender transition is also addressed in Sarah Barczyk's *Nenn mich Kai* (2016), Joris Bas Backer's *Küsse für Jet* (2020), and Peer Jongeling's *"Hattest du eigentlich schon die Operation?"* (2020). In six independent, short scenic chapters and an introduction that adopts an educational approach, Jongeling deals with the socio-political issues of transgender and body politics. Jongeling's comic is productive in that it resists stereotypical binary pictorial realizations of gender and thus does not risk undermining its own critique of stereotypical attributions.

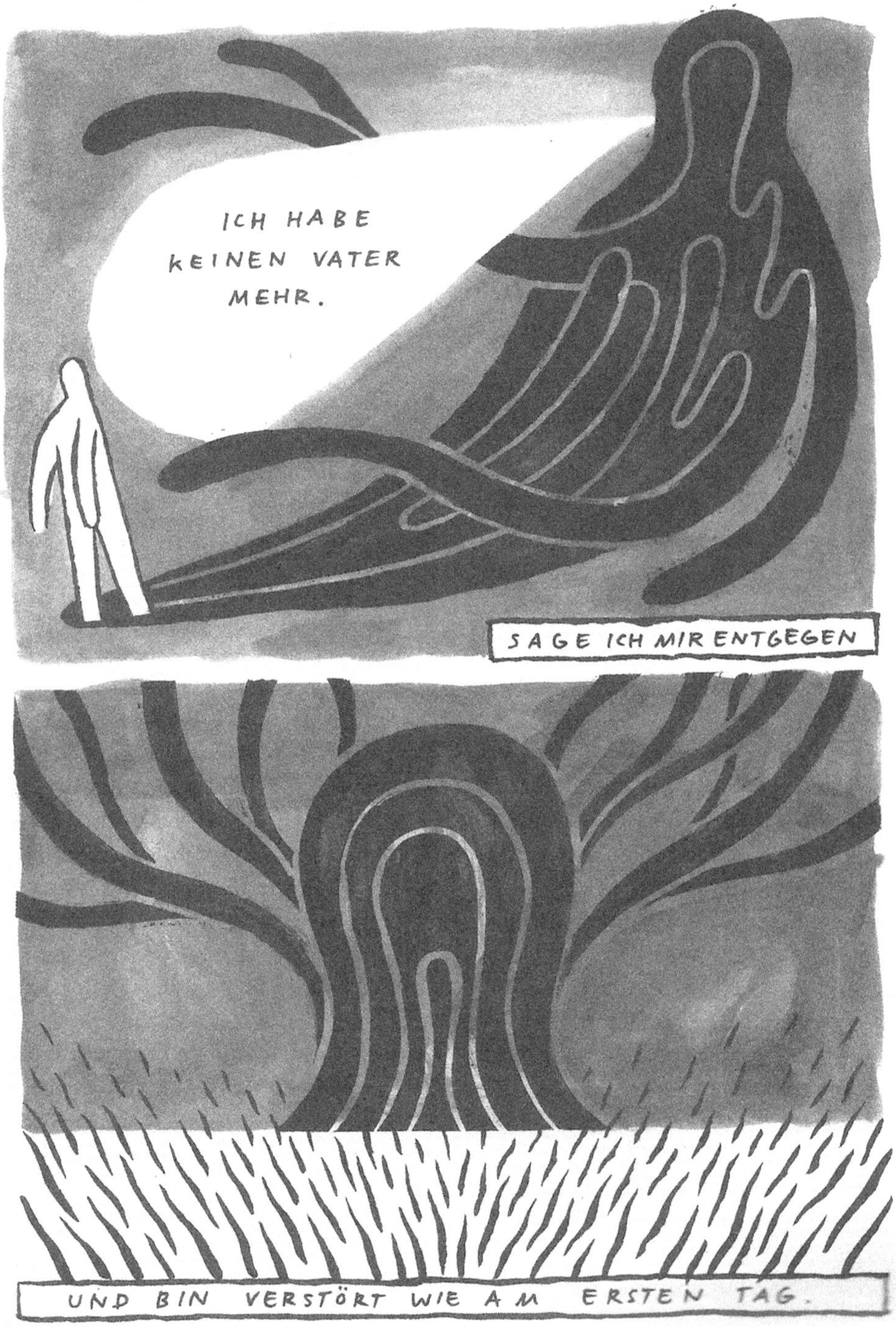
ICH HABE
KEINEN VATER
MEHR.
SAGE ICH MIR ENTGEGEN
UND BIN VERSTÖRT WIE AM ERSTEN TAG.

FIGURE 5.2: The abstraction of bodies and memories. Christine Färber and Markus Färber, *Fürchtetal* (2021): n.p. Kassel: Rotopol. Copyright: Christine Färber and Markus Färber.

Pregnancy, Reproduction, Abortion, and Birth

Comics on pregnancy are not only insightful concerning the associated physiological and psychological processes, but also reflect on gender roles and family concepts, and thus on social expectations and care. Examples are Ingrid Sabisch's *Schwangersschaftsstreifen* (2005), Charles Lewinsky and Andreas Gefe's *Zwei Mal Zwei* (2011), Anna Sommer's *Das Unbekannte* (2018), and Dorothea Huber's autobiographical account *Aus Mutters Mund* (2022). As has already become apparent with Tina Brenneisen's *Das Licht, das Schatten leert* (see section "Death and Dying" in this essay), complications such as stillbirth or—as shown in Verena Weißenböck's autobiographical work *Eine Geschichte vom Kinderkriegen* (2007)—miscarriage are also dealt with. Moreover, concerning regressive, conservative tendencies, the discussion of abortion, such as in Julia Zejn's *Andere Umstände* (2021), is of core political importance. A critical-parodistic examination of reproduction (and sexual norms) is sketched out in Katharina Greve's *Frau Doktor Waldbeck näht sich eine Familie* (2011) (Krüger-Fürhoff 2019a and 2019b).

In *Andere Umstände*, Zejn discusses an unwanted pregnancy and the decision to have an abortion through the lens of the young sociologist Anja and her partner, Olli. Zejn provides contexts for the decision-making process in detailed drawings and differently colored chapters, such as an insight into the pair's relationship, the division of gender roles in Anja's friendship group, and her employment situation. In addition, the aesthetic reflection on medical representations is of particular interest: Zejn visualizes embryonic development in drawings and thus also reflects on the protagonist's perspective on the fetus (152).

Huber's *Aus Mutters Mund* has a playful and humorous approach as the title already demonstrates through the use of a pun on the German word *Muttermund* (i.e., cervix). Using single- and double-sided brightly colored depictions, Huber visualizes the course of a pregnancy, considering the physical changes, fears, and expectations, as well as social constraints concerning pregnant bodies. The often grotesque, alienated depictions of bodies succinctly highlight these moments while simultaneously resisting idealizing notions of pregnancy and motherhood.

Further Psychological Diseases and Mental Health

As has already become apparent—especially concerning eating and addiction disorders—different psychological diseases and mental health are frequently thematized.

Widely discussed and of central educational significance are the works on autism and mental health by Daniela Schreiter: the autobiographical trilogy *Schattenspringer* (2014–18) and the strip collection *Die Abenteuer von Autistic Hero-Girl* (2017). In the latter, Schreiter creates a superhero avatar who goes through various adventures together with their sidekick, a fox. Schreiter dedicates each strip playfully to a specific topic and introduces the everyday experience of people with an autism spectrum disorder.

In the context of coming-of-age, the topic of deliberate self-harm is addressed in Melanie Gerland's *Offene Arme* (2010) and, marginally, in Joris Bas Backer's *Küsse für Jet* (see section "Gender Transition and the Medical System" in this essay).

Julia Bernhard's *Wie gut, dass wir darüber geredet haben* (2019), Simone F. Baumann's *Zwang* (2021), and Anja Wicki's *In Ordnung* (2022) are dedicated to the subject of depression, and, in Baumann's case, also to compulsion and trauma. *Zwang* is characterized by an oppressive visual atmosphere through black hatching and grotesque bodies. While Bernhard and Baumann prioritize an approach to the protagonist's perception over an explicit thematization of these topics, Wicki discusses the illness (e.g., 42). In *Burnout* (2018), Larissa Bertonasco talks about her exhaustion depression, its causes, and the healing process.

Raphaela Buder's *Die Wurzeln der Lena Siebert* (2017) is about a young girl called Lena, whose mother suffers from a schizophrenic disorder. In subtly black-and-white drawings, Buder depicts Lena's conflicted relationship with her mother and its effects on the child's experience. The comic is characterized by detailed shapes, focusing repeatedly on geometric forms that are distinctly elaborated and completed by the precise panel structure. Lena's disorientation in the face of her mother's symptoms is thus made clear, above all, by the contrast with spatial, geometric structures: streetscapes, diverse interior spaces—especially the asylum where her mother is taken into care.

Schizophrenia is also a topic in Stefan Haller's autobiographical work *Schattenmutter* (2021). Using his mother's diaries from the 1970s and 1980s, Haller attempts to reconstruct her mental illness, her schizophrenia diagnosis and depression, and his childhood, while also criticizing the medical system and psychiatric care at the time. To this end, he contrasts different perspectives and creates two narrative levels: While the excerpts from the mother's diary are realized in distinctly structured six-page panels, the narrator's accompanying texts and conversations with third parties do not follow a consistent structure. The diary panels are dense in that they offer detailed, high-contrast black-and-white representations and include a considerable amount of text, yet the other passages are arranged more openly. Also, Pirmin Beeler's *Hat man erst einmal angefangen zu reden, kann alles Mögliche dabei herauskommen* (2018) deals with a mother's mental illness and the search for explanations.

Comics about trauma and post-traumatic stress disorder are a broad area of interest in mental health. Several topics in the context of which trauma is discussed have already been covered; in addition, sexualized violence against children, other traumatic experiences in childhood, violence, flight, and war are of particular interest. Examples are Ulli Lust's autobiographical comic *Heute ist der letzte Tag vom Rest deines Lebens* (2009) (Hochreiter 2014; Rauchenbacher and Serles 2020), which elaborates on sexualized and gender based violence, and Lust's adaptation of Marcel Beyer's novel *Flughunde* (2013), in which childhood trauma is discussed through the character of a fictionalized Magda Goebbels (Rauchenbacher 2022a).

Other Topics

Renate Mowlam's comics, some of which have already been mentioned, are of vital importance in the low-key communication of complex medical topics, for example, her work on *Global Health* (2021) for the Vienna General Hospital and the educational comic *Was ist ein Schlaganfall und wie wird er behandelt?* (2022) for the Viennese Klinik Favoriten.

Another vital topic is physical and mental dis_ability. In *Wirbelsturm* (2017), Roland Burkart tells of a swimming accident that results in the autobiographically inspired protagonist, Piedro, suffering paralysis of all four extremities. Burkart's drawings are sketchy and he utilizes the possibilities of an interlinear reading. There are no panels; instead, the depicted impressions are spread across either a single or double page. The comic adaptations of Johanna Spyri's novels, *Heidis Lehr—und Wanderjahre* (1880) and *Heidi kann brauchen, was es gelernt hat* (1881), from the 1970s and 1980s are also instructive for discussing paralysis by means of the character Klara and, beyond that, psychosomatics, homesickness, blindness, and—above all—the social dispositions of illness (Rauchenbacher 2023).

Mikael Ross provides a vital contribution in terms of inclusion and social concepts of dis_ability in *Der Umfall* (2018). Ross conducted research in Neuerkerode in Germany, a Protestant work and housing project for people with mental disabilities. *Der Umfall* tells the story of Noel, who is placed in a care facility after his mother dies of a stroke.

With regard to an explicit examination of an autobiographical claim, Reto Gloor's *Das Karma-Problem: MS—eine unheilbare Krankheit übernimmt die Kontrolle* (2015) is insightful insofar as Gloor explicitly reflects on his own story. His multiple sclerosis diagnosis meant he could no longer draw by hand, so he learned to work digitally: "Die Arbeit am Bildschirm und die digitale Präzision der Maschine erleichterten mir, den nötigen Abstand zum autobiografischen Inhalt zu finden." (3) Gloor's work addresses the diagnosis, the course of the disease, and the psychological and social consequences in black-and-white images that are repeatedly accentuated by a deliberately applied blue tone. An approach to MS for children and teenagers is offered in *Ich, mein Schatten und das volle Leben*: *Ein Buch über Multiple Sklerose* (2019) by children's author Brigitte Endres, for which Ingrid Sabisch produced individual strips.

A humorous approach to the symptom of stutter is provided in Mawil's *Schtttotttern* (2006/7), where the author also elaborates on coping strategies.

An unusual example in the context of Health Humanities is Ursula Fürst's historical comic *Die Ballade von der Typhoid Mary* (1990), an adaptation of Jürg Federspiel's eponymous novel (1982), in which the spread of typhus around 1900 is the subject.

CONCLUSION

Graphic medicine contributes significantly to a diversified understanding of different health conditions and diseases. Comics and the pedagogical, media- and culture-theoretical, as well as philological analyses of these comics offer diverse perspectives on healthcare systems and work against what Deborah Lupton already criticized in 1997 through her elaborations on public health (research), namely that humanities are not appropriately included in the examination of health, illness, and the healthcare system: "Due to its links with biomedicine, which favours positivistic forms of inquiry based on the gathering of empirical quantifiable data, public health research has tended to undervalue the more humanistic, critical, theoretical and interpretive approaches." (Lupton 1997, 1).

As the above examples show, comics offer many possibilities for this, beginning with the fundamental structural characteristics of the medium, such as hybridity, interlinearity, and the central function of body representations, and ending with the diversity of aesthetic approaches. Moreover, as a narrative medium, comics allow for a comprehensive contextualization; thus, the different topics can be told as non-fiction comics to convey knowledge and science or as individually experienced—be it (auto)biographical or not, thereby embedded in socio-political contexts.

A paradigmatic example for these possibilities of contextualization is Maki Shimizu's *Über Leben* (2021), in which various themes relevant to graphic medicine, such as aging, depression, traumatization (e.g., due to sexualized violence), chronic illness, cancer, death, and a confrontation between conventional medicine and alternative methods of healing, are episodically woven into the experience of, and living in, Berlin and linked with other topics, such as anti-Semitism, gentrification, and racism. Of particular interest is that Shimizu does not deal with these themes in terms of bodies that can be identified as human, but in terms of animalistic bodies, especially the tomcat Adagio and Maki Maus. By doing so, Shimizu also emphasizes the artificial-symbolic dimension of comic bodies, thus identifying them as discursive areas and, simultaneously—in the sense of critical posthumanism—also withdraws the focus on human bodies.

Bodies, as has been made clear by the various examples, are not only of particular structural relevance to the medium of comics, but also to the genre of graphic medicine. They oscillate between their use as a means of identification for pedagogical-didactic teaching and an abstracting, deconstructive, and thus meta-reflexive approach. They are pictorial elements through which emotions, suffering, and pain are realized aesthetically in different ways and are thereby externalized. Depending on the focalization, external or internal perspectives on these bodies are depicted; the more an internal perspective is functionalized, the more the theme of body perception comes to the fore. This is particularly evident, for example, in the topic of eating disorders. Finally, bodies are embedded in the plot differently depending on whether they are used to create a coherent "narrative arc" (Couser) or narrate more episodically.

In any case, comics from the field of graphic medicine—precisely in the overview of such different (aesthetic) concepts—offer new approaches to the understanding of illness, health, and related topics, and thereby also contribute significantly to the formation of visual literacy insofar as they provide a variety of offerings, taking up and criticizing culturally and medically shaped visual discourses.

NOTES

1. The underscore in *dis_ability* (e.g., Köbsell 2016) refers to in-between spaces and—following the established meaning in Gender Studies—to a subversion of binary constructs. Dan Goodley's notation *dis/ability* also emphasizes "the interplay between 'normality' and 'disability'" (Waldschmidt 2017, 26; Goodley 2014) and between connection and separation.
2. The didactic-educational approach is evident—as far as the German-speaking world is concerned—in an exhibition project by the Medical University of Vienna/Vienna General Hospital, which has been

running since 2019 (e.g., Masel and Praschinger 2020; Masel et al. 2020; Rauchenbacher 2020). In addition to the 2020/21 exhibition, Renate Mowlam created a comic dedicated to the question why comics are so applicable in the medical-didactic field (Mowlam 2020).

3. See also: https://www.graphicmedicine.org/.
4. In the German-speaking realm, the Berlin research project *Pathographics* (Krüger-Fürhoff et al. 2017; Krüger-Fürhoff 2019a; Squier and Krüger-Fürhoff 2020) was pioneering in this field of research. See also: https://www.geisteswissenschaften.fu-berlin.de/friedrichschlegel/assoziierte_projekte/Pathographics/index.html.
5. Due to the editorial process of this volume, only comics published until approximately mid-2022 have been included.
6. Unless, of course, comics are abstract-experimental, in which case the omission of the body requires considerable effort.
7. For further elaborations on the aspect of "difference," see Frahm (2010) (following Gilles Deleuze) and Rauchenbacher (2022b).
8. "Blad" is a pejorative Austrian colloquial term for "fat."
9. Rodes and Cacciapaglia, who are not native speakers of German, worked in cooperation with translators and proofreaders.

WORKS CITED

Barczyk, Sarah. 2016. *Nenn mich Kai*. Köln: Egmont.

Bas Backer, Joris. 2020. *Küsse für Jet: Eine Coming-of-Gender Geschichte*. Berlin: Jaja Verlag.

Bauer, Jutta. 2021. *Corona Diaries*. Hamburg: Kibitz Verlag.

Baumann, Simone F. 2021. *Zwang*. Zürich: Edition Moderne.

Beeler, Pirmin. 2018. *Hat man erst einmal angefangen zu reden, kann alles Mögliche dabei herauskommen*. Zürich: Edition Moderne.

Bernhard, Julia. 2019. *Wie gut, dass wir darüber geredet haben*. Berlin: avant-verlag.

Bertonasco, Larissa. 2018. *Burnout*. [Self-published].

Brenneisen, Tina. 2019. *Das Licht, das Schatten leert*. Zürich: Edition Moderne.

Buder, Raphaela. 2017. *Die Wurzeln der Lena Siebert*. Hamburg: Edition Mairisch.

Burkart, Roland. 2017. *Wirbelsturm*. Zürich: Edition Moderne.

Butschkow, Peter. 2018. *Was geht'n im Alter so ab, Alter? Cartoons & Texte*. Oldenburg: Lappan Verlag.

Cacciapaglia, Federico. 2022. *Impfland*. Translated and proofread by Oskar Köhn, Annette Köhn, and Alexandra Weyrich. Berlin: Jaja Verlag.

Chute, Hillary. 2010. *Graphic Women: Life Narrative and Contemporary Comics*. New York: Columbia University Press.

Couser, Thomas G. 2009. *Signifying Bodies: Disability in Contemporary Life Writing*. Ann Arbor: University of Michigan Press.

Couser, Thomas G. 2016. "Body Language: Illness, Disability, and Life Writing." *Life Writing* 13, no. 1: 3–10. doi: 10.1080/14484528.2016.1132376

Czerwiec, MK, Ian Williams, Susan Merrill Squier, Michael J. Green, Kimberly R. Myers, and Scott T. Smith. 2015. *Graphic Medicine Manifesto*. University Park, Pennsylvania: The Pennsylvania State University Press.

DeFalco, Amelia. 2016. "Graphic Somatography: Life Writing, Comics, and the Ethics of Care." *Journal of Medical Humanities* 37: 223–240. doi: 10.1007/s10912-015-9360-6.

Dinkel, Sabine. 2018. *Meine Arschbombe in die Untiefen des Lebens: Comic-Tagebuch einer Krebserkrankung*. Raubling: Hawewe Media.

Domingo, Sheree. 2019. *Ferngespräch*. Zürich: Edition Moderne.

Donovan, Courtney. 2014. "Representations of Health, Embodiment, and Experience in Graphic Memoir." *Configurations* 22: 237–253. doi:https://doi.org/10.1353/con.2014.0013.

El Refaie, Elisabeth. 2012. *Autobiographical Comics: Life Writing in Pictures*. Jackson: University Press of Mississippi. doi:https://doi.org/10.14325/mississippi/9781617036132.001.0001.

Endres, Brigitte and Ingrid Sabisch. 2019. *Ich, mein Schatten und das volle Leben: Ein Buch über Multiple Sklerose*. Leverkusen: Bayer Vital GmbH.

Eshrat, Hamed. 2022. *Coming of H*. Berlin: avant-verlag.

Färber, Markus and Christine Färber. 2021. *Fürchtetal*. Kassel: Rotopol.

Faroqhi, Anna. 2017. *Krebs Kung Fu: Eine Geschichte vom Kampf gegen den Krebs*. Berlin: be.bra verlag.

Flix. 2012. *Don Quijote*. Hamburg: Carlsen.

Frahm, Ole. 2010. *Die Sprache des Comics*. Hamburg: Philo Fine Arts.

Fürst, Ursula. 1990. *Die Ballade von der Typhoid Mary: Nach einem Roman von Jürg Federspiel*. Zürich: Edition Moderne.

Gerland, Melanie. 2010. *Offene Arme*. Bonn: BALANCE buch + medien verlag.

Gloor, Reto. 2015. *Das Karma-Problem: MS – Eine unheilbare Krankheit übernimmt die Kontrolle*. Zürich: Edition Moderne.

Goodley, Dan. 2014. *Dis/ability Studies: Theorising Disablism and Ableism*. London/New York: Routledge.

Green, Michael J. 2015. "Graphic Storytelling and Medical Narrative: The Use of Comics in Medical Education." In *Graphic Medicine Manifesto*, edited by MK Czerwiec, Ian Williams, Susan Merrill Squier, Michael J. Green, Kimberly R. Myers, and Scott T. Smith, 67–86. University Park: The Pennsylvania State University Press.

Green, Michael J. and Kimberly R. Myers. 2010. "Graphic Medicine: Use of Comics in Medical Education and Patient Care." *British Medical Journal* 340: 1–8. doi: 10.1136/bmj.c863.

Greve, Katharina. 2011. *Patchwork: Frau Doktor Waldbeck näht sich eine Familie*. Gütersloh: Gütersloher Verlagshaus.

Grünewald, Dietrich. 2022. "'Jeder wehrt sich gegen die Zeit': Zum Thema Alter im Comic." In *Alter(n) in der Populärkultur*, edited by Henriette Herwig and Mara Stuhlfauth-Trabert, 195–215. Bielefeld: transcript.

Haller, Stefan. 2021. *Schattenmutter*. Zürich: Edition Moderne.

Hawkins, Anne Hunsaker. 1999. *Reconstructing Illness: Studies in Pathography*. 2nd ed. West Lafayette: Purdue University Press.

Heidi. Die schönsten Geschichten nach dem berühmten Roman. 1976–7. 21 Issues. Köln: Bastei.

Heidi. 179 Hefte. *Mit neuen Geschichten zur Fernseh-Serie* (1–168); *Ganz neue Geschichten zur Fernseh-Serie* (169–179). 1977–81. Köln: Bastei.

Heidi. Die schönsten Geschichten nach dem berühmten Roman. 1987–8. 28 Issues. Köln: Bastei.

Heger, Illi Anna. 2016. "Minicomic 05: Laborlüftung." https://www.annaheger.de/minicomic05.

Hochreiter, Susanne. 2014. "Heldinnen und keine: Zu Genre und Affekt in Ulli Lusts *Heute ist der letzte Tag vom Rest deines Lebens*." In *Bild ist Text ist Bild: Narration und Ästhetik in der Graphic Novel*, edited by Susanne Hochreiter and Ursula Klingenböck, 233–256. Bielefeld: transcript.

Hochreiter, Susanne, Marina Rauchenbacher, and Katharina Serles. 2022. "Queer Visualities – Queer Spaces: German-Language LGBTQ+ Comics." In *The LGBTQ+ Comics Studies Reader: Critical Openings, Future Directions*, edited by Alison Halsall and Jonathan Warren, 114–133. Jackson: University Press of Mississippi.

Hofer, Regina. 2018. *Blad*. Wien: Luftschacht. (i.e. Borretsch. 2008. *Blad*. Part 1 and 2. Accessed July 13, 2022. https://www.electrocomics.com; engl.: 2021. *Fat*. Translated by Natascha Hoffmeyer. University Park: The Pennsylvania State University Press/Graphic Mundi.)

Hommer, Sascha. 2009. *Vier Augen*. Berlin: Reprodukt.

Huber, Dorothea. 2022. *Aus Mutters Mund*. Berlin: Jaja Verlag.

Interactive Media Foundation. 2017. *Ninette: Dünn ist nicht dünn genug. Ein interaktives Comic in 11 Folgen*. Accessed July 12, 2022. https://ninette.berlin.

Jongeling, Peer. 2020. *"Hattest du eigentlich schon die Operation?"* Berlin: Jaja Verlag.

Jüliger, Lukas. 2013. *Vakuum*. Berlin: Reprodukt.

Kilic, Ilse and Fritz Widhalm. 2005. *Ein kleiner Schnitt: Unser Krebsjahr*. Wien: Das Fröhliche Wohnzimmer.

Kilic, Ilse and Fritz Widhalm. 2012. *Kann ich solange zeichnen, bis alle Ängste verfliegen? Auf Nimmerwiedersehen, Krebs!* Wien: Das Fröhliche Wohnzimmer.

Klar, Elisabeth. 2011. "Wir sind alle Superhelden! Über die Eigenart des Körpers im Comic – und über die Lust an ihm." In *Theorien des Comics: Ein Reader*, edited by Barbara Eder, Elisabeth Klar, and Ramón Reichert, 219–236. Bielefeld: transcript.

Klar, Elisabeth. 2014. "Transformation und Überschreibung: Sprache und Text in ihrer Beziehung zum Körper-Zeichen in den Comics von Alfred." In *Bild ist Text ist Bild: Narration und Ästhetik in der Graphic Novel*, edited by Susanne Hochreiter and Ursula Klingenböck, 169–189. Bielefeld: transcript.

Klingenböck, Ursula. 2022. "'Ich bleibe hier': Alter(n)sdarstellung und -konzepte in Thomas von Steinaeckers und Barbara Yelins Comic *Der Sommer ihres Lebens*." In *Alter(n) in der Populärkultur*, edited by Henriette Herwig and Mara Stuhlfauth-Trabert, 217–233. Bielefeld: transcript.

Köbsell, Swantje. 2016. "Doing Dis_ability: Wie Menschen mit Beeinträchtigungen zu 'Behinderten' werden." In *Managing Diversity: Die diversitätsbewusste Ausrichtung des Bildungs- und Kulturwesens, der Wirtschaft und Verwaltung*, edited by Karim Fereidooni and Antonietta P. Zeoli, 89–103. Wiesbaden: Springer.

König, Ralf. 2017. *Herbst in der Hose*. Reinbek bei Hamburg: Rowohlt.

König, Ralf. 2021. *Vervirte Zeiten*. Reinbek bei Hamburg: Rowohlt.

Krämer, Karin. 2016. *SIE*. Berlin: Reprodukt.

Kreisl, Jana. 2015. *Ton und Scherben*. Berlin: Jaja Verlag.

Krüger-Fürhoff, Irmela-Marei. 2024. "Alter, Demenz, Körperlichkeit: Gender und Sorgearbeit im Comic." In *Comics Studies x Gender Studies: Schnittmengen von Forschung, Lehre und Praxis – Intersections of Research, Teaching, and Practice*, edited by Naomi Lobnig, Marina Rauchenbacher, and Katharina Serles. Berlin, Boston: de Gruyter [in progress].

Krüger-Fürhoff, Irmela-Marei. 2021. "Entfaltungen: Alternde Körper in Comics." *Closure: Kieler e-Journal für Comicforschung* 7, no. 5. http://www.closure.uni-kiel.de/closure7.5/krueger-fuerhoff. Accessed July 5, 2022.

Krüger-Fürhoff, Irmela-Marei. 2020. "Illness narratives in Comics: Using Graphic Medicine in the Medical Humanities." *Wiener Medizinische Wochenschrift* 132: 44–47.

Krüger-Fürhoff, Irmela-Marei. 2019a. "Narrating the Lived Reality of Illness in Comics and Literature: Research by the PathoGraphics Team at Freie Universität Berlin." *DIEGESIS: Interdisciplinary E-Journal for Narrative Research/Interdisziplinäres E-Journal für Erzählforschung* 8, no. 1: 109–120.

Krüger-Fürhoff, Irmela-Marei. 2019b. "Zitat, Schnitt, Naht: Ästhetische Strategien der Transplantation in David Wagners Roman *Leben* und Katharina Greves Comic *Patchwork: Frau Doktor Waldbeck näht sich eine Familie*." In *Kulturwissenschaftliche Konzepte der Transplantation*, edited by Ottmar Ette and Uwe Wirth, 147–165. Berlin, Boston: de Gruyter.

Krüger-Fürhoff, Irmela-Marei, Uta Kornmeier, stef lenk, Nina Schmidt, and Susan Merrill Squier. 2017. *Sick! Kranksein im Comic – Reclaiming Illness Through Comics*. [Exhibition Catalogue]. Berlin.

Krüger-Fürhoff, Irmela-Marei, and Nina Schmidt. 2021. "Konstruktion und Subversion von Körperbildern im Comic: Über diese Ausgabe." *Closure. Kieler e-Journal für Comicforschung* 7, no. 5. http://www.closure.uni-kiel.de/closure7.5. Accessed July 1, 2022.

Krüger-Fürhoff, Irmela-Marei, Nina Schmidt, and Sue Vice, eds. 2022. *The Politics of Dementia: Forgetting and Remembering the Violent Past in Literature, Film and Graphic Narratives*. Berlin, Boston: de Gruyter (Media and Cultural Memory).

Kühn, Antonia. 2018. *Lichtung*. Berlin: Reprodukt.

Leder, Drew. 1990. *The Absent Body*. Chicago and London: The University of Chicago Press.

Lewinsky, Charles and Andreas Gefe. 2011. *Zwei Mal Zwei*. Zürich: Edition Moderne.

Lexe, Heidi. 2015. "Coming of Age vor dem Hintergrund der Apokalypse: Zu Lukas Jüligers Graphic Novel *Vakuum*." *kjl&m* 15, no. 3: 27–35.

Lobnig, Naomi. 2021. *Alternative Krankheitsnarrative in den Comics "Vergiss dich nicht" (2018) von Lika Nüssli und "Aliceheimer's: Alheimer's Through the Looking Glass" (2016) von Dana Walrath*. Masterarbeit. Wien 2021. https://utheses.univie.ac.at/detail/61875

Lötzerich, Suskas. 2014. *Hexenblut*. Wien: Luftschacht.

Lupton, Deborah. 1997. *The Imperative of Health: Public Health and the Regulated Body*. London, Thousand Oaks, and New Delhi: SAGE Publications.

Lust, Ulli. 2009. *Heute ist der letzte Tag vom Rest deines Lebens*. Berlin: avant-verlag (engl.: 2013. *Today Is the Last Day of the Rest of Your Life*. Translated by Kim Thompson. Seattle: Fantagraphics.)

Lust, Ulli and Marcel Beyer. 2013. *Flughunde*. Berlin: Suhrkamp (engl. 2017. *Voices in the Dark*. Translated by John Brownjohn. Translation adapted by Nika Knight. English Lettering by Kevin Cannon. New York: New York Review Comics.)

L'Arronge, Lilli. 2021. *Das geheime Tagebuch eines miesen Virus*. Berlin: Jacoby & Stuart.

Marijpol. 2013. *Eremit*. Berlin: avant-verlag.

Mark, Josephine. 2022. *Trip mit Tropf*. Hamburg: Kibitz Verlag.

Masel, Eva Katharina, Andrea Praschinger, Marina Rauchenbacher, and Ruth Kutalek. 2020. *Art Action Attitude: Körper – Body*. [Booklet accompanying the exhibition at the Allgemeines Krankenhaus Vienna 2020/2021]. Medizinische Universität Wien.

Masel, Eva Katharina and Andrea Praschinger. 2020. "Using Comics to Teach Medical Humanities." *Wiener Medizinische Wochenschrift* 132: 47–50.

Mawil. 2007. "Schtttotttern." [2006]. In *Action Sorgenkind*. Berlin: Reprodukt.

Mowlam, Renate. 2021. *Global Health*. Concept: Renate Mowlam and Ruth Kutalek. Wien: Medizinische Universität Wien.

Mowlam, Renate. 2019. *Off the Blob: Gespräche mit Frauen über den Wechsel – Ein Comic*. [Self-published].

Mowlam, Renate. 2022. *Was ist ein Schlaganfall und wie wird er behandelt?* Wien: Klinik Favoriten.

Mowlam, Renate. 2020. *What Is a Comic?* Concept: Renate Mowlam and Marina Rauchenbacher. Wien: Medizinische Universität Wien.

Mowlam, Renate. 2020/2021. "Wir bleiben zuhause – Corona-Comics." Accessed July 1, 2022. https://www.renatentwurf.at/?page_id=657.

Müller, Eva. 2017. *Sterben ist echt das Letzte!* Weimar: Schwarzer Turm.

Nüssli, Lika. 2018. *Vergiss dich nicht*. Berlin: Vexer Verlag.

Die Original-Heidi nach Johanna Spyri. 1978–81. 4 Vol. Frankfurt am Main: Condor.

Rauchenbacher, Marina. 2020. "Comics – Graphic Medicine – Comics." In *Art Action Attitude: Körper – Body*. [Booklet accompanying the exhibition at the Allgemeines Krankenhaus Vienna

2020/1], edited by Eva Katharina Masel, Andrea Praschinger, Marina Rauchenbacher, and Ruth Kutalek, 12–13. Medizinische Universität Wien.
Rauchenbacher, Marina. 2022b. "Comics – posthuman, queer-end, um_un-ordnend." *Genealogy+Critique* 8, no. 1: 1–27.
Rauchenbacher, Marina. 2023. "Das 'Wunder an unserem Kinde': Körper, Dis_ability, Krankheit in Heidi-Comics – am Beispiel Klara." In *(Re)Reading Heidi*, edited by Linda Leskau and Sigrid Nieberle, 311–326. Bielefeld: transcript.
Rauchenbacher, Marina. 2024. "Psyche zeigen: Comics über Essstörungen." In *Comics Studies x Gender Studies: Schnittmengen von Forschung, Lehre und Praxis – Intersections of Research, Teaching, and Practice*, edited by Marina Rauchenbacher, Katharina Serles, and Naomi Lobnig. Berlin, Boston: de Gruyter [in progress].
Rauchenbacher, Marina. 2022a. "] [: Verstummen und Stille in Ulli Lusts Comic-Adaption von Marcel Beyers Roman *Flughunde*." In *Jahrbuch Musik und Gender: Laute(r) Bilder: Musik in Manga, Comic & Co.*, edited by Melanie Unseld and Akiko Yamada [in press].
Rauchenbacher, Marina and Katharina Serles. 2020. "Fragmented and Framed: Precarious 'Body Signs' in Comics by Regina Hofer, Ulli Lust, Barbara Yelin and Peer Meter." In *Spaces Between: Gender, Diversity, and Identity in Comics*, edited by Nina Eckhoff-Heindl and Véronique Sina. 79–93. Wiesbaden: Springer. doi:https://doi.org/10.1007/978-3-658-30116-3_6.
Richthofen, Greta von. 2021. *Das Gute am Ende des Tages*. Berlin: Jaja Verlag.
Rickenbach, Kati. ["COVID-19 cartoons"]. Accessed July 1, 2022. https://www.instagram.com/katirickenbach.
Rickenbach, Kati. 2007. *Filmriss*. Zürich: Edition Moderne.
Rodes, Josep. 2021. *Corona Go Home: Tagebuch aus Varanasi*. Translated by Elena Botica. Berlin: Jaja Verlag.
Ross, Mikael. 2018. *Der Umfall*. Berlin: avant-verlag.
Sabisch, Ingrid. 2005. *Schwangerschaftsstreifen: Abenteuer Schwangerschaft – ein Erlebnisbericht*. Heroldsberg: Die Heldin.
Sabisch, Ingrid. 2011. *41,3 kg – Magersucht?* Gütersloh: Gütersloher Verlagshaus.
Schmidt, Nina. 2020. "Beyond the Personal: The Systemic Critique of German Graphic Medicine." *Seminar: A Journal of Germanic Studies* 56, no. 3–4: 368–388.
Schreiter, Daniela. 2017. *Die Abenteuer von Autistic Hero-Girl*. Stuttgart: Panini Comics.
Schreiter, Daniela. 2014. *Schattenspringer*: Vol. 1: *Wie es ist, anders zu sein*. Stuttgart: Panini Comics.
Schreiter, Daniela. 2015. *Schattenspringer*: Vol. 2: *Per Anhalter durch die Pubertät*. Stuttgart: Panini Comics.
Schreiter, Daniela. 2018. *Schattenspringer*: Vol. 3: *Spektralfarben*. Stuttgart: Panini Comics.
Shimizu, Maki. 2021. *Über Leben*. Berlin: Jaja Verlag.
Schreiter, Daniela and Friedrich W. Zimmermann. 2018. *Liebe Lust Prostata*: *Der Comic*. Norderstedt: BoD.
Sina, Véronique. 2016. *Comic – Film – Gender: Zur (Re-)Medialisierung von Geschlecht im Comicfilm*. Bielefeld: transcript.
Sommer, Anna. 2018. *Das Unbekannte*. Zürich: Edition Moderne.
Squier, Susan Merrill and Irmela Marei Krüger-Fürhoff. 2020. *PathoGraphics: Narrative, Aesthetics, Contention, Community*. University Park: The Pennsylvania State University Press.
Steinaecker, Thomas von and Barbara Yelin. 2017. *Der Sommer ihres Lebens*. Berlin: Reprodukt (2015/16. *Der Sommer ihres Lebens*. https://www.fischerverlage.de/magazin/extras/der-sommer-ihres-lebens).
Steiner, Elke Renate. 2010. *Risiken und Nebenwirkungen*. Gütersloh: Gütersloher Verlagshaus.
Strapazin 2015, no. 121: *Alter*.
Szép, Eszter. 2020. *Comics and The Body: Drawing, Reading, and Vulnerability*. Columbus: The Ohio State University Press. doi: 10.26818/9780814214541.

Waldschmidt, Anne. 2017. "Disability Goes Cultural: The Cultural Model of Disability as an Analytical Tool." In *Culture – Theory – Disability: Encounters between Disability Studies and Cultural Studies*, edited by Anne Waldschmidt, Hanjo Berressem, and Moritz Ingwersen, 19–27. Bielefeld: transcript.

Wegner, Gesine. 2020. "Reflections on the Boom of Graphic Pathography: The Effects and Affects of Narrating Disability and Illness in Comics." *Journal of Literary & Cultural Disability Studies* 14, no 1: 57–74.

Weißenböck, Verena. 2007. *Eine Geschichte vom Kinderkriegen*. [Self-published].

Wicki, Anja. 2022. *In Ordnung*. Zürich: Edition Moderne.

Williams, Ian. 2015. "Graphic Pathography in the Classroom and the Clinic: A Case Study." In *Graphic Medicine Manifesto*, edited by MK Czerwiec, Ian Williams, Susan Merrill Squier, Michael J. Green, Kimberly R. Myers, and Scott T. Smith, 87–114. University Park: The Pennsylvania State University Press.

Winkelmann, Jutta. 2016. *Mein Leben ohne mich: Ein Bericht*. Frankfurt am Main: Weissbooks.

Winter, Florian. 2020. *XES*. Berlin: avant-verlag.

Wolsch, Jürgen. 2007. *Drogen: Ein Wissenscomics*. Frankfurt am Main: Eichborn.

Wunder, Eric. 2019. *Rauschgift*. Berlin: Edition Error.

Zejn, Julia. 2021. *Andere Umstände*. Berlin: avant-verlag.

CHAPTER SIX

Disability and Embodiment in Contemporary German Comics

KATJA HERGES

Scholarship at the intersection of literature and disability studies has critiqued the medicalized model of disability and argues for a politicized approach that emphasizes the sociocultural aspects of embodiment and disability, taking assumptions about class, gender, race, age, health, and beauty into account. However, in addition to literature, embodiment, illness, and disability are also key themes of many works of comics. According to Hillary Chute (2010), in the US, formative works in the field of comics were generated out of experiences with illness and disability; for instance, the first autobiographical work in comics was Justin Green's pathbreaking book *Binky Brown Meets the Holy Virgin Mary* (1972) about a young man with debilitating obsessive-compulsive disorder. In the introduction to *Disability in Comic Books and Graphic Narratives* (2016), Chris Foss, Jonathan Gray and Zach Whalen argue that it is therefore "crucial to begin to apply disability studies approaches to a wide variety of comic forms and then to theorize multiple potential paradigms for how we can initiate a generative critical articulation of disability and sequential art" (1–2). To exclude graphic narratives from the realm of disability studies is to neglect a substantial resource from which insights can be gained. This chapter takes up this call and analyzes the representation of dis/abled bodies in contemporary (autobiographical) German-language comics from a disability studies perspective, arguing that the comics represent both cognitive and physical disabilities in mostly affirmative ways and contribute to diversify and individualize cultural narratives and medial imagery of being dis/abled. In doing so, the comics not only reflect existing imagery about disability, but also produce new models for representations of dis/abled bodies.

Comics scholarship has highlighted the possibilities of the medium in representing dis/abled embodiments. In contrast to written texts, autobiographical comics use a range of aesthetic and visual strategies to highlight the corporeality of the protagonists and of the body as location of disability. In the *Graphic Medicine Manifesto* (2015) Susan Squier argues that the visual medium of comics directs our attention to the body and its movements, postures and gestures; it can "incorporate the representations of medical treatment or the experiences of disability without framing the narrative or protagonist entirely within that category" (49). Irmela Krüger-Führhoff and Nina Schmidt (2021) argue that comics can address both the lack of visibility of dis/abled embodiments in cultural representations and the hypervisibility of dis/abled bodies in public spaces. Comics, Krüger-Führhoff and Schmidt contend, can become "a space for the narration of dis/abled lives," and reach for a large audience beyond the dis/abled community, thereby intervening in these representational politics of disability (20). By creating tensions between images and texts, they can challenge preconceived ideas about dis/abled bodies.

This chapter builds on comics and disability scholarship to examine how the comic protagonists are marked as disabled through their bodily representations, how these constructions of disability intersect with other identity markers (such as sexuality and gender), and how performative and aesthetic strategies subvert normative imagery of dis/abled bodies. While the field of graphic medicine has focused on English language comics, recently, comics about embodiment, disability, and illness have also increased in popularity in Germany; however, they have received limited attention in scholarship. In the following, I will sketch how a variety of strategies in contemporary German comics construct and challenge images of the dis/abled body.

MOVING BODIES: VISUALIZATION OF DIS/CONTINUITIES

In the past decade, several German-language comics have been published that focus on autobiographical experiences of disability of movement, including two comics by Swiss artists, Reto Gloor's *Das Karma-Problem* (2015, the karma problem) and Roland Burkart's *Wirbelsturm* (2017, in English as *Twister*, 2021). Both narratives focus on the narrators' experiences of moving dis/abled bodies and the impact of disability on their lives, but they also draw attention to the continuities of movement and the creation of new (crip) temporalities.

Das Karma Problem describes Gloor's life from his diagnosis with multiple sclerosis in 2010 to the time of finishing the comic in 2014. The first image foregrounds the comic's tension between the disruption and continuity of bodily movements. The image, which is dated May 2013, shows the narrator standing in the pouring rain, reflecting on the gloomy stagnation and immobility of his life: "Alles in meinem Leben scheint zum Stillstand gekommen zu sein. Alles scheint fest, unbewegt, die Außenwelt ist in Stagnation, lange, lange Zeit." (Everything in my life seems to have come to a stand. Everything seems fixed, inert; the world is in stagnation, for a long, long time (Gloor 2015, 5).[1] However, in the next paragraph, he recognizes: "Doch ... Es gibt **etwas**, das nicht stehengeblieben ist." (But ... There is **something** that hasn't stopped, 5, emphasis in original.) This tension between immobility and the moving "etwas" is reflected in the image's contrasting white and turquoise background. The "etwas" in the initial panel could refer to the pouring rain in the image, but, also to the fact that his body and life are still moving. Indeed, despite his increasing difficulties of moving, the comic features many detailed image sequences in which Gloor moves in the city, in nature, on vacations or on the way to different healers, in public transportation and with assistive devices like a cane. In many of these moving images, the color-coding highlights and interrelates movement and technology: While Gloor uses mainly black, white, and shades of grey, all structures related to transportation including ticket counters, buses, trains, and planes are emphasized through the hopeful turquois color. Moreover, by referencing this exact same image in smaller size, the last image of the comic (before the epilogue) adds another layer of significance to the question of the moving "etwas." Dated a month earlier, the commentary explains how he decided to draw and write this story, after finding new ways to draw digitally, highlighting the continuity of moving and narrating.

The epilogue, dated to August 2014, takes up the comic's ambivalence of stagnation and movement and disrupts normative time of illness and recovery. In a one-page sequence of small panels, the narrator walks with a cane, falls, and continues walking with his cane beyond the panel border only to return two pages later, where he is shown walking, jumping, and happily throwing his cane in the air. Like a slow film sequence, this "moment-to-moment" panel series (Mc Cloud 1994, 70) highlights the disruption and continuity of movement by giving the reader a detailed sensuous and embodied understanding of falling and continuous walking. Most interestingly, the imaginary movements—the jump and the walking beyond the rigid panel structure—indicate how (moving) disabilities are not mere *loss* of movements. In transgressing the panel, the image challenges and transcends "restrictive categories of disability experience" and envisions a hopeful future which is often denied to people with disability (Kafer 2013, 2). (Squier 2016, 49).

The textual commentary adds to this gesture towards the future. While the narrator first laments his "failure" to document his "Heilung" (recovery) and to follow what Arthur Frank has described as "restitution narrative" (1995, 75), he also describes how he has shifted towards a subtly ironic acceptance of life as is and points jokingly at the future healing by love. In addition, the narrator points toward the future beyond the story time: "Ich habe meine Geschichte zu Ende erzählt. Die Geschichte ist zu Ende, doch mein Leben geht weiter." (I have finished narrating my story. My story has ended, but my life goes on, Gloor 2015, 91). By subverting the plot of the restitution narrative, the comic envisions new narrative possibilities and futurities for dis/abled lives. The epilogue also references another fall sequence, which further disrupts normative temporality of illness and narration (Gloor 2015, 42). In the earlier sequence, going back to February 2011, an animated "stroboscopic image" (with two bodies within one frame in different positions in the process of falling) (El Rafaie 2012, 118), highlights the embodied experience of falling. And the commentary expresses feelings of failure and depression after this fall (also indicated through repeated rain). Like in the epilogue, the following panels show him walking again in the rain. The images thus create "visual echoes" (El Rafaie 2012, 129) between repeated panels of walking, falling, and raining at different, non-chronological moments in time, creating associative connections across the story. Through repetitions, disruptions, and continuities of dis/abled movement, narration, and life, non-linear temporalities emerge in the comic—reminiscent of what disability theorists have defined as "crip time." (Samuels 1997, Kafer 2013) Ellen Samuels highlights the ambivalent and challenging aspects of disability and crip time, how it "requires to break in our bodies and minds to new rhythms, new patterns of thinking and feeling and moving through the world" (2017, para. 13). By developing non-linear, circular and imaginary forms of narration, *Das Karma-Problem* crips conventional illness narration and visualizes the multiple times and futures of dis/abled experiences.

Similar to Gloor's falling and walking sequences, Burkart's autofictional comic *Wirbelsturm* features sequences that juxtapose Piedro's current morning routine as a person with tetraplegia with his routine right before the disabling accident, highlighting continuities and disruptions. The sequence of his earlier morning routine shows how he wakes up, walks to the bathroom, washes his hands, brushes his teeth, shaves, makes coffee, smokes a cigarette on the balcony, and drives off (Burkart 2017, 7–13). While these actions are told and drawn over eight consecutive pages, the narrative of his current morning routine covers double the number of pages and is continuously disrupted through the fragmented memories of the accident. The longer duration reflects the additional time he needs to complete the same tasks with the support of an assistant. The home nurse wakes him up, empties his catheter, transfers him out of the bed into the wheelchair and gives him a suppository to induce a bowel movement. However, despite the comparatively lengthy and strenuous routine, the overlapping of both narratives, the similar tasks, and the textual statement "er ist eigentlich noch fast derselbe wie früher" (he is almost the same person as before, Burkart 2017, 5) foreground the continuities between his life prior to and after the accident. Schmidt and Krüger-Führhoff argue that the narrator's statement might "surprise some nondisabled readers, as they may expect a more drastic distinction between life and embodiment before and after the accident" (2021, 20). This tension between image and text and between the image series before and after the accident highlights the continuities and discontinuities of life with disabilities.

The continuity is further highlighted through different aesthetic strategies that detail and highlight all movements in the comic. Both morning routine sequences show "action-to-action images" (Cloud 1994, 70) that visualize his movements step by step; for instance, how he brushes his teeth with his functional hand or how he shaves himself before the accident. Each sequence features abstract close-up images of his body or body parts in black ink on a white background, which magnifies the moving body rather than any context. In addition to serialization and magnification, Burkart uses strategies of animation by drawing two or three short parallel, wave-shaped "motion lines" next to the edges of head, hands, finger, wrist, and shoulder, which imitates the kinesthetic experience of moving articulations (El Rafaie 2012, 118). Finally, the use of onomatopoeic language gives further insight into the subjective, sensory experience of embodied movements and memories: After the accident, the discharge of urine from the catheter makes "RaschelRaschel" (rustling, rustling, Burkart 2017, 4), his bowel movements "toc!toc!toc!" (33), and his wheelchair is introduced with "clapclap" (44) before we see it moving into the image. Similarly, Piedro's narrative of the morning before the accident is accompanied by loud background noise of the neighbor's lawn mower that is indicated by "RRRRRRRRMMMM," written in wavy lines and capitalized letters across several page that span the duration of his morning preparations, only to be followed by lyrics and musical notes he listens on the radio while driving to the swimming pool. Burkart's use of multimodal elements creates a sensory and embodied perspective of all dis/abled movements and subverts the common tragic juxtaposition of life narratives before and after disability.

These movement sequences with implied sounds, close-ups, and animations give insight in the continued mobility of the dis/abled experience and convey a subjective duration of diachronic time. In contrast, and affective the overlapping of the morning narratives at different moments in time opens a synchronic perception of time, an impossible at-onceness that is often used in comics to capture the unique qualities of traumatic memory, when the past intrudes the present "in the form of flashbacks, hallucinations and dreams" (El Rafaie 2012, 129). Indeed, the narrative of his current morning routine shifts into a flashback of the accident, a jump into the swimming pool, where he hits his head and loses consciousness. In addition, the narrative of the accident itself reinforces a synchronic experience of timelessness: it is represented through visual fragments of memory on the same page, of the springboard, of his upper body, and of his legs in an upside position that are "cut off" at the middle fold, only to be followed by rough strokes of black color that run off the edges of the next page and almost completely cover the following several pages. The bodily fragmentation and disappearance reflect not only the memory gaps of the experience but remove the pages from any specific time span and create the feeling of time passing. In contrast to traditional comics, where panels fracture both time and space, offering a "jagged staccato rhythm of unconnected moments," Mc Ćloud suggests that "borderless panels" can take on a "timeless quality" (1994, 67, 102):

> Because of its unresolved nature, such a panel might linger in a reader's mind and its presence might be felt in the panel which follows it. When such 'bleeds' are used—i.e. when a panel runs of the edges of the page, this effect is compounded. Time is no longer contained by the familiar icon of the closed panel, but instead hemorrhages and escapes into timeless space. Such images can set the mood or a sense of place for whole scenes through their lingering timeless presence.
>
> (103)

In these black borderless pages without diachronic "action," time seems to "hemorrhage" into a timeless or synchronic presence, reinforced by the depicted fluid element of water that "runs" off the page. The impression of free-floating time is reinforced by Burkart's style that does not separate text and image through thought and speech bubbles (based on his tetraplegia and his difficulties to draw straigtht lines with his technical hand after reconstructive surgery). Texts and images, like the body fragments, float in the space of the page in no particular order, creating simultaneity and dreaminess. The borderless, fragmented and fluid images of the accident open a timeless space that captures feelings of sadness, grief, anger, isolation, and hope and that set the mood throughout the narrative. In addition to fragmentation and disembodiment, Burkart uses fantastical animal metaphors to convey the experience of timeless floating. After the jump, Piedro's body is shown floating from the deep darkness of the ground to a white circular area at the surface of the swimming pool. In the following, his body transforms into an abstract wavy fish-like shape, a merman in a hospital bed that is surrounded not only by a swarm of many very small floating fish, but also by the captain of a submarine, in the shape of his physician, and his family as a group of singing seamen. The narrator comments how "eine unheimliche Ruhe breitete sich aus. Ich schwebte einsam durch die Meere." [An uncanny silence spread. I was floating lonely through the ocean, Burkart 2017, 31.] The oceanic and fish metaphor transgresses the borders between reality and dream, human and non-human and visualizes in a poetic way the inevitable gaps in the recollection of memory, the hallucinations during the coma and embodied feelings of silence, loneliness, and timelessness. Beyond Gloor's strategies of repetition and disruption, *Wirbelsturm* experiments with juxtaposition, fragmentation, sensory modalities, (metaphorical) embodiment, and borderless panels to highlight multiple sensory and affective experiences and continuous and synchronic (crip) temporalities across dis/abling trauma.

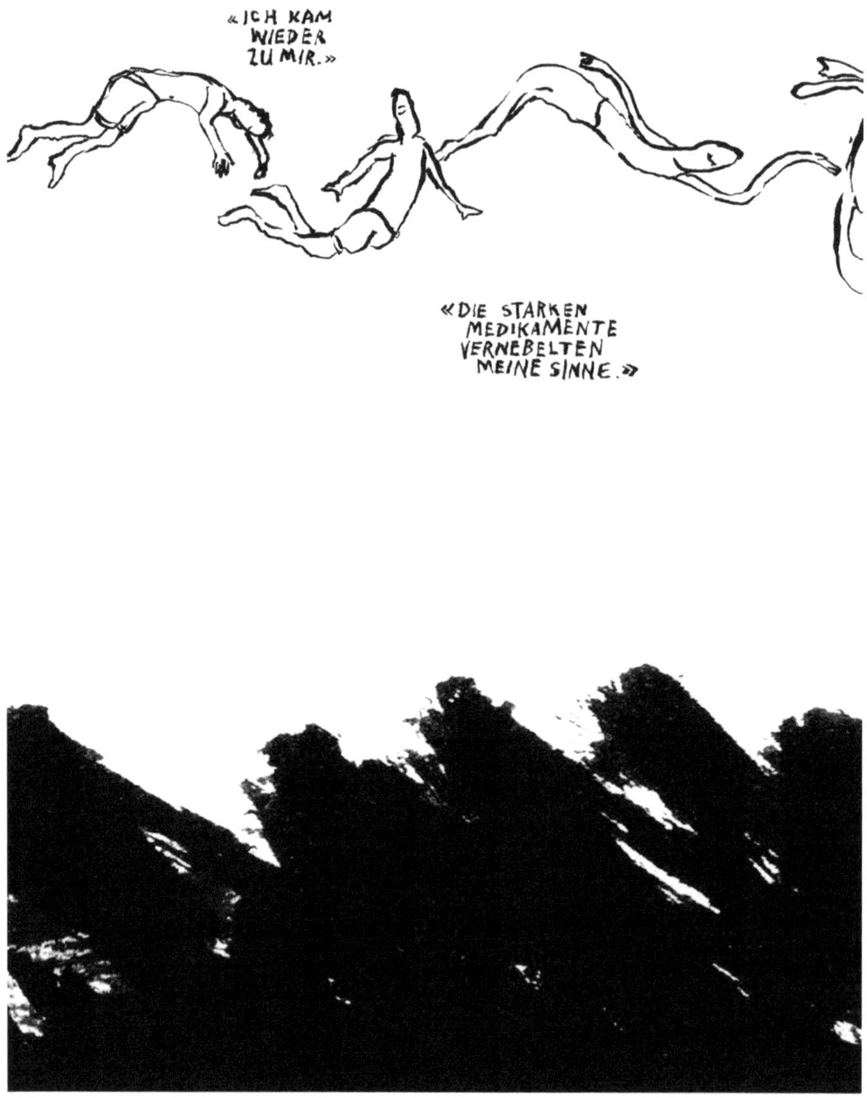
«ICH KAM WIEDER ZU MIR.»
«DIE STARKEN MEDIKAMENTE VERNEBELTEN MEINE SINNE.»

FIGURE 6.1: Roland Burkart, *Wirbelsturm* (2017). Copyright: Zurich: Edition Modern.

DESIRING BODIES: SEX, GENDER, AND DISABILITY

In addition to questions of mobility, German comics by dis/abled artists address issues of gender, sexuality, and dis/ability, often through humor. For instance, Phil Hubbe, who himself has multiple sclerosis, engages satirically with the experience of being dis/abled in cartoons and short comics for newspapers, journals, and the book series *Behinderte Comics* (Disabled Comics, 2004–21). One instance of the book series, Hubbe's *Das Leben des Rainer* (2009, Rainer's Life), deals with questions of access and language and stigmatization of people with disabilities (in particular, people in a wheelchair). In the book, one two-image cartoon addresses the intersections of disability, masculinity, and sexuality. While the first image shows a man standing in the ocean, counting the seconds that another person stays invisibly under water, the second image on the beach reveals the violent context of the situation: The man under water is now shown sitting in a wheelchair on the beach with his body and mouth covered with fish, algae, and sea fruit. A conversation between the first able-bodied man and his female partner on the beach further explains why he aggressively pushed the other man under water. Even though the woman indicates how the man in the wheelchair "only" smiled at her, the man's statement "Wer weiß, was er als nächstes getan hätte" (Who knows what he would have done next, Hubbe 2009)[2] indicates how he fears and suspects the disabled man to be sexually aggressive and threatening. Margrit Shildrick explains how in the West the intercorporeality of sexuality is perceived as a "possible threat to the integrity of the self," and even more so if the other already "breaches normative standards of embodiment" (2009, 84). As a result, representations of disabled sexuality "veer between the asexual and the hypersexual" (Shildrick 2009, 84). Through strategies of (violent) exaggeration, the cartoon critiques the widespread (able-bodied) perception of the disabled male body as sexually threatening and perverse. It also debunks imaginaries of hegemonic masculinity that provide the entitlement to aggressively "protect" women from the imagined threat. However, the exaggeration also risks reinforcing stigmatizing narratives of disability and gender. By juxtaposing the upright, strong, aggressive, and desirable male body in the center of the image with the body of the man in the wheelchair that is sitting alone, silenced, and visibly disabled at the corner of the image, the image reiterates representations of disabled people as helpless and undesirable victims. In addition, the woman is not only shown in a sexualized position on the beach, but she is also stripped of any agency that would allow her to act on her own behalf, limiting her to a sexual spectacle and a caricature of female fragility.

The short five-page comic "Schtttotttern" (Stuttering) in the comic book *Aktion Sorgenkind*[3] (2007, campaign for the problem child) by Berlin comic artist Marwil also uses hyperbolic humor in contrasting imaginaries of the disabled and able-bodied body. In contrast to Hubbe, Marwil addresses his own experience of speech disability and growing up. In a two-image panel about a date, the first image entitled "vorher: verkrampft" (before: tense, Marwil 2007, 27) shows a woman and the narrator in a bar, with his body bent, gesturing, sweating, and stuttering during their conversation. The image recalls Michail Bakthin's description of the distressful stuttering body as example of the "grotesque life of the body" that is degraded to the lower part of the body by struggling to give "birth to the word" (1984, 309–310).

In the second image "nachher: entspannt" (after: relaxed, 27), both are shown lying in bed and smoking, seemingly after having had sex. In contrast to the first image, his body is naked and relaxed, and he gives fluent speeches about Nietzschean philosophy, performing the role of the bohemian intellectual. By juxtaposing the grotesque leaking and degraded body with the classic ideal of the confident and intellectual and virile male body the panels construct the disabled body as emasculated, undesirable, and embarrassing. However, by drawing on the subversive aesthetics of grotesque exaggeration, the comic playfully subverts these stereotypes. El Rafaie argues that the popular medium of the comic with its inherent tendency toward the carnivalesque hyperbole "can provide a poetic means of conquering through humor the cosmic terror we all experience in the face of the limitless vulnerability of the self" (2012, 71). Through exaggeration, the panel ridicules the idealized character of the second panel and gives voice to the uncontrollable vulnerable body. By drawing the grotesque body as male, the images not only humorously undermine the female and maternal body as the icon of the abject and grotesque but also the traditional image of the male body as closed and abstract (Russo 2012, 1–3). The panel thus draws attention to how cultural stereotypes of the disabled body are "particularly difficult for men to contend with, as dominant definitions of masculinity are based on the ideal of a strong, autonomous body" (El Rafaie 2012, 91). In addition to the grotesque, Marwil uses an extradiegetic commentator and additional alter ego of the author to ambiguously point at the idealized character. Situated in miniature at the edges of the panel, the bunny narrator makes fun of the imaginary character of the able-bodied, voiced, and potent male body, which another disembodied speech bubble (seemingly the author himself) attempts to silence with "Ksch!" (Marwil 2007, 27). Through "multiple playful self-portraits," El Rafaie explains, comics offer a "way of constantly inventing and reinventing themselves" (2012, 71). In contrast to Hubbe's cartoon, Marwil's multiple levels of self-portraits and different versions of the self and the staged dialogues among them underscore a self-reflective and continuous process of constructing the dis/abled male self between abjection and idealization.

In contrast to Hubbe's and Marwil's cartoons that address how norms of masculinity intersect with the disability experience, Daniela Schreiter creates episodic cartoons and comics about her female experience of being autistic, in particular in her *Schattenspringer* triology (2014–2018, translated as The World Beyond My Shadow, 2020). In *Die Abenteuer von Autistic-Hero-Girl* (2020, the adventures of autistic hero girl), Schreiter draws on the genre of the superhero comic to narrativize autism from a female perspective and thereby undermines the traditional male and able-bodied dominance that Chute finds in the superhero comic genre (2010). Like Hubbe's one-page cartoons, Schreiter's comic features short humorous one-to-two-page cartoons. They stage dialogues between her alter ego avatar "Autistic hero girl" and a friendly and speaking fox figure named "Superfox" that engage with political questions of inclusion and cultural stereotypes about disability. While she draws on the simplified aesthetics of a traditional superhero comics with traditional panel structure and bright colors, in contrast to ableist superheroes, Autistic hero girl is often overwhelmed by the seemingly simple challenges of the ableist world, for instance, with small talk at parties, shopping, phone calls, and appointments. However, in contrast to Hubbe and Marwil, who foreground nostalgia about the lost able body, Schreiter affirms being an autistic woman that prefers intimacy beyond heteronormative relationships. El Rafaie explains how female comic artists increasingly challenge traditional gendered and sexualized norms of the body and represent their bodies on their own terms, often overturning the stereotypical notion of the (disabled) woman as powerless and asexual victim (2012, 80). For instance, the one-page cartoon "Lesetarier"[4] (reading monster) aligns intimate and embodied relations not with sexual encounters but with reading books. The images of her encounter with a book satirically imitate heteronormative dating practices; they show how she holds the book tight to her body, how she focuses single-mindedly on her body and her book, how she tends to sensuous details of smell and texture, and how she starts reading it precociously on the train. In addition to the dating rituals, the pink-colored thought bubbles adopt heterosexualized and gendered language and imaginary to ironically address the object of desire. For instance, she calls the book "mein Schatzzz [sic]," (my darling) or "meine Beute" (prey) and thinks about where to indulge in it: "Im Bett? Auf der Couch? In der Badewanne?" (In bed? On the couch? In the bathtub?, Schreiter 2020). Drawing humorously on normative practices of romance, the cartoon productively queers heteronormative intimacy and allows for representation of female agency and other forms of desire, for dis/abled women. Most interestingly, the last image shows her metamorphosis into a green dinosaur-shaped creature, a "Lesetarier," that is shown to devour the book. In experiences of illness or disability, Krista Quesenberry argues, "comics artists are compelled to self-represent in 'freaked and Othered bodies' that highlight particular aspects of their experiences not easily accessed by more normatively encoded bodies" (2017, 417). Thus, the animal metaphor not only highlights her desiring engagement with the book, but also marks visually her invisible disability as Otherness.

COGNITIVE DISABILITY, EMBODIED GAZE, AND TRAUMA IN INSTITUTIONAL COMMUNITIES

Like Schreiter's comic, Mikael Ross' comic *Der Umfall*[5] (2018) addresses cognitive disability. It tells the autofictional narrative of the main character Noel, a young man with an unknown cognitive disability, who is forced to move to an inclusive community after his mother had a stroke. Neuerkerode is a village near the German city of Braunschweig, where citizens with and without disabilities are living together. The comic's short conclusion, written by the director of the Protestant foundation Neuerkerode, Rüdiger Becker, explains that the book was commissioned by the Foundation for the celebration of its 150th birthday. Based on the extended time that Ross spent as guest in Neuerkerode, *Der Umfall* is inspired by people's lived experience in the community. Together with Schreiter's work on autism, the comic can be situated within the shift in disability scholarship from the focus on physical disability to what Benjamin Fraser calls a "second-wave disability studies" that is more centered around the (in)visibility of cognitive disability and constructions of able-mindedness in the theoretical, historical, and cultural realms (2018, 3). Acknowledging that not all people with disabilities can represent themselves according to norms of individuality, the comic underscores the "collaborative context" (Fraser 2018, 97) of cognitive disabilities as it emerged in response to the author's stay in the community and in collaboration with the artists Jean-Baptiste Coursaud and Claire Pay. Narrated from a dis/abled perspective but by an able-bodied author, the comic mainly features episodes that foreground the tolerant and reciprocally supportive community of care and the "normal" life within it. While this representation of Neuerkerode also fulfills the goal of the commissioned work to portray the community in a positive way, it also destigmatizes unusual behaviors and dis/abled bodies and expands the genre of the coming-of-age narrative against the background of institutional living. However, in contrast to works that include dis/abled co-authors, *Der Umfall* does not fully address the collaborative potential between the material practices of the arts and the experience of disability, thereby partially maintaining the tension of representation and being represented, looking at and being looked at throughout the work. Nevertheless, the comic foregrounds how the body and the gaze construct and challenge invisible cognitive disability and disability history.

The comic's prelude narrates the "Umfall" of Noel's mother and Noel's arrival in Neuerkerode, and construct him as disabled. A panel series visualizes how he finds his mother unresponsive on the bathroom floor, is frightened and doesn't know what to do, but finally calls the neighbor and the ambulance to get help. In these scenes, his body is visualized as disproportionate with short legs and a plump figure, and while he attempts to call the ambulance under visible duress, his body movements are drawn as ungraceful with excessive, grotesque gestures and facial expressions. His mouth is wide open, and his eyes are rendered big, thereby highlighting anger and frustration about his difficulties. By visualizing a groteque and excessive body, the comic embodies and visualizes cognitive disability and marks the protagonist as disabled. In addition to the body language, his language speaks to his cognitive disability. For instance, his thoughts in the commentary resemble spoken child-like language in short sentences, in the third person, or with spelling and grammar mistakes ("Und Blut ... Da is Auch Blut ... Blut Auf Dem Boden .... Gehört Da Nich Hin," And blood ... There is also blood ... blood on the ground ... does not belong there, Ross 2018, 9). Later, when he calls the ambulance, his speech is written in large letters with exclamation marks and wavy lines that highlight the high volume and his difficulty speaking. Finally, the scene is represented in slow speed with small transitions between the panels. For instance, after he finds his mother, he first walks in circles with a frightened face, then repeats "schlecht" (bad, Ross 2018, 9) to himself in next panel and even takes a plant out of a pot and throws the flowerpot over his head in order to be able to think. These visual and textual strategies allow the reader not only to get an understanding of a cognitively disabled perspective, but also to stare at what Elisabeth Garland-Thomson has called an "extraordinary body" (1997, 7) that shows "fascinating" behavior (2005, para. 3). Garland-Thomson relates the practice of staring back to the history of disabled people displayed in freak shows, which, by the mid-twentieth century, have been replaced by the medicalization and the sequestering in mental institutions and hospitals.

While the prelude partially reinforces cultural practices of looking at disabled bodies, at the same time, Ross uses strategies to challenge the othering. For instance, the comic draws on common conventions in superhero comics, similar to Marwin's use of the hyperbolic grotesque. The images in the prelude exaggerate emotions, body shapes, and movements for readability, entertainment, and suspense, which undermines the construed excessiveness and otherness of Noel's body and gesturing. In addition, a scene inverses the gaze of staring at the disabled body. In a two-panel image the viewer first looks at a close-up of Noel's invisible head hidden under a flowerpot with the background disappearing, which foregrounds his isolation, helplessness, and separation from the able-bodied world. In contrast, in the next image, the nightly background of the previous images reappears and situates him within the image world. Most importantly, the pot becomes transparent, and the reader faces Noel's direct gaze with large bright white eyes. This illuminated gaze not only illustrates his revelation that he might need to call the doctor, as indicated in the comment under the image, but it also allows a reciprocal gaze between the (supposedly) able-bodied reader and the disabled protagonist. The reader not only stares at the disabled body, but engages in what Eszter Szép has called the "reader's embodied participation with comics (2020, 3): The disabled body looks back at the reader, who is encouraged to change perspectives and to create interconnections across disability. The pot becomes a metaphor for the limiting aspects of cognitive disability, but at the same time it also politicizes the gaze and endows dis/abled bodies with agency.

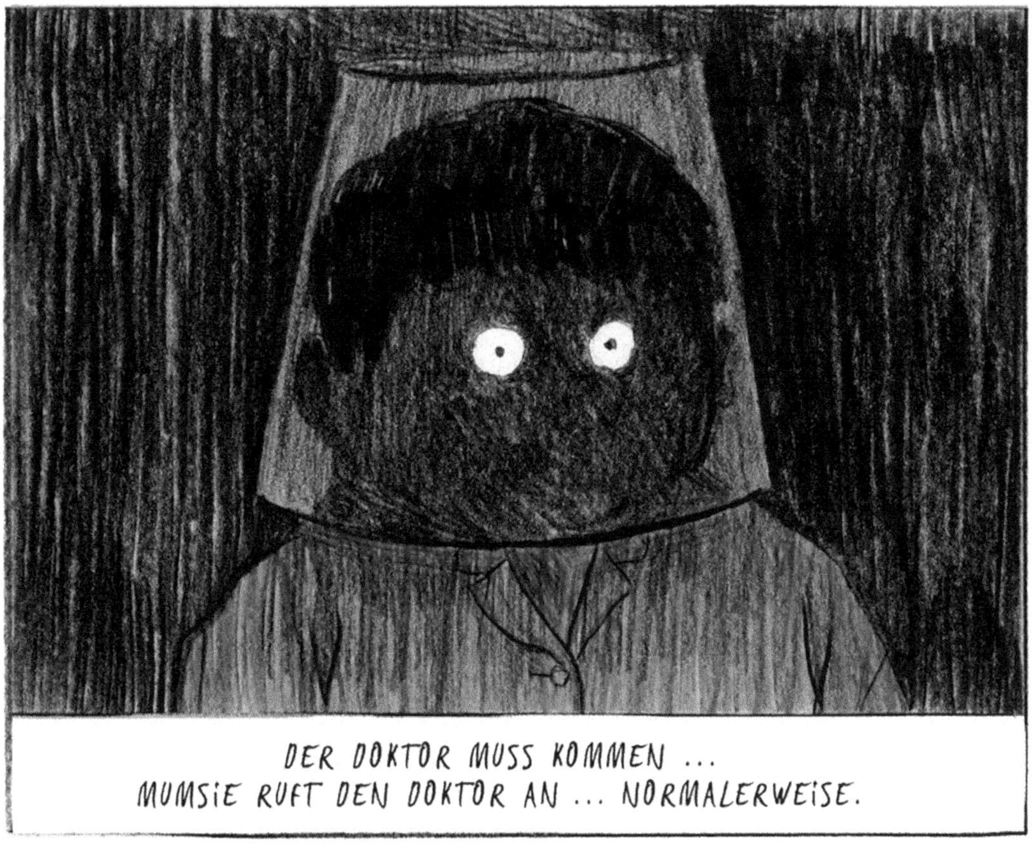
DER DOKTOR MUSS KOMMEN ...
MUMSIE RUFT DEN DOKTOR AN ... NORMALERWEISE.

FIGURE 6.2: Mikael Ross, *Der Umfall* (2018)—Flower Pot Episode. Copyright: Berlin: Avant.

Beyond Noel's dis/abled perspective, in one of the most interesting episodes in the second part of the comic, *Der Umfall* shifts perspective and gaze to make visible Neuerkerode's participation in institutional violence during National Socialism. In an interview, Ross explains how the episode is based on the testimony of an old woman in Neuerkerode that he spoke to during his stay (Hartung, para. 17). The image series starts with a nightly encounter between Noel and another older inhabitant of Neuerkerode, Irma, who randomly meet at the village's bus stop. Triggered by the fence next to the stop, Irma narrates her fragmented memories of her experiences in Neuerkerkode during National Socialism when a high fence separated girls and boys within the institution. Like a (cinematic) flashback, the images shift to Irma's perspective and into the past and the viewer first sees her as an older lady with a walker in front of the high wall and then as a young girl in the same position. The images stage repeated secret dialogues between Irma and her brother Erwin across the fence and in church, in which they wonder why children suddenly have to go "auf Reise" (on a trip, Ross 2018, 68) in winter in grey buses and fear that they are actually getting killed. In the final images of this episode, Irma narrates how she has survived by hiding in the forest, while she still grieves the death of Erwin who did not come back, seemingly still waiting at the bus stop during some nights. The fragmentary flashback scene reminds us how comics have the potential to represent trauma. Chute explains how "[i]mages in comics appear in fragments, just as they do in actual recollection; this fragmentation, in particular, is a prominent feature of traumatic memory" (2010, 4). By taking what Chute calls the "risk of representation" of trauma (2019, 5), the episode foregrounds the perspective of a disabled person and a victim of National Socialism in narratives of euthanasia, giving epistemic justice and narrative agency to the affected community, which has often been considered unreliable narrators. While Noel does not follow the historical details of Irma's narration, he affectively witnesses her grief and testimony. The scene highlights how witnessing is possible across divides of generations, dis/abilities, and perspectives and invites the reader to join. *Der Umfall* thus not only constructs and looks at dis/abled bodies but also allows dis/abled bodies to look back and gain agency in political and historical discourses of disability.

This brief discussion of contemporary German comics has shown how the works represent disabilities in mostly affirmative ways and individualize cultural and historical narratives and imagery of disability. The medium of the comic can make visible different forms of disability and thereby counters the historical invisibility of populations with disabilities. The comics not only reflect dis/abled embodiments in activities like gestures, expressions, and movements that are recognizable from the outside, but they also convey feelings and inner processes about what it means to live in a dis/abled body. By using a wide range of aesthetic strategies, including bodily metaphors, changes in gaze and perspectives, animation, fragmentation, grotesque, and exaggeration German language comics about disability rethink more inclusive models of representation and embodiment against the backdrop of the continued invisibility and stigmatization of dis/abled bodies in German-language public spheres.

NOTES

1. All translations are mine.
2. There are no page numbers.
3. "Aktion Sorgenkind" was the title of a German non-profit organization for disability and inclusion that is financed through lottery. The name has been changed to "Aktion Mensch" (campaign for humans) in 2000 based on the pejorative term "Sorgenkind" (problem child).
4. There are no page numbers.
5. The word "Umfall" is a neologism that is composed of "Unfall" (accident) and "Umfallen" (falling over).

WORKS CITED

Bakhtin, Mikhail. 1984. *Rabelais and His World*. Translated by Hélène Iswolsky. 1965. Bloomington: Indiana University Press.
Burkart, Roland. 2017. *Wirbelsturm*. Zurich: Edition Moderne.
Burkart, Roland. 2021. *Twister*. University Park: Graphic Mundi.
Chute, Hillary. 2010. *Graphic Women: Life Narrative and Contemporary Comics*. New York: Columbia University Press.
Chute, Hillary. 2019. *Disaster Drawn: Visual Witness, Comics, and Documentary Form*. Cambridge: Harvard University Press.
El Rafaie, Elisabeth. 2012. *Autobiographical Comics: Life Writing in Pictures*. Jackson: University Press of Mississippi, 2012.
Foss, Chris, Jonathan W. Gray, and Zach Whalen, eds. 2016. *Disability in Comic Books and Graphic Narratives*. London: Palgrave Macmillan.
Frank, Arthur. 1995. *The Wounded Storyteller: Body, Illness and Ethics*. Chicago: The University of Chicago Press.
Fraser, Benjamin. 2018. *Cognitive Disability Aesthetics: Visual Culture, Disability Representations, and the (In)Visibility of Cognitive Difference*. Toronto: University of Toronto Press.
Garland-Thomson, Rosemarie. 1997. *Extraordinary Bodes: Figuring Physical Disability in American Culture and Literature*. New York: Columbia University Press.
Garland-Thomson, Rosemarie. 2005. "Staring at the Other." *Disability Studies Quarterly* 25, no. 4: https://doi.org/10.18061/dsq.v25i4.610
Gloor, Reto. 2015. *Das Karma Problem*. Zurich: Edition Moderne.
Hartung, Andreas. 2018. "Comic 'Der Umfall:' 'Ich hasse Mensch ärgere Dich nicht.'" *Tagesspiegel*, https://www.tagesspiegel.de/kultur/comics/ich-hasse-mensch-argere-dich-nicht-4003279.htm
Hubbe, Phil. 2009. *Das Leben des Rainer: Behinderte Cartoons 3*. Oldenburg: Lappan.
Kafer, Alison. 2013. *Feminist, Queer, Crip*. Bloomington: Indiana University Press 2013.
Krüger-Fürhoff, Irmela Marei, and Nina Schmidt. 2021. "Constructions and Subversions of the Body in Comics– About This Issue." *Closure: Kieler e-Journal für Comicforschung* 7: 16–30.
Mawil. 2007. "Schtttottern." *Action Sorgenkind*, 25–30. Berlin: Reprodukt.
McCloud, Scott. 1994. *Understanding Comics: The Invisible Art*. Kitchen Sink Press.
Ross, Mikael. 2018. *Der Umfall*. Berlin: Avant.
Russo, Marie. 1995. *The Female Grotesque: Risk, Excess, and Modernity*. New York: Routledge.
Quesenberry, Krista. 2017. "Intersectional and Non-Human Self-Representation in Women's Autobiographical Comics." *Journal of Graphic Novels and Comics* 8, no. 5: 417–432.

Samuels, Ellen. 2017. “Six Ways of Looking at Crip Time.” *Disability Studies Quarterly* 37, no. 3: https://doi.org/10.18061/dsq.v37i3.5824
Schreiter, Daniela. 2020. *Die Abenteuer von Autistic Hero-Girl*. Stuttgart: Panini Books.
Schreiter, Daniela. 2014. *Schattenspringer 1: Wie es ist, anders zu sein*. Stuttgart: Panini Comics.
Shildrick, Margrit. 2009. *Dangerous Discourses of Disability, Subjectivity and Sexuality*. London: Palgrave Macmillan.
Squier, Susan Merrill. 2016. “The Uses of Graphic Medicine for Engaged Scholarship.” In *Graphic Medicine Manifesto*. State Park: Pennsylvania State University Press.
Szep, Eszter. 2020. *Comics and the Body: Drawing, Reading, and Vulnerability*. Columbus: Ohio State University Press.

CHAPTER SEVEN

Drawing on Pain: Depicting Disability and Trauma in Mikael Ross' Graphic Novel *Der Umfall*

PRISCILLA LAYNE

When it comes to representing trauma, comics and graphic novels, due to their combination of text and image, have often been praised for achieving what text alone cannot. In *Comics, Trauma, and the New Art of War*, Harriet Earle writes that the "comics form is not simply visual but aspects of the form can be used to reproduce and mimic the experience of a traumatic rupture, thus acting as a representation of so-called 'authentic social history'" (Earle 2017, 11). In *Disaster Drawn: Visual Witness, Comics and Documentary Form*, Hillary Chute argues that comics can be uniquely capable of documenting traumatic historical events because "graphic narratives that bear witness to authors' own traumas or to those of others materially retrace inscriptional effacement; they repeat and reconstruct in order to counteract" (Chute 2016, 4). What Chute gets at is that comics do not just have a unique capability of conveying traumatic experience visually, they are also a good medium for "mak[ing] visible fragments of traumatic experience that formerly have been neglected, repressed or censored" (Ulanowisz 2011, 8); thus, making it an especially useful medium for conveying the experiences of people whose trauma often goes unrecognized due to their marginalization in society. In the German context, a perfect example is people with disabilities, a group that suffered targeted discrimination and systematic murder under the Nazis and whose history of suffering is not often acknowledged.

Comics present a unique opportunity to address the experience and trauma of people with disabilities, due to the unique subcategory of comics referred to as graphic medicine. Nina Schmidt defines graphic medicine as "comics speaking to or engaging with the discourses of illness and disability, medicine, health, and well-being (including the end of life)" (Schmidt 2020, 368). Thanks to the growing popularity of this medium, there have been increasing numbers of comics "dealing with the themes of illness and disability from a personal, often auto/biographical stance" (Schmidt 2020, 369). Autobiographical comics like Regina Hofer's *Blad* (2018), which deals with eating disorders, E. T. Russian's *Ring of Fire Anthology*, which deals with her use of prosthetics, and Pina Varnel's ADHD alien comic, which she distributes on social media via Twitter and Instagram, are each examples of artists with disabilities using the comics medium to convey their own experiences. Thus, the democratizing nature of the comics medium allows people with disabilities to generate their own representations and counter the lack thereof in mainstream media. In *Demystifying Disability*, Emily Ladau writes:

> Truly good representations of disability in any form of media can be hard to come by. There are many common ways disability is depicted in media that reduces disabled people to one-note caricatures rather than portraying them as multidimensional human beings. Even more striking is that people with disabilities often aren't represented *at all* in the media, let alone accurately and authentically.
>
> (Ladau 2021, 121)

Mikael Ross' *Der Umfall*, published in English as *Thud*, presents a unique opportunity to discuss both personal and historical trauma and it does so via a character who is a person with a disability. It offers a chance to look at, in the words of Jay Dolmage and Dale Jacobs, the "knowledge and meaning which disability *generates*, moving beyond policing negative portrayals of disability to recognizing disability as an engine of innovation and rhetorical invention" (Dolmage and Jacobs 2016, 15).

Der Umfall was published in 2018 and nominated for a Max und Moritz German comic prize in 2020. The protagonist of *Der Umfall* is Noel, the adult son of a single mother. The mother and son do not have much money, which is emphasized by their apartment in a Berliner *Plattenbau* (industrial apartment block). Noel's specific intellectual disability is never explicitly stated, nor is it depicted as the sole, all-encompassing part of his identity. Near the beginning of the graphic novel, Noel's mother experiences a medical emergency in the middle of the night, which causes her to fall in the bathroom and slip into a coma. Such an event would be devastating for anyone, but for Noel it is even more difficult, because his intellectual disability requires him to have a caretaker, who until now has been his mother. While his mother stays in the hospital, Noel is taken to live at *Villa Luisa*, an assisted living facility in the village of Neuerkerode.

Although, as Schmidt points out, most graphic medicine comics are autobiographical, Noel's story is entirely fictional. Schmidt argues that it is important to recognize that "Graphic medicine from German-speaking Europe also encompasses entirely fictional—even wildly fantastic—treatises on matters of life, death, and social cohesion" (Schmidt 2020, 369). Because Ross does not have an intellectual disability himself and has created a fictional character with Noel, there is a particular danger that he might take an ableist approach to the story, thereby othering people with disabilities. In their overview of representations of intellectual disability on television, Vertoont et al. remark that scholarship has "disclosed that people with disabilities are predominantly portrayed as 'victims of their condition' or as 'superheroes who undertake extraordinary measures to overcome their condition'" (Vertoont 2021, 4). I would argue, however, that Ross' depiction of disability does not fall into the same stereotypes. Ross' comic resulted from an invitation he received, to observe how a community of people with and without disabilities live together in Germany. Neuerkerode is an inclusive village in Lower Saxony with a population of 1,300 people, 800 of whom have disabilities. Ross spent time living in Neuerkerode, getting to know its inhabitants, in order to write *Der Umfall*. At the end of the graphic novel, Ross includes photos and information about Neuerkerode. Thus, Ross uses the qualitative information he gathered from visiting Neuerkerode in order to create this fictionalized story. For this reason, rather than presenting an exploitative depiction of people with disabilities, one could best describe Ross' project as an example of "community comics creation," which Sarah McNicol describes as:

> engag[ing] groups in a process of discussion and dialogue about themselves: their "culture," in the widest sense; their ways of life, which might include family, neighborhood, and personal relationships; and wider issues such as employment and education. In this approach, the emphasis is not so much on action and explicit policy-related outcomes, but on assisting people to become engaged in a process of reflection on the major themes in their lives.
>
> (McNicol 2021, 90)

The respect which Ross has for the community of Neuerkerode is reflected in his depiction of Noel. First of all, Ross does not *ablesplain* Noel. Dolmage and Jacobs describe ablesplaining as "ways that disability gets confidently explained and defined by people who have no experience of the disability. In fact, ablesplaining also encapsulates the fact that most people with disabilities are not seen as authorities about their own minds and bodies" (Dolmage and Jacobs 2016, 26). Ablesplaining Noel's disability would require an authoritative, narrative voice that does not belong to Noel. By contrast, *Der Umfall* is entirely told from Noel's perspective and none of the medical authorities within the text ablesplain Noel's disability.

In addition to not being ablesplained by a medical authority, Noel's disability is also not portrayed as something negative. Noel understands the world differently than most, often escaping into a realm of fantasy. In fact, Noel's perspective of the world is often depicted as something magical, which is partly made possible by the comics genre. This is an example of how comics can "*become a form of prosthesis themselves*, an additional tool in making meaning accessible and for intervening in and interrogating disability" (Domage and Jacobs 2016, 14). *Der Umfall* also offers a critical perspective on disability by showing the care work that goes into taking care of Noel. We see how frustrated his mother becomes going grocery shopping with him or responding to his repetitive questions. But despite the challenges that caring for him brings, Noel's mother clearly loves her son and loves spending time with him.

And because Noel has a different way of seeing the world, he does not understand what has happened to his mother or why he cannot remain with her or remain in their home.

Because Noel's mother was his primary caretaker and Noel no longer has anyone to fill that role, he is taken to *Villa Luisa*. While living in Neuerkerode, he becomes infatuated with a woman, whom he believes to be a princess. The rest of the narrative follows his pursuit of her, during which he gets to know several other inhabitants of the village. I see trauma as being central to understanding *Der Umfall* for two reasons. First of all, Noel experiences his mother's accident as a traumatic event that fundamentally changes his life. He is ripped out of the comfort of his daily routine and forced to adapt to an entirely new living situation. Suddenly, he must become more self-reliant *and* learn to rely on and trust an entirely new group of people. And ultimately his mother passes away, closing off the possibility of ever returning to his former life. But *Der Umfall* does not just grapple with Noel's personal trauma. Rather, it places his trauma and his experience of living in Germany as a person with a disability into conversation with the trauma of the Holocaust and the Nazis' treatment of people with disabilities. *Der Umfall* thereby contributes both to disability studies and trauma studies, by moving beyond negative portrayals of disability and showing what kinds of knowledge and meaning disability *generates*. Noel's experience causes us to question not only how his disability makes grappling with trauma more difficult, but also shows how it sometimes helps him develop coping mechanisms to deal with trauma. Furthermore, Ross' ability to tie past and present discourses about disability together via personal and historical trauma not only warns us about the dehumanization caused by certain discourses on disability, but also gives us a model for a more respectful, humanizing depiction of disability.

The manner in which Ross introduces Noel as a character is an example of a humanizing portrayal of disability. When we first encounter Noel, he is at the store shopping. He is staring at several dolls of royal characters. When he says, astonished, "Oh [...] der Prinz und die Prinzessin" (3) ["Oh [...] the Prince and the Princess"] (1), this expression does not at all seem strange. We do not yet know how old he is. He may be a child who has been searching for these particular dolls. In the next panel, a worker happens to be stocking shelves nearby. Here we learn that it is Noel's birthday and assume he might be looking for a potential present. It is only when Noel and the worker have difficulty communicating that we realize Noel does not think like most adults. When the worker asks him "Wie alt wirst du denn" ["How old are you?"] Noel responds, "Hää? [...] wie, alt werden? ich werde doch nich alt!" (4) ["Huh? What do you mean, how old? I'm not old!"] (2). We can glean two things from this comment. First, Noel misunderstands the salesman's question. The salesman tries to clarify by asking "[...] der wievielte Geburtstag meinte ich" (4) ["Which birthday is it?"] (2). Second, regardless of his age, Noel identifies as young. The way Noel is drawn in relation to the worker and his mother makes him appear small and childlike. Although Noel is at least twenty, as is revealed at the end of the novel, the salesman is standing on a ladder, which makes him tower over Noel. Also, Noel's mother is drawn in the foreground with Noel in the background, which also affects the perspective and possibly distorts his height. This makes him appear smaller than his mother and suggests that he might still be a child. We do not see Noel as a man who acts like a child. And Noel's age will remain a mystery until the very end of the graphic novel, when we learn he was twenty-one when his mother had her accident. What is clear is Noel's distance from the real world. Noel yells to his mother "Mumsie! Der Weihnachtsmann fragt, wievielter Geburtstag heute is!" (4) ["Mumsie! Santa's asking which birthday this is?"] (2). The employee, likely someone working at a big box store like Walmart, as suggested by the smiley face he is wearing on the back of his vest, is presumably wearing a Santa hat because it is the Christmas season. But Noel has trouble separating fantasy from reality and for him, this man is the real Santa Claus, just like there are real princes and princesses in the world.

We soon learn how the world of fantasy functions as a kind of refuge for Noel, when he is confronted with his mother's harrowing accident. Noel is awakened that night by a loud noise. He peeks into his mother's bathroom and sees her lying on the floor wearing just a towel, bleeding from her head. Noel's description of the situation gives us a window into his thought process: "Mumsie schläft da auf dem Boden. Schlafen tut man aber im Bett!" (9) ["Mumsie's sleeping on the floor. But sleeping happens in bed!"] (7). Noel's rationalization of the scene is further proof that he cognitively cannot understand what has happened. The next panel indicates how Noel's mental state begins to unravel. Noel appears three times in different positions, which conveys that he is pacing in a circle. The dashes separating incomplete sentences show that Noel does not know what he should do. He says, "Und Blut [...] da is auch Blut [...] Blut auf dem Boden [...] gehört da nich hin" (9) ["And blood [...] there's blood too [...] blood on the floor [...] blood shouldn't be there"] (7). Noel knows that in this situation, he must take control. He tells himself that he must stop pacing and calm down. But several of the next panels show him wearing a plant pot on his head, which indicates Noel's need to escape difficult situations. Noel is eventually able to draw on what his mother has taught him and calls for help. Despite his difficulty remembering the correct number to dial for emergency assistance, he eventually calls 112, which his mother taught him to visualize as a fish (Figure 7.1). This sequence of panels provides us with some insight into the coping mechanisms necessary for taking care of someone with cognitive or developmental disabilities. But outside support is also necessary. When Noel cannot remember the house number, he ultimately seeks the help of a neighbor.

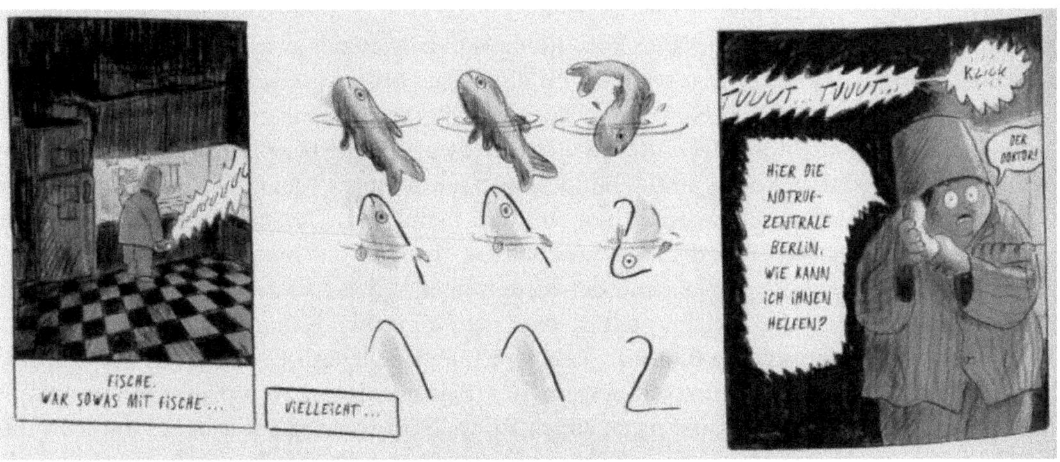

FIGURE 7.1: Mikael Ross, *Der Umfall* (2018)—Fish Episode. Copyright: Berlin: Avant.

The traumatic effects of the accident on Noel become clearer after the ambulance brings him and his mother to the hospital. The hospital is a frightening place for Noel. He imagines the doctors as giant ducks who storm past him quacking. He imagines their speech is quacking, because he does not understand the medical terminology they are using. Noel only catches a few words: in German they are *Koma* (coma) and *Schlaganfall* (stroke). *Schlaganfall* is a compound word, consisting of *Schlag* (hit) and *Anfall* (seizure). Noel grasps on to the one word he does understand, *Schlag*. Due to his failure to comprehend the compound word, Noel can only understand the circumstances on a simpler level, stating in the German version "und dass Mumsie einen Schlag wegbekommen hat. Schlag von wem denn?" ["and that mother got hit. Hit by whom?," my translation] (19).[1] But the doctors do not try to explain to Noel what is happening. Thus, this scene demonstrates in what ways medical staff can fail to communicate with people with disabilities; they do not even try to adjust their language so that he might be able to understand.

To cope with his fear and confusion, Noel finds solace in fantasy. He imagines that the gold emergency blanket they have given him is really a cape. When he runs from the hospital out of fear, he imagines an entirely different world, one in which he encounters a horse standing alone in the woods. He mounts the horse and finds a pond, where he sees a white ballerina dancing on its surface. This ballerina, who reoccurs several times during the narrative, has two reference points. First, there was a large image of a ballerina hanging in the family apartment. And we will later learn that his mother had also been a dancer once. Thus, he likely envisions his mother this way, because of an old picture of her in which she is dressed as a ballerina. These stories help make Noel feel more in control of his environment. Diane Wiener describes graphic medicine as "address[ing] issues of power in the silencing of disability and the 'voices' of those who experience barriers in healthcare and healthcare education and practice" (Syracuse University Humanities Center 2019). Wiener describes how a symposium on Graphic Medicine and disability, held at Syracuse University in October 2019, hoped to "address how disabled people's 'voices' are sometimes silenced in graphic medicine, the comics industry and beyond, thus demonstrating why adaptations are necessary to (re)fashion a primarily visual medium so that it is consistently accessible to a spectrum of creators and audiences." It is through these narrative strategies and aesthetics that Ross attempts to convey things from Noel's perspective, thus countering the silencing that people with disabilities otherwise experience.

In *Der Umfall*, the only person in the hospital who seems concerned with how Noel is coping is a nurse. She finds Noel cowering in the hallway, hiding beneath the gold emergency blanket. She senses that Noel is afraid, but despite her attempts to get more information from him, all he can utter is a few words, "[...] will jetzt heim" (21) ["want home now"] (19). In order to calm him down, she distracts him, stating that she has noticed something special about his hands: "dein Ringfinger und der Mittelfinger [...] die sind gleich lang [...] da wo ich herkomme, ist das ein Zeichen dafür, dass man au seiner Königsfamilie stammt" (22) ["your ring finger and middle finger [...] they're the same length [...] where I come from, that's a sign that someone's of royal descent [...] that means you're a prince young man"] (23). The final panel on this same page, which shows Noel wearing the same costume as the prince doll from the beginning of the book, reinforces our understanding that seeing himself as a prince makes Noel feel better (Figure 7.2). But the very next page depicts Noel still in his

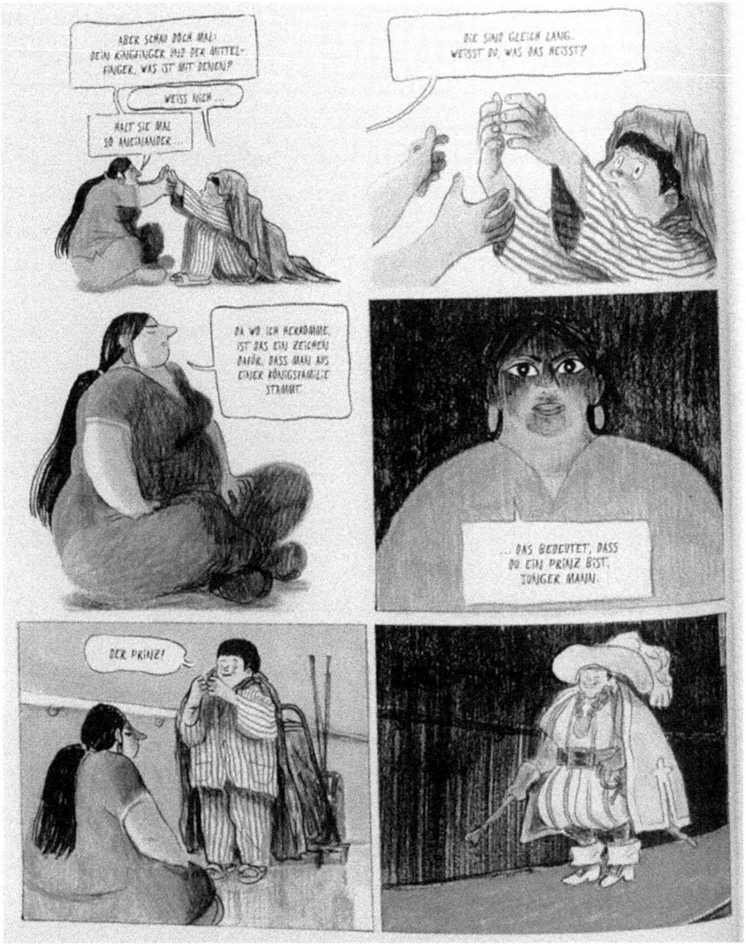
ABER SCHAU DOCH MAL:
DEIN RINGFINGER UND DER MITTELFINGER. WAS IST MIT DENEN?
WEISS NICH...
HALT SIE MAL SO ANEINANDER...
DIE SIND GLEICH LANG. WEISST DU, WAS DAS HEISST?
DA WO ICH HERKOMME, IST DAS EIN ZEICHEN DAFÜR, DASS MAN AUS EINER KÖNIGSFAMILIE STAMMT.
... DAS BEDEUTET, DASS DU EIN PRINZ BIST, JUNGER MANN.
DER PRINZ!

FIGURE 7.2: Mikael Ross, *Der Umfall* (2018)—Prince Episode. Copyright: Berlin: Avant.

princely garb, cowering in a castle [the hospital], which is being bombarded by knights with swords and arrows. This conveys that his mother falling into a coma is too traumatic for Noel and that he does not feel that the hospital is a safe space. As he narrates what has occurred, he states "Schlag, Koooma, Umfall [...] ich versteh nix mehr. Ein Mann mit Bart ist jetzt der Chef" (23) ["thud, stroke, coooma [...] I don't understand anything anymore. A man with a 'stache is the boss now"] (21). This man with a moustache is the man who drives him to *Villa Luisa*, the assisted living facility to which he is taken while his mother is in the hospital.

His mother's accident has a lasting, traumatic effect on Noel. Afterwards, whenever he encounters illness or death, he rationalizes what happens by insisting that the person must be in a coma. This occurs when he and a friend from *Villa Luisa* named Valentin encounter a dead bird in the woods. Noel takes it home and places it in the freezer because he believes it is only in a coma and will reawaken soon. For Noel, a coma is a state of sleep that is temporary.

He cannot fathom that his mother might not wake up, and, therefore, he cannot accept the bird's death either. Even after the caretaker at *Villa Luisa* insists Noel dispose of the dead bird and they bury it in the woods, Noel holds on to the fantasy that it will return. When he sees a bird of the same kind flying away later, he insists that the bird he buried must have awoken from its coma. In another scene, when his friend Alice has an epileptic seizure and falls to the floor, he immediately thinks she has gone into a coma, until her father comes and explains her condition. In this particular scene, Noel uses the play on words from the book's German title, *Der Umfall*, which relates to Noel's misunderstanding. The noun *Unfall* with an "n," means an accident. But the verb *umfallen*, with an "m," means to fall down. Noel creates a new word, *Umfall*, to describe both what happened to his mother and to Alice. Just like when his mother had her accident, Noel attempts to hide from this frightening experience by placing a bucket on his head.

Despite his hesitation about living in a new place, Noel quickly becomes adjusted to life in *Villa Luisa*. He finds new friends who live in the facility, like Valentin, who is obsessed with order and death. But there are also people with disabilities who live outside of the facility, like Alice who has epilepsy and lives with her father on a farm. The assisted living facility seems to stress independence for its inhabitants, as they are free to come and go as they please. We see residents going to concerts and fairs and engaging in a multitude of activities ranging from drawing to watching pornography. The counselors on site only intervene when someone has a problem. We never learn why the other characters are living at *Villa Luisa* and the book never differentiates between people with and people without disabilities. What also contributes to the graphic novel's diverse cast of characters is that there seem to be fewer barriers between different generations. Noel does not only spend time with young people. On several occasions, older residents of Neuerkerode give him advice and invite him to participate in various activities.

One older woman, named Irma, who plays a unique role in the narrative, is someone Noel meets when he and Valentin find the dead bird in the woods. Irma asks Noel to help her home, because one of the wheels on her walker is damaged. Irma and Noel have what is, at first, a puzzling exchange. As Noel walks her to her apartment building, she asks whether Valentin always acts so strangely. Noel simply replies "Nich immer. Er mag nur Ordnung halt" (44) ["Not always. He just likes everything in order"] (42) presumably referring to Valentin's neurodiversity. Irma then sighs and repeats the word "order" (42). When she tells him that they have now reached her apartment building, Noel responds "is schön hier" (44) ["it's nice here"] (42). Though Noel is referring to her residence, Irma seems to interpret his statement as describing Neuerkerode more generally because she says in response, "[...] aber war nicht immer so schön" (44) ["but it wasn't always so nice"] (42). We will only later learn that her comment refers to what occurred in Neuerkerode during the Third Reich.

During a second encounter, Irma gives Noel advice regarding his unrequited love for a girl named Penelope. Noel first encounters Penelope at a concert. Penelope has a boyfriend and she does not appreciate it when Noel, in a jealous rage, loses his cool and assaults him. Noel becomes infatuated with Penelope, convinced that she is a real princess. This is, in fact, how he first meets Alice. Alice promises him she can give him access to the "princess." But, in fact,

Alice has a crush on Noel and is hoping to win him over so he will forget Penelope. One day, Alice lures Noel to the bus stop, with the promise that the princess will be coming there to meet him. While Alice hides in the bushes, observing Noel at the bus stop, Noel and Irma run into each other again.

Irma tells Noel that it is best to stay single and that she has never been in a romantic relationship. She insists this is, in part, a personal choice, because she likes her freedom. However, she admits that this decision was also forced upon her, because of the fence that once cut through the entire town, separating men from women. Her seemingly simple advice about relationships reveals a legacy of persecution against people with disabilities during the Third Reich. As it turns out, Irma and her brother, who both have disabilities, lived in Neuerkerode when they were younger and when the Nazis took over the village, one of the changes they made was separating the men from the women. Irma could not even be with her brother; they were only allowed to see each other in church. A flashback reveals what that time was like for her. We see Irma and her brother Erwin sitting at church, while a pastor installed by the Nazi party claims that people with disabilities should not procreate, thus explaining the wall running through the village. Irma and Erwin's treatment at the hands of the Nazis transitions from gender-based segregation to genocide as a number of people from the area were sent on an alleged "trip" from which they never returned. It is only because Irma's brother warned her and instructed her to hide that she survived the Nazi period. His final words to her were "Irma, du musst mir versprechen nie in so einen Bus einzusteigen" (70) ["Irma, you must promise me to never get on such a bus"] (68). Irma has since realized that everything her brother said was true and he likely perished with the others. Irma's presence as one of the sole survivors of the Nazi genocide allows her to be a constant reminder of this devastating past. This is an example of how, according to McNicol, comics help us "becom[e] aware [that] normally invisible social ghosts can help us make sense of the more visible, yet fragmented, present" (McNicol 2021, 86).

People with disabilities are one of the many groups that were targeted by the Nazis during the Third Reich. Because Hitler framed "all domestic policies around preparing the nation for war," a key factor of that ideology was that anyone who would be "useless" during a war was a detriment to Nazi German society (Gellately and Stoltzfus 2018, 4). People with disabilities were the first ones targeted for the Nazis' trials with the agent *Zyklon B*, before officials decided, at the Wannsee Conference in 1942, to use the agent to systematically murder millions of Jews, Sinti and Roma, political opponents, gay people, and other groups the Nazis condemned as being a detriment to Nazi society:

> We know from other sources that Nazi medical officials who toured some parts of the country wanted to sterilize whole villages when the people (all "ordinary Germans") did not appear well-kept or tidy enough. At the very least sterilization, forced and otherwise, would mean that the people who had "infirmities" and other problems would not be able to pass them on. In the event, an estimated 400,000 people were sterilized in Germany. The exclusionary polices that aimed to cleanse the Fatherland of chronic-care cases and the mentally ill became more radical with the coming of the war. Hitler backdated to

> September 1, 1939 his authorization (not order) for doctors to begin the "mercy killing" operation, as if to symbolize that war made it possible at last to put aside mere civilian considerations in the creation of the "community of the people." When the public got wind of what was happening there was some unrest, but no open protest. Some, but not all, local residents near the killing sites were appalled. One woman wrote to the hospital where her two siblings reportedly died within a few days of each other. She said she accepted the Third Reich, and hoped to "find peace again" if doctors could assure her that her siblings had been killed by virtue of some law that made it possible to "relieve people from their chronic suffering."
>
> (Gellately and Stoltzfus 2018, 11)

Ross' insertion of the past into Noel's story has several functions. First, Ross' ability to tie past and present discourses about disability together warns us about the effects of dehumanizing discourses around disability. Moving away from a genocidal, dehumanizing, and ableist understanding of disability toward a humanizing understanding that fosters respect and communal living between people with and without disabilities necessitated a shift in thinking about disability, one that made a community like Neuerkerode's current iteration possible. Despite the Nazis' defeat in 1945 and the founding of a new, democratic Federal Republic of Germany in 1949, it still took several decades before Germany adopted specific rights accommodating citizens with disabilities:

> During the 1950s it was primarily the organizations of the war dis-abled that achieved the first postwar improvements for disabled people. In the late 1950s and early 1960s, several advocacy organizations, such as Life Help for the Mentally Handicapped Child (Lebenshilfe für das geistig behinderte Kind) and the Spastics' Association (Spastikerverein), were formed. These were run mostly by parents and professionals. In connection with the far-reaching, democratic, social transformations of the late 1960s, however, some younger disabled and nondisabled people became dissatisfied with this arrangement. They began to critique these organizations for advocating the segregation of disabled people in many types of special institutions and for pressuring disabled people to con-form to unquestioned standards of normality in many ways.
>
> (Poore 2007, 274)

It was beginning in the 1970s that "disability rights activists, along with some professionals, also began to critique how these normalizing rehabilitation practices had supported the segregation of disabled people in the broadest sense" (Poore 2007, 274). Neuerkerode began in the nineteenth century as one of the many "religious institutions [that] cared for people with epilepsy, chronic mental disorders, physical handicaps and ID" (Elstner and Theil 2018). Founded by Gustav Stutzer, Neuerkerode began as a home for "girls and boys with disabilities" (neuerkerode.de). Today, however, more than 150 years later, "Neuerkerode [is] a place where inclusion is not just a word. Here, people work together to produce slatted frames in the workshops, prepare meals for schools, grow vegetables, and create sculptures and paintings" (neuerkerode.de). Thus, *Der Umfall* does not just challenge us to remember the trauma of the past, but also to recognize how much things have changed.

By spending time in Neuerkerode and drawing inspiration from the community to write *Der Umfall*, Ross creates a narrative set in what seems like a haven for people of all ages with varying degrees of (dis)ability. It is a place where people with disabilities are not judged and can lead ordinary lives filled with the everyday activities that we witness in the comic: going to a dance, falling in love, and watching pornography, the latter of which may seem insignificant, but it resists past media representations of people with disabilities as without love or desire. For the narrative, Irma's story serves as a bridge that helps Noel ultimately understand that some people do, in fact, never wake up. Several additional incidents lead him to this personal growth. He gets over his infatuation with Penelope after he learns she has a boyfriend named Kevin.

After physically attacking Kevin, one of the older residents suggests that Noel take a judo course, a course where Alice is also a student, so that he can learn how to deal with his anger in a more productive way. During his first lesson, the instructor emphasizes the importance of learning how to fall above anything else. The notion that one must learn how to fall functions as a metaphor for Noel's journey over the course of the narrative, which is also a reason for its title *Der Umfall* (*Thud*), something I will return to below. Initially, Alice is angry to see him turn up at Judo, because she is still hurt over his crush on Penelope. But the two reconcile and Alice becomes one of the consistent people Noel can count on. She even accompanies him to Berlin, when he is convinced that if he just returns to his apartment, he will be reunited with his mother.

However, once he arrives there, he learns that a new family has moved in, closing the door to the past. It is during this trip to Berlin that Noel has his final imagined encounter with his mother in the form of the white ballerina. In this fantastical form, she tells him it is time for her to leave and he has to let her go, promising him "Alles wird gut, mein Noel" (116) ["Everything will be well"] (114). Noel does not want her to leave. But thanks to the support system he has found in Neuerkerode, he is able to weather this devastating loss. The book ends with Alice surprising Noel on his birthday, bringing the narrative full circle; exactly one year has passed since his mother's accident. After Alice playfully tackles Noel, the book ends with Alice praising him for his falling, which has gotten much better since his first Judo class. This brings us back to the graphic novel's title. At the start of the graphic novel, Noel's mother's "thud" is the cause of fear and stress, disrupting his entire life. By the end of the book, falling is no longer scary, because Noel learns how to brace himself. Noel's final words are "Kann man lernen" (125) ["I'm learning"] (123). Ross' narrative does not focus solely on the protagonist's disability. Instead, he centers the narrative around a life-changing incident that does not have anything to do with his disability. Thus, we get to know Noel at a moment in his life when he is faced with an experience that would be challenging for anyone—namely, a parent falling ill and losing a parent; it is simply that his mental developmental disability changes how he copes with this event. With these final words, "I'm learning," Ross stresses that Noel is able to adapt to a new life and work through the trauma of his mother's accident and her subsequent death.

NOTE

1. In the English publication, the play on words of *Schlaganfall* (stroke) and *Schlag* (hit) are lost because Noel's words are translated as "mumsie had a stroke. A stroke from who?" (17).

WORKS CITED

Chute, Hillary. 2016. *Disaster Drawn: Visual Witness, Comics and Documentary Form*. Cambridge: Harvard University Press.

Dolmage, Jay and Dale Jacobs. 2016. "Mutable Articulations: Disability Rhetorics and the Comics Medium." In *Disability in Comic Books and Graphic Narratives*, edited by Chris Foss, Jonathan W. Gray, and Zach Whalen, 14–28. New York: Palgrave Macmillan.

Earle, Harriet E. H. 2017. *Comics, Trauma, and the New Art of War*. Jackson: University Press of Mississippi.

Elstner, Samuel and Michael-Mark Theil. 2018. "The Health and Social Care of People with Disabilities in Germany." *Advances in Mental Health and Intellectual Disabilities* 12, no. 3/4: 99–104.

Evans, Richard J. 2018. "Social Outsiders in Germany History: From the Sixteenth Century to 1933." In *Social Outsiders in Nazi Germany*, edited by Robert Gellately, Nathan Stoltzfus, 20–44. Princeton: Princeton University Press.

Gellately, Robert and Nathan Stoltzfus. 2018. "Social Outsiders and the Construction of the Community of the People." In *Social Outsiders in Nazi Germany*, edited by Robert Gellately, Nathan Stoltzfus, 1–19. Princeton: Princeton University Press.

Ladau, Emily. 2021. *Demystifying Disability: What to Know, What to Say and How to Be an Ally*. Berkeley: Ten Speed Press.

McNicol, Sarah. 2021. "Exploring Trauma and Social Haunting Through Community Comics Creation." In *Documenting Trauma in Comics: Traumatic Pasts, Embodied Histories and Graphic Reportage*, edited by Dominic Davies and Candida Rifkind, 85–102. London: Palgrave.

Poore, Carol. 2007. *Disability in Twentieth-Century German Culture*. Ann Arbor: University of Michigan Press.

Ross, Mikael. 2018. *Der Umfall*. Berlin: Avant-Verlag.

Ross, Mikael. 2021. *The Thud*, translated by Nika Knight. Seattle: Fantagraphics.

"Syracuse University Humanities Center and the Burton Blatt Institute Host 'Cripping' Graphic Medicine: Psychiatric Disability, 'Crip' Culture and the Humanities." *News Bites – Private Companies*, Oct 23, 2019, http://libproxy.lib.unc.edu/login (accessed July 17, 2022).

Ulanowicz, Anastasia. 2010–11. Review of *Graphic Women: Life Narrative and Contemporary Comics*, by Hillary Chute. *ImageText* 5, no. 4. http://www.english.ufl.edu/imagetext/archives/v5_4/ulanowicz.

Vertoont, Susan et al. 2021. "Un/recognisable and Dis/empowering Images of Disability: A Collective Textual Analysis of Media Representations of Intellectual Disabilities." *Critical Studies in Media Representation* 39, no. 1: 1–14.

CHAPTER EIGHT

"Thinking in Comics": Representing Autism Spectrum Disorder in Autobiographical Graphic Narrative

ELIZABETH "BIZ" NIJDAM

In her autobiography *Thinking in Pictures* (1995), American academic, animal behaviorist, and autism spokesperson Temple Grandin writes about her intellectual processes:

> I think in pictures. Words are like a second language to me ... When somebody speaks to me, his words are instantly translated into pictures. Language-based thinkers find this phenomenon difficult to understand (3).

This difference between language-based and image-based thinking has been the subject of much scholarship in the field of autism studies, with Grandin's book foundational in helping people understand the spectrum of neurodivergent intellectual processing and, specifically, that of visual thinking. Grandin's emphasis on how words are a "second language" that are "translated into pictures" echoes the experience of many neurodivergent thinkers. Yet her own autobiography does not contain more than a few images. While words are essential for articulating the experience of children and adults with autism spectrum disorder (ASD), even this essential treatise of autistic thinking reveals how language alone might struggle to represent autistic cognitive processes, such as visual thinking.

Comics and graphic novels, however, with their combination of word and image, present new opportunities for communicating certain kinds of autistic experience. Visual tools have been used in behavior modification for children and adults with autism for decades, but it is only recently that comics have become an important element for autism outreach, autism awareness, and biographical and autobiographical accounts of living on the autism spectrum. In 2000, Keiko Tobe began her series *With the Light: Raising an Autistic Child* (2011) (*Hikari to Tomoni ... ~Jiheishōji o Kakaete~*, 2000–09), depicting the struggles of a young mother, Sachiko Azuma, raising her autistic son, Hikaru, in contemporary Japan. In 2010, John Swogger and Kirsti Evans published *Something Different About Dad: How to Live with Your Asperger's Parent*, examining the difficulties families face when one parent is on the autism spectrum. Then, in 2015 and then again in 2017, Mike Medaglia and Kathy Hoopmann teamed up to produce two graphic novels as part of Hoopman's "Asperger Adventures" series, *Blue Bottle Mystery* (2015) and *Lisa and the Lacemaker* (2017), to help children understand autism spectrum disorder. Since 2017, comics thematizing ASD have continued to appear, demonstrating the appeal of the medium in recounting these stories as much as the increased interest in neurodivergence more broadly.

With the comic form's ability to bring text and image together to illuminate the complexities of human experience, graphic narrative can communicate the experience of individuals living with ASD more holistically than text-reliant media. Yet even with the increase of graphic literature on autism, autobiographical comics on autistic experience have been slow to emerge. Moreover, despite English-language comics domination of the comics market, the earliest example of this trend has come from Germany.

Daniela Schreiter's graphic memoir trilogy *Schattenspringer* (2014–18) explores the author's childhood, adolescence, and adulthood through the context of her ASD diagnosis. Sharing personal experiences alongside her thoughts on neurodivergence and opinions on neuronormativity, Schreiter humorously and adeptly educates people about autism spectrum disorder. Importantly, however, these ruminations on autism are not restricted to the words describing her experience. In this powerfully personal comic, Schreiter's visuals are equally important, bringing the author's thinking in pictures in dialogue with the text.

This essay thus explores the way in which comics are well-positioned to recount neurodivergent experience to both neurotypical and non-neurotypical audiences. Looking at the representation of visual thinking at the intersection of text and image, I argue that comics help to bridge the gap between language-based and image-based thinkers. Moreover, with comics today existing in digital and print spaces simultaneously, *Schattenspringer* is an excellent example of how comics are capable of reaching diverse audiences and building community. Finally, through the author's explicit engagement with histories of ability, disability, and superability embedded in the comics form, Schreiter's work provides an intervention in superhero genres' preoccupation with super-crip narratives.

First and foremost, however, I would like to acknowledge my own positionality in writing this essay. My neurological function is neurotypical, and, as such, I experience neither the marginalization nor the exclusion featured in many of Schreiter's narratives. However, the stories she tells intersect with the lives of many of my closest people, and, as a comics scholar, I wanted to understand what it meant to bring these narratives of ASD experience to life on the comics page.

Moreover, it is essential to acknowledge, as Schreiter herself does (2014, 7), that characterizing people diagnosed with ASD as uniformly the same is highly problematic and unequivocally inaccurate. Much like the experience of neurotypical individuals, the experience of people on the autism spectrum varies widely, as does the way autistic individuals think, make connections, and communicate. My work here specifically focuses on the role of images in patterns of visual thinking that many autistic individuals experience due to the nature of the comics medium and its capacity to communicate through pictures; however, I acknowledge that dividing language-based and image-based thinking in the account of any individual's personal experience of making sense of the world is an arbitrary move since we all think in varying degrees in images, words, and concepts. This, too, is a spectrum. My intention is, therefore, simply to illuminate how the comics form is a valuable tool of self-expression for authors and artists on the autism spectrum and readers interested in learning more about themselves and/or neurodiversity.

AUTISM SPECTRUM DISORDER: VISUAL AND LITERAL THINKING

Autism spectrum disorder—or ASD—is a neurological disorder characterized by its impact on what is considered "normal" human interaction with the surrounding environment (Bystrova et al.), influencing social behavior and how individuals relate to other people as well as how people process information and make sense of the world around them (Dodd 2005, 131). Historically, ASD was considered extremely rare, but recently, more and more children are being assessed for neurodivergence, and adult diagnoses are also on the rise. Today, the ASD rate is close to 1.5 percent of the population, with some studies indicating that one out of every sixty-eight children is on the autism spectrum (Bystrova et al.). As a spectrum, the experience of individuals with ASD ranges significantly from nonverbal to "high-functioning," the latter of which has been historically identified as Asperger's Syndrome. Recent scholarship, however, has argued that the differentiation in diagnoses between ASD and Asperger's Syndrome is not meaningful, though under some circumstances, the language remains helpful and in use (Hosseini and Molla 2020; Mirkovic and Gérardin 2019). Moreover, many characterizations of high-functioning autistic experience rely heavily on ableist definitions of neurological function, human interaction, and communication. It is useful to understand the difficulties faced by individuals on the autism spectrum, but ASD advocacy groups encourage the identification of high-functioning autism as different and not dysfunctional (Kent 2023).

In addition to idiosyncrasies and delays in normative communicative competencies, often categorized in terms of reduced interest in and increased difficulties with social interaction, the role of visual thinking in comprehending the world is an important characteristic of ASD cognitive processes (Bystrova et al.). Grandin, in particular, has written extensively about her experience as a visual thinker. She asserts that she has "no language-based memory" (1995, 143): "When I hear the word over by itself, I visualize a childhood memory of a dog jumping over a fence" (1995, 143).

This "thinking in pictures" is especially common for individuals on the autism spectrum. Many concepts are initially imagined pictorially instead of verbally—literally, as a picture. These visual thoughts are associated with words, actions, or phrases, which are then communicated verbally to others. For example, when thinking about butterflies, Grandin first sees an image of butterflies that she encountered in her childhood backyard (2009). This is then followed by the metal ornamental butterflies that people use to decorate the outside of their houses, with the third image being a butterfly that Grandin painted herself on a piece of plywood when she was in graduate school (2009). Only through these images does the notion of a butterfly make sense. These visual memories are finally connected to the language-based concept of a butterfly, and once that connection is made, "butterfly" can be expressed verbally.

The visual nature of these thought processes then collides with the neurodivergent predisposition to understand abstract concepts literally. Also sometimes referred to as concrete thinking, literal thinking refers to the way objects are not perceived as representations of something else, as in, for example, a metaphor. A cardboard box is exactly that to a person who thinks concretely—and not, for example, a pretend house or spaceship. It can therefore be difficult for some individuals with ASD to understand idiomatic expressions that rely on metaphor, simile, or synecdoche to impart their meaning. Idioms are thus often understood literally, with visualizations of their literal understanding further reinforcing their concrete meaning. Moreover, abstract concepts such as good, bad, peace and honesty, for example, might be difficult for concrete visual thinkers to conceptualize and often require a mnemonic device, such as an image, to aid in interpretation.

VISUAL AND LITERAL THINKING AS A REPRESENTATIONAL STRATEGY IN *SCHATTENSPRINGER*

In light of their combination of image and text, comics offer unique opportunities for the visual representation of these thought processes that are difficult to express in words alone, as they circumvent the very process of this kind of language-based communication. Turning to Schreiter's autobiographical trilogy *Schattenspringer,* therefore, demonstrates this important avenue for imparting autistic experience, which not only articulates but *shows* readers how visual thinking operates. Furthermore, Schreiter's thematization of these cognitive processing on the level of form transcends the graphic memoir's content and clarification on neurodivergent thought processes to become, as I argue, a representational strategy for autistic experience.

In Schreiter's first volume of *Schattenspringer* (2014), subtitled "wie es ist anders zu sein" ["how it is to be different"], the author recounts her childhood experience of unknowingly living with autism spectrum disorder. Many of her anecdotes are playful and humorous musings on neurodivergent perceptions of living in a neuronormative world, but Schreiter does not shy away from the darker side of trying to masquerade as neurotypical, discussing the deep depressions, social alienation, and even suicidal ideation she experienced. Schreiter thus offers her subjective experience of living with ASD in a way that helps readers understand the difficulties the author encounters daily while simply trying to fit in, setting it in dialogue with other examples of graphic medicine, the genre of comics that thematize healthcare discourses, on ASD.

However, in terms of unique visual-verbal aesthetic strategies, Schreiter's engagement with specifically neurodivergent thought processes sets her work apart from other comics on autism. Series such as Keiko Tobe's *With the Light* (2000), Kirsti Evans and John Swogger's *Something Different About Dad* (2010) and, more recently, Carlton and Bridget Hudgens' *Brother: A Story of Autism* (2019) and Yvon Roy's *Little Victories: Autism Through a Father's Eyes* (2021) all explore autism from the vantage point of family members. Schreiter's *Schattenspringer* series, on the other hand, features a first-person insider perspective that depicts the unique effects of visual and literal thinking for an audience that is potentially unfamiliar with such characterizations—or is perhaps incapable of imagining them. Schreiter's literal imaginings of common idiomatic expressions, for example, are both amusing and enlightening: when interpreting the expression "Abends werden die Bürgersteige hochgeklappt," which means "there's not much to do in the evening because everything shuts down early," she attempts to reconstruct the mechanics of the sidewalks actually folding up on themselves. And instead of understanding that "Mit dem ist nicht gut Kirschen essen" means that "an individual is not an easy person to deal with," she starts avoiding eating cherries with certain people.

While it is not unusual to see comics artists engaging with this form of wordplay—in Emil Ferris's first volume of *My Favorite Thing Is Monsters* (2017), for example, the young protagonist often imagines the literal versions of her mother's superstitious sayings—as a move to communicate a different kind of cognitive processing, it is meaningful. Other comics might mobilize this strategy as an indication of childish naiveté, but Schreiter's representation of these types of misunderstandings as a personal challenge links to her neurodivergence. It thereby illuminates an important barrier she faces in understanding certain concepts to her neurotypical audience and connects with her neurodivergent readers, who, in turn, feel seen and might come to better understand their own concrete thinking through her playful combination of word and image.[1]

Schreiter's engagements with the processes of visual thinking, on the other hand, are subtler. At the same time, however, they are substantially more linked to the author's artistic voice and the affordances of the comics medium in general. After all, the project itself began as a result of the author's inability to articulate her neurodivergence with words; she needed to draw it with the images she herself used to reflect on her own experience. Here, Schreiter's visual thinking manifests on multiple levels. First, the way the author depicts the world around her directly mobilizes the very idea of thinking in pictures. She walks the reader through her experience of space and time via images. This transcends the content of her panels that map onto real-world settings to her identification and description by way of captions of the various stimuli she encounters that agitate her, combining word and image to clarify the discomfort she feels under certain conditions and in certain places.

Then, in accordance with the specific definition of visual thinking, Schreiter also depicts specific words as visual concepts, demonstrating how she imagines words, actions, or phrases pictorially. This is particularly salient in how she visually constructs meaning for herself and her readers. For example, in a panel where she feels especially nervous about ruining a potential date, she depicts herself as a pig as she comments, "Ich hatte Angst wieder alles zu versauen," visually representing the "Sau"—or pig—particle of the word.

Beyond individual panels and words, Schreiter's use of visualization to comprehend abstract concepts also relates to her book project in its entirety, which emerges via metaphors that act as leitmotifs throughout the series. The trilogy's title itself, *Schattenspringer*, is an excellent example of the intersection of concrete and visual thinking. As the nominalization of the idiom "über seinen Schatten springen," which describes someone doing something that contradicts their own beliefs or character and thereby surmounts or transcends their own personal difficulties, this metaphor for Schreiter's daily life is visually referenced on the covers of each of the three volumes.

Within the trilogy as well, Schreiter turns to the visualization of "wrong-planet-syndrome," a playful way of describing autism spectrum disorder, to construct the overarching theme of her graphic autobiography. While the adjective "alienated" is typically not identified with the state of being extraterrestrial, Schreiter represents Dani, her narrative version of herself, as a literal alien, "extraterrestrischer Besucher" (2014, 8). In many panels, we see the protagonist with a pair of antennae. These antennae are imperceptible to every other individual in the comic, with the exception of those acquaintances also on the autism spectrum. They simultaneously signal Dani's outsider status in the larger society and her insider status in the autistic community in which she feels like she belongs. Thus, what the reader perceives as the metaphor of being alien is, in fact, Schreiter's visualization of her sense of self, the meaning of which neurological readers can also access through metaphor. It is thus only when Schreiter depicts Dani with antennae that the author is representing the real version of herself.

In *Thinking in Pictures*, Grandin observes how words become subjective visualizations; all nouns and verbs for Grandin have specific memories associated with them: "The easiest words for an autistic child to learn are nouns, because they directly relate to pictures" (2008, 13–14). While the integration of this type of verbal-visual convergence in the comics form emerges as playful visual manipulations to humorous ends, I argue that this strategy of representation mobilizes and renders neurodivergent cognitive processes legible to a neurotypical audience. Schreiter thereby encodes visual thinking into the very core of her system of representation.

This function of subjective representation extends to the role of the comics medium in general in Schreiter's work. She writes in her foreword to *Schattenspringer,* vol. 1:

> Comics haben eine großen Vorteil: Sie bieten dem Leser einen leichten und sofortigen Zugang zu Themen, mit denen er sich vielleicht sonst nicht beschäftigt hätte. Viele Situationen lassen sich durch die Zuhilfenahme von Bildern auch plastischer darstellen. Bilder sind direkter und offener, gleichzeitig aber auch viel intimer. Der Leser identifiziert sich schneller mit den Figuren und versetzt sich so in die dargestellten Situationen, er kann sie nun auf einmal viel besser nachvollziehen. (2014, 6)

> [Comics have an immense benefit: they offer the reader easy and immediate access to a subject, with which they would otherwise not engage themselves. Many situations are also better represented with the help of images. Images are more direct and open, while simultaneously much more intimate. Readers identify much faster with the characters and

positions themselves in the presented situations in such a way that they can suddenly understand them better.]

However, beyond each panel being a subjective visualization of Schreiter's experience of a situation or understanding of a subject, comics in general are an expression of subjectivity. As Douglas Wolk comments, cartooning is "inescapably, a metaphor for the subjectivity of perception"; just as no two individuals experience the world in the same way, no two cartoonists depict it in the same fashion (Wolk 2008, 21). Consequently, what a cartoonist or illustrator draws brings the reader closest to being able to experience these events through the author's eyes (Wolk 2008, 21). Schreiter's ability to depict her experience of stimuli that neurotypical individuals rarely even notice helps readers understand the daily struggles of individuals living on the autism spectrum, while also demonstrating to other members of the autistic community that they are not alone.

SCHATTENSPRINGER'S RECEPTION AND COMMUNITY BUILDING

Looking at the reception of her work, it is clear how essential the community building aspect of Schreiter's graphic autobiography has been to her success: Mirian, mother of a ten-year-old with ASD, writes to thank Schreiter for helping individuals with ASD feel less alone and neurotypical individuals better understand autistic experience. Similarly, a seventh-grade class writes that *Schattenspringer* taught them that there are many sides to ASD and that being different is entirely okay and something for which people should not be judged. Christian writes that even his therapist commented on how Schreiter's description of the intrinsic aspects of living with ASD goes beyond what any scientific study can demonstrate. And psychologist Heike S. writes that she intends on suggesting Schreiter's comic to parents and youth with an ASD diagnosis. Then, Claudia from Stuttgart writes that *Schattenspringer* even helped her come to her diagnosis, recognizing herself in many of the situations that Schreiter describes. Christoph from Vienna writes that in Schreiter's comic, he finally found himself and he thanks the artist for giving him hope, while another reader writes that *Schattenspringer* helped not only her to understand herself, but also her parents, who finally understood and accepted her for who she was. Finally, Eva, newly diagnosed with ASD at fifty-five, writes how she read the entire first volume of the trilogy with tears in her eyes, finding herself in 95 to 100 percent of all the situations Schreiter described (Schreiter, Email Correspondence 2018).

AUTISTIC-HERO-GIRL TAKES ON SUPERCRIP CONVENTIONS

In addition to these personal correspondences, the publication of many pages of readers' comments on Schreiter's website (www.fuchskind.de), Facebook (https://www.facebook.com/Fuchskind.de), and Instagram (www.instagram.com/fuchskindsfuchsbau/) demonstrates the strength of the trilogy and its webcomic versions for graphic medicine: its ability to build community. Even though all three volumes are available in print, *Schattenspringer* began as a webcomic and still, I would argue, functions largely within the parameters of the webcomic format. Not only does Schreiter continue to publish panels and pages through social media, but readers also continue to participate online in the discourse surrounding Schreiter's project, while contributing ideas for her to represent as future comic strips.[2]

At the same time, however, the media format through which Schreiter explores autistic experience also brings with it some problematic associations. In particular, the close relationship between comic books and superheroes, which has a fraught history but also offered Schreiter a unique opportunity to explore neurodiversity. While the trilogy's autobiographical explorations of autistic experience are firmly situated within the genre of graphic memoir, Schreiter's later work also takes advantage of comic arts' inclination to thematize superpowers. In particular, her 2017 publication *Die Abenteuer von Autistic-Hero-Girl* turns to superhero comics to examine living in a neuronormative world. However, while the rhetoric of this gesture feels uncomfortably close to disability studies discourses on the "super-crip," Schreiter, instead, empowers young readers through her adoption of a superhero persona to undermine the pop-culture convention of equating disability with super-ability.

Historically, superhero comics have always served as "a disability and death-denying representation practice which privilege[d] the healthy, the hyper-powered, and immortal body over the diseased, debilitated, and defunct body" (Alaniz 2014, 6). However, even before disability became an explicit theme in modern comics, this attention to hyper-able-bodiedness signaled comics' preoccupation with its antithesis, disability. And by the Silver Age of superhero comics, from the mid-1950s to the 1970s, depictions of disability and death were widespread in the medium (Alaniz 2014, 18). Through a comics studies lens, disability in comics typically figures as a mechanism "to construct and normalize a particular kind of ideal man" (Carpenter 2011, n.p.).

The classic example here is *X-Men* by Marvel Comics, in which a genetic abnormality, the X-gene, gives the mutants their superhuman powers. While the term "mutant" suggests that these humans are essentially flawed, they are, in fact, presented as superhumans (Carpenter, n.p.). Instead of being characterized as abnormal, they are presented as "the new-and-future normal, more normal than normal" (Carpenter 2011, n.p.). They are essentially "supercrips." According to Jose Alaniz, "supercrip" defines the type of disabled person typically visible in mainstream media (Alaniz 2014, 31). It characterizes a kind of disabled body or neurodiversity that reads as inspirational in ways that do not map onto most disabled experience. It is thus a "model deeply moving to most non-disabled Americans and widely regarded as oppressive by most disabled ones" (Shapiro 1994, 16). Ultimately, disability in comics and graphic novels is rarely about disabled bodies and neurodiversity.

Turning to Schreiter's *Die Abenteuer von Autistic-Hero-Girl*, however, we see a different intersection between discourses of neurodivergence, ability, and superability. At the very beginning of the short volume, which features no page numbers and is comprised of forty-nine short comics of four to twelve panels each, Schreiter recounts the origin of her superhero identity in a two-page comic by the same name. Describing her day to her fox friend, she enumerates the many ways in which she struggles in a neuronormative world: "Hände schütteln, versuchen Augenkontakt zu halten, auf das Gespräch zu konzentrieren …" ["Shake hands, try to maintain eye contact, focus on conversation"] (n.p). She explains that this process of suppressing her neurodivergence is exhausting. She "konnte … schon kaum [ihre] Gedanken sortieren" ["could barely organize [her] thoughts"] (2017, n.p); she was totally overstimulated ("Völlige Reizüberflutung") (n.p.). She then concludes aloud that "[d]ie Leute wissen überhaupt nicht, welche Kräfte ich als Autistin mobilisieren muss, um den Alltag zu überstehen" ["people don't know at all what strengths I have to mobilize as an autistic person to get through everyday life"] (n.p.).

Here, the fox interjects with admiration, observing that Schreiter clearly possesses a kind of superpower that not everyone is capable of. This, in turn, sets them off on their new adventure: as Autistic-Hero-Girl and Sidekick Superfox. On the subsequent pages, we witness Schreiter's protagonist overcoming obstacles, such as bureaucratic requirements for registering as a superhero, navigating the necessity for fine motor skills while designing and producing a costume, and avoiding small talk and phone calls. In each of these scenarios, Autistic-Hero-Girl is depicted in a situation that is designed for or benefits from neurotypical capacities. Each short comic thus demonstrates how neurodiverse individuals might struggle with what many neurotypical individuals consider the humdrum of daily life.

In the cartoon "Alltag," however, the reader sees the protagonist's true superpower on display. Surrounded by speech balloons from shadowy figures parroting many of the comments that individuals with ASD face daily: "Reiss dich zusammen!" ["Pull yourself together!"]; "Mich stört XY auch und ich bin kein Autist" ["XY also bothers me and I'm not autistic"]; "Du kannst doch normal sein, wenn du nur willst!" ["You could be normal if you wanted to be!"]; "Du bemühst dich nur nicht genug!" ["You just do not try hard enough!"]; "Du benutzt deinen Autismus doch nur als Ausrede!" ["You are just using your autism as an excuse!"] (n.p.). However, instead of avoiding confronting these problems, which is how the protagonist dealt with the issues presented to her and her sidekick before, we see the first panel of the short comic featuring the iconic onomatopoeia of the comics form: "Smash," "Bam!," "Pow!," and "Boom!" The team takes on biases directly and defeats the pretenses in a symbolic battle that concludes with a consideration of their impact on the lives of the ASD community: "Wenn wir unsere Kraft nicht für diesen Blödsinn aufwenden müssten, könnten wir uns um echte Probleme kümmern!" ["If we didn't have to spend our energy on this nonsense, we could take care of real problems!"] (n.p.).

Die Abenteuer von Autistic-Hero-Girl ultimately plays with reader expectations cultivated by supercrip narratives that neurodiversity itself might be reinterpreted as a superpower. Schreiter's protagonist, however, deconstructs these notions, offering a corrective to discourses of ability and disability in the superhero genre. Instead of her neurodiverse perception of the world offering her avenues for super-human feats, it is her ability to navigate a society constructed by and for neuronormativity that makes her a superhero. Her superpowers are thus her toolkit for navigating daily life (the premise of "Every-Day-Hero"), overcoming sensory overloads ("Overload-Overlord" and "Overload-Overlord (Nachspiel)"), and promoting awareness for ASD and invisible disabilities ("Inklusion" and "Reflektieren").

CONCLUSION

Grandin's 1986 autobiography, *Emergence: Labeled Autistic,* provided an unprecedented insider perspective on neurodivergent cognitive processes (Sacks 2008, xiii). For the first time ever, neurologist Oliver Sacks writes, autistic experience had a voice—and one that articulately pushed back on the *Rain Man* stereotype, offering insight into autistic ways of thinking, communication, and interpretation. However, explaining visual thinking through its very antithesis—words—presented an interesting conundrum. So, while Grandin's writing, which includes her later *Thinking in Pictures* (1995), certainly opened up an understanding of how some individuals on the autism spectrum process information, it did so in terms counterintuitive even to the author. Moreover, the countless scientific assessments and research studies on neurodivergent cognition that similarly attempt to explain the thought processes of individuals on the autism spectrum in writing alone are likewise insufficient in fully representing neurodivergent experience.

Comics, on the other hand, unite visual and verbal ways of thinking and self-expression. Through the combination of word and image, they are able to depict some of the complicated cognitive processes, conceptual relationships, and visual and literal thinking of some individuals with ASD, which, in turn, facilitates awareness, empathy, and understanding for neurodivergent experience.

According to the introduction to the *Graphic Medicine Manifesto* (2015), this is the power of comics in the discourses of the health sciences. Here, the authors argue that comics about illness and disability disrupt the balance of power: "We believe those best positioned to represent illness and caregiving are those living with it" (Czerwiec et al. 2015, 20). Graphic medicine thereby offers the stories of individuals, patients, family members, and healthcare professionals, giving voice to the marginalized lives of individuals living with illness, chronic disease, and disability in a way that both modern medicine and contemporary literature do not—by visualizing it. With regards to the autistic community, Schreiter and others have stepped up to do the work of visualizing a way into this world for diverse audiences, helping her readership understand neurodivergent ways of navigating ableist environments as well as familiarizing neurotypical individuals with autistic experience through an engagement with supercrip cultures and the artist's own thinking in pictures.

NOTES

1. Similarly, in the sense that concrete thinking is the mind's way to understand abstraction through reference to known objects, Schreiter's visualization of Dani's struggle to make sense of decorative patterns also applies here.
2. While autobiographical graphic narratives on autism spectrum disorder are rare (though Rees Finlay's *Reaffirmation: Coming to Terms with an Autism Diagnosis* (2019) and Bex Ollerton's *Sensory: Life on the Spectrum: An Autistic Comics Anthology* (2022) are two important recent examples), webcomics on ASD are less unusual. Rebecca Burgess' webcomic "Understanding the Spectrum," for example, went viral and has since been translated into Spanish, French, German, and Indonesian (https://the-art-of-autism.com/understanding-the-spectrum-a-comic-strip-explanation/).

WORKS CITED

Alaniz, José. 2014. *Death, Disability, and the Superhero: The Silver Age and Beyond*. Jackson: University Press of Mississippi.

Bystrova, Tatiana, Ludmila Tokarskaya, and Darko B. Vukovic. 2017. "Visual Perception Specifics of Shildren with ASD as a Determinant for Educational Environment Outlinetimes." *International Journal of Cognitive Research in Science, Engineering and Education* 5, no. 1: 75.

Carpenter, Rick. 2011. "Disability as Socio-Rhetorical Action: Towards a Genre-Based Approach." *Disability Studies Quarterly* 31, no. 3: n.p.

Czerwiec, MK, et al. 2015. *Graphic Medicine Manifesto*. University Park: Penn State University Press.

Dodd, Susan. 2005. *Understanding Autism*. Sydney: Elsevier.

Grandin, Temple and Margaret Scariano. 1986. *Emergence: Labeled Autistic*. Novato, CA: Arena Press.

Grandin, Temple. 1995. In *Learning and Cognition in Autism: Current Issues in Autism*, edited by E. Schopler and G. B. Mesibov, 137–156. Boston: Springer.

Grandin, Temple. 2008. *Thinking in Pictures, Expanded Edition: My Life with Autism*. New York: Vintage.

Grandin, Temple. 2009. "How Does Visual Thinking Work in the Mind of a Person with Autism? A Personal Account." *Philosophical Transactions of the Royal Society B: Biological Sciences* 364, no. 1522: 1437–1442.

Hosseini, S. A. and M. Molla. 2022. "Asperger Syndrome." In StatPearls [Internet], n.p. Treasure Island: StatPearls Publishing.

Kent, Annie. 2023. "Autism Advocacy: Inclusion, Empowerment, and Human Rights." *Autism Spektrum News*. Winter Issue. https://autismspectrumnews.org/autism-advocacy-inclusion-empowerment-and-human-rights/.

Mirkovic, B. and P. Gérardin. 2019. "Asperger's Syndrome: What to Consider?" *L'Encéphale* 45.2: 169–174.

Sacks, Oliver, "Foreword." 2008. In *Thinking in Pictures, Expanded Edition: My Life with Autism* by Temple Grandin, xiii–xviii. New York: Vintage.

Shapiro, J. P. 1994. *No Pity: People with Disabilities Forging a New Civil Rights Movement*. New York: Random House.

Schreiter, Daniela. 2014. *Schattenspringer: Wie es ist, anders zu sein*. Hamburg: Panini Comics.

Schreiter, Daniela. 2017. *Die Abenteuer von Autistic-Hero-Girl*. Hamburg: Panini.

Schreiter, Daniela. 2015. *Schattenspringer: Per Anhalter durch die Pubertät*. Hamburg: Panini.

Schreiter, Daniela. 2018. *Schattenspringer: Spektralfarben*. Vol. 3. Hamburg: Panini.

Wolk, Douglas. 2008. *Reading Comics: How Graphic Novels Work and What They Mean*. Boston: Da Capo Press.

PART III

Disability

CHAPTER NINE

Disability = *Behinderung*? The Conceptual History of a Social Category in Germany from a Disability Studies Perspective

ANNE WALDSCHMIDT

INTRODUCTION[1]

When it comes to disability, German discourses tend to be rather idiosyncratic. This applies both to the conceptual history of the term *disability*—or, in German, *Behinderung*[2]—and to the respective academic fields. For example, there is no equivalent translation for either *Heilpädagogik* [curative or remedial pedagogy] or *Sonderpädagogik* [special needs pedagogy], which are the traditional disciplines that claim to treat and educate children with disabilities as their domain and whose roots go back to the late nineteenth and early twentieth centuries. While two other fields, *Soziale Arbeit* [social work] and *Rehabilitationswissenschaft* [rehabilitation sciences] that also provide relevant knowledge for persons with disabilities[3] and their families, are known in other countries as well, the new interdisciplinary *Teilhabeforschung* [participation research] does not translate adequately in English either. This is all the more remarkable as the latter branch of research was introduced in the 2010s with explicit reference to the United Nations' Convention on the Rights of Persons with Disabilities (UN CRPD). To cut a long story short, in Germany there is a whole host of "medicalized applied fields" (Linton 1998, 525) that claim competence for *Behinderung*. At the same time, these "Not Disability Studies" (ibid.) imply that disability exists as a fact, and they tend to deny or ignore that disability is a social category in need of explication and critical reflection.

The international field of Disability Studies, however, has also developed and flourished in German-speaking countries over the past decades (for an overview see Brehme 2020; Köbsell/Waldschmidt 2006; Pfahl/Powell 2014; Waldschmidt 2020; 2022; Waldschmidt/Berressem/Ingwersen 2017; Waldschmidt/Karim 2022). It postulates that *Behinderung* is a social, political, and cultural phenomenon characterized by stigmatization, deviation, and otherness. As a driver for new analytical perspectives, Disability Studies takes as its starting point the contingency of difference, interrogating the historically, culturally, and socially specific understandings from which the notion of disability arises. In German-speaking contexts, Disability Studies thus always involves a critical inquiry of disability, ability, and impairment (Klein 2022; Waldschmidt 2019).[4]

This essay draws on Disability Studies in this sense and intends to examine the German term *Behinderung* by applying different angles. First, the etymology of the word and its current usage are considered. Second, it traces the *Begriffsgeschichte* [conceptual history] and describes how this simple word has developed into an indicator for human difference and a distinct category relevant for social policy that leads to the recognition of a need for assistance and a resulting entitlement to social benefits. Third, recent trends in *Behinderung* related discourses are discussed, and current debates about language and politically correct words are addressed.

As there are still major gaps in research in all these areas, it is not possible to cover the entire spectrum of German-language contexts. For one, the countries of Austria, Switzerland, Luxembourg, and Liechtenstein must be passed over. The following attempt of tracing the genealogy of *Behinderung* concentrates on Germany, and specifically on West Germany, during the period 1949–89.

ETYMOLOGY AND CURRENT USAGE

From an etymological perspective, *Behinderung* is a nominalization of the verb *behindern* [to hinder] and synonymous with words such as *Hindernis* [hindrance] or *Blockade* [blockade, barrier].

First, a look at the *Deutsches Wörterbuch* [German Dictionary] written in the 1830s by the brothers Jacob (1785–1863) and Wilhelm (1786–1859) Grimm, the world-famous philologists and publishers of children's stories and folktales, substantiates this reading. In the first volume of their German-language lexicon, the following definition is given for *behindern*: "verhindern: wart ich daran behindert" [to impede: I was prevented (*behindert*) from doing so]. A second example phrase conveys a similar meaning: "um uns das vorrücken zu behindern" [to prevent (*behindern*) our advance] (Grimm and Grimm 1854, 1341). The entry for the noun *Behinderung* offers only a brief elucidation: "Häusliche Behinderung" [domestic hindrance] (ibid.). All these examples share that they do not fit into the current understanding of disability as a separate social category.

Second, more than 160 years later, the electronic version of the *Duden*, the authoritative German-language dictionary since 1880, gives various definitions for the noun *Behinderung* and the verb *behindern* (Duden Online 2018, n.p.). The following definition is provided for *behindern*: "jemandem, einer Sache hinderlich, im Wege sein; hemmen, störend aufhalten" [to make something difficult for somebody, to be in the way; to hamper, to prevent something in a disruptive manner] (ibid.). Example usages include "die Verletzung behindert ihn" [he is hampered (*behindert*) by the injury], "Nebel behinderte die freie Sicht" [the view was obstructed (*behindert*) by the fog], "den Gegenspieler durch Festhalten behindern" [to impede (*behindern*) one's opponent by holding them down], "sich [gegenseitig] behindern/(gehoben): einander behindern" [to impede (*behindern*) each other (elevated usage)], and "behinderndes Parken" [disruptive (*behinderndes*) parking] (ibid.).

Two possible meanings are given for *Behinderung*: "das Behindern; das Behindertwerden" [the act of impeding or being impeded] and "etwas, was jemanden behindert" [something that functions as an impediment] (ibid.). The list of synonyms is particularly telling (ibid.): *Beeinträchtigung* [impairment], *Erschwerung* [restriction], *Hemmung* [constraint], *Hinderung* [hindrance], *Komplizierung* [difficulty], *Störung* [disruption], *Unterdrückung* [oppression], *Verkomplizierung* [complication], *Verzögerung* [setback], *Obstruktion* [obstruction] (scholarly usage), *Barriere* [barrier], *Erschwernis* [obstacle], *Fesseln* [shackle], *Handicap* [handicap], *Hemmnis* [restraint], *Hemmschuh* [inhibition], *Hindernis* [impediment], *Hürde* [hurdle], *Schwierigkeit* [challenge], *Stolperstein* [stumbling block], *Widerstand* [resistance], *Klotz am Bein* [a ball and chain] (colloquial).

The Grimms' dictionary indicates that until the middle of the nineteenth century, the meanings of the noun *Behinderung* and the verb *behindern* in the German context were largely concrete and not used in a figurative sense. It also seems that the adjective form was more common than the noun. Present trends, as illustrated by *Duden Online*, favor the verb for concrete uses, while the noun, with its many synonyms, often refers to various impairments.

Even if a comprehensive overview is still lacking, studies in Disability History (see, e.g., Diehl/Hansen 2017; Fuchs 2012; 2022; Poore 2007; Schmuhl 2007; 2010) have shown that from before the Middle Ages through the end of the nineteenth century, neither the word *Behinderung* as an indicator of physical, psychological, or cognitive difference nor the word *Behinderte* as name for the classified persons existed in the German language. In its place were various other designations, such as *Blinde* [blind persons], *Epileptische* [epileptic persons], *Idioten* [idiots], *Invalide* [invalids], *Irre* [lunatics], *Krüppel* [cripples], *Schwachsinnige* [imbeciles], and *Taubstumme* [deaf-mutes]. These terms made reference to specific impairments and abnormalities; they functioned, on the one hand, as objective descriptors but also, on the other, as highly discriminatory and demeaning designations. It was not until the rise of late modern society, particularly at the turn of the twentieth century, that a change took place in the way that these limitations and differences were labeled and conceptualized.

In this context, the word *Behinderung* has experienced a remarkable career. In everyday speech, it still has a variety of meanings, many of which are general in nature and do not immediately call to mind a category of human difference. At the same time, the use of *Behinderung* in contemporary German frequently suggests precisely such an association. The so-called word clouds[5] found on *Duden Online* point to precisely this narrowing of meanings in current linguistic practice (Duden Online 2018, n.p.). These computer-generated statistical models show the contexts in which specific vocabulary is favored and used most often. Looking at the word clouds for *Behinderung*, one notices that adjectives (such as bodily, emotional, mental, and difficult), verbs (such as live, suffer, and disadvantage), and nouns (such as impairment, dependency, illness, and age) shape much of the linguistic environment in which *Behinderung* exists today (ibid.).[6]

In sum, we can see that a diverse array of figurative connotations has developed around the word *Behinderung*, but also that the term's connections to health conditions and bodily attributes are the strongest. In addition, the current list of *Behinderung*'s synonyms [impairment, disorder, handicap] indicates that the vocabulary is used increasingly as a means of differentiating between people. In short, the word's literal meaning—a hindrance, blockade, or barrier—which was still dominant during the nineteenth century, has now clearly faded into the background.

NINETEENTH AND EARLY TWENTIETH CENTURY

How did this linguistic practice develop? In the following, the research findings on this question (e.g., Fuchs 2022; Schmuhl 2007; 2010) can only be presented in summarized form. They offer the following insights: During the course of the nineteenth century, terms such as *Idioten* [idiots], *Schwachsinnige* [feeble-minded persons], and *Schwachbegabte* [retarded persons] became commonplace when describing people who would later come to be labeled as "mentally handicapped," and who refer to themselves today as "individuals with learning difficulties" (Leidmedien.de 2023, n.p.). In the case of sensory impairments, terms such as *Blinde* [blind persons] or *Taubstumme* [deaf-mute persons] (hearing impaired or D/deaf,[7] in modern parlance) were common in earlier periods. Those with perceptible physical abnormalities were referred to as *Krüppel* [cripples].

After the birth of the German welfare state, i.e., the introduction of mandatory social insurance for illness (1883), work-related accidents (1884), old age, and invalidity (1889) in the German Empire, the so-called *Krüppelfürsorge* [literally: cripple care] emerged at the beginning of the twentieth century (Osten 2004; Thomann 1995; 2000). This program dates back to the Berlin-based pediatrician, surgeon, and orthopedist Konrad Biesalski (1868–1930), who was convinced that *Krüppel* could be "healed" and transformed from "Almosenempfängern zu Steuerzahlern" ["alms recipients to taxpayers"] (Fuchs 2012, 136). His *orthopädische Krüppelfürsorge* [orthopedic cripple care] treated physical impairment as a social and economic problem to be addressed or even resolved through medical treatment, vocational training, and inpatient care of affected individuals. The main focus of Biesalski's approach lay on the restoration of bodily function and, in turn, individual self-sufficiency and the ability to work that was connected to it.

In 1906, the *Reichskrüppelzählung*, the first national census of "crippled" persons, was conducted in Prussia, which actually focused on *jugendliche Krüppel* [crippled youth]; the results indicated that the majority of young people with physical impairments lived in poverty (Thomann 2000). On this occasion, as a tool for data collection, the word *Krüppel* [cripple] came to be defined as "ein in dem Gebrauch seines Rumpfes oder seiner Gliedmassen *behinderter* Kranker" ["an individual afflicted by an illness *hindering* the use of his torso or limbs"] (Biesalski 1911, 13; emphasis mine). It was here that *behindert*—in its adjective form—made its entry into the vocabulary of demographic statistics and social policy. However, as shown above, *Krüppelfürsorge* did not focus on people who were *behindert*, but on "cripples," despite the increasingly pejorative usage of this term as early as 1900.

WEIMAR REPUBLIC (1919–33)

As shown above, the adjective *behindert* was introduced into German disability-related discourse in the early 1900s, but it was not until the 1920s that its use became gradually more common. Initially, *behindert* appeared typically in combination with words such as *körperlich* [physical, bodily] or *Körper* [body], which limited its application to a broad spectrum of impairments. This usage was promoted by the *Bund zur Förderung der Selbsthilfe der körperlich Behinderten* [League for the Promotion of the Self-Help of the Physically Disabled] (Fuchs 2001). Founded in Berlin in 1919, this organization saw itself as an advocate for physically disabled persons, who were born with impairments or had acquired them in early life. Its activists considered the term *Krüppel* to be demeaning and proposed the nominalization of the adjective *(körperlich) behindert* [(physically) disabled] in its place. They hoped to gain greater social recognition by using this new, seemingly neutral term.

At the same time, *Krüppel* continued to dominate the official language of Weimar's welfare policies (Fuchs 2001, 20–65; Schmuhl 2010, 50–60). In 1920, the *Preußisches Krüppelfürsorgegesetz* [Prussian Cripple Welfare Act] came into effect; clearly built on Biesalski's work, it defined *Verkrüppelung* as a significant impairment of an individual's "Erwerbsfähigkeit auf dem allgemeinen Arbeitsmarkte" ["ability to earn a living on the general labor market"], stemming from "nicht nur vorübergehenden" [non-transitory] limitations to the "Gebrauch von Rumpf oder Gliedmaßen" ["use of the torso and the limbs"] (Osten 2004, 220). In the same year, social policy support for wounded soldiers as well as those afflicted by occupational and other injuries was expanded. The term *Krüppel* was largely avoided in this context; the target group of victims of war and occupation-related accidents was referred to as gravely injured persons and the *Schwerbeschädigtengesetz* [Federal Assistance Act for the Gravely Injured] was enacted specifically for them.

NATIONAL SOCIALIST DICTATORSHIP (1933–45)

In the time of German fascism, when the concept of "racial hygiene" wielded significant influence in national politics, individuals with disabilities were often subject to the so-called *Vernichtung lebensunwertem Leben* [extermination of lives not worth living]; these measures included forced sterilization, gruesome experiments, and, within the framework of Aktion T4, a systematic mass-murder campaign, referred to by the euphemism "euthanasia" and directed mainly against disabled people living in institutions (Schmuhl 1987). Simultaneously, the adjective *behindert* appeared for the first time in the state's official legal language.

The *Gesetz über die Vereinheitlichung des Gesundheitswesens* [National Healthcare Standardization Act] of 1934 defined "körperlich Behinderte" [physically disabled individuals] as a group whose care had been transferred to the national health authorities (Schmuhl 2010, 68). In addition, the *Reichsschulpflichtgesetz* [National Compulsory Schooling Act] of 1938 introduced a new section 6, entitled "Schulpflicht geistig und körperlich behinderter Kinder" ["compulsory schooling for mentally and physically disabled children"], which imposed a national regulation requiring all disabled children to attend a specialized school (ibid., 72). Section 3 of the same act made it possible to hold back children, "die geistig und körperlich nicht genügend entwickelt sind, um mit Erfolg am Unterricht teilzunehmen" ["who exhibit insufficient mental and physical development to participate successfully in classroom instruction"] (Edelstein/Veith 2017, 1217). Stigmatized with the inability to learn and be educated, countless children were segregated into so-called "Sammelklassen" [classes reserved for children seen as ineducable] (ibid., 1216) and residential homes.

In its social and educational policies, the National Socialist regime probably used *Behinderung*, as it was a rather abstract term and easier to apply to large groups of people than impairment-specific vocabulary was. Moreover, *Krüppel* and *Idioten*, who were considered as inferior and largely useless, were deliberately differentiated from *Behinderte*, whose education was seen as possible and for whom effort was deemed worthwhile, because they were likely to succeed on the labor market. After the notion *Behinderung* had found its way into the vocabulary of healthcare and education, it quickly began to appear in other fields as well, such as special needs pedagogy. It was also increasingly applied to greater numbers of impaired persons, making it a collective term—albeit one without clear borders.

GERMANY DIVIDED: 1945 THROUGH THE 1960S

After the end of the Second World War, the Allied occupation (1945–9), and the founding of the Federal Republic of Germany (FRG) and the German Democratic Republic (GDR) in 1949, language usage began to split in different directions, determined to a large extent by the opposing ideologies of the two German states.

While the term *Schädigung* [injury, damage, impairment] was preferred in the GDR, and the development of a "sozialistische Persönlichkeit" [socialist personality] was seen as the official goal of so-called *Rehabilitationspädagogik* [rehabilitation pedagogy] (Barsch 2016, 192–193), FRG specialists in social welfare, orthopedics, and *Heil-* and *Sonderpädagogik* [curative and special needs pedagogy] continued to use the term *Krüppel* well into the 1950s. As in the 1920s, this practice was met with criticism from disability advocacy organizations, which preferred the term *Behinderung*. "[V]on der Verbannung des Wortes 'Krüppel' aus der Fach-, Amts- und Umgangssprache" ["From the banishment of the word 'cripple' from technical, official, and everyday language"] they hoped for a "Statusaufwertung" ["an elevation of social status"] and a closer proximity to the comparatively privileged *Kriegsbeschädigte* [gravely injured war veterans]. They also sought "eine deutliche Abgrenzung" ["a clear distancing"] from people with mental disabilities or psychological disorders (Schmuhl 2010, 85).

In the FRG, victims of war and occupational accidents continued to be referred to as *Schwerbeschädigte* [the gravely injured]; the former *Schwerbeschädigtengesetz* [Federal Assistance Act for the Gravely Injured] from the Weimar Republic was reinstated for them in

1953. In contrast, those who were born with impairments or had acquired them later in life and had not suffered war or occupational injuries continued to be subject to poverty law, which in Germany was called *Armenfürsorge* [poor relief]. In the late 1950s the aforementioned *Preußisches Krüppelfürsorgegesetz* [Prussian Cripple Welfare Act], which also dated from the Weimar Republic, was amended, and this time the voices of disability advocacy organizations were actually heard. To counter their criticism of the pejorative term *Krüppel*, the legislature now chose *Körperbehindertengesetz* [Act for the Physically Disabled] as the new name for the law. It was enacted in 1957, but remained in force for only a few years. In 1961, this law was integrated into the *Bundessozialhilfegesetz* [Federal Social Assistance Act] (BSHG) as part of a comprehensive social policy reform.

The BSHG included the so-called *Eingliederungshilfe für Behinderte* [Integration support for the disabled] as a subsection of *Hilfen in besonderen Lebenslagen* [Assistance for special circumstances] (Rößler 2022; Rudloff 2019). The *Eingliederungshilfe für Behinderte* primarily addressed the needs of disabled children and their families, when no other forms of private or public assistance were available. Within this revised legal framework of social welfare, the concept *Behinderung* remained ambiguous and largely tautological: Those considered *behindert* were those with significant impairments. At the same time, though, the BHSG played a driving role in the incorporation of *Behinderung* into legal parlance as well as in its dissemination into other discourses and fields of practice. From the 1960s, the term was increasingly used to refer to disabled persons [*die Behinderten*] as a social group.

WEST GERMANY (1969–99)

For the history of the concept *Behinderung* in West Germany, the political reforms in the late 1960s and early 1970s were also of great importance (Bösl 2009). After two decades of conservative governments, the Social Democratic Party of Germany (SPD) came to the helm for the first time. In his first parliamentary statement as the new Chancellor, Willy Brandt explicitly spoke of "Alte, Kranke, körperlich oder geistig Behinderte" ["the elderly, the sick, and the physically or mentally disabled"], who "in ihrer Not nicht nur materielle Unterstützung, sondern auch menschliche Solidarität brauchen" ["in their distress need not only material support but also human solidarity"] (Brandt 1969, 3). He went on to call for the comprehensive integration of disabled individuals: "Wir werden [...] besonders für die Mitbürger sorgen, die trotz Hochkonjunktur und Vollbeschäftigung im Schatten leben müssen [...]. Die Bundesregierung wird um verstärkte Maßnahmen bemüht sein, die den Benachteiligten und Behinderten in Beruf und Gesellschaft, wo immer dies möglich ist, Chancen eröffnen" ["We will take special care of our fellow citizens who, despite economic prosperity and a booming job market, must live in the shadows. The federal government will take measures, wherever possible, to open up occupational and societal opportunities for the disadvantaged and disabled"] (ibid., 24–25).

With the *Schwerbehindertengesetz* [Federal Act for the Severely Disabled] of 1974, which supplanted the *Schwerbeschädigtengesetz* of 1953, *Behinderung*, or *Schwerbehinderung* [severe disability], was redefined. In the course of modernizing the rehabilitation system, the old "causality principle" was replaced by an orientation toward "finality:" It was no longer the origin of the impairments—for instance, war injury, accident at work, "birth defect," or domestic accident—that mattered but the fact that chronic health problems existed in the first place. Whether physical, mental, or psychological, the fact of an impairment warranted sociopolitical aid and support (Rößler 2022, 189–190). With this development, the hierarchical valuation and grading of various impairments became less common; subsequently the term *Schwerbeschädigung* [grave injury] fell out of use.

At the same time, disability was conceptualized in social policy as *Minderung der Erwerbsfähigkeit* [reduction in earning capacity]—or, in its more neutral formulation in the 1986 amendment to the *Schwerbehindertengesetz*, the so-called *Grad der Behinderung* [degree of impairment]. In order to obtain legal recognition and an official disability status, individuals had to undergo a medical examination. The physician's report was the basis for the administrative decision that there was "ein *regelwidriger* körperlicher, geistiger oder seelischer *Zustand*" ["an *abnormal* physical, mental, or psychological *state*"] which could not be attributed to age and lasted at least six months (Der Bundesminister der Justiz 1986, 1423; emphasis mine).[8]

With the broadening of access to rehabilitation services to include those who were not yet disabled but—perhaps due to a chronic illness—were at risk of becoming disabled, the spectrum of the target group was also expanded. Thus, on the one hand, the use of rehabilitation services became "normal" in the statistical sense, but on the other hand those labeled as *Behinderte* [the disabled] remained a marginalized group. Ultimately, the concept *(Schwer-)Behinderung* [(severe) disability] became something of a "Universalkategorie" [universal category] (Lindmeier 1993, 28), finding widespread use not only in social law but also in science, the mass media, and everyday culture.

At the end of the 1970s, the disability rights movement emerged in West Germany (Fischer 2019; Lingelbach/Stoll 2013; Stoll 2017). Its strands included, among others, the local *Clubs Behinderter und ihre Freunde* [Clubs of the Disabled and Their Friends], which sought to promote the social integration of disabled persons, as well as the *Krüppelgruppen* [Cripple Groups], which had a decidedly radical and critical orientation. In contrast to the clubs, the groups formed the *Krüppelbewegung* [Cripple Movement] and consisted exclusively of persons with disabilities—anyone who did not self-identify as disabled was not welcome (Mürner/Sierck 2009; Köbsell 2012; 2022). They resorted to the old term *Krüppel*, transforming it into a provocative means of self-stigmatization that called attention to the persistent exclusion of and discrimination against people with disabilities. The activists also criticized the prevailing concept of "integration" at the time, problematizing the fact that it frequently consisted of some half-hearted, patronizing attempts to initiate social contact between people with and without disabilities, while social distance, prejudices, denigration, and institutionalization, in short, exclusion continued. With their formulation of their own *Krüppelstandpunkt* [cripple perspective] (Köbsell 2022, 57) and their early insistence on self-advocacy and a critical stance in relation to mainstream society, their positions resembled those of the early disability rights movements in Britain and the United States.

After its first phase in the 1980s, which was characterized by substantive debates and attention-grabbing protest events, the West German disability rights movement shifted its focus to fostering mutual support and addressing everyday problems (Mürner/Sierck 2009; Köbsell 2012). Activities ranged from creating opportunities for personal assistance, ensuring mobility, and removing barriers to establishing centers for self-determined living. These self-organized services were oriented toward the principle of *Betroffenenberatung* [peer counseling] as well as the concept of independent living, taking their inspiration from the American disability rights movement.

Following Germany's reunification, in 1990, the country entered a new phase of disability policy (Welti 2019), during which disability advocacy organizations also emerged in the former GDR. At the same time, efforts to achieve equal rights and to combat discrimination continued to gain ground. In 1994, the German disability rights movement effected an amendment to the *Grundgesetz*, the German constitution (Grundgesetz, n.d.; Welti 2019, 20–21). The *Bundestag* [Federal Parliament] and *Bundesrat* [Federal Council] ratified the addition of the sentence "Niemand darf wegen seiner Behinderung benachteiligt werden" ["No person shall be disfavoured because of disability"][9] to paragraph 3 of Article 3 "Equality before the law" of the *Grundgesetz*, thus establishing a constitutional right to equality for disabled persons. In 2002, the *Behindertengleichstellungsgesetz* [Equality act for the disabled] additionally came into effect at the federal level, and was followed by similar laws in the sixteen *Bundesländer* [states] over the ensuing years (Welti 2019, 22–23).

REUNIFIED GERMANY IN THE 2000s

In the early 2000s, German activists were increasingly influential on the international stage, playing a leading role in the development of the already mentioned UN CRPD. Even before the enactment of this disability rights convention by the UN General Assembly, in 2006, however, reunified Germany experienced yet another wave of sweeping disability rights reforms (Rößler 2022).

In 2001, the *Schwerbehindertengesetz* of 1974, which had been amended in 1986, underwent a complete revision, yielding the *Sozialgesetzbuch für die Rehabilitation und Teilhabe von Menschen mit Behinderungen* [Social Code Book for the Rehabilitation and Participation of Persons (individuals, people) with Disabilities] (hereafter SGB IX). The new law was also accompanied by a new definition of the term *Behinderung*. Section 2(1) of the SGB IX stated: "Menschen sind behindert, wenn ihre körperliche Funktion, geistige Fähigkeit oder seelische Gesundheit mit hoher Wahrscheinlichkeit länger als sechs Monate von dem für das Lebensalter typischen Zustand abweichen und daher ihre Teilhabe am Leben in der Gesellschaft beeinträchtigt ist" ["Individuals are disabled when their bodily function, mental capacity, or psychological health deviate from the condition typical for their age, when this condition is predicted to last longer than six months, and therefore their participation in society is impaired"] (SGB IX Alte Fassung 2017, n.p.). This formulation, which remained in effect until 2017, made no mention of the earlier *regelwidriger Zustand* [abnormal state] and thus reflected an attempt to loosen normative dimensions and to acknowledge the decisive role of society in shaping the living situations of persons with disabilities.

A few years later, the influence of international politics also became more apparent. Germany's signing of the UN CRPD (2007) and subsequent ratification of it (2009) were important milestones in disability policy that have since guided the national debate and the shaping processes in politics and law (UN-Behindertenrechtskonvention 2017; United Nations, n.d.). This international document also represents a key step in modernizing the concept of disability. The wording of the UN CRPD deliberately avoids a narrow definition; instead, the Preamble sets forth that "disability is an evolving concept and [...] results from the interaction between persons with impairments and attitudinal and environmental barriers that hinders their full and effective participation in society on an equal basis with others" (UN CRPD, Preamble e). In addition, Article 1 lays out that "persons with disabilities include those who have long-term physical, mental, intellectual or sensory impairments" (ibid., Article 1). These formulations help to understand disability as a dynamic process and emphasize the complex interplay of impairments and barriers that lead to disability. Additionally, they acknowledge that people can be affected by a variety of "dis-abling" circumstances at different times, in different situations, and in different ways.

The challenge of defining the term disability is that while countries like Germany have signed and, indeed, ratified the UN CRPD, thereby accepting it as legally binding framework, these same countries additionally have laws and regulations that define disability in very narrow, static, and even medical terms. Nevertheless, in the case of Germany there has been a trend in recent years to suspend strict definitions of *Behinderung* in national discourse, suggesting that international developments can and do have a considerable impact on a country's conception of disability.

As a final milestone—at least for now—in the history of *Behinderung* comes yet another reformulation of disability law in the mid-2010s, one that appears almost identical to the definition put forth in the UN CRPD. Section 2(1) of the current SGB IX offers the following definition of the target group: "Menschen mit Behinderungen sind Menschen, die körperliche, seelische, geistige oder Sinnesbeeinträchtigungen haben, die sie in Wechselwirkung mit einstellungs- und umweltbedingten Barrieren an der gleichberechtigten Teilhabe an der Gesellschaft mit hoher Wahrscheinlichkeit länger als sechs Monate hindern können. Eine Beeinträchtigung nach Satz 1 liegt vor, wenn der Körper- und Gesundheitszustand von dem für das Lebensalter typischen Zustand abweicht" ["Persons with disabilities are those who have physical, mental, intellectual or sensory impairments which—in interaction with attitudinal and environmental barriers—hinder their participation in society on an equal basis with others for a period of longer than six months. An impairment in the sense of sentence 1 is present if a person's bodily state or health condition deviates from the condition typical for their age"] (Sozialgesetzbuch Neuntes Buch 2022, n.p.).

This definition reads like an echo of both the UN CRPD's Preamble and Article 1 in English and the Convention's official German-language translation (UN-Behindertenrechtskonvention 2017), which was prepared and agreed upon in a joint effort by Austria, Germany, Liechtenstein, and Switzerland. In Germany today, the presence of barriers and the interaction between an individual and their environment, the deviation from the condition typical for a person's age, a duration of more than six months, and difficulties to participate in society on an equal footing are now recognized parameters of *Behinderung*. Compared to the 2001 version, the new regulations not only show continuity, given that the old components of the definition are retained, but also a willingness to innovate, as evidenced by the consideration of attitudinal and environmental barriers and the emphasis on equal participation in society, both of which stem from the UN CRPD. As a result, the interactions between individuals, their living conditions, and positions in society have become significantly more important in German disability policy and discourse.

BEHINDERUNG IN THE PRESENT: TRENDS

From the above discussion, we can conclude that *Behinderung* has had a long history as a marker of difference and social category in the German-language context. This has been accompanied by a gradual and continuous change in meaning. The following five trends can be observed in the concept's more recent history.

First, barriers and environmental factors have made marked gains in significance and recognition. The emphasis on medical factors, conversely, has gradually moved into the background—without becoming completely irrelevant, however—and has been replaced by a focus on societal participation. Put another way, instead of viewing disability as a purely "natural" phenomenon, there is increasing acceptance of the condition as "social" and as subject to continuous construction and reinterpretation. There is now also a consensus that the question of "nature versus nurture"—that is, whether disability is best understood in terms of heredity and pathology or as the result of environmental and sociocultural factors—can ultimately not be answered.

Second, considerable effort has been made toward a neutral terminology that avoids pejorative connotations as much as possible. While historical discourse made frequent use of terms such as *Krüppel* [cripple], *Invalidität* [invalidity], *Schwerbeschädigung* [grave injury], and *Regelwidrigkeit* [irregularity, abnormality], recent debates have centered on avoiding normative language and recognizing the necessity of inclusion and participation. As a result, three different approaches to disability can currently be observed. On the one hand, there is the normalization approach, which involves a growing awareness of the need to avoid labeling disability as a deviation from norms and "a diminished state of being human" (Campbell 2009, 16). Instead, it emphasizes that we should acknowledge the fact that impairment and vulnerability are essential parts of the human condition. However, "full" normalcy on an equal footing with others continues to feel out of reach for persons with disabilities. Problematization as another approach is also frequently used because it serves to consider disability as a "social problem" (Groenemeyer 2014), in other words, as a means to justify the provision of welfare services for disabled individuals. Further, the strategy of neutralization stands out as an additional option. From this perspective, *Behinderung* can be understood as a category of difference that gives "deviations" attributed to health, body, mind, psyche or behavior "einen begrenzten legitimen Platz" ["a limited legitimate place"], but "ohne sie zur dauerhaften 'Normalität' werden zu lassen" ["does not allow them to be absorbed into 'normalcy' in the long run"] (Stehr 2013, 195). Although neutralization seems to be a current approach along with problematization and normalization, one must concede that *Behinderung* is still a stigma in everyday life, and the adjective *behindert* continues to be used as a swearword—especially by young persons when they want to insult each other.[10]

Third, there has been a decided push toward "Ausweitung der Behinderungszone" ["widening the zone of disability"] (Felkendorff 2003, 25). More and more groups have been included in this zone by adding further forms of impairment, which, moreover, are not precisely defined: first physically perceptible differences, such as paraplegia, and sensory impairments, such as blindness and D/deafness, followed by cognitive impairments, and finally, long-term mental illnesses—all of which are now subsumed under the generic term *(Schwer-)Behinderung* [(severe) disability]. The UN CRPD provides guidance for the future here by expanding the definition of disability to allow for future additions: for example, individuals grappling with addiction, those who identify as intersex, or those who are overweight.

Fourth, the line between disability and non-disability has become more and more elastic over time. The core of this differentiation is ultimately, it seems, the distinction between the "normal" and the "non-normal" (Link 2006; Waldschmidt 2009). There are two ways of thinking in this context. The first assumes that there is a qualitative difference between disability and normalcy, and that this difference can be clearly defined and diagnosed in medical, psychiatric, or psychological terms. From this perspective, the conception of disability as a marker of deviation or abnormality is justified. The other position advocates for a field of gradual differentiation in which the conditions traditionally labeled as disabilities may well belong to the spectrum of the normal. Thus, it acknowledges that these conditions have different effects depending on situational and functional circumstances and on the different phases of life or also in the interplay with other (e.g. gender- or age-specific) attributes. Looking back, we can see, especially in light of the UN CRPD, that the latter perspective, which asserts the permeability of the boundary between the "normal" and the "non-normal," has been quite successful in gaining acceptance in official politics—even if it remains unclear whether this will also be the case in the long term. Moreover, everyday language still seems rather hesitant to accept or even embrace the widening of the disability field. In any case, if there is a danger that the entire "normal field" will break apart in the case of too great an expansion, there may again be a shift toward rigidity—toward "ein *Einziehen* […], *Festklopfen*, *Verdicken* der Normalitätsgrenze zu einer neuerlichen *Stigma*-Grenze" ["a renewed *stigma boundary*, through *a constriction* (…), a *hardening*, and a *thickening* of the boundary that demarcates the normal"] (Link 2006, 356–357; author's emphasis).

Fifth, practices of universalization and worldwide standardization of disability terminology can be observed. As disability has become the subject of international politics and the United Nations has developed its own terminology with the UN CRPD, a process has been set in motion that makes persons with disabilities a global category (Bennani/Müller 2018). The United Nations' Convention has created a common starting point for categorizing and grouping individuals with impairments on a global level. One possible effect of these universalization efforts could be a move toward homogenization. Practices and experiences of being and becoming disabled, which have so far functioned very differently in various cultures, societies, regions, and countries, will possibly converge in the future. It remains to be seen to what extent this development, which is certainly also to be viewed critically, will prove constructive. Good or bad, however, the influence of the global norms resulting from the UN CRPD is already evident in Germany's reformulation of its legal language to accord with international standards.

BEHINDERUNG VS. *DISABILITY*

As a result of the above-mentioned trends, as well as the increased prominence of the English language in disability-related discourses, such as Disability Studies, the use of the word *disability* in the German context has become more widespread, at least among researchers and activists. However, even though the terms are generally understood as synonyms from a definitional perspective, it is important to highlight the etymological and connotative differences of *Behinderung* and *disability*.

While the German *Behinderung* implies a process—namely, that of *behindert werden* [being impeded], with the nominalization pointing to the evolution of this process into a permanent and seemingly unalterable condition—the English *disability* arises from the negation of functioning, i.e., the ascription of *inability*. Thus, while in the English context, those with disabilities are seen as lacking certain (cap)abilities, the German *Behinderung* connotates relationships that are hindered by specific actions, whether it is a relation between an individual and their environment (in which concrete barriers may be present) or a social relationship (in the sense of two or more people interacting). In comparison to its English counterpart, the German *Behinderung* tends to include external factors and processes of hindrance in its definition. This is because barriers, obstacles, and limitations can only exist in the context of relationships, either between individuals and their surroundings or between several individuals. In other words, the development of *Behinderung* as a concept has by now come nearly full circle, that is, back to the roots of its etymology, the literal meaning of *Hindernis* [hindrance] or *Blockade* [blockade, barrier].

Comparing the German and English terms supports the idea that *Behinderung* is actually more closely aligned with the ideas of the disability rights movement and the UN CRPD than *disability* is, taking into account its literal meaning. Instead of adopting *disability* into German, then, it might be useful to consider *Behinderung* as a potentially relevant term for international discourse. It bears emphasizing at this point, however, that the history of the two words has not yet been fully explored. In particular, there is a lack of comparative studies in different linguistic and cultural contexts.

THE POLITICS OF NAMING

The next section of this essay takes a brief look at recent developments in the story of *Behinderung*, which have been marked by debates about "the power of naming" (Zola 1993, 167). When talking about *Behinderung* and addressing persons with disabilities, avoiding neutral, non-valuing diction is currently a major concern (Leidmedien.de 2023). As in similar debates, there are also different positions and conventions.

Just as terms such as *Ausländer* [foreigner, migrant] and *Flüchtling* [refugee] are now avoided, since they substantivize certain person characteristics and thus elevate them to "master status," the German *die Behinderten* [the disabled] is also considered outdated and unacceptable from the perspective of critical disability discourse. It reduces affected individuals in an objectifying way to a single characteristic, their impairments, thus emphasizing their differences and making them into Others in society. Other relevant facets of a person such as gender, family origin, or profession disappear behind it.

The two expressions *behinderte Menschen* [disabled persons] and *Menschen mit Behinderung(en)* [persons with disabilities/disability] are preferred in contemporary use of non-discriminatory vocabulary. The first phrasing is used in German-language Disability Studies, because it refers to one of the core arguments of the social model of disability: The passive adjective *behindert* [disabled] suggests that people are not inherently disabled but are *behindert* [hindered] by the society, culture, and environment in which they live. It also implies that disability is only one aspect of any individual's complex life story. The version *Menschen mit Behinderung(en)* is also frequently used; here it is argued that the noun *Mensch* [person] emphasizes belonging to the greater family of *Menschheit* [mankind]. While the first option is preferred in British Disability Studies, in the USA it is "persons with disabilities" that has garnered the widest acceptance—in line with People First Language. The mention of *Mensch* as the initial word is to offset *Behinderung*, thereby weakening the stigma and making it fade into the background. Accordingly, the English version of the UN CRPD also uses the formulation "persons with disabilities" (United Nations, n.d.).

However, in the official German translation of the Convention, the English "persons" has been replaced by *Menschen* [human beings] rather than *Personen* (UN-Behindertenrechtskonvention 2017). Accordingly, since the adoption of the UN CRPD into German law, the term *Menschen mit Behinderungen* has found increasing use. The use of the plural—*Behinderungen* and not *Behinderung*—in this context is worth emphasizing, as it points to the multiplicity of barriers that people with disabilities have to overcome on a daily basis. Even if a person has only one impairment, they may encounter a range of challenges and difficulties. For this reason, the variant *Mensch mit Behinderung* should be avoided, it is better to opt instead for the plural *Menschen mit Behinderungen*.

Other frequently used formulations in the German-language are *Menschen mit Handicap* [persons with handicap] and *Menschen mit Beeinträchtigung* [persons with impairment]. In both cases, however, the expressions *mit Handicap* or *mit Beeinträchtigung* attached to *Menschen* [persons, people] seem like a "rucksack"—something affected persons have to carry around with them all the time. Moreover, for reasons of linguistic policy, the word *handicap*, which originated in English, is also avoided in Disability Studies in Germany (Karpa 2019). The newer version *Menschen mit Beeinträchtigung(en)* again revives associations with (physical) deficits, defects, and damage. Even though there is a clear differentiation between *Behinderung* [disability] and *Beeinträchtigung* [impairment], in the sense of the social model of disability, this formulation should also be avoided, as it reduces those affected to their impairments and hides their social situation, which is characterized by barriers.

This also applies—especially applies, in fact—to the term *geistige Behinderung* [mental disability], the use of which the advocacy group *Mensch zuerst—Netzwerk People First*

Deutschland e.V. [Mensch zuerst—A People First Network in Germany e.V.] directly combats. The group's preferred alternative phrasing is *Menschen mit Lernschwierigkeiten* [people with learning difficulties] (Leidmedien.de 2023, n.p.). However, this term lacks broad recognition and also evokes associations with the outdated *Lernbehinderung* [learning disability], which stems from special needs pedagogy. The alternative *Menschen mit intellektuellen/kognitiven Behinderungen/Beeinträchtigungen* [people with intellectual/cognitive disabilities/impairments] is therefore used as well, which is generally perceived as less oppressive.

As a final note on language use, it is important to apply period-appropriate terminology in historical analyses, even if such vocabulary might be seen as offensive and pejorative in a modern-day context. Otherwise, it is impossible to depict and analyze historical facts accurately (Frohne 2017; Metzler 2017). For example, in the literature of *Heilpädagogik* [remedial pedagogy] and psychiatry until the early twentieth century, people with learning difficulties were commonly referred to as *Idioten* [idiots] or *Blödsinnige* [imbeciles] (Schmuhl 2010, 28–45). Today, these terms are considered highly derogatory.

In the context of these linguistic discussions, one needs to be aware that language acts represent only one level of reality among many. In essence, language conventions always remain inadequate, as they must mediate between the rights of inclusion, appreciative addressing, and general comprehensibility. The conceptual history of *Behinderung* demonstrates, on the one hand, how important language is, and how seemingly innocuous words can carry normative assumptions, thoughts, ideas, and narratives. On the other hand, it shows how often denigrations and stigmas reassert themselves "behind the backs" of those who sought to eliminate them. Initially, *Behinderung* was introduced as a fairly value-neutral means of distinction, with the intention of destigmatizing. Over time, however, it acquired increasingly negative connotations and gradually reverted to a term with devaluing meanings.

In Disability Studies, therefore, there is both language advocacy and critical reflection. As Michael Zander, an activist of the disability rights movement and a university professor, puts it, the desire for "correct" language is welcome in principle, but the struggle for non-discriminatory terminology steers away from discussions that deal with "hard," material discrimination, "etwa Armut, Ausgrenzung und schlechte Arbeitsbedingungen in sogenannten Behindertenwerkstätten" ["such as poverty, exclusion, and poor working conditions in so-called sheltered workshops"] (Zander 2016, n.p.).

BEHINDERUNG: AN EMPTY SIGNIFIER?

From a historical perspective, it can be concluded that the term *Behinderung*, which now encompasses a wide range of physical, sensory, cognitive, and psychological conditions, is closely tied to the development of the welfare state and the paradigm of rehabilitation in Germany. The most decisive transformations in this context took place during the nineteenth and early twentieth centuries, but to this day, there are visible efforts to keep conceptualizing and changing the term and its meanings. Social policy, in particular, has contributed to the use of disability as a designation for special life situations; however, German social law continues to rely largely on medical expertise when defining the category. It is important to note here that social policy, with its efforts to use clear-cut *and* flexible terminology, not only serves to allocate social support and resources, but is also always part of social technologies that make fixed or permeable boundaries between "normal" and "abnormal."

The intricate ways in which *Behinderung* has become the focus of scientific, political, and legal discourse, and has been used in business, mass media, and everyday life, have not yet been sufficiently investigated. We can assume, however, that an important factor in the term's success is its indeterminacy. To a far greater degree than the older, impairment-specific designations—such as *blind* [blind], *idiotisch* [idiotic], *taub* [deaf], *verkrüppelt* [crippled]—*Behinderung* can be applied to a wide variety of situations.

From a theoretical standpoint, this term can be considered as an "empty signifier." This concept was coined by Ernesto Laclau and Chantal Mouffe (1985); it implies that the signifier (the word) and the referent (the content evoked by the word) are in a contingent relationship and that a term does not necessarily represent reality. Instead, it represents what the user intends it to represent. By speaking or writing about *Behinderung*, we implicitly connect it to existing ideas while, at the same time, contributing to the body of knowledge associated with it. Moreover, our collective understanding and knowledge are subject to constant battles over content and meaning. Empty signifiers such as *Behinderung* are open to a variety of meanings; they are "filled" and "refilled" through discursive processes shaped by hegemonic and subjugated positions. The case of *Behinderung* illustrates that persons with disabilities and their advocacy organizations play a central role in influencing the word's meaning, even though its use ends up being determined by the fields of medicine, politics, statistics, and law.

CONCLUDING REMARKS

In conclusion, the genealogy of *Behinderung* shows that many discourses, actors, and practices, such as the institutions and laws of the welfare state, international politics, and disability advocacy groups, are necessary to transform a general word into a marker of difference—one that, even today, is often associated with inability, weakness, suffering, and hardship. At the same time, this marker of difference legitimizes medical, political, legal, and educational measures that involve not only social assistance, services, and support for people with disabilities, but also their discrimination, exclusion, and marginalization.

The successful "career" of *Behinderung*, that is, the widely accepted use of this term as a designation for a multifaceted category of difference, was, however, not without purpose and direction: "[Es] schlich sich *nicht* [...] gleichsam beiläufig in den Sprachgebrauch ein, sondern war—ganz im Gegenteil—Resultat eines komplexen und konfliktgeladenen Interaktionsprozesses, an dem eine Vielzahl von Akteuren mit [...] häufig gegenläufigen Interessen und Motiven bewusst und mit klarer Zielsetzung mitwirkte" ["It did *not* creep into language use casually. Quite the opposite, actually: It was the result of a complex and conflict-laden process of interaction, involving an array of different players with (...) often-conflicting interests and motivations, all of whom worked with intention and clear goals in mind"] (Schmuhl 2007, 23; author's emphasis).

Today, *Behinderung* is established as an umbrella term, used to call attention to life situations in which impairments and barriers play a determining role—situations that require public assistance and social political regulation. Belonging to this category allows those with disabilities to receive access to educational and social support, accommodation, and entitlements. Increasingly, however, *Behinderung* also plays a role in other areas of life, such as culture, art, and sports; it is frequently thematized in literature, theater, film, and television, and paralympic athletes are celebrated for their accomplishments. In the end, the existence of a category of difference such as disability affects the lives, worlds, and experiences of people who fall into it as well as people who do not. The story of *Behinderung*, as this essay has attempted to show, is far from over—rather, we can call it a "never-ending story."

NOTES

1. My special thanks go to Jeffrey Daniel Castle and Stephanie Hilger for the translation of this essay. I am also grateful to Peter Meyns for reading my text with a critical eye.
2. Translator's note: This article traces the development of the German concept *Behinderung* through history. Though conventionally translated into English as "disability," the social and linguistic resonances of this term make it distinct and, indeed, utterly specific to the German context. Thus, instances of *Behinderung* in the original text have been left untranslated. Italics are also used for other German words that do not translate well into English.
3. My own diction is influenced by both British and US-American Disability Studies and the United Nations' Convention on the Rights of Persons with Disabilities (UN CRPD). I use the two options "persons with disabilities" and "disabled persons," but avoid the version "the disabled," because it is now outdated. In this essay, translations of quotations use the latter expression when the original refers to "die Behinderten" [the disabled], a term that was and is still frequently heard and read in German-language disability-related discourses.
4. In Germany the English term Disability Studies (with capital letters) is used for the corresponding field of research, which is often also written Disability Studies in English. When I use the capital letters in this essay, I refer to German-language Disability Studies. The same applies to Disability History.
5. The word clouds are created using the *Dudenkorpus* [*Duden* corpus], which consists of over four billion word forms drawn from current texts. The texts range in genre from newspapers and magazines to novels to scholarly and technical documents. Word clouds allow users to visualize the degree of relatedness between a central term and contextual terms based on how frequently they appear together. Contextual terms written in larger font have a stronger degree of relatedness, whereas contextual words written in smaller font have a weaker degree of relatedness. See https://www.duden.de/hilfe/typische-verbindungen.
6. The three word clouds for Behinderung (see https://www.duden.de/rechtschreibung/Behinderung) contain a total of sixteen words, of which eleven relate directly to categorization based on difference. For four others—namely, the adjectives *unbillig* [inequitable] and *massiv* [massive] and the verbs *rechnen* [to calculate] and *einstellen* [to adjust, to cease, or to stop something, also to employ staff]—the connections are ambiguous. Of the sixteen, only *Stau* [traffic jam] clearly resists association with *Behinderung* in its narrowed sense.
7. The term D/deaf is used to describe persons who are Deaf (sign language users) and deaf (who are hard of hearing and lipread and/or use hearing aids; usually they have spoken language as their first language); see for German Deaf Studies Rombach/Kellermann (2022).

8. *Regelwidriger Zustand* can also be translated with "irregular state," which is a slightly less normative term than "abnormal state."
9. I use here the official English translation of the *Grundgesetz* (Basic Law for the Federal Republic of Germany, n.d.; Grundgesetz, n.d.). In the literature one also finds different translations of this sentence, for example, "Nobody may be discriminated against on the basis of disability" or "No person shall be put at a disadvantage because of disability."
10. Translator's note: One might liken the pejorative use of *behindert* to the use of *retarded* in American English.

WORKS CITED

Barsch, Sebastian. 2016. "Der 'geschädigte' Mensch in der Rehabilitationspädagogik der DDR – Entfaltung und Wirkung eines sozialistischen Modells von Behinderung." In *Kontinuitäten, Zäsuren, Brüche? Lebenslagen von Menschen mit Behinderungen in der deutschen Zeitgeschichte*, edited by Gabriele Lingelbach and Anne Waldschmidt, 191–213. Frankfurt am Main, New York: Campus.

Basic Law for the Federal Republic of Germany. No date. "Basic Law for the Federal Republic of Germany in the revised version published in the Federal Law Gazette Part III, classification number 100-1, as last amended by the Act of 28 June 2022 (Federal Law Gazette I p. 968)." Translated by Professor Christian Tomuschat, Professor David P Currie, Professor Donald P. Kommers, and Raymond Kerr, in cooperation with the Language Service of the German Bundestag. In *Gesetze im Internet*, edited by Bundesministerium der Justiz, and Bundesamt für Justiz, Berlin, no pages. https://www.gesetze-im-internet.de/englisch_gg/englisch_gg.html (February 16, 2023).

Bennani, Hannah and Marion Müller. 2018. "'Making Up People' Globally: Die Institutionalisierung globaler Personenkategorien am Beispiel Indigener Völker und Menschen mit Behinderungen." *Zeitschrift für Soziologie* 47, no. 5: 306–331.

Biesalski, Konrad. 1911. *Leitfaden der Krüppelfürsorge: Im Auftrage der deutschen Vereinigung für Krüppelfürsorge gemeinverständlich dargestellt*. Leipzig: Verlag von Leopold Voss.

Bösl, Elsbeth. 2009. *Politiken der Normalisierung: Zur Geschichte der Behindertenpolitik in der Bundesrepublik Deutschland*. Bielefeld: transcript.

Brandt, Willy. 1969. "Regierungserklärung von Bundeskanzler Willy Brandt vor dem Deutschen Bundestag in Bonn am 28. Oktober 1969." In *Willy Brandt: Biografie. Quellen/Bedeutende Reden*, edited by Bundeskanzler-Willy-Brandt-Stiftung, and Die Norwegisch-Deutsche Willy Brandt-Stiftung, Berlin, Oslo, 35 pages. https://www.willy-brandt-biografie.de/wp-content/uploads/2017/08/Regierungserklaerung_Willy_Brandt_1969.pdf.

Brehme, David, Petra Fuchs, Swantje Köbsell, and Carla Wesselmann. 2020. *Disability Studies im deutschsprachigen Raum. Zwischen Emanzipation und Vereinnahmung*. Weinheim/Basel: Beltz Juventa.

Campbell, Fiona K. 2009. *Contours of Ableism: Territories, Objects, Disability and Desire*. Houndmills, Basingstoke, New York: Palgrave Macmillan.

Der Bundesminister der Justiz, ed. 1986. Bekanntmachung der Neufassung des Schwerbehindertengesetzes vom 26. August 1986. *Bundesgesetzblatt Teil I* (No. 45, Z 5702 A, issued September 2, 1986): 1421–1443. Bonn: Bundesanzeiger.

Diehl, Gerhard and Nils Hansen. 2017. "Historische Semantik: Zur terminologischen Unbestimmtheit mittelhochdeutscher Texte." In *Dis/ability History der Vormoderne: Ein Handbuch/Premodern Dis/ability History: A Companion*, edited by Cordula Nolte, Bianca Frohne, Uta Halle, and Sonja Kerth, 97–99. Affalterbach: Didymos.

Duden Online. 2018. Behinderung. In *Duden Online*, edited by Bibliographisches Institut GmbH, no pages. Berlin: Verlag Bibliographisches Institut GmbH. https://www.duden.de/rechtschreibung/Behinderung.

Edelstein, Benjamin, and Hermann Veith. 2017. "Schulgeschichte bis 1945: Von Preußen bis zum Dritten Reich." In *Dossier: Bildung*, edited by Bundeszentrale für politische Bildung, 1206–1219. Bonn: Bundeszentrale für politische Bildung. https://www.bpb.de/gesellschaft/bildung/zukunft-bildung/229629/schulgeschichte-bis-1945.

Felkendorff, Kai. 2003. "Ausweitung der Behinderungszone: Neuere Behinderungsbegriffe und ihre Folgen." In *Wie man behindert wird: Texte zur Konstruktion einer sozialen Rolle und zur Lebenssituation betroffener Menschen*, edited by Günther Cloerkes, 25–52. Heidelberg: Universitätsverlag Winter.

Fischer, Jonas. 2019. "Umstrittene Interessenvertretung von Menschen mit Behinderungen: Zur Geschichte von Kriegsopferverbänden, Elterninitiativen, Clubs, VHS-Kursen und Krüppelgruppen." In *Aufbrüche und Barrieren: Behindertenpolitik und Behindertenrecht in Deutschland und Europa seit den 1970er Jahren*, edited by Theresia Degener and Marc von Miquel, 213–242. Bielefeld: transcript.

Frohne, Bianca. 2017. "Moderne Begriffe und Definitionen – so unentbehrlich wie problematisch." In *Dis/ability History der Vormoderne: Ein Handbuch/Premodern Dis/ability History: A Companion*, edited by Cordula Nolte, Bianca Frohne, Uta Halle, and Sonja Kerth, 52–58. Affalterbach: Didymos.

Fuchs, Petra. 2001. *"Körperbehinderte" zwischen Selbstaufgabe und Emanzipation: Selbsthilfe – Integration – Aussonderung*. Berlin: Luchterhand.

Fuchs, Petra. 2012."'Behinderung' in Deutschland: Aspekte der Kultur und Geschichte des Umgangs mit physischer, psychischer und mentaler Differenz." In *Wege zur Kultur: Barrieren und Barrierefreiheit in Kultur- und Bildungseinrichtungen*, edited by Anja Tervooren and Jürgen Weber, 133–151. Vienna/Cologne/Weimar: Böhlau.

Fuchs, Petra. 2022. "'Behinderung' – eine bewegte Geschichte." In *Handbuch Disability Studies*, edited by Anne Waldschmidt, 35–53. Wiesbaden: Springer VS.

Grimm, Jacob and Wilhelm Grimm. 1854. *Deutsches Wörterbuch: Erster Band. A–Biermolke*. Leipzig: Verlag von S. Hirzel.

Groenemeyer, Axel. 2014. "Soziale Praxis – Institutionen – Diskurse – Erfahrung. Behinderung im Problematisierungsprozess." *Soziale Probleme: Zeitschrift für Soziale Probleme und Soziale Kontrolle* 25, no. 2: 151–172.

Grundgesetz. No date. "Grundgesetz für die Bundesrepublik Deutschland. Art. 3." In *Gesetze im Internet*, edited by Bundesministerium der Justiz, and Bundesamt für Justiz, Berlin, no pages. https://www.gesetze-im-internet.de/gg/art_3.html (February 16, 2023).

Karpa, Jonas. 2019. "Warum 'Handicap' das falsche Wort für Behinderung ist." *Leidmedien.de. Ein Projekt des Berliner Vereins SOZIALHELDEN e.V.*, no pages. https://leidmedien.de/aktuelles/warum-handicap-das-falsche-wort-fuer-behinderung-ist/.

Klein, Anne. 2022. "Gesellschaftskritik: Wie kritisch können, sollen oder müssen die Disability Studies sein?" In *Handbuch Disability Studies*, edited by Anne Waldschmidt, 471–484. Wiesbaden: Springer VS.

Köbsell, Swantje and Anne Waldschmidt. 2006. "Disability Studies in Austria, Germany and Switzerland." *Disability Studies Quarterly* 26, no. 2: n.p. http://dsq-sds.org/issue/view/33.

Köbsell, Swantje. 2012. *Wegweiser Behindertenbewegung: Neues (Selbst-)Verständnis von Behinderung*. Neu-Ulm: AG SPAK.

Köbsell, Swantje. 2022. "Entstehung und Varianten der deutschsprachigen Disability Studies." In *Handbuch Disability Studies*, edited by Anne Waldschmidt, 55–71. Wiesbaden: Springer VS.

Laclau, Ernesto and Chantal Mouffe. 1985. *Hegemony and Socialist Strategy: Towards a Radical Democratic Politics*. London/New York: Verso.

Leidmedien.de. 2023. Begriffe über Behinderung von A bis Z. *Leidmedien.de. Ein Projekt des Berliner Vereins SOZIALHELDEN e.V.*, no pages. https://leidmedien.de/begriffe/.

Lindmeier, Christian. 1993. *Behinderung – Phänomen oder Faktum?* Bad Heilbrunn: Klinkhardt.

Lingelbach, Gabriele and Jan Stoll. 2013. "Die 1970er Jahre als Umbruchsphase der bundesdeutschen disability history? Eine Mikrostudie zu Selbstadvokation und Anstaltskritik Jugendlicher mit Behinderung." *Moving the Social: Journal of Social History and the History of Social Movements* 50: 25–52.

Link, Jürgen. 2006. *Versuch über den Normalismus: Wie Normalität produziert wird*. Göttingen: Vandenhoeck & Ruprecht.

Linton, Simi. 1998. "Disability Studies/Not Disability Studies." *Disability & Society* 13, no. 4: 525–540.

Metzler, Irina. 2017. "Modern versus Historical Vocabulary." In *Dis/ability History der Vormoderne: Ein Handbuch/Premodern Dis/ability History: A Companion*, edited by Cordula Nolte, Bianca Frohne, Uta Halle, and Sonja Kerth, 58–59. Affalterbach: Didymos.

Mürner, Christian and Udo Sierck. 2009. *Krüppelzeitung: Brisanz der Behindertenbewegung*. Hamburg: AG SPAK.

Osten, Philipp. 2004. *Die Modellanstalt: Über den Aufbau einer "modernen Krüppelfürsorge" 1905–1933*. Frankfurt am Main: Mabuse.

Pfahl, Lisa, and Justin J.W. Powell. 2014. "Subversive Status: Disability Studies in Germany, Austria, and Switzerland." *Disability Studies Quarterly* 34, no.2: no pages. https://dsq-sds.org/article/view/4256.

Poore, Carol. 2007. *Disability in Twentieth-Century German Culture*. Ann Arbor: University of Michigan Press.

Rombach, Fabian and Gudrun Kellermann. 2022. "Deaf Studies und Disability Studies." In *Handbuch Disability Studies*, edited by Anne Waldschmidt, 417–434. Wiesbaden: Springer VS.

Rößler, Carl-Wilhelm. 2022. "Rechtswissenschaft in den Disability Studies." In *Handbuch Disability Studies*, edited by Anne Waldschmidt, 183–200. Wiesbaden: Springer VS.

Rudloff, Wilfried. 2019. "Die Eingliederungshilfe: Lückenbüßer, Kernbestand, Auslaufmodell der Hilfen für Menschen mit Behinderungen?" In *Aufbrüche und Barrieren: Behindertenpolitik und Behindertenrecht in Deutschland und Europa seit den 1970er Jahren*, edited by Theresia Degener, and Marc von Miquel, 107–139. Bielefeld: transcript.

Schmuhl, Hans-Walter. 1987. *Rassenhygiene, Nationalsozialismus, Euthanasie: Von der Verhütung zur Vernichtung "lebensunwerten Lebens," 1890–1945*. Göttingen: Vandenhoeck & Ruprecht.

Schmuhl, Hans Walter. 2007. "Schwer behindert, schwerbehindert, schwerstbehindert: Begriffsgeschichtliche Betrachtungen zu den feinen Unterschieden in der Benennung von Menschen mit Behinderungen." In *Herausforderungen: Mit schwerer Behinderung leben*, edited by Markus Dederich, and Katrin Grüber, 23–37. Frankfurt am Main: Mabuse.

Schmuhl, Hans-Walter. 2010. *Exklusion und Inklusion durch Sprache – Zur Geschichte des Begriffs Behinderung*. Berlin: Institut Mensch Ethik Wissenschaft.

SGB IX Alte Fassung. 2017. "SGB IX in der [vom 01. Juli 2001] bis zum 31.12.2017 geltenden Fassung: Neuntes Buch Sozialgesetzbuch – Rehabilitation und Teilhabe behinderter Menschen. Teil 1 Regelungen für behinderte und von Behinderung bedrohte Menschen (§§ 1–67), Kapitel 1 Allgemeine Regelungen (§§ 1–16)." *dejure.org Rechtsinformationssysteme*, Mannheim, no pages. https://dejure.org/gesetze/SGB_IX_a.F./2.html (February 16, 2023).

Sozialgesetzbuch Neuntes Buch. 2022. "Sozialgesetzbuch Neuntes Buch – Rehabilitation und Teilhabe von Menschen mit Behinderungen – Neuntes Buch Sozialgesetzbuch - SGB IX – vom 23. Dezember 2016 [BGBl. I S. 3234], das zuletzt durch Artikel 4 des Gesetzes vom 20. Dezember 2022 [BGBl. I S. 2560] geändert worden ist." In *Gesetze im Internet*, edited by Bundesministerium der Justiz, and Bundesamt für Justiz, Berlin, no pages. https://www.gesetze-im-internet.de/sgb_9_2018/BJNR323410016.html (February 16, 2023).

Stehr, Johannes. 2013. "Normalität und Abweichung." In *Soziologische Basics: Eine Einführung für pädagogische und soziale Berufe*, edited by Albert Scherr, 191–197. Wiesbaden: Springer VS.

Stoll, Jan. 2017. *Behinderte Anerkennung? Interessenorganisationen von Menschen mit Behinderung in Westdeutschland seit 1945*. Frankfurt am Main/New York: Campus.

Thomann, Klaus-Dieter. 1995. *Das behinderte Kind. "Krüppelfürsorge" und Orthopädie in Deutschland 1866–1920*. Stuttgart: G. Fischer.

Thomann, Klaus-Dieter. 2000. "Die Geschichte der Reichskrüppelzählung von 1906." *Der Orthopäde* 29, no. 12: 1055–1066.

UN-Behindertenrechtskonvention. 2017. *Die UN-Behindertenrechtskonvention: Übereinkommen über die Rechte von Menschen mit Behinderungen. Die amtliche, gemeinsame Übersetzung von Deutschland, Österreich, Schweiz und Lichtenstein*. Berlin: Bundesministerium für Arbeit und Soziales.

United Nations, Department of Economic and Social Affairs, Disability, ed. No date. *Convention on the Rights of Persons with Disabilities (UN CRPD)*. https://www.un.org/development/desa/disabilities/convention-on-the-rights-of-persons-with-disabilities.html.

Waldschmidt, Anne. 2009. "'Normalität' und 'Behinderung' im Alltagswissen: Diskursanalyse eines Internetforums." *SWS-Rundschau: Zeitschrift der Sozialwissenschaftlichen Studiengesellschaft* 49, no. 3: 314–336.

Waldschmidt, Anne. 2019. "Why Critical Disability Studies Needs a Cultural Model of Dis/ability." In *Interdisciplinary Approaches to Disability: Looking Towards* the Future. Volume 2, edited by Katie Ellis, Rosemarie Garland-Thomson, Mike Kent, and Rachel Robertson, 71–79. Abingdon, New York: Routledge.

Waldschmidt, Anne. 2020. *Disability Studies zur Einführung*. Hamburg: Junius.

Waldschmidt, Anne, ed. 2022. *Handbuch Disability Studies*. Wiesbaden: Springer VS.

Waldschmidt, Anne, Hanjo Berressem, and Moritz Ingwersen, eds. 2017. *Culture – Theory – Disability: Encounters between Disability Studies and Cultural Studies*. Bielefeld: transcript.

Waldschmidt, Anne and Sarah Karim. 2022. "Was sind Disability Studies? Profil, Stand und Vokabular eines neuen Forschungsfeldes." In *Handbuch Disability Studies*, edited by Anne Waldschmidt, 1–15. Wiesbaden: Springer VS.

Welti, Felix. 2019. "Zwischen unteilbaren Menschenrechten und gegliedertem Sozialsystem: Behindertenpolitik erster und zweiter Ordnung von 1990 bis 2016." In *Aufbrüche und Barrieren: Behindertenpolitik und Behindertenrecht in Deutschland und Europa seit den 1970er Jahren*, edited by Theresia Degener and Marc von Miquel, 15–42. Bielefeld: transcript.

Zander, Michael. 2016. "Neue Wörter, neue Gesellschaft?" *Hintergrund. Das Nachrichtenmagazin* 2: no pages. https://www.hintergrund.de/soziales/reformen/neue-woerter-neue-gesellschaft/.

Zola, Irving K. 1993. "Self, Identity and the Naming Question: Reflections on the Language of Disability." *Social Science & Medicine* 36, no. 2: 167–173.

CHAPTER TEN

A New View of an Old Prosthesis: Creating a Digital 3D Model of a Sixteenth-Century Iron Hand

HEIDI HAUSSE

There are few objects that illustrate so well the intersections of medicine, technology, and culture as early modern mechanical hands. My book, *The Malleable Body: Surgeons, Artisans, and Amputees in Early Modern Germany*, uses them to explore how surgical and artisanal interventions in the sixteenth and seventeenth centuries created a growing perception, essential to biomedicine today, that humans could alter the body. These artifacts, I argue, reveal that the driving force behind the ideas and development of mechanical limb technology were not surgeons, but amputees and artisans. Bringing them out of the shadowy corners of armor exhibits and into the light of historical analysis suggests how amputees took inspiration from art and craft to manage new body shapes and shape the perceptions of others in powerful ways. Over the course of research and writing, in fall 2017, I hired an architect to create a digital 3D model of one sixteenth-century mechanical hand and produce diagrams of its mechanisms. By the time the model and diagrams were completed, in summer 2018, my working relationship with the architect, Ben Tulman, had become a collaboration, and the process of digitally modeling had turned into an experimentation that created new knowledge about premodern prosthetic technology. There was no road map for us to follow in this undertaking, but the experience was intellectually enriching and creatively stimulating. Sharing about our process and its trials and errors may prove useful to other scholars in the health humanities exploring themes in material culture, technology, or disability. Far from a straightforward illustration of what is already known, 3D modeling is an epistemic exercise that requires one to continually reassess and rearrange different pieces of information to render increasingly complex understandings of an object. It requires constant communication with others, bringing vastly different skillsets together in ways that generate new questions, new theories, and new opportunities to explore them through the act of creating.

Mechanical hands like the example I asked Tulman to model were singular objects of artifice designed to supplement the natural body in early modern Europe. They represent a form of prosthetic technology that first appeared in the late fifteenth century and continued into the sixteenth and seventeenth. With moveable fingers and flesh-toned paint, they incorporated practical and aesthetic functions in ways impossible with other kinds of prostheses. After all, silver noses could not smell, nor enameled eyeballs see. Mechanical hands, by contrast, could hold things. Wearers operated them passively, pressing down on artificial fingers to lock them into various positions and activating a release button to free them. While there is no comprehensive list of artifacts, I am familiar with approximately thirty-five. These survived when upper limb prostheses made entirely of wood or leather—options more affordable for the majority of the population—did not. Most are made of iron, a more durable material that allowed some to withstand the ravages of time in a riverbed or field. Some were buried with wearers of high social status in well-preserved tombs, only to be uncovered during church renovations. Still others were held as keepsakes, passed from one generation to the next, maintained in private collections.

Though these objects have sparked modern imaginations for over two centuries, surprisingly little is known about their makers, wearers, and significance. Written sources concerning them are scarce. Even the autobiography of Götz von Berlichingen, the sixteenth-century knight who inspired Goethe's influential play *Götz von Berlichingen mit der eisernen Hand* (1773), only mentions his prosthesis in passing (Berlichingen 1981, 118). While the appearance of a mechanical hand design in an early modern surgical treatise led to a thread of scholarship crediting its author, the surgeon Ambroise Paré (1510–90), as the inventor of such objects, the reality is that early modern surgeons and physicians had little to do with limb prostheses (Hausse 2019, 36). In the United States today, one needs a medical prescription to obtain an artificial limb. In early modern Germany, artificial limbs had yet to be medicalized, and obtaining prostheses was, as one scholar recently described it, a "private affair" (Heide 2019, 341). As our main surviving source, the objects themselves must be carefully analyzed. My research into their materiality shifts attention to processes of making and questions of intended functions. This approach not only removes romanticized lenses of heroic knights or ingenious surgeons, but also recovers the vital roles of amputees and artisans in the development of a new prosthetic technology.

The Kassel Hand, a sixteenth-century artifact in the collections of Museumslandschaft Hessen Kassel in Germany, was the ideal choice among the objects in my source base for detailed internal diagramming, for two reasons. First, the number and clarity of the photographs I took of its interior were exceptional. No two mechanical hands are the same, but one thing most do share: it is hard to see their mechanisms without taking the hands apart, which aside from an early nineteenth-century episode has not been attempted in modern times (Mechel 1815). Some interiors are concealed completely by a solid plate positioned over the wrist opening of the hand's hollow shell. The shell's shape, such as a narrow wrist, also affects what one can see. The dimensions involved are small, too, with mechanisms in most of these objects spanning 10 centimeters or less. The angle is difficult as well. Peering through a wrist (or forearm) opening presents a foreshortened perspective that distorts the shape of mechanisms. Finally, their interiors are dark, caked in dust, and obscured by corrosion. To photograph them, one needs to use the camera's flash or, ideally, to shine a flashlight into the wrist opening without casting shadows—a tricky feat as a one-person operation. When museum specialists allowed me to examine the Kassel Hand, they let me position its wide wrist opening in a way that made the most of the light in the room. At one point, one of them also shined a small flashlight into the hand while I took photographs. The resulting images are remarkably clear.

The second reason I chose the Kassel Hand was because its mechanical layout was similar to that of the famous artificial hand woodcut in Ambroise Paré's surgical treatise. This suggested that the printed image was a viable design recording a form of prosthetic technology that artisans in different craft groups were producing. Closely studying the Kassel Hand's interior allowed me to use material culture to anchor the woodcut image in ongoing craft practices and demonstrate that the source of the image's design was, as Paré himself acknowledged, an artisan (Hausse 2019, 44–45). But to make that case clearly, I needed diagrams that would illustrate my explanations of how the object worked.

In spring 2017, toward the end of my first year at the Society of Fellows in the Humanities at Columbia University, colleagues who saw my attempt at a crude diagram smartly suggested that I commission a professional. By happy chance, I mentioned this to an early modern historian who had recently published a book with illustrations by an architect, with whom she promptly put me in touch (Wunder 2017). After a brief consultation, that individual recommended making a digital 3D model as the best way to create the desired diagrams and introduced me virtually to Ben Tulman, an architect based in Cambridge, Massachusetts, who had experience with the digital tools needed. By October, Tulman and I were discussing the terms of the project. Using research funds from the Society of Fellows, I hired him as an independent contractor to create an accurate and impactful illustration—both as a digital 3D model and as diagrams drawn from that model—of the Kassel Hand's internal mechanisms. We set a start date for early December. Neither of us had experience modeling a sixteenth-century artifact, but we were confident it could be done by summer 2018, when my fellowship (and therefore my funding) would end.

The modeling process, as I experienced it, unfolded in three phases: passive and reactive, active and collaborative, and collaborative and experimental. In the initial phase, I entered into the endeavor with the naïve notion that I could simply share my files about the artifact and Tulman—who was not an early modern European historian and had never seen the artifact in person—would have everything needed to digitally recreate it. I shared approximately 185 photographs of the artifact, my own rough diagram of its mechanisms, written explanations of the object and its components, and an image and explanation of the sixteenth-century woodcut from Paré's surgical treatise for historical comparison. Through this first phase, in which Tulman focused on the shell of the hand, the shared files and photographic evidence provided enough data for him to recreate the object's shape without significant input from me. Using the modeling software Rhinoceros 3D, Tulman imported different views from the photographs and scaled them to map out the object's exterior. Crucial to this was a photograph I had taken showing the object at full length with a measuring tape beside it. Communicating via email, Tulman sent views of his progress as he mapped out geometric shapes to create the hand's shell and fingers. Our first exchanges focused on what visual style would best convey the information I wished to illustrate. Thus, in mid-December, we discussed turning the simplified geometry with its faceted appearance into a smooth-surfaced object. Doing so would better illustrate the shape of the Kassel Hand's wrist, a valuable detail to capture because the wrist's shape affected how it attached to its wearer. Executing this was, as Tulman later explained, an additive process of modeling in which he "manipulated the surface typology to make a more organic looking form rather than adding and subtracting shapes from each other" (Ben Tulman, conversation with author, July 8, 2022).

Phase two began in February 2018, after Tulman shifted from the shell of the hand to its internal mechanisms. In this phase, I became an active participant and our exchanges were increasingly collaborative. We each had specialized knowledge and skills that needed to be brought into conversation to successfully tackle the interior. As Tulman reflected later, his task was to recreate a three-dimensional object in three-dimensional space filtered through the language of two-dimensional representation. This was made all the more challenging by relying solely on photographs. "I never saw the object, held it, looked at it ... [and] no matter how great the photo documentation is, it can be hard to assess what is happening in 3D from a photograph" (Ben Tulman, conversation with author, July 8, 2022). By contrast, my understanding of the object was based not only on data I accumulated from examining other artifacts and broader historical research, but most important on an examination of the Kassel Hand itself. This took place in April 2013 in the presence of a curator and a restorer at the restoration workshop of Museumslandschaft Hessen Kassel. They allowed me to handle the object (with gloves, of course) to see how it felt, weighed, and moved. When I asked whether the mechanisms still functioned, they suggested we find out together. The thumb mechanism was broken, but we counted seven positions that the four fingers could be locked into and then freed by pulling a release trigger on the outside of the wrist. To our collective surprise, when I measured it, I discovered that it was 23.5 centimeters in length from finger to wrist, contrary to an exhibition catalog that had described it as 30 centimeters (author's field notes, April 23, 2013; Burhenne 2003, 110). All the while I snapped hundreds of photographs, took detailed notes, asked questions, and looked at documents they generously shared. My first-hand encounter with the object lasted a little over an hour and a half, and in the hours immediately afterward I took copious additional notes and sketched what I had seen. My photographic and written records of that day formed the core source material I used to further study the object. Yet simply sharing those records with Tulman could not fully convey the physicality of the object and its motion as I had experienced it. Asking the architect to create without that historical and experiential knowledge of the artifact led to a deeply flawed model of its interior.

I came to this realization in late February, when Tulman sent a progress update showing a diagram draft based on the model that missed some internal components entirely and portrayed the main release lever inaccurately. Until that point, the only progress images of the model's interior I had seen were from the perspective through the wrist opening. This imitated the artifact photographs, which are all, by necessity, from that view. The foreshortened perspective distorts the components' shapes and some components are only partially visible. The result is that from this view, one cannot see how several of the components interface with one another, nor their real shapes. Thus, the problems with the model only became visible to me when Tulman sent the draft diagram showing all of the mechanisms. In the draft, there were no flat springs to act on the pawls that lock into the toothed wheels at the base of the fingers. The horizontal portion of the release lever was a T-shape: a shaft ending in a narrow perpendicular bar stretching along the proximal ends of all four pawls. This contradicted what I knew of the object's interior, which had two pairs of flat springs exerting pressure on four pawls and a release lever that branched out horizontally in a V-shape.

Replicating the hand's internal mechanisms proved to be a different sort of challenge than recreating its exterior not only because of the foreshortened perspective in photographs, but also because these components *move*. Each one acts upon another. To map them, one must understand how they move and act in relation to every other part. One can have a general sense of how, in principle, the mechanism operates. For example, a pawl locks a finger wheel, a flat spring applies pressure to a pawl, and a release lever unlocks a pawl from a finger wheel by countering the pressure exerted by a flat spring. It is one thing to broadly describe such relationships. It is another thing entirely to visually render every component involved in them in 2D, let alone 3D, because one cannot see the full shape and movement of *any* individual interior component, creating gaps in our knowledge of their construction. Tulman and I had to start working together to make several informed decisions about how to render these relationships.

It is no exaggeration to say that on the very day I became an active participant in the process, I discovered that modeling was itself a tool for learning more about an object. The first surprise came from a flurry of emails about the main release lever in the draft diagram. I insisted that the full lever was a Y-shape: a shaft that came down vertically from the exterior release trigger and then branched out horizontally in a V-shape stretching toward the pawls (Figure 10.1). Sketches from the day I examined the object in person demonstrate that I had interpreted the horizontal portion of the release lever as two arms branching outward. Tulman held firm that the lever ended in a line that touched the proximal ends of all four pawls, and he pointed out that there was no other apparent means by which the middle and ring fingers, which the two middle pawls locked, could be unlocked. The back-and-forth led me to ask him if we were talking about a solid plate rather than a "T" or a "V." There is a great deal of dust and decay inside iron hands, and I paused to consider whether this could have obscured the lever's shape, causing a plate to seemingly blend into the interior surface with only its outermost edges—the "V"—clearly visible. Thinking through Tulman's reasoning, I combed through all my photographs, scrutinizing them anew for signs of a solid plate. I was shocked to find evidence of it, most clearly captured in one particular snapshot when the flashlight illuminated a portion of the component just right. I then corroborated this finding using other photographs. Tulman agreed that upon review, the lever possessed, as he coined it, "a solid triangular plate" (Ben Tulman, email to author, February 27, 2018). My vision of a "V" and

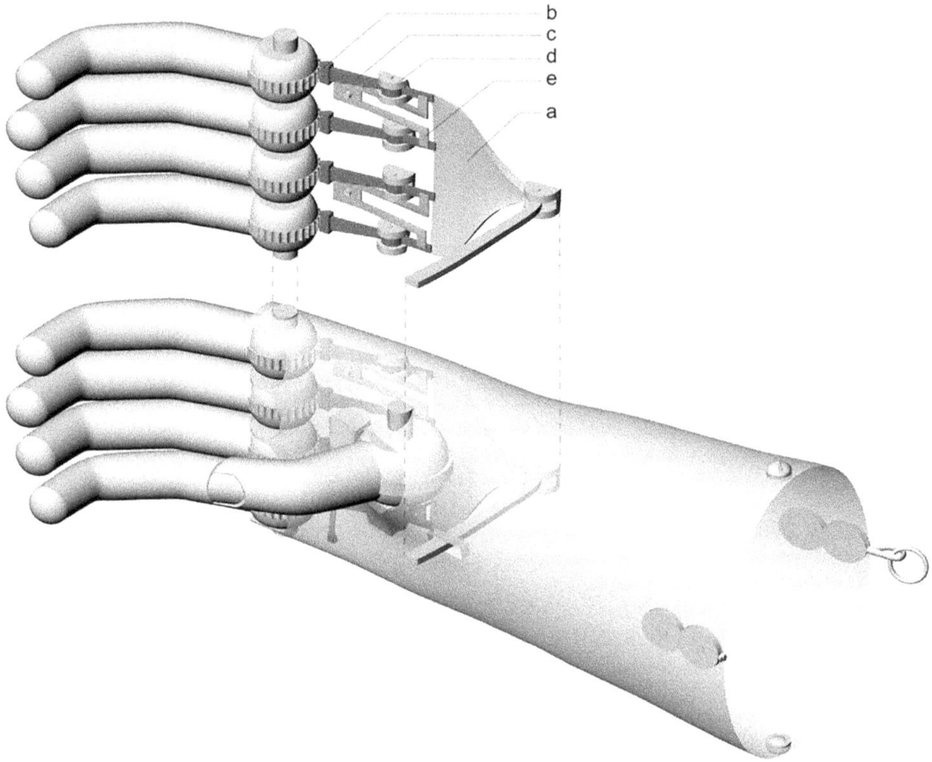

FIGURE 10.1: Diagram of Kassel Hand Mechanisms: a. Main release lever. b. Toothed wheel. c. Pawl. d. Base of pawl. e. Flat spring. Source: Drawing and 3D model by Ben Tulman. Credit: Heidi Hausse.

his vision of a "T" merged into a coherent component shape—a triangle—that made greater sense of how the lever acted on all four pawls at once (Figure 10.1).

This proved to be the beginning of an exciting new dynamic in which we worked through ideas in a constant exchange, applying our different skillsets in a coordinated effort to extrapolate more information about how the object worked. Our methods of communication reflected the shift. As Tulman was in Massachusetts and I was in New York, we were rarely able to meet in person. During the first phase we relied almost exclusively on email correspondence. In the second phase, phone calls and virtual meetings that enabled Tulman to share his screen became crucial for brainstorming and discussing ideas while looking at the model. In early March, we met using Google Hangouts for the first time to plan how we would revise the internal layout. By the end of that meeting, we had agreed on the external reference points for the spatial dimensions of the interior, talked through each component in the four fingers' mechanism, and decided to pause work on the thumb until these revisions were complete.

The March meeting was particularly productive in part because I had spent the days prior developing a more precise verbal and visual language. I had prepared by consulting with

María González Pendás, who was then my colleague at the Society of Fellows and is now at Cornell University. As an architectural historian and a former architect, she possessed skillsets that overlapped with both the humanities and design. She looked at my photographs, Tulman's draft diagram, and a progress snapshot of the digital model's interior, and she listened carefully as I described the situation. Several things happened over the course of our discussions. First, she explained I needed to shift away from the perspectival view of the photographs that look through the wrist opening. My emphasis on it had created the conditions for Tulman to accurately recreate *that* view in the model, without accurately recreating the *actual* layout of the mechanisms. I had falsely assumed that one would follow from the other. After showing me the error of my ways, González Pendás then had advice for how to move forward. She recommended I ask Tulman for three orthogonal views each time he shared a snapshot of his progress: a top view (resembling a bird's-eye-view) and two side views. These would better convey the state of the model's interior. The advice proved invaluable and led to clearer communication when Tulman sent images of his progress from that point onward.

Next, González Pendás advised me to become directly involved in determining the spatial layout of the interior and offered to sketch views of it to share with Tulman before our meeting. This meant indicating to Tulman how details on the artifact's exterior corresponded to its interior. I had documented the signs of nails and bolts apparent on the external surface of the iron hand, but it had not occurred to me to systematically map them to the interior mechanisms. We began by printing several full-page images of the artifact, circling and highlighting details with clear correlations. We focused on three in particular: two rivets that corresponded to each pair of boot-shaped flat springs and a square-shaped bolt that indicated the position of the main release lever. She then grabbed tracing paper, placed it over a bird's-eye-view photograph of the artifact, and marked those reference points from the exterior to map out the spatial layout of the interior. My basic sketches of the interior had been limited to the foreshortened perspective through the wrist opening. González Pendás showed me how to move beyond that by using information I already had in a new way. As soon as she marked the approximate places where the two rivets and square bolt corresponded to the interior, it was obvious that the pawls of the four fingers were much longer than the short, stubby tabs that Tulman and I had interpreted from the photographic evidence. The way that the pawls locked on the toothed wheels of the fingers was the same, but the *shape* of the pawls was dramatically different, as Figure 10.1 clearly shows.

González Pendás turned her sketches into one sheet of paper with three views of the four fingers' mechanisms reminiscent of plan and section drawings. I shared this with Tulman before our virtual meeting to facilitate a conversation about revising the model. Conveyed in the drawing was a demonstration of the three orthogonal views to focus on moving forward, the external reference points to establish the spatial dimensions of the interior, and a numbering of each component that the model should include. Reflecting back, Tulman pointed to this document as a pivotal moment in modeling the mechanisms of the four fingers (Ben Tulman, conversation with author, July 8, 2022). He incorporated the sketch's reference points, which González Pendás drew as dashed lines, to create "guide planes" for the model. These appeared in top view progress snapshots he shared of the model as three vertical lines used to determine the placement and size of individual components (Ben Tulman, email to author, March 22, 2018). The result transformed the model's interior. In the revised internal layout, the two rivets of the flat spring pairs and the square bolt of the release lever are anchors for the entire spatial configuration.

The third phase of the process marked a deliberate shift in approach as we turned our attention to the thumb in mid-April. Mapping the thumb mechanism was a new frontier. The unique challenges it posed introduced me to the experimental possibilities modeling allows as we used it to theorize about what could not be known with complete certainty. Unlike the Kassel Hand's four fingers, the thumb is currently inoperable. No living person has seen it function. When I examined it, I recorded that it was "loose and cannot be locked into different positions" (author's field notes, April 23, 2013). Not only is it impossible to see the thumb work, it is also unclear *why* it is not working. The cause could be damage to existing components, a missing component, or even the remote possibility that it never functioned. In addition, in contrast to the four fingers' mechanisms, which are mostly visible, much of the thumb mechanisms are only partially visible. When one looks through the wrist opening, the toothed wheel at the base of the thumb blocks the view of the components behind it and how they interact with each other and the wheel itself. As Tulman later pointed out, there is "more of a 2D aspect to the [four] fingers, but the thumb you can only understand in 3D." Referring to González Pendás's sketch of the four fingers, he explained that for the thumb mechanism, "plan and section wouldn't be enough" (Ben Tulman, conversation with author, July 8, 2022). Its components traverse the space of the hand's interior in a more complex way in how they are positioned and presumably once moved (Figure 10.2). In a two-dimensional diagram, it would have been simple to omit the thumb. By pursuing a 3D model, we were moving toward as total an understanding of the object's layout and construction as possible. Addressing this challenge resulted in the first detailed theory of how the thumb could have operated.

Tulman and I embarked on this new stage informed by what we had learned so far. Work on the thumb began with a phone call, which over the course of a lengthy discussion switched over to Google Hangouts so that we could share screens. We looked at photographs of the artifact's interior and talked through every component related to the thumb, identifying each and discussing its shape and its relationship to the others. I sketched out the mechanism in a notebook as we spoke, coloring and numbering the individual parts with highlighters and red and blue pens within reach on my desk and scribbling in names for them as we developed our own shared vocabulary. These included a "release arm" that ended in a "curly-cue," a "curved tab" that seemed to act as a pawl on the thumb's toothed wheel, and a "flat spring—lateral through the hand" that ended somewhere behind the toothed wheel (author's notes, April 14, 2018). After the meeting, I consolidated and polished the information. Using Microsoft Paint, I annotated a photograph of the artifact's interior with bright yellow arrows and numbers, and then in a separate document I typed up descriptions of each numbered part. I emailed these to Tulman to check that it accurately reflected what we had agreed upon. Once he confirmed we were on the same page, those numbers and terms became a shorthand, our own unofficial jargon that we subsequently used to discuss the thumb mechanism. This included a component we had described as a "tab" in our virtual meeting that we believed acted as a pawl to lock the thumb wheel. In lengthy email chains that followed, we referred to it simply as "#6."

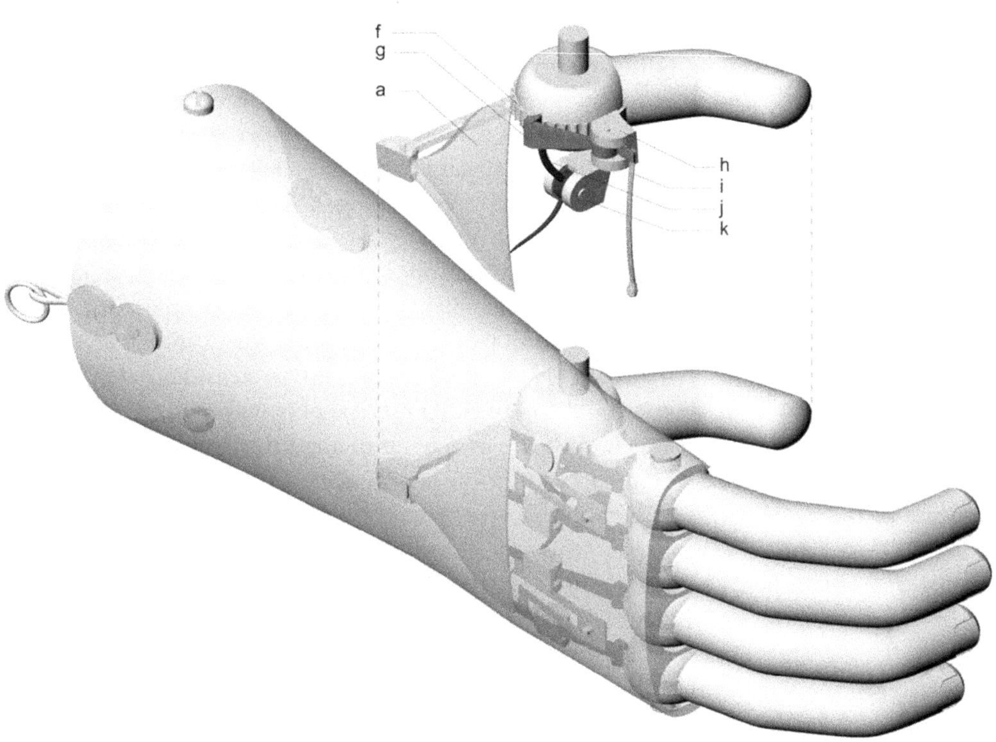

FIGURE 10.2: Diagram of Kassel Hand Thumb Mechanism: f. Toothed wheel. g. Pawl. h. Pawl base. i. Flat spring. j. Thumb release lever. k. Thumb lever mount. a. Main release lever. Source: Drawing and 3D model by Ben Tulman. Credit: Heidi Hausse.

Creating three-dimensional versions of these components allowed for a visual assessment of our theories about them. An element that seemed sound in the abstract could appear specious when mapped out in the model, leading to further dialogue and revision. These were experiments with geometry and space that were informed by, and in turn also themselves informed, how we understood the physical forces at work in the mechanism. Our greatest point of speculation concerned the thumb's pawl and how it interfaced with a long flat spring than runs laterally near the hand's interior surface (Figure 10.2). In photographs, most of the pawl and the entire area where it interacts with the flat spring are hidden behind the thumb's toothed wheel (Figure 10.2). We initially conjectured that the pawl's distal end rested between the flat spring and the interior surface of the hand. This imitated the positioning of the four fingers' pawls in relation to their two pairs of boot-shaped flat springs (Figure 10.1). Yet we acknowledged it was unclear what the flat spring's role was in this case, and that it might be acting on an unknown component. Tulman sent the first progress views of the thumb a few days after our mid-April meeting. While all of the pieces we discussed were there and arranged as we had hypothesized, the interface of those located behind the toothed wheel struck me as unsound. Having learned the importance of using visuals, I opened Tulman's progress screenshot of the flat spring and pawl configuration in Paint and inserted arrows indicating how I understood the pawl would pivot, adding a question mark next to the arrow where the pawl's distal end met the flat spring. I emailed this to ask whether I understood the configuration correctly and expressed concern with our theory of the pawl, though I could not identify clearly what the precise problem was. After a few more days of looking at the progress views, thinking about it, and time and again balancing a pen on my index finger and moving it in a see-saw motion to better visualize the pivoting movement of the pawl and how different directions of pressure affected the movement, I had gone from uneasy to absolutely certain that something was missing from our equation.

I sent Tulman an email explaining that our configuration did not account for the force needed to keep the thumb's pawl at tension to lock the thumb wheel in a fixed position. Thinking about the object as a prosthesis that someone wore, it was clear there was nothing in our working model to keep the proximal end of the thumb pawl from pivoting away from the toothed wheel any time the wearer moved the iron hand in any direction. Our configuration was not functional. I asked for Tulman's input on how this could have worked, noting that the thumb in the artifact was broken and so we were "moving into the realm of judicious speculation." As I put it at the time, "this is a question of what force (and in the shape of what material component) is keeping #6 [i.e. the pawl] from swiveling when it *isn't* being acted on" by the thumb's curly-cue release lever (Heidi Hausse, email to Ben Tulman, April 24, 2018). Tulman responded that my questions pointed back to his initial confusion about the direction of the flat spring's force in the area hidden in photographs. In the four fingers, the boot-shaped flat springs operated on pawls to keep them locked in a finger wheel. Yet, in our configuration of the thumb, "the flat spring would be producing a rotational force on the pawl in the same direction as the force from the arm [i.e. thumb release lever]." He pointed to the arrows I had previously annotated over the progress screenshot indicating the pawl's pivot in relation to the flat spring. "The spring," Tulman wrote, "somehow needs to counteract the force from the arm [i.e. thumb release lever]" (Ben Tulman, email to author, April 24, 2018). Tulman pinpointed the issue, identifying why the current configuration was unsound and, by doing so, also addressing the missing application of force needed for the thumb's pawl to lock the toothed wheel. We reassessed the interface of the flat spring with the thumb's pawl so that instead of mirroring the positional relationship of the boot-shaped flat springs in the four fingers, it mirrored their technical one. The long flat spring in our model simply needed to be moved *between* the thumb's pawl and the interior surface of the hand (Figure 10.2). This relocation of the flat spring then explained its slightly curved shape, which allowed the pawl to move enough to free the toothed wheel when the release lever was activated (Heidi Hausse, email to Ben Tulman, April 24, 2018). All the components in view or partial view from photographs now made sense in a configuration accounting for the lock and release of the thumb. The revised configuration, seen in Figure 10.2, remains to my knowledge the first and only detailed theory on the workings of the Kassel Hand's inoperable thumb mechanism.

My experience working with Tulman was transformative. Digital 3D modeling of a complex artifact like an early modern mechanical hand requires collaborative problem-solving to overcome the limitations of photographic evidence. It is a process that constantly generates new questions, invites creativity, and puts discrete pieces of information about an object together into a relational whole. It allows for a continuous evolution of concepts as participants theorize, assess, revise, and tweak. Fundamental to the endeavor is the bringing together of a humanities-based skillset with a technical-based one. In the case of the Kassel Hand, this was Tulman's expertise in digital tools and technical knowledge of design and construction with my historical knowledge of early modern prosthetic technology and material culture research. Rather than a straightforward process of imitation, creating a digital 3D model proved to be one of experimentation. This was recursive: our ideas influenced the shapes he rendered, and the shapes he rendered influenced our ideas. The challenge of working through the total object of the Kassel Hand in a model let us experiment to come to a speculative configuration of the known components that is impossible to know without disassembling the artifact itself.

The impact of the experience has reverberated through my work as a historian in several ways. Most evident, perhaps, is that I learned more about the Kassel Hand. The process created a more precise grasp of the components and the object's overall construction, reframing what I thought I knew and at points contributing entirely new knowledge. Even the thumb mechanism, which I deemed unknowable in 2017, now is tentatively knowable. More broadly, the project influenced my approach to material culture. Consulting with an architect introduced me to new ways of thinking about the artifacts I study. I learned how to connect my knowledge of their exteriors and interiors into a comprehensive whole. This is an invaluable tool that allows scholars to utilize available information in a way that overcomes the limitations of what the eye can see, a photograph can show, or even an X-ray can suggest.

Conceptually, the experience encouraged me to think more deeply about the processes of design and the implications of these for mechanical hands. Pursuing this thread eventually led to my engagement with the design model of disability, in which design—defined as "processes of planning and making the material world"—has "played an active role in shaping the meaning of disability" in modern society (Guffey and Williamson 2020, 1). Drawing on this notion in the early modern European context highlights the role of amputees and artisans in developing a new prosthetic technology and, as my research argues, in altering perceptions about surgical and artificial intervention in the body in Western medicine. Those who commissioned artisans to make mechanical hands exerted far more control over the design process than is possible for most amputees today because these early modern objects were custom orders produced by different craft groups on an ad-hoc basis.

A final way in which the modeling experience was particularly impactful was discovering how interdisciplinary collaboration begets further collaboration, taking research in delightfully unexpected and fruitful directions. Recently I began a dialogue with a mechanical engineer specializing in wearable robotics and assistive devices at Auburn University to explore developing Tulman's digital 3D model into a functioning 3D printed object, an incredibly complicated undertaking that would require printing all components individually and assembling them together. Should there prove to be a way forward, it would present an opportunity for a university robotics lab to assess a 3D printed model of the Kassel Hand. Determining how to study this technology in a lab in ways that are useful for members of two different disciplines working together—one interested in its relationship to modern prosthetic technology and the other concerned with its potential to shed light on the experiences of early modern prosthesis wearers—holds the potential to break new ground in historical analysis of early modern prosthetic technology. Fascinating work on another early modern artifact has been done in a neuroscience lab at Offenburg University in Germany, where in 2017 medical engineers were creating a 3D model and printed replica of a mechanical hand purportedly worn by Götz von Berlichingen at the same time as Tulman and I were mapping out the Kassel Hand. The Offenburg team based their design on a written description and diagram drawn by a historian in 1982, but they did not work with the original material culture or collaborate with a humanities-based scholar during the process (Otte 2020, 305). Their efforts demonstrate that there is an appetite for exploring historical medical objects among STEM researchers. My experience has taught me that humanities scholars should be involved in this kind of endeavor and stand to gain immensely from such collaboration. It presents an excellent opportunity not only to contribute our expertise, but also to enhance our work.

WORKS CITED

Berlichingen, Götz von. 1981. *Mein Fehd und Handlungen*. Edited by Helgard Ulmschneider. Sigmaringen: Thorbecke.

Burhenne, Verena, ed. 2003. *Prothesen von Kopf bis Fuß: Katalog zur gleichnamigen Wanderausstellung des Westfälischen Museumsamtes, Landschaftsverband Westfalen-Lippe*. Münster: Landschaftsverband Westfalen-Lippe.

Guffey, Elizabeth and Bess Williamson. 2020. "Introduction: Rethinking Design History through Disability, Rethinking Disability through Design." In *Making Disability Modern: Design Histories*, edited by Bess Williamson and Elizabeth Guffey, 1–13. London: Bloomsbury.

Hausse, Heidi. 2019. "The Locksmith, the Surgeon, and the Mechanical Hand: Communicating Technical Knowledge in Early Modern Europe." *Technology and Culture* 60, no.1: 34–64.

Heide, Mareike. 2019. *Holzbein und Eisenhand: Prothesen in der Frühen Neuzeit*. New York: Campus Verlag.

Mechel, Christian von. 1815. *Die eiserne Hand des tapfern deutschen Ritters Götz von Berlichingen, wie selbige noch bei seiner Familie in Franken aufbewahrt wird*. Berlin: Decker.

Otte, Andreas. 2020. "3D Computer-Aided Design Reconstructions and 3D Multi-Material Polymer Replica Printings of the First 'Iron Hand' of Franconian Knight Gottfried (Götz) von Berlichingen (1480–1562): An Overview." *Prosthesis* 2: 304–312.

Wunder, Amanda. 2017. *Baroque Seville: Sacred Art in a Century of Crisis*. University Park: Penn State University Press.

CHAPTER ELEVEN

Rewriting Illness from the Turkish German Margins: Eating Disorders in Narratives by Renan Demirkan and Yade Yasemin Önder

HEIKE BARTEL

Narratives describing experiences of eating disorders have to rise to the challenge of representing highly complex and multifactorial health conditions. This includes the thematic, formal, and aesthetic challenges of conveying a deeply problematic relationship with the body, a disturbed self-perception and feelings of inadequacy, disgust, or guilt that can cause great distress and may spiral out of control, even become self-destructive and violent. In addition, eating disorder narratives have to engage with the transgression or confirmation of numerous and complex orders dictating who eats what, when, how, and how much.

Yet literature is also uniquely equipped to explore eating disorders both thematically and with regards to representations of the topic through textual form, its language, structures, and imagery. After all, the arts and humanities in general and literature in particular have the ability to reflect critically and imaginatively on orders proposed by history, culture, class, gender, ethnicity, religion, socio-economic, and other factors that shape eating and feeding behavior. Furthermore, literature can give unique personal insights into a life, body, and mind affected by mental disorders and take us "*outside* and *beyond* the biomedical gaze" (Crawford, Brown, Baker, et al. 2015, 59), the statistics, diagnostic criteria, and quantitative analyses that dominate empirical and biomedical research. This is one of the reasons why Health Humanities and related interdisciplinary approaches award literature a privileged position particularly when it comes to articulating, communicating, and understanding complex mental disorders such as eating disorders.[1] The context of migration that is central to this chapter adds further strands to the literary engagement with experiences of eating disorders. Here, literature can also amplify previously unheard voices by individuals or groups affected by the topic and provide a space for their expression.

The two novels at the center of this chapter deliver each a unique narrative about food, eating, and its orders and disorders in the context of Turkish German migration: Renan Demirkan's *Schwarzer Tee mit drei Stück Zucker* [Black tea with three pieces of sugar] (1991) and Yade Yasemin Önder's *wir wissen, wir könnten, und fallen synchron* [we know, we could, and we fall in sync] (2022). The following two parts investigate via close readings how these novels interlink problematic experiences around eating and body image with the key themes of growing up, family life, migration, integration, and identity formation. The conclusion will return to addressing the relationship between literature and health and use the framework of health humanities to outline three core areas emerging from the engagement with these texts.

Written nearly thirty years apart, in very different styles and by authors separated by a thirty-year age gap and with different biographies, each text needs to be acknowledged in its own right. Their family stories of migration differ and the problematic relationships with food and the body depicted show distinct variations. This underlines that there is not one universal experience of migration and not one universal experience of mental disorder. The latter applies in particular to eating disorders which are highly complex forms of psychiatric illness interlinked with biological, genetic, and socio-cultural factors that are differently experienced by each individual. Whilst acknowledging the specificity of each novel, there is, however, also generic potential in the thoughts and themes developed through close readings of both. This needs to be undertaken in full recognition of the limits presented by working with only two texts which, in addition, focus on women only, and I have argued elsewhere for the need to open research into eating disorders to include men, boys, and individuals from LGBTQ communities (Bartel 2020).

The texts by Demirkan and Önder describe the attempts by young female protagonists with Turkish heritage to integrate into a German community and link these attempts to extreme food regulation and manipulation expressed through two types of eating disorder. Önder's text deals throughout with bulimia nervosa characterized by episodes of eating large amounts of food mostly rapidly and alone (binging). Release for resulting feelings of disgust and guilt regarding the digested food is then sought in hidden practices of self-induced vomiting (purging), followed by further attacks of binging and purging. Food consumption and the regulation of emotions are closely interlinked. In contrast, Demirkan's text alludes in one particular episode in the novel to severe restriction, even rejection of food inherent in anorexia nervosa. The Diagnostic and Statistical Manual of Mental Disorders (DSM V) sets out the following three criteria to describe anorexia nervosa: restriction of energy intake relative to requirements leading to a significantly low body weight; an intense fear of gaining weight or becoming fat, even though underweight; and a disturbance in the way in which one's body weight or shape is experienced (APA, 2013). However, in reality, the picture is much more complex and different for each individual.[2]

Historically and culturally, the configuration of women's identities has been closely associated with food, eating, and the body. Since the 1970s feminist scholarship has produced seminal studies that have shaped critical cultural engagement with eating disorders linking them to sexual politics, gendered power hierarchies, and prevailing concepts of femininity. Including Susie Orbach's pioneering *Fat Is a Feminist Issue* (1978), these studies emphasize that eating disorders are intrinsically linked to norms and expectations women are subjected to. Anorexia in particular has become a powerful signifier in this context with Orbach reading the female "anorectic's struggle as a metaphor for our age" (1986). Other key contributions to scholarship in the field emphasize the necessity of *Reflections on the Tyranny of Slenderness* (Chernin 1981) and women's and girls' struggle under the *Unbearable Weight* (Bordo 1993) of expectations regarding their body shape, size, and looks.

The topic has also increasingly found expression in literature, particularly in North American and European women's writing, even leading to a reworking of Hélène Cixous' notion of "écriture feminine" as "écriture feminine" (see Jordan and Still 2020, 12). Most of these eating disorder narratives focus on young White middle-class women with a particular focus on anorexia as the dedicated "girls" illness that is deemed to affect this cohort.[3] There are as yet relatively few literary explorations of eating disorders as experienced by individuals and groups with lesser visibility and audibility in society. Susan Bordo highlights this gap regarding African American women by emphasizing "Fat is a black woman's issue, too" in a critical take on Orbach's dictum (1993, 63). Furthermore, the editors of a collection of scholarly essays engaging with French, Italian, and German literary narratives of eating disorders point out the sparsity of references to experiences by working class individuals and "other than white women" (Jordan and Still 2020, 15). Against this backdrop, the narratives by Demirkan and Önder with their representations of anorexia and bulimia in females from the largest German minority group, Turkish Germans, form a considerable contribution to the field.

SCHWARZER TEE MIT DREI STÜCK ZUCKER (RENAN DEMIRKAN)

It is befitting for this chapter on health and migration that the first text in our focus is set in a hospital. *Schwarzer Tee mit drei Stück Zucker* [Black Tea with Three Pieces of Sugar], the 1991 debut novel of the author, journalist, and actress Renan Demirkan, is one of the first novels by an author with a Turkish background writing in German to head the best-seller lists in Germany. The novel is written from the perspective of a female third-person narrator whose life-story has some parallels with Demirkan's own. In 1962, the author moved with her family from Turkey to the Federal Republic of Germany at the age of seven.

The frame narrative situates the protagonist Maika in the present time in the labor and delivery ward of a German hospital awaiting the birth of her first child. Alone and confined to bed she is anxiously waiting for the anaesthetist to start procedures for her C-section and for the arrival of the child's German father who is stuck somewhere in transit. This situation of crisis triggers a narrative of episodic flash-backs (Fachinger 2001, 15) of the narrator's childhood and youth in Germany in the 1960s as the oldest daughter of Turkish parents and of her family in Turkey. I have written elsewhere on the role of memory, food, and identity in this and other Turkish German novels (Bartel 2019, 335–359) and have argued that Demirkan's text, despite having drawn criticism for delivering "exotic commonplaces" (Teraoka 1997, 529) or for "affirming only the readily acceptable, picturesque elements of Turkishness" (Cheesman 2007, 60), deserves more scholarly attention.

In particular, Demirkan's portrayal of the protagonist's struggle with food allows the unfolding of new perspectives on health and Turkish German identity. Eating—or, rather, not eating—illuminates the mechanisms of Demirkan's second generation Turkish-German protagonist Maika to cope with the socio-cultural challenges of migration during her teenage years. From her hospital bed, ordered not to eat anything due to her scheduled C-section, the grown-up Maika reflects back on a time in her life "in der sie sich nur untergewichtig im Spiegel betrachten mochte" ["when she could only stand looking at herself in the mirror when she was underweight"] (Demirkan 1991, 26):

> So lange sie sich zurückerinnern konnte, hatte sie Eisenmangel und zu niedrigen Blutdruck. Täglich kämpfte sie morgens mit dem bleiernen Körper. Es bedurfte morgens einer gewaltigen Überwindung, den schwindelnden Kopf in die Senkrechte zu heben, um dann doch zufrieden in die extra engen Hosen zu kriechen.
>
> (Demirkan 1991, 26–27)

> [As long as she could remember, she had an iron deficiency and a blood pressure that was too low. Every morning she fought with a body that felt like lead. It required enormous efforts to lift her dizzy head upright but then she had the satisfaction of slipping into her extra tight trousers.][4]

The biological and psychological symptoms described here bear the hallmarks of anorexia nervosa: deliberate, continuous, and obsessive undereating and avoidance of food that leads to—among other and potentially lethal outcomes—the described chronic iron deficiency, low blood pressure, light-headedness, circulatory problems and, importantly, a fixation on a body that is constantly measured and shrunk. Maika is what Petra Fachinger calls a "second-generation narrator" who looks at Turkey and Turkish traditions through "western eyes" (Fachinger 2001, 64). She perceives her image in the mirror as unacceptable if she is not underweight and rejects attempts by her Turkish family to make her gain weight. The onset of Maika's problematic relationship with eating coincides with puberty which confirms another common—yet not exclusive—marker of an eating disorder (Beat, n.d.).

In her work on body image, *The Beauty Myth*, Naomi Wolf links anorexia to "a culture fixated on female thinness" (1991, 187). Demirkan's novel with its particular focus on a migrant context adds a different perspective to this. Schoolgirl Maika is not directly striving to look like ultrathin models shown by the media or a size-zero fashion industry. Maika wants first and foremost to come as close as possible to the look of *German* girls:

> Wenn sie schon nicht so groß und blondig schön war wie die deutschen Mädchen, so zumindest die Dünnste mit der kleinsten Konfektionsgröße.
>
> (1991, 26)

> [Even if she wasn't as tall and blonde-pretty as the German girls, she was nevertheless the skinniest with the smallest dress size.]

Maika's point of orientation is the western beauty ideal of tall blonde female skinniness, an ideal that she identifies with being German. Whilst she succeeds in becoming even thinner than her peers, the look of a tall blonde German remains unattainable for her. She is set up for failure.

Demirkan's text employs the motif of anorexia and the role of food, feeding, and eating to navigate cultural norms and regimes that affect the protagonist from two sides: her Turkish heritage and her new German context. Whilst Maika's mother is portrayed as reverting to the stereotypical gendered realm of food production in an attempt to find a place as a Muslim woman in her new German living environment, Maika herself rejects this realm. Her efforts of integration are expressed through taking control of one of the few areas in her life she has power over: her intake of food. Consequently, she rejects her mother's attempts to feed her food cooked according to Islamic dietary rules, and manipulates her food intake in a futile attempt to fulfil the desired body image of German skinniness.

Anthropologists propose a reading of eating disorders as "culture-bound syndromes" (Littlewood and Lipsedge 1986, 253) reflecting the "efforts of certain individuals of inferiors status—typically defined by age or sex—to protest against or otherwise escape from their oppression by the more powerful" (Gordon 2000, 189). Maika's obsession to become thinner than the thinnest in a society that dictates skinniness for women fits this concept of the "power of the weak" (Littlewood and Lipsedge 1986, 261). It is expressed in Maika's attempt to gain control over processes of assimilations and integration. Squeezing into extra small jeans not only rejects a stereotypical body and fashion image of Turkish women in Germany but also expresses triumph over her German peers. Beating them and gaining the badge of honour "smallest dress size" gives her "auf merkwürdige Weise [...] Selbstvertrauen" ["self-confidence in the strangest way"] (Demirkan 1991, 26). Richard Gordon highlights, though, that such triumph and "rebellion" attributed to eating disorders remains "indirect and unarticulated and does not result in a fundamental change in the status quo and invariably results in the relegation of the deviant to a marginal status or an alternative identity" (Gordon 2000, 190). Being caught in the double-bind of being female *and* of Turkish heritage throws Maika even further off course in the complex balancing act of obtaining power through rejecting food. Ultimately, the control she asserts over her weight and shape, although it brings momentary self-confidence, does not empower her. Moreover, the behavior is ultimately self-destructive as eating disorders, and anorexia in particular, are "problematic, paradoxical, harmful instruments of self-empowerment" (Calamita 2018, 87). Paradoxically, shrinking her body emphasizes adolescent Maika's defiant alterity confirming her position outside the idealized norm of tall blonde German girls.

Moving on to a phase in her life when she allows her (pregnant) body to be bigger also means refusing to take on the identity of victim or sufferer. Both in linguistic and behavioral terms the third-person narrator learns to "talk back" (Fachinger 2001, 65). We can find traces of this empowering future expressed by the present-day narrator who looks back onto her adolescence from a critical distance. The ideal of female Germanness admired by teenage Maika is presented through the neologism "blondig schön." The phrase deliberately alters grammatical and linguistic conventions, adding the suffix "-ig" ungrammatically to the adjective "blond." It invites new semantic readings of the word blonde and its varied associations in German culture and history. These range from the "golden haired" maiden in German fairy tales and folklore, to the "Aryan" ideal promoted under German National Socialism, the "Blondine" as the butt of jokes about attractive yet dumb blondes, to blonde German super models like Claudia Schiffer and Heidi Klum. As a reductionist stereotype "blonde" also acts as a reminder that by no means are all German women blonde—or tall. By introducing the phrase "blondig schön," the narrator signals a shift to a position of critical distance from a stereotypical beauty ideal that is unrealistic, unattainable, potentially racist and sexist, and interconnected with contested notions of Germanness.

Changes in her body mark a clear departure from Maika's anorexic behavior: "Die Zeiten waren vorbei gewesen" ["Those times had passed"] (1991, 27). The present sees her embracing her new pregnant body, the swelling of her belly to a "schöne dicke Kugel" ["beautiful round ball"] (Demirkan 1991, 26), putting on weight, and even growing "fett" ["fat"] (Demirkan 1991, 27). Demirkan highlights the complex negotiations of cultural belonging via the female body and the cultural practices of (not) eating and feeding which play out differently over time and over two generations of Turkish German women, Maika and her mother. To (re)create a place of belonging in Germany, the first-generation mother looks to Turkish religion and tradition particularly via food, feeding, and cooking, whilst her second-generation teenage daughter looks to the dictate of Western female skinniness for orientation. Both behavioral patterns trap the individual within established albeit very different cultural boundaries. The arrival of a third generation, a daughter, announces yet a third form of negotiating cultural belonging and identity. Elizabeth Boa sees in the ending of the novel (Boa 1997, 134–135) a transgression of boundaries in the realms of languages and cultures. Tellingly, this is signalled through food: Turkish mulberries eaten with German pancakes (Demirkan 1991, 12) are part of a final tableau that paints a "hybridized future" (Fachinger 2001, 66) for the expected third generation.

WIR WISSEN, WIR KÖNNTEN UND FALLEN SYNCHRON (YADE YASEMIN ÖNDER)

Whilst Demirkan's 1991 novel marks the beginnings of wider public recognition of texts written by Turkish German authors, Önder's novel *wir wissen, wir könnten und fallen synchron* [we know, we could, and we fall in sync] (2022), published almost thirty years later, moves the German literary engagement with migration, integration, identity, and eating disorders into a very different direction.

The debut novel by Wiesbaden-born Önder started out as the author's winning entry for the 2018 Open-Mike-Wettbewerb carrying then the title "Bulimieminiaturen" ["bulimiaminiatures"] (Schellbach 2022). This early title sums up several key elements of the novel: Firstly, the literary processing of the pathology of bulimia depicting a life-disrupting cycle of binging and purging. Secondly, an aesthetic experimentation that pieces together forty-eight chapters over 250 pages. Many are prose-miniatures of great intensity often connected to others by association only, the shortest being a mere two lines, the longest forty-three pages. Thirdly, a style that plays imaginatively, often with dark comedy, to describe serious, sometimes morbid, and often grotesque events.

The longer title of the 2022 novel, *wir wissen, wir könnten und fallen synchron* [we know, we could, and we fall in sync], reflects too the fragmented character of the text yet also introduces the subjunctive "könnten" ["could"] in central position. The emphasis on the irrealis mood via this *coniuntivus irrealis* fits in with an often-deliberate openness of the narrator's account: The protagonist remains nameless and the narrative changes from the first person to third-person. Events are described in several alternative ways and by mixing dreamlike sequences with childhood memories and report-like descriptions. For example, the death of the father is alternatively introduced as him being gruesomely self-dismembered by a chainsaw in a woodworking accident, as drowning in a public swimming pool, or as simply vanishing. The novel ends with a dreamlike fantasy where the father returns. The author also acknowledges being influenced by Raymond Queneau's seemingly spontaneous yet painstakingly constructed perspectival writing and by Benjamin von Stuckrad-Barre's autobiographical novel *Panikherz* (2016), dealing with the author's bulimia and addiction and part of New German Pop Literature.[5]

Notwithstanding the novel's openness for different readings, its individual miniature stories are by no means vague but present very realistic, sharp, and hard-hitting descriptions of problems surrounding identity, sexual and family relationships, emotional belonging, and mental health. The protagonist looks back onto her childhood of growing up in Germany with a German mother and a Turkish father who dies when she is young, leaving mother and daughter in an increasingly fraught relationship that lasts into adulthood. Tensions within the wider family further complicate the protagonist's biography, particularly the lack of acceptance of her Turkish father, portrayed as grotesquely overweight by her German grandparents who are themselves obsessed with diets and exercise. The deeply unsettling effect of these overwhelming and toxic family relations can be read behind the protagonist's description of herself as a "Mischling aus meiner Mutter und meinem Vater" ["a mix of my mother and my father"] (2022, 21).

Problematic relationships with food and the body are part of this "mix" from the start and intensified by the protagonist's Turkish heritage that shapes how she is seen in society and by her own German grandparents. The pubescent girl is torn between conflicting messages linked to her body. Pointing to what he calls the prepubescent child's "Speckbrüstchen" ["little chubby breasts"] (2022, 21), her German grandfather tells her not to eat too much. Particularly not too much of the fatty foreign food offered proudly by her Turkish father during a tense family outing to a Turkish restaurant. An embarrassment to the child, particularly during sport lessons, the teenage protagonist finds later that these very "Speckbrüstchen" attract attention from boys. Veering between making her body desirable and undesirable, these unsettling experiences prepare the ground for a troubled relationship with her own body and for deeply problematic sexual relationships with men in later life.

Her mixed ethnic background, awakening sexuality that causes both lust and disgust, and the turbulences of a growing body are the unreliable markers for the protagonist's deeply conflicted identity. The perception of female foreignness in modern German society in a particular mix of sexism and racism adds further to this conflict. One minute her "exotic" looks are rated by this society as "French," equalling desirable and attractive. Another minute, when her surname discloses her Turkish background, she is perceived as undesirable and ugly, "Turkish" (2022, 209–210).

The link between food, body, and foreignness plays out in particular in an episode at school. Like Demirkan's text, Önder's novel shows here the longed-for yet rejected integration of the teenage protagonist into her German peer group. Despite being born in Germany and having a German mother, little seems to have changed for Önder's protagonist since the 1960s when Demirkan's Maika and her family were being insulted as "Knoblauchfresser" and "Kümmeltürken" (Demirkan 1991, 21). Önder's protagonist is being publicly humiliated by the coolest boy of her school who reacts "angeekelt" ["with disgust"] (2022, 203) to her presence, loudly shouting: *"Igitt, warum stinkt's denn hier plötzlich so nach Knoblauch?"* ["Yuck, why does is suddenly stink of garlic here?"] (Önder 2022, 203). What Önder's protagonist experiences here—just like Maika thirty years earlier—is the continuation of a long cultural history of xenophobia and racism expressed via associations with particular foods. The texts show how, since the 1960s, Turks as the largest German minority group have become the main target of racism. These racist attitudes are not changed by the blatant fact that "Döner," the food associated with the protagonists' imagined disgusting smell of garlic, has become a staple German fast-food. Önder calls out the hypocrisy of this insult by describing how all pupils—including the peer group who bullies her—eat Döner nearly daily buying it from friendly "Ali" (2022, 204) at their local kebab shop. The popular dish signals superficial multicultural openness, yet only when stripped off any offending foreignness. Even down to its spelling the Döner has been embraced as a German consumer good, and Americanized marketing strategies as e.g. "McDöner"[6] further signal its part of the teenage diet in the text alongside globally branded hyper-processed foods like Twix, Nutella, and McDonald's which are, in turn, essential ingredients in the protagonist's binge eating attacks.

Önder employs food to reflect critically on the façade of German society that superficially embraces foreignness yet only thinly veils its underlying xenophobia. Reducing the protagonist to an ill-fitting racist caricature of a constantly Döner-eating and offensive-smelling foreigner, her peers use food to hatefully mock her and single her out. That the protagonist makes clear that these associations do not have anything to do with her does little to change the insult. Reading the novel as a "Migrationsmemoir" Hanna Engelmeier identifies this as a tension between the protagonist's identification with the German social environment in which she grows up and a (Turkish) difference assigned to her by this very environment (Engelmeier 2022).

The experience of being stigmatized as "stinking of garlic" by the most desirable boy in her school and in the presence of those whom the protagonist considered her best friends delivers one crucial piece in the complex picture of her developing bulimia. The eating disorder fulfils a function that is not predominantly aimed at the desire to look a certain way but at wanting to escape and punish a body that is perceived as offending and causing disgust.

Disgust is a central theme in this text that also plays with the effect that descriptions of dismembered body parts and bodily fluids may have on the reader. Yet disgust also marks xenophobic behaviors in society and is mockingly displayed by the ring-leader at school who reacts to her fictitious offending body odour. His humiliating and hateful reaction is mirrored by her other peers who simulate retching and vomiting. The absence of any real olfactory offense—the protagonist is freshly showered and, above all, Döner with onion and garlic is not in the least offensive to these teenagers—highlights that this scene plays out a symbolic order via food and its associations with foreignness.

Julia Kristeva delivers a cultural and historical definition of disgust beyond alimentary disgust as the reaction to a real or imagined disturbance of an identity, a system, or an order (Kristeva 1982, 2). She highlights the *Powers of Horror* inherent in culturally and historically conditioned fantasies of contamination and shows how the concept of disgust underpins political, cultural, and linguistic practices of exclusion and violence (Sjöholm 2005, 80–82). The long history of insults linked to garlic, e.g. via the term "Knoblauchfresser," illustrates a particular German context for these practices. Since the eighteenth century, foreign foods like garlic have played a role in racist practices. The insult "Knoblauchfresser" has been employed in Nazi Germany to justify the persecution of Jews, associating them with perceived bad odours, "un-German" cultural practices, and contamination (Mandel 2008, 135–137). Since the 1960s the association with garlic has been taken up as a tool of abuse against Turks in Germany, and Önder's novel reflects its still common use.

In a psychological twist that turns the disgust she is objected to by others against herself, Önder's protagonist internalizes the feeling which then becomes central to her self-destructive bulimic behavior. Winfried Menninghaus defines disgust in the context of cultural history and aesthetics as

> die Erfahrung einer Nähe, die nicht gewollt wird. Eine sich aufdrängende Präsenz, eine riechende oder schmeckende Konsumtion wird spontan als Kontamination bewertet und mit Gewalt distanziert.
>
> (Menninghaus 2000, 247)
>
> [the experience of a proximity which is not wanted. An obtruding presence, a smelling or tasting consumption is spontaneously rated as contamination and forcefully pushed away].[7]

Internalizing the disgust expressed by her peers, the protagonist perceives the smell of her own body, intensified by the hormonal changes of puberty, as a contaminating presence that needs to be forcefully eliminated. Continuing the association with "disgusting" food, her own sweat starts to smell for her of "onion and garlic" (2022, 203). Frightened and embarrassed by her developing body, she imagines a disgusting foul smell of fish emanating from her vagina. The pubescent teenager reacts with the futile vow to rid her body of any smell in an attempt to banish any insulting comments as well as negating her developing female sexuality. This manifests in the obsessive and compulsive cleansing and scrubbing of her body—outside and inside. In violent acts of expelling any food on which she has previously binged she scrubs out her inside aiming to become "komplett sauber" ["completely clean"] (207). The fear of contamination and the obsessive desire to cleanse herself signal serious psychological distress further exacerbated by the onset of puberty and culminate in the pathological pattern of bulimia.

It is not only her own smell and body that take on an obtruding presence for the protagonist. In a turn that intermixes the psychological with the fantastic, boys start emanating unbearable smells for her. Their close proximity, sexual interest, and any tentative "*Ich liebe dich*" ["I love you"] (206) are thrilling and wanted, yet at the same time manifest themselves as highly disturbing olfactory invasions.

In line with her developing eating disorder, the protagonist describes her later life as dominated by her "missbräuchliche Beziehung mit der Mikrowelle" ["abusive relationship with the microwave"]: "Reinschieben, rausziehen, reinziehen, rausholen" ["push in, pull out, take in, take out"] (2022, 207). This dark comical play with words describes the bulimic cycle of microwaving food, consuming, and purging it. Here, any cultural or personal order to life through food, e.g., via family meals, celebrations or simply cooking, feeding or eating to give rhythm and regularity to a day, is reduced to a mechanical process. The only order is presented by the destructive pattern of chronic bulimic behavior that sets a mechanism in motion that gains autonomy and ultimately spirals out of control.[8] The image also contains sexual connotations alluding to intercourse as a mechanical act of penetration and withdrawal, an "in and out" void of any emotion and the body resembling an automaton. The image of the penetrating penis becomes interchangeable with that of the ready-to-eat-meal being pushed into a microwave oven or a finger pushed down the throat to self-induce vomiting. Unsurprisingly, many of the protagonist's numerous relationships with boys and men—one chapter lists fifty-one (2022, 135–140)—bear marks of the abusive, destructive, and self-destructive. Particularly in the longest chapter of the novel, the stylistically Queneau-inspired "Hymen II," Önder's repeated yet always different descriptions of one violent/sado-masochistic sexual encounter raise uncomfortable questions around consent and rape. These are being left provocatively open by the author and are expressed in the repeatedly inserted sentence "*So hast du das gewollt?*" ["This is how you wanted it?"] (2022, 189–232). The protagonist is unable to deliver answers as she has lost any sense of feeling and of self.

The tension between "Innen außen" ["Inside outside"], so the title of chapter twenty-two (2022, 86–91), can be seen as driving this text. It finds its graphic culmination in the eating disorder bulimia with its cycle of taking in and expelling. The reader gains insight into a world of mental disorder through a narrative that is deliberately disorientating, fractured, unsettling, and that resists attempts of linear readings. In addition to conveying the feelings, thoughts, and memories of the protagonist, Önder also portrays a surrounding world that is deeply hostile and threatening. Part of this "outside" are social and cultural patterns that are clearly contributing factors to the protagonist's illness, yet they are also deeply troubling in themselves: xenophobic attitudes in German society, hostile peer groups, fractured families, and a cultural history of racism that continues to the present day and shapes particular forms of singling out those with Turkish heritage. However, Önder's text also broadens its focus by moving from Turkish German matters to a much broader global context. The novel starts by dating the protagonist's year of birth with reference to "Tschernobyl" (2022, 5), an unprecedented nuclear catastrophe with lasting effects on lives and the environment. Further global and national events mark a world of rapid political and cultural change, wars, and often disconcerting disorder. The Third Gulf War, Erdoğan becoming prime minister of Turkey, and the Arab Spring are only three examples.

The text ends with an apocalyptic tableau of a comet hitting the earth. Yet the novel that has kept its characters and the world around them on a constant collision course does not end with an ultimate all-annihilating smash-up. Rather, it transports the narrator to an unexpected dreamlike scenario where she falls asleep—seemingly content and at peace—on top of the rough body of the comet that has turned into the large body of a friendly giant resembling her father who stretches out like a new continent. This ending of calm in chaos expresses a tangible yearning to belong, be safe and protected, yet against the backdrop of a novel of disintegration and fragmentation the novel continues to question whether this can ever be fulfilled.

CONCLUSION

The discipline of Health Humanities, alongside related disciplines such as critical medical humanities and narrative medicine, advocates the role of the arts in general and literature in particular to instigate conversation between arts & humanities and biomedical sciences in order to broaden our understanding of health, improve how systems and individuals promote good health, and how we interact with those who are affected by illness.

This volume explores how German Studies and Health Humanities can relate to each other and inform scholarship across and within disciplines. Through the close readings of the two texts by Demirkan and Önder, this chapter has started to unfold the particular contribution that literature written in German dealing with migration and Turkish heritage can make to this exploration. The topics and questions the texts thematize through their different representations of eating disorders open a wide historical, cultural, and political field in which the ordering and disordering of food, eating, feeding is played out. Part of these engagements are also theoretical and historical perspectives ranging from anthropological and linguistic studies and theories of disgust; questions regarding gender, sexual politics; and particularly factors regarding migration, identity, and integration. A Health Humanities-informed approach can highlight three key areas emerging from the analysis of the two narratives in the context of these questions and approaches.

USE OF TEXTS TO ADVANCE HEALTHCARE

Due to their perceived status as a western illness that mainly affects White teenage girls from affluent backgrounds, eating disorders are notoriously missing when it comes to considering health problems of individuals and groups who fall outside these narrow criteria. This is despite recent research highlighting that children and young people with a background in migration are particularly prone to developing an eating disorder (Robert Koch Institute 2020; World Health Organisation 2018; Migrazine 2017). Lack of knowledge of the illness (and life) experiences of minority groups often stands in the way of understanding the needs and problems of individuals and cohorts. Demirkan's and Önder's narratives show the potential of literature to address this lack by portraying eating disorders as experienced by characters with Turkish heritage. Bringing such texts into interdisciplinary conversations with healthcare professionals or use them in training can encourage a re-evaluation of health policies and practices regarding eating disorders concerning under-represented and under-researched groups. In turn, the critical reflections upon prevailing stereotypes around eating disorders from a perspective from the margins can also be fruitful for re-evaluating how eating disorders in general are seen and researched.[9]

More generally, the detailed analysis of textual representations of experiences of illness can advance discussion around the prevalence of people with a background in migration for mental and physical illness. They can add insight into individual experiences but also add a much wider socio-cultural and historic context for what is clinically defined as "idioms of distress" (Nichter 1981, 379) and "ethnopsychiatric phenomena [...] brought on or exacerbated by cultural displacement, migration stress, and sociopolitical marginalization" (Vanderlinden 2009, 45). The texts by Önder and Demirkan with their nuanced and individual reflections on the complex matter of health also remind us to resist labels that pathologize experiences of migration.

WIDENING THE CONTEXT OF HEALTH

Both Demirkan and Önder situate the individual in a life context that outlines in detail how society, family, peer groups, culture, language, history as well as national and global events affect their protagonists' life, identity, and health. This is particularly relevant to understanding eating disorders, which are affected by biological and genetic factors and by socio-cultural influences. There are numerous examples for the latter in the two texts, e.g., in the link between Maika's rejection of food and her complex balancing of her Turkish family background and German assimilation. Such socio-cultural influences are also illustrated in the reaction to insult and humiliation of Önder's protagonist who internalizes emotions of the disgust she is made to feel by others and, in turn, projects these emotions back onto them. With its emphasis on the tense relationship between "Innen außen" ("Inside outside") (2022, 86), Önder's text uses the pathology of bulimia nervosa for a dark portrayal of modern life that puts the individual onto a collision course with others and with itself from birth. The perspective from the margins of society offered by both texts not only gives insight into experiences of living in Germany with a Turkish background but also invites critical reflection about Germany. Both texts raise questions around health, integration, xenophobia, and racism in the historical context of migrant movement to Germany from Turkey since the 1960s and regarding the status of people with Turkish heritage in the first, second, and third generation. As such the texts also contribute to (re)mapping the genre of "Turkish German migrant literature" with Önder's text in particular resisting narrow categorizations.[10]

ILLNESS AND LITERARY FORM

Literature takes us to but also beyond the particular thematic representation of eating disorders. The close readings of both texts show that their style, narrative form, structure, and language are essential in giving expression to complex concerns, emotions and experiences, even to struggles finding language.

In Demirkan's novel, the linear framework narrative that culminates in the birth of a daughter supports the notion that the narrator has moved on from her problematic relationship with food. As such, the novel shows the characteristics of overcoming struggles and emotional growth inherent in the traditional *Bildungsroman* genre or in the "quest narrative," as Arthur Frank calls such stories in his topology of illness narratives (Frank 1995, 115–126). Consequently, food is embraced rather than rejected in Demirkan's final tableau announcing change and the transgression of cultural boundaries. Furthermore, stylistic tools—like the neologism "blondig schön"—are employed to create critical distance from a former self and signal that the grown-up narrator has found her own language.

In contrast, Önder's novel largely resists a linear reading due to its fragmented form and various takes on reality. Form and language are here instrumental in conveying severe bulimia nervosa as an experience of constant mental distress. Like other texts about mental disorder, Önder's novel can be "challenging, even alienating" for the reader through a "destruction of linear narrative form, twisting of narrative time and place, and thematic concerns which emerge as sometimes violent, explicit, and boundary dismantling" (Baker 2022, 143). The representations of sex are particularly disconcerting in Önder's text. The repetition of one sex scene in multiple narrative "takes" in the chapter "Hymen II" robs the woman at its center of agency and identity, destabilizes her position, and leaves her utterly vulnerable for violation. Furthermore, structural and narrative elements emphasize a memory and perception that is not always reliable but can play out events in arrays of different versions. In addition, a darkly humorous episode introducing an elaborate fake story about hosting an invented Christmas dinner party to cover up a massive food binge offers a different take on the concept of the unreliable narrator. Images of the body as a mechanically functioning machine convey the pathology of bulimia nervosa with its repeat cycles of "in and out," yet also signal the dehumanization of the individual in a threatening and disintegrating world and mark the vulnerability of the person who has lost all sense of self. Önder's borrowings from the fantastic and grotesque and her stylistic references to writers like Raymond Queneau contribute to portraying that the familiar can turn utterly unfamiliar in the experience of an individual.

The two narratives encourage us to consider how literature can provide a space for individual, unique, and imaginative expression of experiences of disorder and distress outside a "homogenizing diagnostic framework" (Baker 2022, 143). They portray illness and life experiences in the context of German writings about migration, integration, and identity. These give, in turn, insight into the meaning the orders and disorders around eating carry for the individual and also how this meaning relates to the social and cultural world they inhabit. The scope and potential of the two texts at the centre of this chapter have been unfolded through scholarship grounded in German literary and cultural studies yet with a health humanities-inspired openness to matters of health and healthcare. Such an approach that harnesses the strengths of the individual discipline yet is also open to interdisciplinary thinking and to exploring the use of findings in other contexts may offer new and exciting dimensions to inspire and rethink German Studies.

NOTES

1. See Gammelgaard (2022, 1–20); Crawford et al. (2015).
2. For more details on anorexia and bulimia nervosa see, for example, Gordon (2000, 14–56); Beat (n.d.).
3. Examples of this in the German-language context are: Ulrike Drasener's *Mitgift* (2002); Karen Duve's *Regenroman* (1999), and *Dies ist kein Liebeslied* (2000); Helene Flöss' *Dürre Jahre* (1988); Anna Mitgutsch's *Die Züchtigung* (1985).
4. Unless otherwise stated, translations are the author's own.
5. For an analysis of Stuckrad-Barre's narrative of anorexia and bulimia, see Bartel (2020).
6. "The Döner" remains of interest to writers and scholars engaging with the negotiations of Turkish-German identity. See Cagla (1995, 209–230); Schami (1993, 11–24).
7. Translation by Keyvan Sarkhosh (2014, 102).
8. This subjective account of bulimia finds echoes in accounts by others. See Gordon (2000, 37–50).
9. The author's research in this field has been undertaken as part of the interdisciplinary project EDIFY (Eating Disorders: Delineating illness and recovery trajectories to inform personalized prevention and early intervention in young people) https://edifyresearch.co.uk/. The author acknowledges funding for this work from the Medical Research Council.
10. For most recent research in the extensive field, see Brandt and Yildiz (2022); Gezen, Layne, and Skolnik (2022); and Selfe (2019).

WORKS CITED

Bagley, Petra M., Francesca Calamita, and Kathryn Robson, eds. 2018. *Starvation, Food Obsession and Identity: Eating Disorders in Contemporary Women's Writing*. Berne: Peter Lang.

Baker, Charley. 2022. "Rethinking Clinical and Critical Perspectives on Psychosis in Kathy Acker's Writing." In *Madness and Literature: What Fiction Can Do for the Understanding of Mental Illness*, edited by Lasse R Gammelgaard, 143–163. Exeter: Exeter University Press.

Bartel, Heike. 2020. *Men Writing Eating Disorders: Autobiographical Writing and Illness Experience in English and German Literature*. Bingley: Emerald.
Bartel, Heike. 2019. "Writing Food and Food Memories in Turkish-German Fiction." In *Memory and Postcolonial Studies: Synergies and New Directions*, edited by Dirk Göttsche, 335–359. Oxford: Peter Lang.
Beat, n.d. "Types of Eating Disorders." Accessed January 15, 2023. https://www.beateatingdisorders.org.uk/get-information-and-support/about-eating-disorders/types/.
Boa, Elizabeth Boa. 1997. "Sprachenverkehr: Hybrides Schreiben in Werken von Özdamar, Özakin und Demirkan." In *Interkulturelle Konfigurationen: Zur deutschsprachigen Erzählliteratur von Autoren nichtdeutscher Herkunft*, edited by Mary Howard. 115–138. Munich: Iudicium.
Bordo, Susan. 1993. *Unbearable Weight: Feminism, Western Culture, and the Body*. Oakland: University of California Press.
Brandt, Bettina and Yasemin Yildiz, ed. 2022. *Tales That Touch: Migration, Translation, and Temporality in 20th- and 21st-Century German Literature and Culture*. Berlin/ Boston: De Gruyter.
Cagla, Ayse. 1995. "McDoner: Doner Kebap and the Social Positioning Struggle of German Turks." In *Marketing in a Multicultural World: Ethnicity, Nationalism and Cultural Identity*, edited by Janeen Costa and Gary Bamossy, 209–230. Thousand Oaks: Sage.
Calamita, Francesca. 2018. "On the Verge of Emotional Hunger." In *Starvation, Food Obsession and Identity: Eating Disorders in Contemporary Women's Writing*, edited by Petra M. Bagley, Francesca Calamita, and Kathryn Robson, 67–90. Berne: Peter Lang.
Cheesman, Tom. 2007. *Novels of Turkish-German Settlement: Cosmopolite Fictions*. Rochester: Camden House.
Chernin, Kim. 1981. *The Obsession: Reflections on the Tyranny of Slenderness*. New York: Harper & Row.
Crawford, Paul, Brian Brown, Charley Baker, Victoria Tischler, and Brian Abrams. 2015. *Health Humanities*. London: Palgrave Macmillan.
Engelmeier, Hanna. 2022. "Nach Hause, in klobigen Schuhen. Rezension." *Die Zeit online*. Accessed December 15, 2022. https://www.zeit.de/kultur/literatur/2022-04/wir-wissen-wir-koennten-und-fallen-synchron-yade-yasemin-oender?utm_referrer=https%3A%2F%2Fwww.google.com%2F.
Fachinger, Petra. 2001. *Rewriting Germany from the Margins: "Other" Literature of the 1980s and the 1990s*. London/ Ithaca: McGill-Queens University Press.
Frank, Arthur W. 1995. *The Wounded Storyteller. Body, Illness and Ethics*. Chicago: The University of Chicago Press.
Gammelgaard, Lasse R., ed. 2022. *Madness and Literature. What Fiction Can Do for the Understanding of Mental Illness*. Exeter: Exeter University Press.
Gezen, Ela, Priscilla Layne, and Jonathan Skolnik, eds. 2022. *Minority Discourses in Germany since 1990*. Oxford: Berghahn.
Gordon, Richard A. 2000. *Eating Disorders: Anatomy of a Social Epidemic*. Oxford: Blackwell.
Gorfinkel, Elena. 2012. "Weariness. Waiting: Enduration and Art: Cinema's Tired Bodies." *Discourse* 34, no. 2–3: 311–347.
Jordan, Shirley and Judith Still, eds. 2020. *Disorderly Eating in Contemporary Women's Writing*. Special Issue of *Journal of Romance Studies* 20.2.
Kristeva, Julia. 1982. *Powers of Horror: An Essay on Abjection. Translated from French by Leon Roudiez*. New York: Columbia University Press.
Littlewood, Roland and Maurice Lipsedge. 1986. "The Culture-Bound Syndromes of the Dominant Culture: Culture, Psychopathology and Biomedicine." In *Transcultural Psychiatry*, edited by Jon L. Cox, 253–273. London: Croom Helm.
Mandel, Ruth. 2008. *Cosmopolitan Anxieties: Turkish Challenges to Citizenship and Belonging in Germany*. Durham/London: Duke University Press.

Menninghaus, Winfried. 2000. "'Wir lernen den Ekel um' (Nietzsche). Grundlinien einer Philosophie modernen Ekels." In *Große Gefühle. Bausteine menschlichen Verhaltens*, edited by ZDF-Nachtstudio, 247–264. Frankfurt am Main: Suhrkamp.

Migrazine. 2017. "'Das Leben hat Gewicht!' ein Projekt der Primärprävention von Essstörungen im Kontext von Migration." Accessed December 15, 2022. http://www.migrazine.at/artikel/das-leben-hat-gewicht-ein-projekt-der-prim-rpr-vention-von-essst-rungen-im-kontext-von-migra.

Naiboglu, Gozde. 2018. *Post-Unification Turkish German Cinema: Work, Globalisation and Politics Beyond Representation*. Cham: Palgrave Macmillan.

Nichter, Mark. 1981. "Idioms of Distress: Alternatives in the Expression of Psychosocial Distress. A Case Study from South India." *Culture, Medicine, and Psychiatry* 5, no. 4: 379–408.

Robert Koch Institut. 2020. "Frauengesundheitsbericht." Accessed December 15, 2022. https://www.rki.de/DE/Content/Gesundheitsmonitoring/Studien/Geschlecht_Gesundheit/FP_frauengesundheitsbericht.html.

Sarkhosh, Keyvan. 2014. "'Sick, Sick, Sick'? Pornographie, Disgust, and the Limit Value of Aesthetics." In *Quote, Double Quote: Aesthetics between High and Popular Culture*, edited by Paul Ferstl and Keyvan Sarkhosh, 99–120. Amsterdam/New York: Rodopi.

Schami, Rafik. 1993. "Kebab ist Kultur." In Rafik Schami *Der Fliegenmelker: Geschichten aus Damaskus*, 11–24. Kiel: Neuer Malik Verlag.

Schellbach, Miryam. 2022. *"Twix, Nutella und ich." Süddeutsche Zeitung online*. Accessed December 15, 2022. https://www.sueddeutsche.de/kultur/yade-yasemin-oender-wir-wissen-wir-koennten-und-fallen-synchron-1.5583565.

Selfe, Lauren. 2019. *Representations of Muslim Women in German Popular Culture, 1990–2015*. Berne: Peter Lang.

Sjöholm, Cecilia. 2005. *Kristeva and the Political*. London/New York: Routledge.

Teraoka, Arlene. 1997. "Turkish–German Literature." In *The Feminist Encyclopedia of German Literature*, edited by Friederike Ursula Eigler and Susanne Kord, 528–529. Westport: Greenwood.

Vanderlinden, Lisa K. 2009. "East in West: Turkish Migrants and the Conception of the Ethic Other in Germany." In *Assisting Reproduction, Testing Genes: Global Encounters with New Biotechnologies*, edited by Daphna Birenbaum-Carmeli and Marcia C. Inhorn, 29–60. Oxford: Berghahn.

Wolf, Naomi. 1991. *The Beauty Myth: How Images of Beauty Are Used Against Women*. New York: Morrow & Company.

World Health Organisation. 2018. "Mental Health Promotion and Mental Health Care in Migrants." Accessed December 15, 2022. https://www.euro.who.int/__data/assets/pdf_file/0004/386563/mental-health-eng.pdf

CHAPTER TWELVE

Teaching at the Intersection of German Studies and Disability Studies

ALEC CATTELL

Disability studies scholarship has a long tradition of demonstrating how stories about disability shape how we think about disability and how people with disabilities are viewed and treated (Garland-Thomson 1997). While cultural representations of disability have been used to objectify, exoticize, and silence people with disabilities, they can also serve to empower and enable by giving voice to lived experiences and raising awareness about disabling policies, practices, and discourses (Waldschmidt 2017, 24–25). While representations of disability and narratives about disability abound in the realm of cultural production (Bérubé 2016), those who encounter them are often underequipped to interpret the ways that cultural deployments of disability reflect, shape, and embody discourses that have an impact on lived experiences. Whether consciously or unconsciously, those who create cultural artifacts that deal with disability and those who consume them are involved in a process of negotiating what it is like, and what it means, to live with a disability. From films, novels, and graphic novels to blogs, vlogs, and TikTok videos, ideas about disability are constantly circulated and negotiated, and critical perspectives are needed to help us understand their impact on how we view disability and how our paradigms influence individual and collective actions.

This essay explores how Disability Studies might be taught in a German Studies course with a critical pedagogical approach within a Health Humanities paradigm. The goals of such a course within a higher education curriculum, as Therese Jones et al. (2017) have argued, should be to provide "students and practitioners access to a distinctive point of view about experiences of illness and impairment that may, in turn, change how providers, especially physicians, see patients" (934). The development of such a course might be part of a larger restructuring of the curriculum to make explicit connections between German Studies and health careers. Interdisciplinary connections are not only vital for the continued relevance of German Studies programs in higher education, but they are also essential for equipping future health professionals with the kinds of knowledge and skills that enable them to grapple with the complex ethical dimensions of healthcare. Jones et al. point out that the best course offerings in Health Humanities today are not limited by disciplinary boundaries; rather, they are grounded in a concern for "individual and cultural experiences of illness and disability and with the social/structural/political impediments to health and healing" (934) in a wide range of cultural artifacts from the past and present. This broader lens requires a flexible approach to the selection of content and a thoughtful course design process to ensure that learners are guided through readings, viewings, discussions, and other activities in ways that support their development. While subject-specific knowledge and (transferable) skills will certainly feature as learning objectives, a German Studies/Disability Studies course should also serve to empower students and cultivate attitudes such as curiosity, openness, empathy, and the ability to identify the limits of their knowledge and lived experiences.

This chapter is organized around three central concerns that faculty will likely encounter as they develop a course at the intersection of German Studies and Disability Studies. The first of these—Why is such a course valuable for students and academic programs?—will be taken up in the opening section, while the second question—What theories and primary texts can help to guide the development of this course?—will be taken up in the middle section. The third question—How can faculty make pedagogical choices to ensure that this course is accessible, inclusive, and engaging for all students?—will be addressed in the final section.

A CASE FOR DISABILITY STUDIES IN GERMAN STUDIES

Establishing a rationale for a German Studies and Disability Studies course involves delving into the histories of each discipline to trace their development and identify current issues that may be addressed at their intersection. The emergence of disability studies is marked by a movement from a medical model of disability toward a social model of disability, out of which a cultural branch has emerged. Building on research and social movements in the 1970s, the activist and lecturer Michael Oliver coined the term "the social model of disability" (1981), which Colin Barnes describes as entailing these key principles:

> [...] a social model perspective is not a denial of the importance or value of appropriate individually based interventions, be they medically, re/habilitative, educational or employment-based. Instead, it draws attention to their limitations in terms of furthering disabled people's empowerment. Second, the social model is a deliberate attempt to shift attention away from the functional limitations of individuals with impairments onto the problems caused by disabling environments, barriers and cultures. In short, the social

> model of disability is a tool with which to provide insights into the disabling tendencies of modern society in order to generate policies and practices to facilitate their eradication.
>
> (Barnes 2020, 20)

As Barnes indicates, the medical model defines disability as an individual, biological problem that requires correction or eradication, while the social model views disability as distinct from impairment (a biological phenomenon) and as a product of disabling social environments that require reformation. While the social model continues to be an important and useful tool for social change to remove barriers for people with disabilities, Tobin Siebers (2013) points out that the issue of embodiment remains a "bone of contention in disability studies because it seems caught between competing models of disability" (290). In the context of the debate within Disability Studies regarding how to conceptualize the body, Siebers intervenes to help the field move forward in a productive direction by outlining a theory of complex embodiment, which

> [...] raises awareness of the effects of disabling environments on people's lived experience of the body, but it emphasizes as well that some factors affecting disability, such as chronic pain, secondary health effects, and aging, derive from the body. [...] they belong to the spectrum of human variation, conceived both as variability between individuals and as variability within an individual's life cycle, and they need to be considered in tandem with social forces affecting disability. [...] Complex embodiment theorizes the body and its representations as mutually transformative. Social representations obviously affect the experience of the body, [...] but the body possesses the ability to determine its social representations well, and some situations exist where representation exerts no control over the life of the body.
>
> (290)

Siebers thus provides a powerful conceptual tool for understanding social construction in a radical and politically potent way. Demonstrating that constructions possess both social and physical forms, Siebers helps us to conceive of "reality as a mediation, no less real for being such, between representation and its social objects" (293). This insight resonates with work that disabilities studies scholars in the humanities have done to investigate the ways in which ideas about disability and cultural representations of disability have shaped and been shaped by lived experiences of disability (cf. Rosemarie Garland-Thompson 1997; David T. Mitchell and Sharon L. Snyder 2000; Carol Poore, 2007; Ato Quayson 2007; Jay T. Dolmage 2014).

Engagements with fictional narratives that deal with disability are particularly helpful because they enable us to learn about embodiments that differ from our own and imagine others' experiences without transgressing the boundary of ethical reading (Liu 2009). For instance, a guided reading of a novel that portrays experiences of disability can help readers to acknowledge the difference between *knowing about* disability and *experiencing* disability. Fictional narratives therefore provide opportunities to engage deeply with peripheral embodiments (Mitchell and Snyder 2016) and explore anti-normative narratives of embodiment (Mitchell 2020) without relying on disability simulations that can end up reifying negative myths about disability as loss or lack and tempting participants to compare disabilities to determine "What Is Worse?" (Siebers 2013, 292). In other words, cultural perspectives on disability are useful for advancing the political aims of disability studies while protecting people with disabilities.

A further contribution to the field has been made Anne Waldschmidt (2017), a German sociologist who builds on the work of Anglophone scholars to draft a cultural model of disability. Like Siebers, Waldschmidt posits that neither disability nor impairment should be considered as "clear-cut categories of pathological categorization that automatically, in the form of a causal link, result in social discrimination" (24) and that a cultural model of disability should view impairment, disability, and normality as "effects generated by academic knowledge, mass media, and everyday discourses" (24). Waldschmidt's approach complements Siebers' theory of complex embodiment by accounting for the *cultural construction* of disability in addition to biological and social factors. Waldschmidt's cultural model of disability avoids two pitfalls: the tendency of the medical model to label people with disabilities as defective, and the tendency of the social model to view disability "as a social problem [that] can be 'solved' through accessibility and participation, mainstreaming and human rights policies" (21).

Waldschmidt challenges us to adopt a constructivist approach to investigate how prevailing symbolic orders and institutional practices produce the categories of disability and ability and explore ways to problematize issues of health and normality. In so doing, Waldschmidt argues, "the historical contingency and cultural relativity of inclusion and exclusion, stigmatization and recognition can come into consideration, as well as socio-cultural patterns of experience and identity, meaning-making and practice, power and resistance" (25). Waldschmidt points out that the medical sciences can benefit from cultural model insights to grapple with complex questions such as:

> Why then are certain differences subsumed under the label "disabled" and others considered as "normal" manifestations of diversity? Why do modern societies see the need to categorize people as "normal" and "deviants?" Why and how is disability negatively valued? In which ways is "otherness"—and disability is a form of alterity—(re-)produced in history, society, and cultures?
>
> (19–20)

Humanities disciplines such as German Studies are helpful for investigating such questions through the study of representations of disability in cultural artifacts. In their introduction to the *Edinburgh German Yearbook on Disability in German Literature, Film, and Theater* (2010), Eleoma Bodammer and Michael Schillmeier underscore the fact that "the cultural *is* essentially political" (5, emphasis in original) and demonstrate that "the 'cultural model of disability,' which we define as the analysis of the representations of disabled people in the cultural spaces of art, media, and literature, can assist with the understanding of the history of disability and disabling processes" (Bodammer and Schillmeier 2010, 5). Recent publications such as *Disability in German-Speaking Europe* (2022) have continued in this tradition of mining German-language texts for insights that advance our knowledge about how disability and ability have been represented and deployed in history, memory, and culture.

In turn, Disability Studies presents an opportunity for German programs to reimagine their relevance for twenty-first-century university students. Whether one's specialization lies in past or present cultural production, there are a wealth of artifacts to explore that are valuable for an inquiry into disability *as such* (Bodammer and Schillmeier 2010); that is, as a lived experience that is shaped by and that has the power to shape representation in a range of media and genres. In short, Disability Studies can provide a fresh lens for discovering new and old truths about human experiences. In the current terrain of higher education, German Studies programs are challenged to re-examine assumptions about the aims of studying German language, culture, literature, and film at the postsecondary level. Facing dropping enrollments, some programs have committed to adapting in ways that increase enrollments by reimagining the curriculum and communicating to students and their parents about the value and relevance of a German degree. Notably, the programs that have recently been recognized by the American Association of Teachers of German as College and University Centers of Excellence[1] have all demonstrated a commitment to restructuring their curricula to support access, inclusion, diversity, and justice and to building partnerships with other departments and with community entities beyond the academy.

While it may be rhetorically prudent to frame a German Studies/Disability Studies course in terms of its practical value for specific professions or the survival of an academic program, Kevin Gannon (2020) reminds us of the pitfalls of framing higher education as merely a skills-training venture where education is viewed as a discrete process that can be neatly tracked and measured and that concludes when students graduate with a degree (17). Because "higher education has both a role and a responsibility in creating and sustaining a free, democratic society" (18), Gannon urges practitioners to consider a question that tests the limits of educational instrumentalism: "What is the point of creating new knowledge if we are not teaching students (and ourselves) how to use that knowledge or to inquire into its fundamental nature?" (16). A Health Humanities course that responds to this foundational question can create opportunities for students to consider and discuss what "utility" cultural artifacts such as literature and film might have *beyond* their function as required readings in a course that is required for a degree program, which may be viewed as a steppingstone to a career. For instance, why might it be important to reflect on the disabling effects of the medical gaze, both as a future health practitioner and as a human being whose existence is fragile, interdependent, and finite? It is essential that the skill-training model does not overshadow the transformative nature of education as a dynamic, unpredictable, and never-ending process. In other words, a critical pedagogical approach is necessary for inviting students into an active role as critical producers of knowledge so that the transformative potential of a course in German Studies/Disability Studies can be realized.

For those in the medical field, the intersection of German Studies and Disability Studies is fertile ground indeed for explorations of disabling discourses. Equipped with skills in textual analysis, one can unpack the meanings that disability carries both as a subject (what) and as a strategy (how) to intervene in narratives about the lives of people with disabilities. Health

Humanities is an ideal paradigm within which to explore the productive tensions that reside at the intersection of these fields. To ensure that this interdisciplinary endeavor remains productive, it is imperative that the distinctive quality of each area is preserved, and that equal value is given to their respective contributions to the education of future professionals. What German Studies brings to the conversation on Disability Studies are deep, critical analysis of cultural artifacts that are needed to fully appreciate the cultural contexts, representational modes, rhetorical strategies, aesthetics, and discursive interventions that those who create cultural artifacts enact via their engagement with disability in different times and places.

DISABILITY TEXTS

When selecting texts for a course on Disability Studies in German Studies, it may be helpful to begin by considering the needs of the learners who will be taking this course. For instance, are your students preparing for a health profession? If so, it may be most important for them to gain an appreciation of the power of storytelling as individuals process a diagnosis for themselves or a loved one. They may also benefit from a deeper understanding of the ways in which cultural narratives shape personal and collective experiences of disability and illness. If you are working with future medical professionals, you may decide to focus on comparing the medical, social, and cultural models, and select theoretical and primary texts to explore them further. While students who are primarily studying German and do not intend to pursue a heath career will benefit from these insights as well, they may be more interested in exploring other aspects of disability theory or in analyzing representational or stylistic aspects of primary texts. In short, the makeup of a particular cohort of learners and the learning goals of your course within its curricular context should guide the selection of primary and secondary texts.

A ground-breaking book that continues to be a useful resource for research and teaching in German Studies and Disability Studies is Carol Poore's *Disability in Twentieth-Century German Culture* (2007). This meticulously researched monograph provides an overview of the shifting circumstances and discourses that shaped Germany during the twentieth century and examines a wide range of literary and visual depictions of various forms of disability that were produced between the 1920s and the early 2000s. *Disability in Twentieth-Century German Culture* provides rich material for the discussion of medical and legal texts as well as familiar and lesser-known artifacts from literature, film, and the visual and performing arts. Instructors can draw on this impressive bibliography of twentieth-century texts that thematize disability to compile a list of primary readings for their course. For those seeking to create a specialized course, for example a course on disability in German fairy tales, resources such as Ann Schmiesing's *Disability, Deformity, and Disease in the Grimms' Fairy Tales* (2014) can provide a starting point. Those interested in exploring more recent cultural production and/or life writing genres may wish to consult Nina Schmidt's *The Wounded Self: Writing Illness in Twenty-First-Century German Literature* (2018) for helpful information on this area of inquiry. Schmidt's analysis of five texts published between 2007 and 2013 is especially interesting for interrogating the dividing line drawn between disability and illness and discussing the criteria by which a cultural artifact is deemed worthy of the label "literary." These considerations will certainly arise as one conceptualizes a Disability Studies in German Studies course and begins the process of selecting primary texts to explore with students.

Due to the ubiquity of disability in literary texts (Bérubé 2016), there are nearly endless choices for instructors seeking disability texts. Brueggemann et al. (2001) indicate that a disability text is a text that is "written by a differently abled writer" and "empowers students to see that writing is intimately connected with issues of authority, identity, power, and confidence" (382). Indeed, it is essential to remember that the overarching goal of disability studies is to advance the rights of people with disabilities, whose voices must always be included in discussions of disability; in other words, "Nothing About Us Without Us" (Charlton 1998). Subsequent scholarship on disability rhetoric (Dolmage 2014), disability aesthetics (Siebers 2010), and antinormative narratives of embodiment (Mitchell 2020) seem to indicate that the term "disability text" could be expanded to include cultural artifacts created by authors who have diverse embodiments and neurological functions.

With an expanded notion of what constitutes a disability text, any text (e.g., any cultural artifact such as a poem, a film, a novel, a painting, a play, a blog, etc.) in which disability is a salient feature could be included, regardless of the positionality of its author. The most important consideration, I argue, is that the selected texts are accompanied by disability studies readings as well as discussions and other activities that are designed to guide learners through an analysis of what the text *does* with disability, *for whom* and *for what purpose* it was created, and the potential *effects* it might have on lived experiences. For instance, is disability a phenomenon that is represented, a theme that is explored, a rhetorical technique that is deployed, or an aesthetic quality that is inherent to the text? Was it created by someone with a disability or by a nondisabled person—and how does this influence our reading? For whom was it created? How does this text take up ideas about disability and apply, transform, and leverage those ideas? What are the potential impacts of this representation on the lives of people with disabilities?

If all students enrolled in your course understand German, it will not be difficult to find texts that deal with disability; or, rather, the difficulty lies only in narrowing one's selection and obtaining copies through the university library or bookstore. Some works are in the public domain and are freely available online, for instance via Project Gutenberg, and films may be available free of charge or for a small fee through a streaming service. If the course is taught in English or if the students in your course are at varying stages of learning German, the task of selecting suitable texts becomes more difficult. If you are teaching a graduate course that is cross-listed to include advanced undergraduate students, a unique set of challenges arises in the selection of texts and the activities that will accompany them.

One way to adapt to a mixed-levels context is to select German-language texts for those students who have greater ability in German and assign the same texts in translation to students with lesser German ability. Class discussions could focus on linguistic comparison of the two versions and how the linguistic choices are attached to connotative and symbolic meanings in the German-speaking and English-speaking realms. Another strategy would involve selecting readings that are only available in German for learners with German ability and assigning different, English-language texts that were published around the same time for learners who do not understand German. In that case, one could assign pairs to work collaboratively on oral presentations, reflection papers, or research posters with the goal of bringing these texts into dialogue with one another through the lens of disability theory. Such comparative approaches are one way to leverage a linguistically diverse group of learners to foster fruitful dialogues about the discursive similarities and differences that are negotiated through cultural artifacts in different times and places.

Below is a sample reading list for a fifteen-week course that can serve as a starting point for those seeking to build their own course. The selected primary texts (literary and filmic works) were selected for their suitability for a Disability Studies course that is taught in English and in which the learners' reading and listening comprehension in German ranges from beginner to advanced. While these texts could be paired with the theoretical readings listed in the right-hand column, other pairings are certainly possible. Finally, the primary texts included here provide only a snapshot of texts from the late nineteenth, twentieth, and early twenty-first centuries; there are many more from which to choose, and they need not be taught in chronological order of their publication. The course schedule below integrates three weeks of dedicated time for students to work on research projects during class; this is intended to create space for collaborative work as well as opportunities for students to interact directly with the instructor as they are guided through the research process.

TABLE 12.1 Sample 15-Week Course Schedule with Primary and Secondary Readings.

Week	*Topic*	*Primary Texts*	*Secondary Texts*
1	Introduction to Disability Studies: Anglophone and Germanophone Perspectives	None	"Disability, Identity, and Representation" (Rosemarie Garland-Thompson 1997) "A Short History of the German Disability Rights Movement" (Swantje Köbsell 2006)
2	Introduction to Disability in German Studies	None	"Disability Goes Cultural" (Anne Waldschmidt 2017) "Introduction to the Edinburgh German Yearbook" (Eleoma Bodammer and Michael Schillmeier 2010)
3	The Medical Gaze	Excerpts from *Woyzeck* (Georg Büchner 1836)	"Understanding the Social Model of Disability" (Colin Barnes 2020)
4	Traditions in German Studies	*Little Herr Friedemann* (Thomas Mann 1896)	"Melodrama and the Gaze in Thomas Mann's 'Der kleine Herr Friedemann'" (Ernest Schonfield 2011)
5	The Problem of the Body	*The Metamorphosis* (Franz Kafka 1915)	"Disability and the Theory of Complex Embodiment" (Tobin Siebers 2013)
6	Disability Myths in Literature and Film	*The Hands of Orlac* (Robert Wiene 1924)	"An Archive and Anatomy of Disability Myths" (Jay T. Dolmage 2014)

Week	*Topic*	*Primary Texts*	*Secondary Texts*
7	Dismodern Ethics of the Body	*Mother Courage and Her Children* (Bertolt Brecht 1938/39)	*The End of Identity Politics* (Lennard J. Davis 2013)
8	Research Project 1	*The Man Outside* (Wolfgang Borchert 1946)	"Triangulating Trauma" (Mahan 2017)
9	Euthanasia in the Third Reich	*Daniel the Just* (Heinrich Böll 1955) *Friendship with Adam* (Wolfdietrich Schnurre 1953)	"Toward a Literary Memory of Nazi Euthanasia" (Susanne Knittel 2010)
10	Representing Disability, Writing Alternative Capacities of Living	*Her Happy Eyes* (Ingeborg Bachmann 1972)	"Antinormative Narratives of Embodiment" (Mitchell 2020)
11	Research Project 2	*Chinese Roulette* (Rainer Werner Fassbinder 1976)	"Narrative Prosthesis and the Materiality of Metaphor" (Mitchell and Snyder 2001)
12	Review	*Beyond Silence* (Caroline Link 1992)	"Disability in German Cinema" (Elizabeth C. Hamilton 2004)
13	Research Project 3	*Helmut* (Rachel Seiffert 2001)	"Mētis" (Jay T. Dolmage 2014)
14	Discourses of Access, Inclusion, and Participation	*Children of Utopia* (Hubertus Siegert 2019)	"More than the 'Other'" (Petra Anders 2016)
15	Presentations	None	None

PEDAGOGICAL CHOICES

While the selection of texts is likely the first consideration that comes to mind when planning a German course with a significant Disability Studies component, pedagogical considerations are at least as important in this process. Indeed, deciding how to approach the teaching of Disability Studies in German Studies may be the most transformative element of such a project, as one's choices will have a deep and lasting impact on students' learning. Good course design should therefore consider not only *what* will be learned, but also *how* it will be learned and *why* it should be learned. This section considers three broad pedagogical questions that instructors can ask themselves as they begin to conceptualize a German Studies/Disability Studies course. These macro-level questions set the stage for the micro-level considerations that are discussed in the final paragraphs of this essay.

The first question pertains to the role of the educator and the role of the student. Contrasting metaphors can be helpful for revealing the philosophies of education and approaches to learning that undergird the assumptions that educators and learners bring into instructional settings and which inform their expectations and behaviors. For instance, a professor may see herself as a "sage on the stage" and her students as empty vessels, blank slates, or sponges, which positions them as passive recipients waiting to be filled with knowledge. These metaphors align with an instructivist/instructionist view of learning. Indeed, the very terms *instructor*, *lecturer*, and *professor* imply that "knowledge should be transferred directly into the mind of the learner from the instructor" (Onyesolu et al. 2013, 40).

By contrast, when students are conceptualized as detectives, explorers, or drivers, they are seen (and can see themselves) as active participants in their own learning. This does not render the teacher superfluous, however, as learners still need a "guide on the side" (their professor) to help them understand course material through scaffolded learning activities, timely feedback, and other forms of guidance (Selingo 2018, 27). This set of metaphors aligns with a constructivist approach to learning, which posits that "learning is active, not passive; language is an important element in the learning process; and learning environments should be focused on the learner" (Mattar 2018, 204). While the instructivist/instructionist model may be familiar to both teachers and students, constructivist approaches are arguably better suited to fulfill the mission of a university or college that seeks to provide transformative learning experiences. As Susan Van Schalkwyk et al. (2019) have shown, research on transformative learning pedagogies for students pursuing health professions indicates that the most meaningful and transformative learning occurs when learners are invited into a journey of learning that is "characterized by both a cognitive and affective dimension, an epistemological and ontological position, and these are intertwined" (553).

The constructivist paradigm may be attractive to instructors seeking to design transformative learning experiences for their students, but it may be difficult to translate it into the design of a course. For instance, a professor of German literature might design a course that provides students with an overview of a particular period of literary history and introduces them to the most cherished texts produced during that era. However, the professor may not have articulated *why* students should attain this knowledge, and the course may not have any learning goals beyond the exposure to and mastery of the literary canon for its own sake, where "mastery" is equivalent to a student's ability to recall details about literary texts in the context of a written or oral exam. While such a pedagogical approach may have been acceptable to past generations of learners, it is unlikely to be effective in motivating learners of Generation Z, who desire learning experiences that are valuable in terms of preparing them for a career (Selingo 2018, 29).

Because they are interested in learning experiences that are meaningful as well as practical, these learners need to understand the purpose and value of coursework. This insight addresses a second broad question to consider as one builds a Health Humanities course at the intersection of German Studies and Disability Studies: How will the value of such a course be framed and communicated to others, not only students and their parents but also one's department and university administrators? Professors can begin by thoughtfully choosing content and designing meaningful learning experiences and then explaining to students how these contents and assignments support their personal, academic, and professional goals. By employing backward design (Wiggins and McTigh 2005), instructors can ensure their own clear understanding of what students should be able to know and do by the end of a lesson, a unit, or a course. Having established their own sense of purpose, professors will be better positioned to convey these intended learning outcomes to students and engage in conversations about the role and value of the course within the curriculum.

Once the pedagogical approach and the purpose of the course have been established, it is time to delve into a third question: What kinds of learning experiences will be part of this German Studies/Disability Studies course? Presumably, students will read texts and/or view films and other media throughout the semester, but these activities are surrounded by a series of pedagogical choices that will shape the quality and depth of students' learning. For instance, a course that aims to deepen students' understanding of past and current discourses on disability in the German-speaking world and train their ability to identify, analyze, and communicate about representations and deployments of disability in cultural artifacts might structure activities around questions such as:

- What is going on with disability in this text? In other words, what ideas about disability and people with disabilities are reflected or deployed here? What evidence do you see in the text that points to that conclusion?
- What perspectives influence our reading of disability in this text? How does it relate to the theories about disability we have been learning about?
- What perspectives do you think shaped the depiction or deployment of disability at the time it was created? How did (or how might) this cultural artifact shape the perception and treatment of people with disabilities in the world beyond the text?

Such questions could be used, for example, as recurring writing prompts to accompany assigned readings and viewings. Students could be tasked with submitting their responses before class to ensure they completed the assigned task and with sharing them during class to facilitate synchronous discussion or after class to facilitate asynchronous discussion or support students' progress as they work on individual or collaborative research projects.

Finally, those who teach Disability Studies should engage with the themes of accessibility and inclusive pedagogy in the course design process. To that end, one helpful tool is the Transparency in Teaching and Learning (TILT) framework (Winkelmes et al. 2019), which has been shown to improve learning outcomes when instructors explain the purpose of an assignment, the steps learners need to follow in order to complete it, and the criteria that will be used to evaluate student work. A further tool for those seeking to design courses that are accessible and inclusive of all students is Sheryl Burgstahler's *Universal Design in Higher Education* (2015). The TILT framework and the principles of Universal Design provide support for instructors as they seek to design accessible and inclusive syllabi, learning activities, and assignments. By aiming for accessibility and adopting a mindset of accommodation even before receiving an accommodations letter from the institutional disability services office, instructors can design learning environments and experiences that foster the success of all learners, especially (but not only) students with disabilities.

This chapter set out to address three questions pertaining to the value of a disability studies course for students and academic programs, the theories and primary texts that can shape course development, and pedagogical choices to ensure an accessible, inclusive, and engaging course. The answers sketched in this chapter may be seen as a starting point for others who seek to design a similar course at their own institution. By taking inventory of one's program to assess current challenges and opportunities, and by surveying and taking seriously the needs of the students who could enroll in a course or program, one can work backwards to design courses that meet the needs of these students, thus positioning oneself to justify a course or program to students and their parents as well as colleagues and administrators. In the case of a course in German Studies/Disability Studies, the justification can be summarized as one of academic and professional relevance. One way for German programs to demonstrate their relevance to multiple audiences is to explicitly contribute to the ethical education of future (health) professionals through the study of cultural artifacts in order to grapple with the complexities of being human and of power relationships among populations. While the theories and primary texts discussed in this chapter illustrate some key concepts and influential thinkers whose work can guide the development of a course in German Studies/ Disability Studies, there are many more theoretical and artistic works that have been (and will yet be) created from which one can choose. Therefore, the selection of readings should always be guided by the needs of the students and a thoughtful consideration of curricular goals and objectives. The macro-level and micro-level pedagogical considerations presented in the final section of this chapter serve to affirm practices that foster accessible, inclusive, and meaningful learning experiences so that all students can know that they belong in the German Studies classroom.

NOTE

1. "College and University Centers of Excellence," American Association of Teachers of German. Accessed September 23, 2022. https://www.aatg.org/page/CoE_CollegeandUni

WORKS CITED

Anders, Petra. 2016. "More than the 'Other'? On Four Tendencies Regarding the Representation of Disability in German Film (2005–2010)." *In Cultures of Representation: Disability in World Cinema Contexts*, edited by Benjamin Fraser. New York: Columbia University Press.

Barnes, Colin. 2020. "Understanding the Social Model of Disability: Past, Present, and Future." In *Routledge Handbook of Disability Studies, Second Edition*, edited by Nick Watson and Simo Vehmas, 14–31. New York: Routledge.

Bachmann, Ingeborg. 1972. *Simultan: Erzählungen*. Munich: Piper.

Bérubé, Michael. 2016. *The Secret Life of Stories: From Don Quixote to Harry Potter, How Intellectual Disability Transforms the Way We Read*. NYU Press.

Bodammer, Eleoma and Michael Schillmeier, eds. 2010. *Edinburgh German Yearbook on Disability in German Literature, Film, and Theater*. Vol. 4. Rochester, NY: Camden House.

Böll, Heinrich. 2006. *Kölner Ausgabe, Band 9: 1945–1955*. Cologne: Kiepenheuer & Witsch.

Borchert, Wolfgang. 1947. *Draussen vor der Tür. Ein Stück, das kein Theater spielen und kein Publikum sehen will*. Hamburg/Stuttgart: Rowohlt.

Brehme, David, Petra Fuchs, Swantje Köbsell, and Carla Wesselmann, eds. 2020. *Disability Studies im deutschsprachigen Raum: Zwischen Emanzipation und Vereinnahmung*. Weinheim: Beltz Juventa.
Brecht, Bertolt. 1967. *Gesammelte Werke in acht Bänden*, Vol. I, edited by Elisabeth Hauptmann. Frankfurt am Main: Suhrkamp.
Brueggemann, Brenda Jo, Linda Feldmeier White, Patricia A Dunn, Barbara A Heifferon, and Johnson Cheu. 2001. "Becoming Visible: Lessons in Disability." *College Composition and Communication* 52, no. 3: 368–398.
Büchner, Georg. 1967. *Sämtliche Werke und Briefe: Historisch-kritische Ausgabe mit Kommentar*, Vol. I, edited by Werner R. Lehmann. Hamburg: Christian Wegner.
Burgstahler, Sheryl. 2015. *Universal Design in Higher Education: From Principles to Practice*. 2nd Edition. Cambridge, MA: Harvard Education Press.
Charlton, James I. 1998. *Nothing About Us Without Us. Disability, Oppression, and Empowerment*. Oakland, CA: University of California Press.
Chinesisches Roulette (1976), [Film] Dir. Rainer Werner Fassbinder, Germany: Albatros Production, Les Films due Losange, and Tango Films.
"College and University Centers of Excellence," American Association of Teachers of German. Accessed September 23, 2022. https://www.aatg.org/page/CoE_CollegeandUni
Davis, Lennard J. 2013. "The End of Identity Politics: On Disability as an Unstable Category." In *The Disability Studies Reader*. 4th Edition, edited by Lennard J. Davis, 264–277. New York and London: Routledge.
Die Kinder der Utopie (2019), [Film] Dir. Hubertus Siegert, Germany: S.U.M.O. Film.
Dolmage, Jay T. 2014. *Disability Rhetoric*. Syracuse, NY: Syracuse University Press.
Freire, Paulo. 1994. *Pedagogy of Hope: Reliving Pedagogy of the Oppressed*. Translated by Robert R. Barr. London: Continuum International Publishing Group.
Gannon, Kevin M. 2020. *Radical Hope: A Teaching Manifesto*. Morgantown, WV: West Virginia University Press.
Garland-Thomson, Rosemarie. 1997. *Extraordinary Bodies: Figuring Physical Disability in American Culture and Literature*. New York: Columbia University Press.
Hall, Alice. 2015. *Literature and Disability*. London and New York: Taylor & Francis.
Hamilton, Elizabeth C. 2004. "No Longer Unreasonable: Disability in German Cinema." *Disability Studies Quarterly* 24, no. 3: https://doi.org/10.18061/dsq.v24i3.503
Jenseits der Stille (1996), [Film], Dir. Caroline Link, Germany: Claussen und Wölbke Filmproduktion.
Jones, Therese, Michael Blackie, Rebecca Garden, R., and Delese Wear. "The Almost Right Word: The Move from Medical to Health Humanities." *Academic Medicine* 92, no. 7 (2017): 932–935.
Kafka, Franz. 1935. *Gesammelte Werke: Erzählungen*, edited by Max Brod. Berlin/New York: Schocken.
Knittel, Susanne. 2010. "Bridging the Silence: Towards a Literary Memory of Nazi Euthanasia." In *Edinburgh German Yearbook, Volume 4: Disability in German Literature, Film, and Theater*, edited by Eleoma Joshua and Michael Schillmeier, 72–105. Rochester: Camden House.
Köbsell, Swantje. 2006. "Towards Self-Determination and Equalization: A Short History of the German Disability Rights Movement." *Disability Studies Quarterly* 26, no. 2: 15.
Leskau, Linda, Tanja Nusser, and Katherine Sorrels, eds. 2022. *Disability in German-Speaking Europe*. Rochester: Camden House.
Liu, Sarah. 2009. "The Illiterate Reader: Aphasia after Auschwitz." *Partial Answers: Journal of Literature and the History of Ideas* 7, no. 2: 319–342.
Mahan, William. 2017. "Triangulating Trauma: Constellations of Memory, Representation, and Distortion in Elie Wiesel, Wolfgang Borchert, and W.G. Sebald." *Humanities* 6, no. 94: https://doi.org/10.3390/h6040094
Mann, Thomas. 1965. *Gesammelte Werke: Erzählungen*, Vol. 9. Berlin/Weimar: Aufbau.

Mattar, João. 2018. "Constructivism and Connectivism in Education Technology: Active, Situated, Authentic, Experiential, and Anchored Learning." *Revista Iberoamericana De Educación a Distancia* 21, no. 2: 201–217.

Mitchell, David T. 2020. "Disability and Contemporary Literature: Antinormative Narratives of Embodiment." In *The Routledge Companion to Literature and Disability*, edited by Alice Hall, 167–177. London/New York, NY: Taylor & Francis.

Mitchell, David T. and Sharon L. Snyder. 2000. *Narrative Prosthesis: Disability and the Dependencies of Discourse*. Ann Arbor: University of Michigan Press.

Mitchell, David T. and Sharon L. Snyder. 2016. "The Matter of Disability." *Bioethical Inquiry* 13: 487–492.

Oliver, Michael. 1981. "A New Model of the Social Work Role in Relation to Disability." In *The Handicapped Person: A New Perspective for Social Workers*, edited by J. Campling, 19–32. London: RADAR.

Onyesolu, Moses O., Victor C. Nwasor, Obiajulu E. Ositanwosu, and Obinna N. Iwegbuna. 2013. "Pedagogy: Instructivism to Socio-Constructivism through Virtual Reality." *International Journal of Advanced Computer Science & Applications* 4, no. 9: 40–47.

Orlacs Hände (1924), [Film] Dir. Robert Wiene, Germany/Austria: Pan-Film.

Poore, Carol. 2007. *Disability in Twentieth-Century German Culture*. Ann Arbor: University of Michigan Press.

Quayson, Ato. 2007. *Aesthetic Nervousness: Disability and the Crisis of Representation*. New York: Columbia University Press.

Schmidt, Nina. 2018. *The Wounded Self: Writing Illness in Twenty-First-Century German Literature*. Rochester: Camden House.

Schmiesing, Ann. 2014. *Disability, Deformity, and Disease in the Grimms' Fairy Tales*. Detroit: Wayne State University Press.

Schnurre, Wolfdietrich. 1963. *Funke* im Reisig. Olten: Walter.

Schonfield, Ernest. 2011. "Melodrama and the Gaze in Thomas Mann's 'Der kleine Herr Friedemann'." *Publications of the English Goethe Society* 80, no. 2–3: 153–165.

Seiffert, Rachel. 2001. *The Dark Room*. New York: Vintage.

Selingo, Jeffrey J. 2018. *The New Generation of Students: How Colleges Can Recruit, Teach, and Serve Gen Z. The Chronicle of Higher Education*. 46 pages.

Siebers, Tobin. 2010. *Disability Aesthetics*. Ann Arbor: University of Michigan Press.

Siebers, Tobin. 2013. "Disability and the Theory of Complex Embodiment – For Identity Politics in a New Register." In *The Disability Studies Reader*. 4th Edition, edited by Lennard J. Davis, 278–297. New York/London: Routledge.

Van Schalkwyk, Susan C., Janet Hafler, Timothy F. Brewer, Moira A. Maley, Carmi Margolis, Lakshini McNamee, Ilse Meyer, Michael J. Peluso, Ana M. S. Schmutz, Judy M. Spak, and David Davies. 2019. "Transformative Learning as Pedagogy for the Health Professions: A Scoping Review." *Medical Education* 53, no. 6: 547–558.

Waldschmidt, Anne. 2017. "Disability Goes Cultural: The Cultural Model of Disability as an Analytical Tool." In *Culture – Theory – Disability. Encounters Between Disability Studies and Cultural Studies*, edited by Anne Waldschmidt, Hanjo Berressem, and Moritz Ingwerson, 19–27. Bielefeld: Transcript Verlag.

Wiggins, Grant and Jay McTighe. 2005. *Understanding by Design*. 2nd Edition. Association for Supervision and Curriculum Development.

Winkelmes, Mary-Ann, Allison Boye, and Suzanne Tapp, eds. 2019. *Transparent Design in Higher Education Teaching and Leadership: A Guide to Implementing the Transparency Framework Institution-Wide to Improve Learning and Retention*. Sterling: Stylus Publishing.

PART IV

Race

CHAPTER THIRTEEN

Work, Disability, Race: Toward an Intersectional, "Unsettling" Analysis of German Settler Colonialism

GABI KATHÖFER

This article positions Germans' self-definition as a country of work at the intersection of medical as well as cultural/social definitions of (dis-)ability. As Western understanding of abled-bodiedness has centered on concepts of productivity, autonomy, and agency, the construction of work offered a normative framework for the definition of national cultural identity; however, it also led to the definition and exclusion of presumed disposable, disabled, and worthless bodies, in the German states as well in the context of German settlements abroad. Focusing on German identity construction of the nation as a "fit body" (body politic) in opposition to deviant "Others," this article places discussions on German work in a coordinate system, in which medicine and culture, as well as disability and race served as key coordinates to determine German superiority. Moreover, rejecting the romanticization of German settlements in Brazil, this article examines German settlements as Indigenous spaces and places in which Indigenous lives and bodies were deemed worthless and eliminated. Finally, this article calls for bridges not only between Western Sciences and Humanities Studies, but also, and more importantly, between Western and Non-Western knowledges, especially Indigenous epistemologies.

A PRODUCTIVE, MORAL *KULTURNATION* OF WORK?

In the nineteenth century, the concept of work became a central community-building model for the modern nation state and the definition of modern humanity. European industrialization and globalization depended on an increasing movement of work(ers) across borders. At the same time, it was accompanied by the celebration of national work and productivity as a measurement of national as well as individual value. The nationalization of work played a significant role for national identity constructions, thus counteracting the growing permeability of national borders, restoring difference, and reassuring cultural uniqueness and superiority: "World Exhibitions, international forums for labour and its products, provided regular opportunities for identifying national characteristics and differences" (Conze in Konrad, 338). Nations' self-definition as "countries of work" claims of exceptionalism and superiority and the negotiation of hierarchies became an overarching phenomenon in Europe on which national identity politics increasingly centered.

In the German states, too, work influenced national and cultural self-perception. The transition from an agricultural to an industrialized society changed Germans' living and working conditions as well as their understanding of German cultural uniqueness. As a result, German culture was increasingly defined not only by intellectual and cultural traditions, but also by "German work" as the measure of national strength. By the end of the century, "German work" had become a popular and widely used term, pointing to three phenomena: "the emergence of an increasingly positive connotation assigned to work, a description of Germany as a country of work, and finally an emphasis of the qualitative difference between German work and work done by others" (Conrad 2010, 335). The concept of work thus offered a new criterion to assess cultural superiority; productivity, ability, and diligence signified community-building characteristics. Moreover, the meaning of German work was increasingly equated with the moral and cultural core of its people: "'Soul' and 'moral' were terms that recurred again and again in discussions about 'German work' [...] work was seen as a social activity with moral connotations" (Conrad 2010, 340f). Located in the public sphere, individual productivity was rewarded with social recognition, validation, and appreciation; moreover, work became a cultural virtue, moral obligation, and civil duty in the German *Kulturnation* as a country of work.

The focus on productivity established social hierarchies within the German states, regarding presumed essential cultural and moral abilities of individuals and groups, connecting work to the physical body of workers as well as their contributions to society. Workers were seen as part of the nation's body; thus, work came to define inferior "Others" based on their unfit weakness, abnormality, disability. The celebration of the able, fit body included a growing concern about national fitness and productivity, relying on body politic as a central concept of western modern identity construction. As Andreas Musolff's study on the concept in the context of Nazi propaganda highlighted, German body politic had a long tradition in history, from description of the "monstrous" Holy Roman Empire (Pufendorf 1667) to references to the "state body" and the "Physiologie des ganzen Nationalkörpers" (Herder) in the seventeenth and eighteenth centuries. Interestingly, German body politic changed in age of industrialization, when the term *Volkskörper* "began to replace Nationalkörper, emphasizing the physical presence of the people" (Musolff 2010, 127). Body politic and the concept of work in the nineteenth-century, thus, both shared the centrality of physical bodies for the health of the nation: "if individual citizens are not fit, if they do not fit into the nation, then the national body will not be fit" (Davis 2013, 7). In that vein, the celebration of cultural unity also included the question who would not "fit" into the German *Kulturnation* of work and thus, should be excluded or eliminated.

As work was increasingly attributed with normativity and essential cultural virtue, the physical inability or social unwillingness to contribute to the nation's fitness, in return, stood for a fundamental unworthiness of belonging, justifying the exclusion from the public sphere. Accordingly, the invention of work as a social concept was accompanied by the social construction of disability as its deviant counterpart: "When we think of bodies, in a society where the concept of the norm is operative, then people with disabilities will be thought of as deviants" (Davis 2006, 3). From this perspective, the nineteenth-century European construction of work as a key identity concept can be described as a "social process of disabling [that] arrived with industrialization and with the set of practices and discourses that are linked to late eighteenth- and nineteenth-century notions of nationality, race, gender, criminality, sexual orientation" (Davis 1995, 24). Moral/social as well as physical/medical (dis-)ability, thus, served as pillars for the invention of the nation as well as its deviant "Others."

The European and German obsession with disability manifested itself in the paradox of othering: deviance became both an invisible and hyper visible aspect of identity politics, and it focused not only on the cultural but also on the physical ability of Germans to work. On the one hand, the idea that work was a social and moral duty with a civilizing and educational mission resulted in the establishment of educational institutions, the *Arbeits- und Zuchthäuser*, through which unproductive members, moral deviance, and physical disability could be successfully removed from society (Conze 1972, 173). On the other hand, there was a growing fascination with the extraordinary physical body which resulted in the popularity of freak shows from the mid-nineteenth century on, establishing and enforcing the hegemony of normalcy through hypervisibility of medical abnormalcy[1]; freak shows displayed abnormalities and disability as a spectacle that confirmed the viewer's own normalcy and able-bodiedness: "The show-personas presented communal anxieties and fantasies of Otherness in highly commercialized, fetishized, colonized forms, which served entertainment and educational purposes, conditioned responses of revulsion and pleasure, and consolidated the comforting, illusorily self-same identity of the ordinary average majority populace" (Kérchy and Zittlau 2012, 2). Shows of physical "deviance" were among the most popular attractions for the middle class and were an enormous commercial success. Overall, work became a dominant factor for nineteenth-century constructions of social hierarchies and power structures, in which disability was discussed as a question of medicine and health as well as cultural belonging, developing into a central "question of politics and power(lessness)" (Pothier and Devlin 2006, 2), and serving as justification to exclude bodies that could weaken German national health and wealth.

With the increasing transgression of national borders through work migration and mass emigration in the nineteenth century, German settlements abroad also offered spaces of cultural work and prime examples of the ideological construction of German physical, cultural, and moral superiority by both German as well as Portuguese politicians and intellectuals.

GERMAN SETTLERS IN BRAZIL: DISABLING ELEMENTS OR EXAMPLES OF GERMAN WORK?

As scholars like Klaus Bade, Mack Walker, and Sebastian Conrad have explored in detail, migration and expansionism played a vital role in nineteenth-century German history and national narratives, intensifying discussions on belonging and the nation as an imagined community (Anderson 2006) across and beyond borders. In that vein, scholars like Bradley Naranch have stressed the polycentric structure of German culture and the need to expand the geographical scope of German Studies. The debate on German settlements in Brazil is a key example of nineteenth-century glorification of German culture abroad, and both the German and Brazilian/Portuguese promotion of German settlements in Brazil were closely related to the concept of work productivity as an essential cultural trait. In fact, German immigration to Brazil was encouraged by the Brazilian government. After Brazil's independence in 1822, the first emperor of Brazil, Dom Pedro I (1798–1834), son of King Dom João VI of Portugal and Queen Carlota Joaquina, invited European settlers to populate presumed uninhabited regions in Southern Brazil and to prevent military encroachments by neighboring countries; moreover, his invitation was directly connected to a labor shortage in Brazil and the increasing international pressure on Brazil to abolish slavery.

Although Italian, Spanish, and Portuguese immigrants represented more than seventy percent of the total immigration to Brazil, the German colonist was often portrayed as the ideal settler to fill Brazil's presumed cultural and geographical emptiness. Especially at the beginning of German mass emigration, texts on Brazil portrayed German colonies as idyllic spaces of Germanness and European civilization. The first literary text on Brazil, for example, Amalia Schoppe's *Die Auswanderer nach Brasilien oder die Hütte am Gigitonhonha* (1828), depicted German life in Brazil as a utopia in which settlers lived "wie Vater Adam einst in seinem Paradiese" (58): "eine stattliche Hütte, oder vielmehr ein angenehmes Haus, mit allen europäischen Bequemlichkeiten versehen, erhebt sich am Ufer des schönen, spiegelhellen Flusses; ein trefflich bestellter, großer Garten mit den edelsten und seltensten Früchten angefüllt, liegt neben der Hütte; weiterhin schöne Aecker, die ihnen reichlich alle Bedürfnisse des Lebens, und dies fast ohne alle Mühe, gewähren" ["a stately cottage, or rather a comfortable house, furnished with all of the European comforts rises above the banks of the beautiful, crystal clear river; next to the cottage lies a large, well-appointed garden filled with the most precious and rare fruits, and beyond the garden are splendid acres that provide them almost effortlessly with all of life's necessities"] (132).[2] Throughout the century, German and Brazilian supporters of emigration confirmed and reinforced the idea of superior, moral work as German settlers' essential cultural core: "[t]he aptitude of these settlers for agricultural work, for arts and crafts, and their peaceful and conservative spirit are proven by the most authentic testimony. [...] Love of work and of family, temperance, resignation, respect for authority are qualities which generally distinguish German settlers from those of other origins" (Abrantes 833). Unsurprisingly, until the middle of the 1870s, most of the colonies established in Southern Brazil were German (Seyferth 2003) and were celebrated as spaces of exceptional productivity and cultural purity. The glorification of German settlements in Brazil continued to play a role in national(istic) identity construction in the twentieth century.[3]

The popular auto- and hetero-stereotype of the "upright, physically powerful, and racially pure national pioneer" (Naranch 2005, 33) contributed to nineteenth-century discourses of German exceptionalism and framed how German Studies scholars and historians have conceptualized German settler colonialism in Brazil. Ute Ritz-Deutch rightly points out with regard to the existing scholarly work that efforts "to portray German communities in southern Brazil in the most positive light [...] have a longstanding tradition, carrying forward the momentum of propagandists, economists, politicians and intellectuals who published at the turn of the twentieth century" (Ritz-Deutch 2008, 102). Influenced by Susanne Zantop's ground-breaking study on German colonial fantasies (1997), studies on German settlements in South America often restricted their analysis of German settler colonies to their function as imaginary spaces of essential German culture and productivity that played a crucial role in German nationalism.

Considering the causes of German mass emigration, however, it is evident that German settlements in Brazil provided alternative spaces for the exclusion of unwanted, unproductive others from the German cultural community rather than examples of German exceptionalism, and thus, served similar purposes as the *Arbeits-* and *Zuchthäuser* in the German states. Klaus Bade points out that German mass emigration was a proletarian mass migration: "As a mass movement, it must be viewed against the background of population growth, profound changes in the social institutions and a rapid economic transformation. Hence, the million-fold emigration from nineteenth-century Germany served to relieve widespread social tensions in the home country, with the effect of exporting social problems" (Bade 1995, 512). Nineteenth-century texts on German emigration to Brazil support this evaluation. In fact, emigrating Germans were not celebrated and sent off as German cultural ambassadors to represent the German *Kulturnation* abroad. On the contrary, the majority of emigrating Germans belonged to the lower social stratum (rural peasantry and village artisans), and politicians and economists who supported German settlements abroad saw emigration as a welcome opportunity to dispose of these excess masses ("überflüssige Masse") and lazy people ("müßiges Volk") so that economic strength, morality, and social peace could be restored in the German states: "Nur die Auswanderung kann die unnatürliche Lage, in die die Staaten geraten, ändern. Die überschüssigen Massen müssen fort, um den Zurückbleibenden die frühere Ruhe und das verlorene Glück wiederzugeben" ["Only emigration can change the unnatural situation in which the German states find themselves. The surplus masses have to leave in order to restore peace and happiness to those who stay"] (Ackermann 1834, 15). In the context of national work and German body politic, emigration became a corrective measure with the goal to restore German strength, through a cleansing of the German body from socially marginal groups.

While the removal of certain bodies was justified to heal the German *Volkskörper*, German settlements were also praised as an opportunity for self-improvement; it was proclaimed that emigrating Germans would be transformed to "good German citizens" through physical and cultural work abroad. Stressing the educational benefits and curative power of work, emigration enthusiasts argued that settlements abroad would become spaces for a re-education and betterment for "unproductive," worthless Germans; in the words of Johann Eduard Wappäus: "Even work-shy people or those who here are, so to speak, lost to society [could, through hard physical work] in a foreign country gain a kind of energy and feeling that very often turns them into good citizens" (Wappäus 1846, f5). As life in the settlements centered on agricultural work, German work in Brazil was often glorified as a "back to the roots" movement and a space in which German productivity could be re-established, along with the cultural patterns characteristic of peasant societies—"patterns threatened in Germany by socioeconomic change" (Smith 1986, 25). In the end, the argument came full circle: the rehabilitation discourse allowed for a re-integration in the imagined German community, defining work as good citizenship and an essential cultural trait that German emigrants would represent. Furthermore, Central and South America were declared ideal spaces for German re-education, while it was also claimed that German work would best cultivate Central and South America: "Ist es doch fast, als habe die Vorsehung die reichen Gefilde Mittel- und Südamerika dem deutschen Elemente vorbehalten. Denn während England berühmt ist, mit seinen Auswanderern [...] Australien zu bevölkern, während Nord-Amerika noch lange Zeit zu thun haben wird, die unermesslichen Strecken [...] auch nur mit einem dünnen Ansiedelungsnetze zu überziehen, scheint es, als könne Central- und Süd-America seine Regeneration nur von dem dritten großem Wandervolke, von Deutschlands Söhnen erwarten! ["It is almost as if destiny had reserved the rich climes of Central and South America for the German element. While England is famous for populating Australia with its emigrants [...], while it will still take a long time for North America to develop a settlement network in its vast spaces, it seems as if Central and South America can expect its regeneration only from the third great nomadic people, from Germany's sons"] (Gaebler 1850, 22). This suggested a symbiotic, natural, and mutually beneficial relationship.

In reality, only very few German settlements in Brazil were successful[4]; furthermore, numerous texts and documents presented a critical analysis of the idealized view of German settlers in Brazil. To give but a few examples: Therese Stutzer's short stories in *Am Rande des brasilianischen Urwaldes* (1889) presents an alternative view on German life in Brazil that depicts the settlements as dystopian spaces of immorality, illness, and unproductivity. Autobiographies of immigrants, too, show that the image of German unity, conformity, and cultural isolation was a political invention, as Frederik Schulze has shown: "Germanness was thus a contested category, used as a political argument in nationalist discussions on immigration" (Schulze 2015). Eveline Hasler's novel *Ibicaba, Paradies in den Köpfen* (1985) is an example of a more recent re-interpretation of German-Brazilian pasts. Hasler's *Ibicaba,* based on Thomas Davatz's historical account of the infamous Swiss colony Ibicaba, published in 1858, contains a philosophical as well as gendered discussion on emigration and the growing social inequalities in nineteenth-century Europe. Relating emigration to the ideals of German humanism and the Enlightenment, Hasler questions the ways in which humanness is linked to intersecting discourses of work, gender, and disability as a basis for the definition and exclusion of disposable, replaceable, or unworthy bodies.

A re-examination of German-romanticized settler pasts also calls for a critical analysis of German colonial settler projects that focuses on German settlements not merely as places of German (un-)productivity or "contact zones" (Pratt 1992), but also, and first and foremost, as Indigenous spaces in which German settlers did not only encounter Indigenous people, but in which they also participated in the dispossession, exploitation, and eradication of Indigenous land, people, and cultures.

SETTLER COLONIALISM AS BACTERIAL INFECTION?

The interrelation of work, (dis-)ability, and race was at the center of discussions on German emigration to Brazil, both in the German states as well as in Brazil. German immigration was welcomed by the Brazilian government as Brazil needed to replace slaves; however, it was also part of the deliberate plan to whiten Brazil's population (*branqueamento*). In the German states, however, the intersection of work, disability, and race manifested itself in a different discourse: while advocates for migration celebrated German settlements in Brazil as innocent spaces of German productivity and cultural purity, opponents warned against the exploitation of German settlers, making Brazil the most contested destination for emigrating Germans in the nineteenth-century (Sudhaus 1940, 3). Nineteenth-century reports on German emigration increasingly contained information on the mistreatment of Germans in Brazil, initiating a discourse on white slavery that portrayed Germans as victims and in a triangular relation to Black and Indigenous slaves in Brazil. In that vein, the "Brasilianische Menschenjagd" (1858) ["Brazilian human hunt"], a series of anonymous articles in the *Illustrierte Zeitung*, defined colonization as a disguised form of slavery: "Man taufte den weißen Sklaven 'Kolonist,' die Plantage 'Kolonie,' den Sklavenhandel 'Kolonisationsunternehmung,' den Sklavenhändler 'Kolonisations-unternehmer,' den Sklavenjäger 'Agent'." ["The white slave was christened "colonist," the plantation "colony," the slave trade "colonization enterprise," the slave trader 'colonization entrepreneur,' and the slave hunter 'agent'"] (772, cit. Sudhaus 1940, 95). While discourses on white slavery reflected and participated in the scientific racist discourses of the time, the presumed special bond or shared suffering of Germans and oppressed groups, characteristic for nineteenth-century German armchair colonialism, reconfirmed German-elevated moral status. Settlers were portrayed as "inherently better humans—better than the peoples they have left behind and certainly better than the indigenous peoples they would encounter" (Veracini 2014, 616), while being far removed from both groups.

In studies on nineteenth-century German settlements in Brazil, German settlers' interactions with other cultures have been largely reduced to their importance as role models and their "[b]ringing of the 'saving virtues' of work and discipline to the 'indolent natives' of the extra-European world" (Fitzpatrick 2020, 54). While the German colonial amnesia regarding German colonies in Africa has been overcome (Zimmerer 2013), studies on settler colonialism in Brazil continue to portray settlements as homogeneous, isolated cultural enclaves, presenting "the ultimate anticolonial fantasy" (Naranch 33) of German settlers as cultural cultivators "in the service of others" (33) rather than colonial perpetrators. As Marcos Justo Tramontini points out, studies on German participation in the enslavement, mistreatment, or eradication of Black and Indigenous People in Brazil have been inhibited by two narratives: on the one hand, German emigration to Brazil was generalized and reduced to Brazilian efforts to replace slaves with German settlers; this narrative made it seem inconsequential to even ponder German involvement in slavery. On the other hand, German settlers were continuously described in terms of their presumed essential cultural traits, emphasizing the settlers' moral high ground with respect to slavery as an inhuman institution, as well as the value of (free) labor as a moral and communal obligation and virtue.

A reflection on the difference between colonial and settler colonial systems can help further examine why intercultural conflicts in the context of German settler colonialism abroad have not received sufficient scholarly attention. Here, Lorenzo Veracini's work offers an innovative approach, comparing colonialism and settler colonialism to medical definitions of viruses and bacteria: "While both viruses and bacteria are exogenous elements that often dominate their destination locales, viruses need living cells to operate, while bacteria attach to surfaces and may or may not rely on the organisms they encounter" (616). Building on the definition of viral infections, Veracini explains the fundamental difference between colonizers and settler colonizers that has framed German cultural memory of settler colonialism: while a colonial system of relationships is, like a virus, "premised on the presence and subjugation of exploitable 'Others'" (616), settler collectives, like bacteria, attach to surfaces/land, without being dependent on "living others."

Elaborating on the similarity between bacteria and settler colonialism, Veracini discusses the settlers' elimination or removal of indigenous tribes and their transformation of environments as fundamental elements of settler colonial systems. This could explain why German settlements in Brazil have been discussed as terra nullius. That German settlements did not depend on Indigenous people to survive, however, does not justify that studies on the topic continue to ignore the impact that German immigration had on Indigenous land, people, cultures, and knowledges. On the contrary, it calls for a thorough examination of the processes with which Indigenous presence was eliminated. While "colonialism [...] cannot be reduced to a historically specific and geographically particular articulation of the colonial project" (Bhambra et al. 2018, 5), further studies on German settlements in Brazil would be a crucial step toward the urgent task to account for German settler colonialism in places like Brazil where Germans settled "with a view to eliminating Indigenous societies" (Wolfe 2006, 393). A few, recent studies have started to document and draw attention to settler violence; as Stefan Rinke has shown in his study on settlements in Southern Brazil, Germans "joined other ethnic groups of European origin in the genocidal endeavor against the indigenous population" (Rinke 2020, 21–22). Linking the German settler colonial violence to medical as well as cultural discourses of (dis-)ability and race in the nineteenth century can help carve out the conceptual frame for the definition, exclusion, and eradication of presumed deviant, inferior bodies, and knowledges of "Others" to which the discourses contribute.

DISABLING RACE OR RACIAL DISABILITY?

As the German work concept was exported to spaces beyond the German borders, disability and race discourses became increasingly intertwined. Disability Studies research has pointed out how closely racist theories and the construction of disability in the nineteenth century were interrelated: "By the mid-nineteenth century, non-white races were routinely connected to people with disabilities, both of whom were depicted as evolutionary laggards or throwbacks" (Baynton 2013, 19). Similar to the nineteenth-century obsession with disability, Western preoccupation with race, too, manifested itself in the paradox of othering. Ethnographic shows offered powerful, physical examples of racial deviance as mass entertainment; as racialized "freak shows" they reconfirmed European normalcy at the intersection of disability and race, while at the same time denying presumed inferior races a future.[5] The public discussion of racial otherness in nineteenth-century Brazil also took place in travel literature, a genre that had "become the most important medium of information on foreign countries" (Grosser 1992, 275) in the nineteenth century. As scholars like Mary Louise Pratt (1992) or Birgit Tautz (2006) have shown, German travel writings participated in the European network of knowledge production that reproduced long-passed-down images, preconceptions, stereotypes, and scientific theories of the self and other cultures and races, building on the "fierce debate among scientists and philosophers, many of whom were clustered at universities in German-speaking lands" (Eigen/Larrimore 2006, 1), among them thinkers like Friedrich Blumenbach, Samuel Thomas Sömmerring, Christian Meiners, to name a few. The scientific thought of the Enlightenment was a precondition for the celebration of European whiteness, or, in the words of David Brion Davis, it was "a precondition for the growth of a modern racism" (Brion Davis 2006, 76). Racism became the matrix through which the modern world order was established (Gutiérrez-Rodríguez 2018), and travelogues became a key medium for its spread.

Travel reports on Brazil reflect the German obsession with Indigenous tribes, a phenomenon that Harmut Lutz has described as German Indianthusiasm, the "yearning for all things Indian, a fascination with American Indians" (Lutz 2002, 168) that manifested itself in a "dual stereotype of the Indian as a 'red gentleman' and a 'bloodthirsty red devil'" (173). While nineteenth-century travelogues on Brazil reproduced a positive image of Indigenous tribes to promote "the idea of a special affinity between Germans and Native Americans based on shared experiences" (Zantop 2002, 4), the German scientific inquiries and debates on Brazil that took place in travel reports often focused on Indigenous Cannibalism: "Cannibalism was used from the earliest colonial moment to 'define, qualify, name, and classify' the Brazilians who were otherwise unknown to Europeans" (Myscofski 2007/8, 150). Like other stereotypes in European travel reports, the German imagination of Brazilian cannibalism had a long history, going back to Hans Staden's famous *Warhaftige Historia und Beschreibung eyner Landschafft der Wilden Nacketen, Grimmigen Menschenfresser-Leuthen in der Neuenwelt America gelegen* (1557). While the *Warhaftige Historia* was declared "a fundamental text in the history and discovery of Brazil" (Whitehead 2000, 721), its authenticity has been questioned and its description of cannibalism interpreted as part of the racial invention of Otherness in the context of German colonial history (Ascárate 2004; Schmölz-Häberlein 2001). This critique is in line with postcolonial studies that analyze cannibalism as a myth constructed to justify identity construction and behavior toward the Other. William Arens' ground-breaking *Man-Eating Myth* (1979) was among the first studies to argue that the definition of non-Western "savages" as cannibals was not only a Western fantasy, but also an important prerequisite for colonial conquest, "the projection of western imperialist appetites onto the cultures they then subsumed" (Kilgour 1990, VII). Cannibalism, thus, can be understood as a self-serving colonial form of dehumanization that "involves the removal of qualities especially cherished as human" (Chen 2012, 43): while the white settler introduced and created civilization and humanity, the cannibal devoured it, which made him not only inferior, but also a threat to Western identity.

In nineteenth-century travelogues, the production of scientific and cultural knowledges as a form of control and power played a key role. Many nineteenth-century authors of travel writing were doctors and scientists (Fisch 1989), and they explicitly described the discovery and examination of cannibalistic Indigenous tribes as their "wichtigste Angelegenheit" (Wied-Neuwied 1821, 133), their main goal, while emphasizing the essential inferiority of these indolent, lazy, weak "Menschen, die fast keine Spur von Humanität in ihrem wüsten Aeusseren trugen" ["people whose desolate appearance showed almost no trace of humanity"] (Spix/Martius 480). In depictions of native tribes, medical/scientific and cultural observations become intertwined; physical appearance is frequently related to a presumed lack of morals, productivity and civilization: "Indolenz, Stumpfsinn und thierische Rohheit waren in ihren viereckigen, plattgedrückten Gesichtern, in ihren kleinen und furchtsam stieren Augen; Gefrässigkeit, Trägheit und Schwerfälligkeit in den wulstigen Lippen, in dem Hängbauche, wie in dem ganzen torösen Körper und trippelnden Gange ausgeprägt" ["indolence, dullness and bestial barbarism were in their square, flattened faces, in their small and fearfully staring eyes; gluttony, lethargy and clumsiness were pronounced in their bulging lips, the saggy belly, as well as in the whole fleshy body and tripping gate"] (Spix/Martius II, 480). Offering distinct images of racial inferiority and laziness, travel reports fulfilled several functions: they satisfied their readers' obsession with the exotic Other and provided a confirmation of Western cultural superiority. Frequently integrating racial theories and referring to famous scientists in their travelogues, they "popularized" modern racism. Moreover, they dehumanized Indigenous people to the extent that their cultures as well as their bodies were denied a worthiness or future.

This dehumanization legitimized objectification, curative violence, and eradication. Desecrations of Indigenous graves, the collection of excavated Indigenous remains as well as the captivation of Indigenous people were promoted as important tasks for the advancements of medicine and science: Prince Maximilian of Wied-NeuWied, for example, proudly related his successful hunt for an Indigenous skull to his readers as follows: "Ein zweytes Anliegen, welches mich hier noch einen Tag zu verweilen bewogen hatte, war die Hoffnung, eines Botocuden-Schädels habhaft zu werden. Am Quartel dos Arcos war ich an der zu diesem Zweck beschlossenen Ausgrabung eines Leichnams gehindert worden; hier war ich glücklicher. In geringer Entfernung von den Gebäuden hatte man in dem dichten Urwalde unter rankenden schön blühenden Gewächsen, einen jungen Botocuden von 20 bis 30 Jahren begraben, der einer der unruhigsten Krieger dieses Stammes gewesen war. Wir begaben uns, mit Hacken versehen, zu dem Grabe, und befreyten den merkwürdigen Schädel ["A second matter which made me stay here for another day, was the hope of getting hold of a Botocudo skull. At the Quartel dos Arcos I was prevented from digging up a corpse that had been selected for this purpose. I had more luck here. A short distance from the buildings, in the dense jungle, under vines with beautiful blossoms, a young, 20- to 30- year-old Botocudo man who had been one of the most restless warriors of this tribe, had been buried. We went to the grave with pickaxes and freed he strange skull"] (Wied-NeuWied 1821, 136). In their famous report, Johann Baptist von Spix and Carl Friedrich Philipp von Martius also described the collection of Indigenous skulls, here for the famous scientist Friedrich Blumenbach; moreover, they reported on the capturing of Indigenous people as museum pieces: "Der vormalige Portugiesische Staatsminister, Conde da Barca, hatte nämlich von dem Districtscommandanten der Indianer in Minas Geraës einen indianischen Schädel für unseren Landsmann, Hrn. Hofrath Blumenbach, verlangt; [...] so schickt er dem Grafen zwei lebendige Botocudos [...]; Hr v. Langsdorff erhielt nun den Einen derselben, welcher [...] nicht nur als lebendiges Cabinetstück, sondern auch als Einsammler von Naturalien diente" ["The former Portuguese minister Conde da Barca had, it seems, applied to the district commander of the Indians, in Minas Geraës, for an Indian scull, for our celebrated countryman, Professor Blumenbach; [...] the commandant [...] sent the count two living Botocudos [...]. M. Von Langsdorff obtained one of them, [...] who served him not only as a living cabinet piece, but as a collector of objects of natural history"] (Spix/Martius I, 96–97). Thus, travelogues on Brazil did not merely contain colonial fantasies. They were a key medium for medically trained intellectuals and scientists from various fields to document and participate in Western scientific knowledge production and distribution, and thus an important part of European domination and suppression of Indigenous lives, cultures, and knowledges.

Interestingly, the concept of the cannibal was adapted by Brazilian intellectuals in the early twentieth century to reflect on and protest against European colonization and knowledge production. Instead of merely copying European (French) models, they searched for more authentic Brazilian forms of expression that would incorporate (cannibalize) imported models (e.g. Shakespeare) to produce a local variety. In his famous *Manifesto Antropófago* (1928), the Brazilian modernist poet Oswald de Andrade defined cultural cannibalism, the incorporation of European knowledge and culture, as a counter-colonial project at the core of Brazilian cultural identity, referring to Hans Staden's account as one of the main sources for his theory. Adapting Shakespeare's famous "to be or not to be," the *Manifesto*'s famous slogan, "Tupi or not Tupi: That is the question" defined Brazilian identity as ongoing acts of incorporating/devouring European thought. While the *Manifesto* has long been understood as "a central trope of self-recognition, a model for the incorporation of difference, and a central concept in the definition of Latin American identities" (Jáuregui 2012, 22), recent studies criticize its disconnect from any social movement or actual decolonization effort, interpreting it as yet another form of colonial appropriation and objectification of Indigenous cultures that negates Indigenous people real political presence and agency as producers of knowledge (Madureira 2005; Clavo 2016).

The cruel treatment of Indigenous people by German travelers and scientists that their travel reports document raises questions about the relation between scientific travel (reports) and German settler colonial projects and the elimination of Indigenous populations as one of its key elements in the nineteenth century. On the one hand, the systematic elimination of Indigenous tribes from the settlements as well as the history of German settlements, which were established in the name of science, civilization, and humanity, can be interpreted as a manifestation of European racism. One the other hand, this also points toward the "other side of genocide" (De Sousa Santos et al. 2007, IX), the suppression of Indigenous knowledges; this approach might open paths to find new approaches, for example in Health Humanities, that not only establish bridges between the Humanities and the sciences, but also, more importantly, center on suppressed voices and knowledges.

CONCLUSIONS: TOWARD GLOBAL COGNITIVE JUSTICE

Ideas of work, disability, and race were at the center of German identity constructions as well as debates of German settler colonialism in the nineteenth century. These discourses intersected, providing an ideological and scientific framework for the construction of cultural and racial hierarchies. German body politic relied on the construction of deviant bodies, within the German cultural community as well as regarding other cultures. "Freak shows" and ethnographic *Völkerschauen* were manifestations of a general obsession with disability as well as race; both concepts, disability, and race served as key coordinates in the construction of German physical, moral, and racial superiority. Travel reports, too, became mass entertainment; intertwining observations with references to racial theories and scientific studies, travel writers propagated modern racism; and as travel writers were humanists as well as scientists, travel writings provided a space for knowledge production and distribution, building bridges and interrelations between the Humanities and the Sciences.

The interrelation between nineteenth-century constructions of disability and race can also offer novel approaches to the study of German settler colonialism, rejecting the portrayal of German settlements in nineteenth-century Brazil as isolated cultural spaces and instead focusing on processes of eliminating Indigenous people, cultures, and knowledges, from the locations of German settlements as well as from German cultural memory. Lorenzo Veracini's innovative approach, a comparison of settler colonialism and bacterial infections, places these processes at the core of settler colonialism, allowing for a critical re-examination of German colonial settler projects. Furthermore, his study builds bridges across disciplines to question, revise, or augment national and cultural memories.

Debates on German settlements abroad participated in Western knowledge production about other cultures as well as in the suppression of Indigenous epistemologies. A reflection on German settler colonialism, however, cannot be limited to the past; scholarly work in our field still often "unfolds in a still colonized space, by scholars who themselves are, predominantly, settler colonialists" (Manthripragada and Mušanović 2020, 27), contributing to and upholding settler futurity. Therefore, as research on German-Indigenous relations and the decolonization of German studies emphasize, projects to "unsettle" (Manthripragada and Mušanović 2020) German Studies and German cultural memory require, first and foremost, a (self-)critical reflection of the role of "an invader whose epistemological understanding of the world [...] resembled delusions of grandeur. That is, in the universe of Enlightened rationalism, it was assumed that reason [...] could differentiate between truth and falsehood, and thus, that the world was inherently decipherable, universal, and [...] able to be unidimensionally transcribed" (Hokowhitu 2016, 93). Secondly, it calls for establishing bridges and dialogues not only between Western Sciences and Humanities Studies, but also between diverse knowledges, toward an "equality of opportunities" (De Sousa Santos et al. 2007: XX) for different kinds of knowledge.

I would like to end this article with two examples of recent publications that make space Indigenous voices and epistemologies: The collection of interviews entitled *Indianthusiasm: Indigenous Responses* (2020) aims to bridge "the multidisciplinary field of Indigenous Studies with those of other Western scholarly discourses that are occupied with historical, Eurocentric representations of Indigeneity" (32). With respect to the intersectionality of disability and race, Rachel Presley's work (2019) calls for "the conceptualization of a Native medicine wheel which acts as a collective counter-rhetoric to dominant discourses of ability and impairment" (n.p.). Both studies are examples of "unsettling," non-relativistic dialogues among diverse knowledges that can offer original approaches to keys questions in the Humanities and the Sciences, building transdisciplinary relationships and relational frameworks for an ecology of knowledges and toward global cognitive justice.

NOTES

1. "The normalcy must constantly be enforced in public venues [...], must always be creating and bolstering its image by processing, comparing, constructing, deconstructing images of normalcy and the abnormal" (Davis 2013, 10).
2. All translations are mine, unless otherwise noted.
3. See, for example, Bade (1974); Schulze (2018).
4. See Ritz-Deutch (2008), or Schulze (2016).
5. For information on ethnographic shows, see, for example, Eric Ames (2009), Sierra Bruckner (2003), or David Ciarlo (2011).

WORKS CITED

Abrantes, Visconde de. 1941. "Memória sobre os meios de promover a colonização." *Revista de Imigração e Colonização* 2, no. 2–3: 832–391.

Ackermann, Franz Xavier. 1834. *Das Kaiserreich Brasilien: Beobachtungen und praktische Bemerkungen für deutsche Auswanderer*. Heidelberg: Groos.

Ames, Eric. 2009. *Carl Hagenbeck's Empire of Entertainments*. Seattle: University of Washington Press.

Anderson, Benedict. 2006. *Imagined Communities: Reflections on the Origin and Spread of Nationalism*. London and New York: Verso.

Arens, William. 1979. *The Man-Eating Myth: Anthropology & Anthropophagy*. Oxford: Oxford University Press.

Ascárate, Richard John. 2004. "Translating Cannibalism, or the Possible Politics of Representation in Hans Staden's *Warhaftig Historia* (1557)." *Interdisciplinary Journal for Germanic Linguistics and Semiotic Analysis* 9, no. 2: 301–322.

Bade, Klaus. 1975. *Friedrich Fabri und der Imperialismus in der Bismarckzeit: Revolution – Depression – Expansion*. Freiburg: Atlantis.

Bade, Klaus. 2002. *Europa in Bewegung: Migration vom späten 18. Jahrhundert bis zur Gegenwart*. München: Beck.

Bade, Klaus. 1995. "From Emigration to Immigration: The German Experience in the Nineteenth and Twentieth Centuries." *Central European History* 28, no. 4: 507–535.

Baynton, Douglas. 2013. "Disability and the Justification of Inequality in American History." In *The Disability Studies Reader*, edited by Lennard J. Davis, 17–34. New York and London: Routledge.

Bhambra, Gurminder K., Dalia Gebrial, and Kerem Nişancıoğlu. 2018. "Introduction: Decolonising the University?" In *Decolonising the University*, edited by Gurminder K. Bhambra, Dalia Gebrial, and Kerem Nişancıoğlu, 1–15. London: Pluto Press.

Blackbourn, David. 1998. *The Long Nineteenth Century: A History of Germany, 1780–1918*. Oxford: Oxford University Press.

Brion Davis, David. 2006. *Inhuman Bondage: The Rise and Fall of Slavery in the New World*. Oxford: Oxford University Press.

Bruckner, Sierra. 2003. "Spectacles of (Human) Nature: Commercial Ethnography between Leisure, Learning, and Schaulust." In *Worldly Provincialism: German Anthropology in the Age of Empire*, edited by Glenn Penny and Matti Bunzel, 127–155. Ann Arbor: University of Michigan Press.

Calloway, Colin, Gerd Gemünden, and Susanne Zantop, eds. 2002. *Germans and Indians: Fantasies, Encounters, Projections*. Lincoln: University of Nebraska Press.

Cassidy, Eugene. 2015. "The Ambivalence of Slavery, The Certainty of Germanness: Representations of Slave-Holding and Its Impact Among German Settlers in Brazil, 1820–1889." *German History* 33, no. 3: 367–384.

Chen, Mel Y. 2012. *Animacies: Biopolitics, Racial Mattering, and Queer Affect*. Durham: Duke University Press.

Conrad, Sebastian. 2010. *Globalisation and the Nation in Imperial Germany*. Cambridge: Cambridge University Press.

Ciarlo, David. 2011. *Advertising Empire: Race and Visual Culture in Imperial Germany*. Cambridge/London: Harvard University Press.

Clavo, María Iñigo. 2016. "Is Brazil a Postcolonial Country?" *Paragrana* 25, no. 2: 63–79.

Conze, Werner. 1972. "Arbeit." In *Geschichtliche Grundbegriffe: Historisches Lexikon zur politisch-sozialen Sprache in Deutschland*, edited by Reinhart Koselleck, Otto Brunner, and Werner Conze, 154–215. Stuttgart: Klett-Cotta.

Davis, Lennard. 2013. "Introduction: Disability, Normality, and Power." In *The Disability Studies Reader*, edited by Lennard J. Davis, 1–14. New York/London: Routledge.

Davis, Lennard. 1995. *Enforcing Normalcy: Disability, Deafness, and the Body*. London/New York: Verso.

Eigen, Sara and Mark Larrimore. 2006. "Introduction: The German Invention of Race." In *The German Invention of Race*, edited by Sara Eigen and Mark Larrimore, 1–7. Albany: State University of New York Press.

Feagin, Joe R. 2013. *The White Racial Frame: Centuries of Racial Framing and Counter-Framing*. New York/London: Routledge.

Fisch, Stefan. 1989. "Forschungsreisen im 19. Jahrhundert." In *Der Reisebericht: Die Entwicklung einer Gattung in der deutschen Literatur*, edited by Peter Brenner, 383–405. Baden Baden: Suhrkamp.

Fitzpatrick, Matthew and Peter Monteath, eds. 2020. *Savage Worlds: German Encounters 1798–1914*. Manchester: Manchester University Press.

Flitner, Christine. 1997. "Women's Writing in German-Speaking Switzerland: Engaging with Tradition – Eveline Halser and Gertrud Leutenegger." In *Post-War Women's Writing in German: Feminist Critical Approaches*, edited by Chris Weedon, 305–325. Providence: Berghahn.

Forsyth, Donald. 1985. "Three Cheers for Hans Staden: The Case for Brazilian Cannibalism." *Ethnohistory* 32, no. 1: 17–36.

Gaebler, Ernst Wilhelm Johann. 1850. *Deutsche Auswanderung und Kolonisation: Erster Rechenschaftsbericht des Berliner Vereins zur Centralisation Deutscher Auswanderer und Kolonisation*. Berlin: Schneider & Co.

Gretz, Daniela. 2007. *Die deutsche Bewegung: Der Mythos von der ästhetischen Erfindung der Nation*. München: Fink.

Grosser, Thomas. 1992. "Der mediengeschichtliche Funktionswandel der Reiselektüre in den Berichten deutscher Reisender aus dem Frankreich des 18. Jahrhunderts." In *Europäisches Reisen im Zeitalter der Aufklärung*, edited by Hans-Wolf Jäger, 275–310. Heidelberg: Winter.

Hasler, Eveline. 1988. *Ibicaba: Das Paradies in den Köpfen*. München: dtv.

Hokowhitu, Brendan. 2016. "Monster: Post-Indigenous Studies." In *Critical Indigenous Studies*, edited by Aileen Moreton-Robinson, 83–101. Tucson: University of Arizona Press.
Jáuregui, Carlos. 2012. "Antropofagia." In *Dictionary of Latin American Cultural Studies*, edited by Robert McKee Irwin and Mónica Szurmuk, 22–28. Gainesville: The University Press of Florida.
Kérchy, Anna and Andrea Zittlau, eds. 2012. *Exploring the Cultural History of Continental European Freak Shows*. Cambridge: Cambridge Scholars Publishing.
Kilgour, Maggie. 1990. *From Communion to Cannibalism: An Anatomy of Metaphors of Incorporation*. Princeton: Princeton University Press.
Kim, Eunjung. 2015. "Unbecoming Human: An Ethics of Objects." *GLQ: A Journal of Lesbian and Gay Studies* 21: 295–320.
Kremer, Arndt. 2016. "Transitions of a Myth? The Idea of a Language-Defined *Kulturnation* in Germany." *New German Review* 27, no. 1: 53–75.
Lestringant, Frank. 1997. *Cannibals: The Discovery and Representation of the Cannibal from Columbus to Jules Verne*. Berkeley: University of California Press.
Lutz, Hartmut. 2002. "German Indianthusiasm. A Socially Constructed German National(istic) Myth." In *Germans and Indians: Fantasies, Encounters, Projections*, edited by Colin G. Calloway, Gerd Gemuenden, and Susanne Zantop, 167–184. Lincoln: University of Nebraska Press.
Madureira, Luís. 2005. *Cannibal Modernities: Postcoloniality and the Avant-garde in Caribbean and Brazilian Literature*. Charlottesville: University of Virginia Press.
Manthripragada, Ashwin and Emina Mušanović. 2020. "Accounting for Our Settler Colonialism: Toward an Unsettled German Studies in the United States." In *Diversity and Decolonization in German Studies*, edited by Regine Criser and Ervin Malakaj, 23–40. New York: Palgrave Macmillan.
Menninger, Annerose. 1984. "Hans Stadens Warhaftige Historia: Zur Geschichte eines Bestsellers der Reiseliteratur." *Geschichte in Wissenschaft und Unterricht* 9: 509–523.
Mignolo, Walter. 2000. *Local Histories/Global Designs*. Princeton: Princeton University Press.
Musolff, Andreas. 2010. *Metaphor, Nation and the Holocaust: The Concept of the Body Politic*. London/New York: Routledge.
Myscofski, Carole. 2007/8. "Imagining Cannibals: European Encounters with Native Brazilian Women." *History of Religions* 47, no. 2/3: 142–155.
Naranch, Bradley. 2005. "Inventing the Auslandsdeutsche: Emigration, Colonial Fanatsy, and German National Identity, 1848–71." In *Germany's Colonial Past*, edited by Eric Ames, Marica Klotz, and Lora Wildenthal, 21–40. Lincoln/London: University of Nebraska Press.
Pothier, Diane and Richard Devlin. 2006. *Critical Disability Theory: Essays in Philosophy, Politics, Policy, and Law*. Vancouver: University of British Columbia Press.
Pratt, Marie Louise. 1992. *Imperial Eyes: Travel Writing and Transculturation*. New York: Routledge.
Presley, Rachel. 2019. "Decolonizing the Body: Indigenizing Our Approach to Disability Studies." *The Activist History Review*. https://activisthistory.com/2019/10/29/decolonizing-the-body-indigenizing-our-approach-to-disability-studies/. Accessed 29 September 2022.
Pufendorf, Samuel. 1976. *Die Verfassung des deutschen Reiches*. First edition 1667, translated, notes, and afterword by Horst Denzer. Stuttgart: Reclam.
Raphael-Hernandez, Heike and Pia Wiegmink. 2017. "German Entanglements in Transatlantic Slavery: An Introduction." *Atlantic Studies* 14, no. 4: 419–435.
Rinke, Stefan. 2020. "'No Alternative to Extermination': Germans and their 'Savages' in Southern Brazil at the Turn of the Nineteenth Century." In *Savage Worlds: German Encounters 1798–1914*, edited by Matthew Fitzpatrick and Peter Monteath, 21–42. Manchester: Manchester University Press.
Ritz-Deutch, Ute. 2008. *Alberto Vojtech Fric, the German Disaspora, and Indian Protection in Southern Brazil, 1900–1920: A Transatlantic Ethno-Historical Case Study*. Diss., Binghamton University.
Rodríguez, Encarnación Gutiérrez. 2018. "Conceptualizing the Coloniality of Migration: On European Settler Colonialism-Migration, Racism, and Migration Policies." In *Migration: Changing*

Concepts, Critical Approaches, edited by Doris Bachmann-Medick and Jens Kugele, 193–210. Berlin/Boston: de Gruyter.
Santos, Boaventura de Sousa, João Arriscado Nunes, and Maria Paula Menses. 2007. "Introduction: Opening Up the Canon of Knowledge and Recognition of Difference." In *Another Knowledge Is Possible: Beyond Northern Epistemologies*, edited by Boaventura de Sousa Santos, ix–lxii. London and New York: Verso.
Schmölz-Häberlein, Michaela and Mark Häberlein. 2001. "Hans Staden, Neil L. Whitehead, and the Cultural Politics of Scholarly Publishing." *The Hispanic American Historical Review* 81: 745–751.
Schule, Frederik. 2015. "Von verbrasilianisierten Deutschen und deutschen Brasilianern: 'Deutschsein' in Rio Grande do Sul, Brasilien, 1870–1945." *Geschichte und Gesellschaft* 41, no. 2: 197–227.
Schulze, Frederik. 2016. *Auswanderung als nationalistisches Projekt., Deutschtum' und Kolonialdiskurse im südlichen Brasilien (1824–1941)*. Köln/Weimar/Wien: Böhlau.
Schulze, Frederik. 2018. "German Settler Colonialism in Southern Brazil in German Documentary Films of the 1930s." In *Archiving Settler Colonialism*, edited by Yu-ting Huang and Rebecca Weaver-Hightower, 84–99. London: Routledge.
Seyferth, Giralda. 2003. "German Immigration and Brazil's Colonization Policy." In *Mass Migration to Modern Latin America*, edited by Samuel Baily and Eduardo José Míguez, 227–244. Wilmington: Scholarly Resources Inc.
Smith, Woodruf. 1986. *The Ideological Origins of Nazi Imperialism*. Oxford: Oxford University Press.
Spix, Johann Baptist and Carl Friedrich Phillipp von Martius. (1823–31). *Reise in Brasilien: auf Befehl Sr. Majestät Maximilian Jospeph I., Königs von Baiern, in den Jahren 1817 bis 1820 gemacht und beschrieben*. München: Lindauer.
Sudhaus, Fritz. 1940. *Deutschland und die Auswanderung nach Brasilien im 19. Jahrhundert*. Hamburg: Hans Christians Verlag.
Staden, Hans. 1557. *Warhaftige Historia und Beschreibung eyner Landschafft der Wilden Nacketen, Grimmigen Menschenfresser-Leuthen in der Neuenwelt America gelegen*. Marburg: Andreas Kolbe.
Stutzer, Therese. 1889. *Am Rande des brasilianischen Urwaldes*. Braunschweig: Hellmuth Wollermann Verlagsbuchhandlung.
Tautz, Birgit. 2006. "Cutting, Pasting, Fabricating: Late 18th-Century Travelogues and their German Translators between Legitimacy and Imaginary Nations." *German Quarterly* 79, no. 2: 155–173.
Tramontini, Marcos Justo. 2000. "A escravidão na colonia alemã." *Anais das Primeiras Jornadas de História Regional Comparada*: 1–17.
Veracini, Lorenzo. 2014. "Understanding Colonialism and Settler Colonialism as Distinct Formations." *Interventions* 16, no 5: 615–633.
Walker, Mack. 1964. *Germany and the Emigration 1816–1885*. Cambridge: Harvard University Press.
Wappäus, Johann Eduard. 1846. *Deutsche Auswanderung und Colonisation*. Leipzig: Hinrich.
Wied-Neuwied, Maximilian von. 1821. *Reise nach Brasilien in den Jahren 1815 bis 1817*. Frankfurt: Brönner.
Whitehead, Neil. 2000. "Hans Staden and the Cultural Politics of Cannibalism." *Hispanic American Historical Review* 80: 721–751.
Weber, Klaus. 2009. "Deutschland, der atlantische Sklavenhandel und die Plantagenwirtschaft der Neuen Welt (15. bis 19. Jahrhundert)." *Journal of Modern European History* 7, no.1: 37–67.
Wolfe, Patrick. 2006. "Settler Colonialism and the Elimination of the Native." *Journal of Genocide Research* 8, no. 4: 387–409.
Zantop, Susanne. 1997. *Colonial Fantasies: Conquest, Family, and Nation in Precolonial Germany, 1770–1870*. Durham: Duke University Press.
Zantop, Susanne. 2002. "Close Encounters: *Deutsche* and *Indianer*." In *Germans & Indians: Fantasies, Encounters, Projections*, edited by Colin G. Calloway, Gerd Gemünden, and Susanne Zantop, 1–14. Lincoln/London: University of Nebraska Press.
Zimmerer, Jürgen, ed. 2013. *Kein Platz an der Sonne: Erinnerungsorte der deutschen Kolonialgeschichte*, Frankfurt/New York: Campus.

CHAPTER FOURTEEN

The Post-1945 Eugenics Consensus and the Persecution of Germans of Color in the Third Reich: A Legal Case Study

JULIA ROOS

In the summer of 1937, the Nazi regime forcedly sterilized between 400 and 600 biracial Rhenish children and young adults. These were the German descendants of colonial French soldiers from Madagascar, the Maghreb, Senegal, and Vietnam who had participated in the 1920s Rhineland occupation. The Nazis vilified the children as *Rheinlandbastarde* ["Rhineland bastards"], a derogatory term denoting out-of-wedlock birth as well as "mixed-race" descent (Pommerin 1979; Bock 1986, 354; Campt 2004, 72–80; Aitken and Rosenhaft 2013, 264–266; Tascher 2016a and 2016b; Hohnholz 2017, 62–75; Roos 2023).

The sterilization campaign's prehistory reached into the early Weimar Republic (1919–33), when the racialist propaganda movement against the "schwarze Schmach am Rhein" ["black horror on the Rhine"] fomented hatred of France's colonial troops and their German offspring (Nelson 1970; Koller 2001; Maß 2006; Wigger 2007; Roos 2009 and 2012).[1] To discredit the Versailles Treaty, black horror discourse focused on alleged sexual crimes by African soldiers against white German women. Biracial occupation children (*Besatzungskinder*) featured as symbols of the Rhineland's purported "pollution" through contagious diseases and racial "mixing" (Campt 2004, 58–62; Maß 2006, 206–213). In 1927, Bavarian officials urged the Reich Health Office (*Reichsgesundheitsamt*) to sterilize these children "zur Reinhaltung der Rasse im besetzten Gebiet von farbigem Blut" ["to protect the purity of the race in the occupied territory from colored blood"] (Pommerin 1979, 92). Such proposals initially remained unsuccessful, partly because Weimar Germany lacked a sterilization law. After the Nazi takeover of power, divisions over how best to neutralize the perceived racial "dangers" of the Rhenish children persisted for a while; proposals ranged from forced exile to compulsory sterilization (Pommerin 1979, 71–77). In mid-April of 1937, Hitler personally ordered "die Maßnahmen zur Durchführung der Unfruchtbarmachung der Rheinlandbastarde sofort in Angriff zu nehmen" ["the immediate start of measures for the implementation of the sterilization (*Unfruchtbarmachung*) of the Rhineland bastards"].[2]

POSTWAR INVESTIGATIONS OF DOCTORS COMPLICIT IN THE *RHEINLANDBASTARDE* CAMPAIGN: BACKGROUND AND BROADER SIGNIFICANCE

To date, the problem of physicians' roles during the planning and implementation of the *Rheinlandbastarde* campaign has attracted only limited scholarly attention (Tascher 2016a and 2016b; Hohnholz 2017, 62–75). This chapter explores the hitherto unknown case of Dr. L., a state physician (*Amtsarzt*) in French-occupied Rhineland-Palatinate (Rheinland-Pfalz), who in 1948 came under investigation for a potential crime against humanity.[3] The proceedings against the *Amtsarzt* created unique (albeit temporary) openings for victims of the *Rheinlandbastarde* campaign to tell their stories and confront the medical perpetrators. During the investigation, victims' statements comprised crucial incriminating evidence, forcing the physician to justify his Nazi-era actions. This discursive dynamic in the denazification records sheds fresh light on major aspects of the "on-the-ground" unfolding and radicalization of the 1937 sterilizations. Because Dr. L. belonged to a small minority of doctors investigated for their participation in Nazi-era forced sterilizations of German citizens, his case offers a rare opportunity for examining up-close how medical officials presented (and rationalized) their active support of negative eugenic policies of the Third Reich. The tensions in Dr. L.'s self-exculpatory narrative—which often crystallized around his resentful tone vis-à-vis the victims and his efforts to discredit the latter's moral reputation—point to the important ways in which postwar investigations into the *Rheinlandbastarde* campaign potentially threatened key axioms of apologetic myths embraced by large sections of the West German medical profession after the war (Freimüller 2001; Forsbach 2015).

After 1945, a major element of physicians' apologetic strategies centered on the contention that their own support of eugenic policies aimed at "Aryans" had remained completely disconnected from the Nazi regime's crimes against Jews and other "non-Aryans" (Hahn 2000, 52–56; Herzog 2018, 4). The debate over the Law for the Prevention of Hereditarily Diseased Progeny (*Gesetz zur Verhütung erbkranken Nachwuchses*, or, GzVeN) of 14 July

1933 shows that this line of argumentation ultimately proved successful in shielding the vast majority of West German doctors from negative sanctions. The GzVeN permitted forced sterilization of people (allegedly) suffering from certain congenital conditions (Bock 1986, 88; Weindling 1989, 522–525).[4] As historians have shown, the law greatly enhanced the power of physicians, who made a range of key decisions: they identified and reported "hereditarily ill" patients, served on the hereditary health courts (*Erbgesundheitsgerichte*) ruling on cases of sterilization, provided expert testimonials to these courts, and performed the surgical procedures (Bock 1986, 184; Labisch and Tennstedt 1991, 38, 44; Vossen 2006). Gisela Bock estimates that between 1933 and 1945, up to 1 million individuals (or, around 3 percent of the population between 16 and 50) were reported for sterilization and roughly 400,000 were sterilized (Bock 1986, 232, 238).

By paving the way for the "biological filtering" of the entire population, Alfons Labisch and Florian Tennstedt have argued, the 1933 sterilization law was essential to the goals of National Socialist health policy to create a "rassenreiner, erbgesunder, großer 'arischer Volkskörper'" ["racially-pure, hereditarily-healthy greater 'Aryan people's body'"] (Labisch and Tennstedt 1991, 62). In the immediate aftermath of the Second World War, few viewed the GzVeN in critical terms. The Nuremberg Doctors' Trial of 1946–7 included the forced mass sterilizations of Jews and Romani among the medical crimes (Mitscherlich and Mielke 1949, 131–145; Forsbach 2015, 105). Yet, the Allies decided that the 1933 sterilization law was not a true "Nazi law," because it contained (nominal) provisions for a right of appeal (Weindling 2008, 249; Westermann 2010, 60; Tümmers 2011, 43). Several western democracies, including the U.S., also had laws permitting compulsory sterilization of certain groups (e.g., the mentally disabled, criminals, and individuals accused of "antisocial" behavior) (Kluchin 2009, 11–19). The vast majority of German doctors who had performed forced sterilizations in the Third Reich never experienced any legal or economic sanctions, and most victims remained unsuccessful in their efforts at compensation (*Wiedergutmachung*) (Weindling 2008; Westermann 2010, 88).

For a brief historical moment during the interregnum of 1945–9, the eugenics consensus that helped shield many German doctors from prosecution seemed somewhat less impermeable. Physicians implicated in the *Rheinlandbastarde* campaign had reason to worry that they might not receive impunity. For a person's racial descent was *not* among the official diagnoses listed in the 1933 sterilization law. The systematic sterilizations of biracial Rhenish children during the summer of 1937 occurred in secret and without even the pretense of a judicial process (Pommerin 1979, 77–78). Postwar investigations into the *Rheinlandbastarde* campaign potentially affected physicians who had participated in "legal" Nazi-era sterilizations, as well. As we will see, evidence gathered during the proceedings against Dr. L. revealed significant affinities and overlap between the physician's official tasks in the context of the 1933 sterilization law and related eugenic public health measures, on the one hand, and his actions in connection with the *Rheinlandbastarde* campaign, on the other hand. In this way, postwar scrutiny of the forced sterilizations of biracial Rhenish Germans had the *potential* to pierce the myth of the existence of "impartial" Nazi-era policies of negative eugenics whose medical practitioners had remained entirely disconnected from—and, hence, "untainted" by—Nazism's racial crimes. This also means that we need to reconsider the considerable degree to which the resilience of eugenic discourse in postwar West Germany depended on processes of the obfuscation and denial of black Germans' persecution in the Third Reich.

ANATOMY OF AN INVESTIGATION: THE MILITARY GOVERNMENT INTERVENES

On July 12, 1948, Governor Claude Hettier de Boislambert, head of the French military government of Rhineland-Palatinate (Rheinland-Pfalz), shared evidence of a Nazi-era crime with the civilian German state government.[5] Three women had testified that Dr. L., the former deputy director of a state health bureau (*staatliches Gesundheitsamt*), was responsible for the forced sterilizations of several biracial children. The events had occurred in 1937, when the youngest victim was nine years old. Hettier de Boislambert stressed that "les enfants en question n'étaient d'ailleurs même pas atteints d'une maladie ou infirmité quelconque, leur seul tare était d'être nés de père non aryans" ["the children in question did not suffer from any disease or infirmity, their only flaw was to be born of a non-Aryan father"]. He drew attention to the "gravité de ces actes qui constituent en raison du motif racial de ce traitement un crime contre l'humanité parfaitement caractérisé" ["seriousness of these acts, which due to their racial motivation fit perfectly the characteristics of a crime against humanity"]. In mid-June of 1948, a German denazification tribunal (*Spruchkammer*) had reclassified the physician a "follower" (*Mitläufer*), the second-lowest level of culpability. However, the *Spruchkammer* had failed to consider the evidence of the three women's testimonies. The Governor demanded "d'avoir à nouveau une instruction contre le docteur L. ... et événtuellement contre tout autre médicin qui y aurait participé" ["to reopen the investigation of Dr. L., and possibly any other doctor who might have participated"]. In the following months, the Mainz chief state prosecutor (*Oberstaatsanwalt*) investigated the physician, Dr. L., along with his former superior at the health bureau, for a potential crime against humanity as specified by Allied Control Council Law No. 10.[6]

Hettier de Boislambert's emphasis on the retrieval of new evidence against Dr. L. was purposeful. The State Ordinance for the Political Purification of Rhineland-Palatinate (Landesverordnung zur politischen Säuberung im Lande Rheinland-Pfalz) of April 17, 1947, granted German courts significant authority over matters of denazification (Möhler 1992, 279–280). It established the new civilian German office of the State Commissioner for Political Purification (Landeskommissar für politische Säuberung). The Landeskommissar appointed the "public plaintiffs" (*öffentliche Kläger*) who initiated proceedings against specific individuals. District examination committees (*Untersuchungsausschüsse*) conducted the investigations and recommended sanctions to the denazification tribunals in Koblenz, Mainz, Montabaur, or Trier. The *Spruchkammern* then ruled on a person's denazification status (Groups I–V: Major Offenders, Offenders, Lesser Offenders, Followers, Exonerated) and potential penalties. At the time of Hettier de Boislambert's letter, the military government could appeal a *Spruchkammer* decision only if new facts or evidence had transpired, or if there existed proof that a witness had committed perjury (Möhler 1992, 346).

THE WOMEN'S TESTIMONIES

The case against Dr. L. hinged significantly on the evidence of witness testimonies given by three women: a female victim of the 1937 sterilization campaign, her mother, and the mother of another (male) victim. The district *Untersuchungsausschuß* likely solicited the three women's statements sometime in January or February of 1948.

On February 27, 1948, A. H. (born 1925) and her mother signed two separate affidavits.[7] H.'s biological father was a colonial French soldier from Tonkin (present-day northern Vietnam). Because the young woman had been only twelve at the time of her forced sterilization, her mother, M. R., recounted the events. During 1935–6, the health bureau repeatedly summoned Frau R. and her daughter. On one occasion, Dr. L. severely reproached Frau R. "bezüglich meines Verkehr mit einem artfremden Menschen, zumal dieser die Uniform einer fremden Macht getragen habe" ["for having had relations with a man of an alien race, who, to make matters even worse, had been wearing the uniform of a foreign power"]. Health bureau personnel photographed mother and daughter and took samples of their blood and hair. Dr. L. told Frau R. that her daughter "daß meine Tochter keine Kinder zur Welt bringen dürfe, da sie fremdes Blut in den Adern hätte" ["must never bear children, since she has foreign blood in her veins"]. When she protested that her child was only ten years old, the *Amtsarzt* responded that this was "das richtige Alter um eine solche Operation zur guten Heilung zu bringen" ["the right age for this kind of surgery to make a good recovery"].

In 1937, Frau R. received a letter from the health bureau telling her to bring her daughter to the municipal hospital. When she arrived on the specified day, Frau R. encountered two other mothers and their biracial children. Under false pretenses, nurses separated the three women from their children. Only now did the mothers learn that their children would be undergoing (unspecified) surgery. Frau R.'s own daughter spent ten days confined in the hospital. When she finally found out that her daughter had been sterilized, a doctor told Frau R. that "die Operation sei halb so schlimm gewesen, es handele sich ja nur um eine Kürzung der Eierstöcke, was jederzeit wieder behoben werden könnte" ["the procedure had been minor, since it involved only a shortening of the ovarian tubes, which was easily reversible at any time"]. Frau R. remembered, "auch nach der Operation meiner Tochter hatte ich keine Ruhe von Seiten des Gesundheitsamtes. Wiederholt wurde ich von Dr. L. bestellt, der mir erklärte, daß meine Tochter keinen deutschen Wehrmachtsangehörigen heiraten dürfte. Eine Heirat sei nur möglich zwischen meiner Tochter und einem ebenfalls unfruchtbar gemachten Manne" ["even after the surgery, the health bureau did not leave me alone. Repeatedly, Dr. L. reminded me that my daughter was not allowed to marry a member of the German military, and that she could only marry a man who also had been sterilized"].

In her own statement, A. H. confirmed, "pour autant que je puisse m'en souvenir, les déclarations faites par ma mère sont bien exactes" ["as far as I can remember, my mother's account of events is accurate"].[8] The young biracial woman mentioned a subsequent encounter with Dr. L. that had occurred late in 1944. On this occasion, the physician administered an intelligence test to her. Dr. L. posed a series of questions, including "où en etait l'invasion, que signifiait l'expression, 'der Apfel fällt nicht weit vom Stamm,' ce que je pensais de la guerre et de la fin qu'elle aurait, si j'ecoutais la radio, si je lisais les journaux pour me tenir au courant, en un mot si je m'intéressais à la politique" ["where did the invasion occur, what is the meaning of the phrase, 'the apple does not fall far from the tree,' what do you think about the war and its probable outcome, do you listen to the radio, do you read magazines to keep up with current affairs, in a nutshell, if I was interested in politics"]. A. H. told Dr. L. that "ça m'est bien egal de savoir comment la guerre finira, car de toute façon je n'aurais pas d'enfants" ["the outcome of the war does not matter at all to me, since in any event, I will be unable to have children"]. In response, the *Amtsarzt* accused her of being "hostile à l'état" ["hostile towards the state"]. In February of 1945, the police arrested Frau H. She claimed that a prison officer told her that someone had reported her for listening to enemy radio. In mid-March, the young woman managed to escape from a prisoner transport to Bensheim (possible destination was the forced laborers' camp at Auerbach, a satellite [*Außenlager*] of Natzweiler-Struthof concentration camp) and went into hiding. She was convinced that it was Dr. L. who had denounced her to the Gestapo (Geheime Staatspolizei, or, Secret State Police), since he was the only person who had quizzed her about her political views and listening to the radio.

The third witness against Dr. L. was Frau K. R., one of the three mothers who met at the hospital.[9] Frau R.'s son K. (born 1928) descended from a Moroccan French soldier. In her affidavit of March 15, 1948, Frau R. mentioned that she had met Dr. L. during a mandatory visit to the health bureau in 1937. She recalled, "mein Sohn wurde von Dr. L. untersucht und auf seinen Geisteszustand geprüft" ["Dr. L. examined my son and tested his mental capacities"]. A few months later, the health bureau informed Frau R. that her son had an urgent appointment at the municipal hospital. During the appointment, the boy was examined yet again, as well as "von allen Seiten photographiert" ["photographed from all sides"]. Frau R. identified Dr. L. as one of the physicians who had participated in her son's exams; another man, she learned later, was Eugen Fischer of the Kaiser Wilhelm Institute in Berlin. After the doctors had finished examining the boy, they told Frau R. that "ich nach Hause gehen könne, dass das Kind aber im Krankenhaus verbleiben müsse" ["that I could go home, the child, however, had to remain at the hospital"]. No one, the mother insisted, had told her beforehand that her son would be sterilized.

Frau R.'s sighting of Eugen Fischer, the director of the Kaiser Wilhelm Institute for Anthropology, Human Heredity, and Eugenics (KWI-A) in Berlin and one of the leading race scientists of the Third Reich, was a major discovery. It provides proof that the anthropologist's personal involvement in the mass sterilizations of biracial Rhenish children was significantly more substantial than historians hitherto have realized (Lösch 1997, 231–305; Schmuhl 2008, 117–135; Weiss 2010, 69–110). During the 1937 sterilization campaign, Fischer and other scientists affiliated with the KWI-A conducted the final round of anthropological exams that determined whether a child was indeed a biracial *Besatzungskind* and hence would be sterilized (Pommerin 1979, 78; Lösch 1997, 344–348; Schmuhl 2008, 224–230; Roos 2023). Frau R.'s testimony forced Dr. L. to explain his relationship to Fischer. We will return to this aspect, below.

"ICH ERGRIFF DEN ARZTBERUF, UM ZUR LINDERUNG DER NOT BEIZUTRAGEN:" A PHYSICIAN'S SELF-EXONERATION

For Dr. L., the July 1948 intervention by the French military government occurred at a crucial juncture in his personal battle against denazification measures. The *Amtsarzt* had joined the Nazi paramilitary, Sturmabteilung (SA), in June of 1933.[10] In May of 1937, he became a member of the Nazi Party. In addition, Dr. L. had belonged to various other Nazi organizations, including the official representation of Nazi doctors, the NS-Ärztebund. During his tenure as deputy director of the district state health office, he had been a voting member of the hereditary health court which ruled on cases of compulsory sterilization. In 1946, the Central Purification Commission (Zentrale Säuberungskommission, or, ZSK) in Neustadt an der Haardt classified the *Amtsarzt* an "offender" (*Belasteter*, or, Group II), barring him from private and public employment as a physician, and imposing a monetary penalty of 25,000 Reichmarks. Although the 1946 ZSK ruling formally required his immediate dismissal, Dr. L. continued to work intermittently at a local tuberculosis clinic.

Taking advantage of the reforms of the April 1947 State Ordinance for the Political Purification of Rhineland-Palatinate, Dr. L. filed an appeal against the 1946 denazification verdict in early June of 1947 (Möhler 1992, 280). His efforts temporarily succeeded on June 17, 1948, when the Mainz *Spruchkammer* reclassified him a "follower" (*Mitläufer*, or, Group IV).

Before we examine Dr. L.'s behavior during his investigation for a potential crime against humanity, it is useful first to get a better sense of how the physician presented himself and his motivations in his 1947 appeal. Dr. L. claimed to have joined the NSDAP reluctantly, and only because membership in the SA required simultaneous membership in the Party.[11] He had joined the SA not out of strong ideological conviction, but because "ich glaubte dann allerdings an die Ehrlichkeit der propagierten sozialen Ziele, ebenso wie Millionen anderer Menschen auch" ["like millions of others, I initially believed in the propagated social goals"]. The *Amtsarzt* emphasized his altruistic and religious reasons for entering the medical profession: "als Sohn eines praktischen Arztes mit großer Stadtpraxis hatte ich schon in früher Jugend Einblick in die sozialen Nöte. Aus innerer Berufung und in dem Bestreben, durch meine Tätigkeit zur Linderung der Not beizutragen, ergriff ich späterhin selbst den Arztberuf" ["As the son of a general practitioner with a large urban practice, I was aware from early youth of the extent of social misery. Later on, an inner sense of calling and the urge to contribute to the alleviation of poverty led me to become a physician myself"]. He had taken significant risks in openly resisting Nazi Party attacks on his local Lutheran congregation. Although the mayor had threatened to dismiss him from the position of *Amtsarzt*, Dr. L. had continued to attend Lutheran church services (he was not dismissed). The physician underlined his rejection of the Nazi regime's official "Rassenlehre" ["racial doctrine"]. According to affidavits by health bureau staff, Dr. L. had criticized the antisemitic attacks of *Kristallnacht*. A number of prominent members of the Lutheran congregation—including a leading industrialist whom occupation authorities had appointed mayor after the war—vouched for the doctor's moral and political integrity.

In a statement addressed to the Mainz denazification tribunal during May of 1948, Dr. L. denied any knowledge at the time of the "euthanasia" murders of mentally and physically disabled patients.[12] The *Amtsarzt* admitted to having served on the district hereditary health court. However, he always had adhered strictly to the rules and procedures of the 1933 Law for the Prevention of Hereditary Progeny, and his actions therefore had been perfectly legal. Dr. L. reminded the *Spruchkammer* of the July 1947 decision by the American Military Tribunal that "support, proclamation, or promulgation of laws concerning the sterilization of mentally ill persons or of persons afflicted with a hereditary disease do not constitute crimes in the purview of this court if these laws include legal provisions protecting the rights of the persons in question." As a member of the *Erbgesundheitsgericht*, the physician underlined, he had been discriminating and impartial; medical-scientific, not ideological, considerations had guided his decisions. He even had voted in favor of sterilizing a Nazi Party member. According to Dr. L., his principled actions showed that "die Annahme einer politischen Belastung oder eines Nazi-Aktivismus wegen der Mitwirkung am Erbgesundheitsgesetz dürfte nach dem Gesagten hinfällig sein" ["any claims that my participation in the hereditary health law constitutes proof of political culpability or Nazi activism are baseless"].

Dr. L. drew a categorical line between "legal" Nazi-era negative eugenics, support of which he admitted, and the forced sterilizations of the biracial descendants of colonial French soldiers, involvement in which he denied. The latter cases, he insisted, "liefen nicht über das Erbgesundheitsgericht. ... Ärzte des Gesundheitsamtes waren hieran *nicht* beteiligt. Die in Frage stehenden Personen wurden aufgrund der Akten des Jugendamtes durch die Sonderkommission I in Berlin unter Führung von Prof. Eugen Fischer vorgeladen und untersucht, ohne dass die Gesundheitsämter vorher vom Zwecke der Untersuchung unterrichtet waren" ["did *not* go through the hereditary health courts. ... Physicians at the state health bureaus were *not* involved in this. Special Commission I in Berlin, which was chaired by Professor Dr. Eugen Fischer, used the records of the youth bureau to identify the persons in question and subsequently examined them without informing the health bureaus of the purpose of these examinations"]. Those children whom the Special Commission determined to be "farbige Mischlinge" ["mixed-race coloreds"] were subsequently sterilized: "die Gesundheitsämter wurden erst nachträglich über die getroffenen Maßnahmen unterrichtet" ["only after the fact did the health bureaus find out about the measures taken"].[13]

"DENUNZIATION ÜBLER ELEMENTE:" DR. L.'S ATTACKS ON THE VICTIMS

In March of 1948, Frau K. R. testified that she had witnessed an amiable conversation between Dr. L. and racial anthropologist Eugen Fischer. The conversation occurred while Fischer was examining her son K. at the municipal hospital. Immediately thereafter, the boy was forcedly sterilized. Frau R.'s observation potentially cast doubt on Dr. L.'s profession of ignorance (and innocence) of the plan of the *Rheinlandbastarde* sterilization campaign.

Dr. L.'s own depiction of his relationship to Fischer is missing from the archival record. However, the Mainz chief state prosecutor's report of September 17, 1948 fills in some of the gaps. According to the *Oberstaatsanwalt*, Dr. L. admitted to having met Fischer. This meeting, however, had been completely unconnected to Fischer's work as "Kommissionsmitglied für die zu sterilisierenden Rassemischlinge" ["member of the commission in charge of the mixed-race children who were going to be sterilized"].[14] Apparently, the *Amtsarzt* contended that his conversation with Fischer had been of a purely personal nature. The state prosecutor noted that "Dr. L., der ein Schüler Professor Fischers gewesen ist, hatte damals von dessen Anwesenheit in [der Stadt] erfahren und mit Dr. S. zusammen die Gelegenheit wahrgenommen, seinen früheren Lehrer zu begrüßen. Dieser nur kurze Besuch fand statt im Stadtkrankenhaus ... Bei der Gelegenheit der kurzen Unterhaltung der Beschuldigten mit Professor Dr. Fischer befaßte sich dieser gerade mit der Untersuchung des Sohnes R. In dieser Zufälligkeit liegt keine strafbare Handlung ..." ["Dr. L., who had been a student of Professor Fischer's, had heard that Fischer was in town and together with Dr. S. took the opportunity to welcome his former teacher. The brief encounter took place in the municipal hospital ... On the occasion of the short exchange between the defendants and Professor Dr. Fischer, the latter happened to be engaged in the exam of Frau R.'s son. This coincidence does not constitute a criminal offense"]. An affidavit by Fischer confirmed Dr. L.'s account.

To prove that neither he nor anyone else at the *Gesundheitsamt* had been involved in the sterilizations of the biracial children, Dr. L. submitted a piece of "exonerating" evidence that was more ambiguous than he seemed to think. This was a letter of mid-June of 1937 the *Amtsarzt* had received from Walter Albath, a high-ranking Gestapo officer who played a key role in coordinating the 1937 sterilization campaign (Pommerin 1979, 78–79; Klee 2003, 11). In his letter, Albath mentioned that Dr. L. had contacted Fischer on June 1, 1937, to inquire about the anthropologist's exam of Frau R.'s second son, A. K. According to Albath, Dr. L. had asked whether the boy was eligible for children's allowance (*Kinderbeihilfe*), or if this child, too, was descended from a colonial soldier. Only "Aryan" children were eligible for *Kinderbeihilfe*; the health bureaus were in charge of ascertaining "Aryan" descent. Albath told Dr. L., "ich bin vom Reichs- und Preussischen Ministerium [des Innern] angewiesen, eine derartige Bescheinigung nicht auszustellen. Dagegen ist vorgesehen, dass nach Beendigung der Arbeiten der Kommissionen den Gesundheitsämtern mitgeteilt wird, welche Personen sterilisiert sind und bei welchen wegen ihrer Zugehörigkeit zum europäischen Rassekreis von einer Sterilisation abgesehen wurde ... Bezüglich des hier in Betracht kommenden ... A. K. teile ich Ihnen zur schnellen Erledigung der Angelegenheit schon jetzt mit, dass der Genannte nach dem anthropologischen Gutachten zum europäischen Rassekreis gehört" ["[t]he Reich and Prussian Ministry of the Interior has instructed me not to issue any such confirmations at this point. After completion of the work of the commissions, we will inform the health bureaus which individuals were sterilized, and which ones were not, due to their membership in the European racial category ... However, to expedite matters, I can tell you already that according to the anthropological assessment, the boy in question, A. K., belongs to the European racial category"].[15]

Dr. L.'s correspondence with Fischer and Albath did not prove that he had known in June of 1937 what *exactly* would happen to children who did *not* fit the criteria of "European racial category." However, the physician's letter to Fischer suggested that he may have helped identify children in his district (like A. K.) who might be descendants of colonial French soldiers. Moreover, the *Amtsarzt* clearly had been ready to exclude a child from *Kinderbeihilfe* who did not qualify as "Aryan." That Dr. L. submitted Albath's letter as "exonerating" evidence during an investigation of his own potential complicity in a racial crime is somewhat surprising—as well as disturbing. Evidently, the physician was not worried that his correspondence with Fischer and Albath might shed negative light on his own active support of policies excluding "non-Aryans" from child welfare benefits.

Vis-à-vis A. H. and her mother, Dr. L. adopted an openly aggressive strategy centered on attempts to discredit the women's moral reputations. In October of 1948, when the *Amtsarzt* was being investigated for his potential role in Frau H.'s 1944 arrest, he told the district *Untersuchungsausschuß* that it was H. and her mother, not he, who deserved to be prosecuted for knowingly lying under oath and defaming a civil servant. The women's baseless accusations, Dr. L. complained, rendered him incapable of providing for his family. "Ich stehe also mit 6 unversorgten Kindern nach 20 Jahren aufopfernder ärztlicher Tätigkeit vor der schwersten wirtschaftlichen Not und Sorge um das tägliche Brot ohne die Möglichkeit, meinen Kindern eine ihrer Begabung entsprechende Ausbildung zu gewähren" ["After twenty years of dedication and sacrifices in my work, I cannot provide for my six children, face the most severe destitution and worry about the daily bread, and lack the means to grant my children an education commensurate with their talents"]. French officials had barred him from employment as a physician, "da ich auf Grund einer Denunziation gerichtsbekannter und vorbestrafter übler Elemente in ein Verfahren wegen Verbrechens gegen die Menschlichkeit verwickelt wurde" ["since due to denunciations by sinister elements with a criminal record, I was ensnarled in legal proceedings for a crime against humanity"]. Dr. L. insisted, "die Anzeigerin ist nicht von mir aus politischen Gründen ins Gefängnis gebracht worden, sondern rechtskräftig von der Strafkammer wegen eines üblen Betrugsdelikts bestraft worden. Ich selbst habe lediglich im Verfahren ein Gutachten über den Geisteszustand abgeben müssen" ["I did not get the plaintiff arrested for political reasons. Rather, she was properly sentenced in a court of law for committing the most repugnant fraud. All I had to do during the trial was to provide testimony concerning her mental state"].[16]

What was the nature of the alleged fraud committed by the young woman, and what had been Dr. L.'s role in connection with her arrest? To shed light on these questions, we need to look at sources outside of the physician's denazification records. One key task of the health bureaus focused on the creation of "family registers" (*Sippentafeln*) which recorded information deemed relevant for assessing the racial "value" of individuals and families. The extant *Sippentafel* for Frau H.'s family sheds light on Dr. L.'s actions.

Affixed to Frau H.'s name on her family's *Sippentafel* was the comment, "artfremd, Unfruchtbarmachung durchgeführt; Geheimakten" ["racially alien; sterilization has been implemented; secret records"]. Several handwritten annotations bore Dr. L.'s initials, among them a note of 10 May 1943, which read, "die H. wurde in Gegenwart ihrer Mutter darüber unterrichtet, dass sie die Genehmigung zur Eheschliessung nur mit einem unfruchtbaren Ehepartner erhalten könne" ["[i]n the presence of her mother, H. was told that she will get permission to marry only if the marital partner is sterilized, as well"].[17] On October 1, 1944, Dr. L. submitted a report marked, "Ermittlungssache gegen A. H." ["criminal investigation of A. H."][18] The *Amtsarzt* described the young woman, "H. ist voreheliches Kind ihrer Mutter und Bastard eines Angehörigen der Besatzungstruppe und zwar eines Anamiten" ["H. is her mother's illegitimate daughter and the bastard of a member of the occupation troops who was an Annamite"]. The young woman had worked as a maid, agricultural laborer, and worker in a chemical factory: "1936 mußte über sie Schutzaufsicht verhängt werden, da sie gemeinsam mit einem anderen Mädchen einen Diebstahl begangen hatte. Bei einer … Begutachtung durch Medizinalrat Dr. S. … wurde festgestellt, daß es sich um ein intellektuell normal entwickeltes, charakterlich aber minderwertiges Mädchen handelt" ["In 1936, she was taken into protective custody, because she and another girl had committed theft. The medical exam conducted by Dr. S. … showed that although the girl's intellectual faculties are normally developed, she is of inferior moral character"]. In the fall of 1944, Frau H. was charged with defrauding two German soldiers to gain "finanzielle Vorteile" ["financial advantages"]. She allegedly had told the men that "sie erwarte ein Kind von ihnen bzw. sie habe ein Kind geboren" ["she was pregnant with their child and had given birth to a child, respectively"]. Since Frau H. was sterilized, Dr. L. stressed, she knew that her sexual relations with the two soldiers were against the law.

The physician posited a causal link between H.'s racial descent and her allegedly deceitful behavior: "Die körperliche Untersuchung ergibt deutliche Zeichen eines fremdrassischen, mongolischen Einschlags" ["The physical exam shows clear signs of racially alien, Mongol influences"]. He conceded that the girl's academic and practical knowledge was good, and that letters she had written "zeigen sogar eine gewisse Gewandtheit im Stil" ["even show a certain nimbleness of style"]. Dr. L. asserted, "die H. ist über ihre Umwelt und die gegenwärtige Lage in vollem Umfang unterrichtet" ["H. is fully informed about her social environment and current affairs"]. She clearly had been aware of the wrongfulness of her actions: "Es handelt sich bei ihr lediglich um eine charakterliche Minderwertigkeit, die aus der Tatsache der Zwiespältigkeit ihrer Abkunft zu erklären ist. Sie ist der typische Bastard, der unausgeglichen zwischen des Rassen steht" ["Her case is merely an example of an inferiority of character, which stems from the ambiguity of her descent. She is the typical bastard, who stands moodily between the races"].

Dr. L.'s 1944 report does not contain clear evidence that he suspected Frau H. of subversive political activities, or that he reported her to the Gestapo. What the report *does* show is that the physician shared the belief of Nazi "race experts" like his former teacher, Eugen Fischer, that persons of "mixed-race" descent (*Mischlinge*)—even if they occasionally displayed above-average intellectual abilities—were morally and physically "inferior" to "racially pure" whites and thus posed a danger to the *Volk* (Fischer 1913, 292–304; Lösch 1997, 65–75). The physician's critical report likely further diminished H.'s chances of receiving any consideration of mitigating circumstances (she was nineteen at the time).

CODA

On September 17, 1948, the Mainz *Oberstaatsanwalt* terminated the investigation of Dr. L. and his superior Dr. S. for a crime against humanity. The chief state prosecutor's report endorsed key elements of the physicians' own self-exculpatory narrative: "Im Jahre 1937 waren Dr. S Leiter und Dr. L. stellvertretender Leiter des Staatlichen Gesundheitsamtes … Es ist bekannt, daß in diesem Jahre allenthalben in Deutschland, so auch in [dieser Stadt] alle sogenannten Rassemischlinge sterilisiert worden sind …" ["In 1937, Dr. S. was the director, and Dr. L., the deputy director, of the district state health bureau … It is well-known that in this year, the so-called racial mixed-bloods were sterilized throughout Germany, including in [this city] …"]. The *Oberstaatsanwalt* dismissed the victims' testimonies implicating the physicians in the *Rheinlandbastarde* campaign, "da nach den angestellten Ermittlungen feststeht, daß nirgends in Deutschland, also auch nicht in [dieser Stadt], die Staatlichen Gesundheitsämter zu der Aktion zur Sterilisierung der Rassemischlinge herangezogen worden sind. Hiermit befaßte sich ausschließlich eine vom Reichsminister des Innern eingesetzte Sonderkommission, deren ärztliches Mitglied Professor Dr. Fischer aus Berlin gewesen ist" ["since our investigations have ascertained that neither in Germany as a whole, nor in this specific city, did the state health bureaus participate in the measure of the sterilization of the mixed-bloods. This measure was the sole responsibility of a special commission convened in the Reich Ministry of the Interior and on which Professor Dr. Eugen Fischer served as chief medical expert"]. It was true that Dr. L. had examined Frau H. in 1944. Yet, the exam occurred in the context of the woman's arrest for a criminal activity; she was not a victim of political persecution. In his conclusion, the *Oberstaatsanwalt* referred to Walter Albath's letter of June 1937, which he argued proved "mit absoluter Sicherheit …, daß die Gesundheitsämter weder mit der Aktion selbst noch mit deren Vorbereitungen irgendwie befaßt waren" ["with absolute certainty that the *Gesundheitsämter* were never involved in the measure itself, nor in any of the preparatory work for it"].[19]

For a while, the French military government continued to oppose Dr. L.'s reclassification of "follower." Only in December of 1948 did Governor Hettier de Boislambert reluctantly agree to Dr. L.'s placement in Group IV.[20] Internally, French officials were hopeful that they would be able to resume proceedings against the *Amtsarzt* in the coming year. Testimony by two additional female victims of the *Rheinlandbastarde* campaign directly implicated Dr. L.'s former superior, Dr. S., in the crimes. Yet this attempt to indict the two physicians ultimately failed, as well. After the founding of the Federal Republic in May of 1949, denazification was rapidly losing momentum. Dr. L. and Dr. S. retained the status of *Mitläufer*. By the end of 1950, the two men once again worked as a team of directors of another *Gesundheitsamt* in Rhineland-Palatinate. French authorities never identified the surgeon who had sterilized the local group of biracial children.

Despite formal admission of his own leading role during the 1937 *Rheinlandbastarde* campaign, Eugen Fischer never faced criminal charges for facilitating the forced sterilizations of hundreds of biracial children.

In November of 1949, Frau H. underwent re-fertilization (*Refertilisierung*) surgery.[21] The regional Office for Restitution (Amt für Wiedergutmachung) covered the costs. It is unclear whether Frau H.'s surgery was successful, enabling her to have children; historians emphasize the low rate of success of refertilization surgery (Westermann 2010, 123–124).

K. K., the biracial son of Frau R., spent over twenty-five years applying unsuccessfully for *Wiedergutmachung* for his forced sterilization and wartime incarceration in the youth concentration camp at Moringen, Lower Saxony (Niedersachsen).[22]

* * *

What did the proceedings against Dr. L. and Dr. S. achieve? Although the two physicians ultimately were rehabilitated, for a brief moment during 1948–9, their careers seemed to hang in the balance. The victims' testimonies did not lead to a formal indictment; there never was an actual trial. And yet, there arguably *were* costs for the two *Amtsärzte*. Dr. L. stressed the financial difficulties he faced due to the loss of employment. Within their Lutheran congregation and social circles, it was known that the men were being investigated by the Mainz chief state prosecutor. Many of the details of the case probably seeped out into the wider public sphere. Interestingly, despite the support they received from the town's social elites, the two *Amtsärzte* moved away soon after they had been exonerated.

To a great extent, it was the determination of the victims and their families to tell their stories and seek justice that allowed representatives of the French military government to launch multiple proceedings against Dr. L. and Dr. S. The victims' testimonies drew attention to the important ways in which employees of the *Gesundheitsamt* had contributed to enabling the 1937 sterilizations. That the Mainz chief state prosecutor decided to endorse unblinkingly the physicians' tension-ridden version of events points to the problematic ways in which a shared sense of social status (*Standesbewußtsein*) among civil servants—which was infused with authoritarian attitudes toward the working-class poor—hindered a more consistent and thorough denazification of medical officials. The chief state prosecutor's decision to terminate the investigation into a crime against humanity also suggests the resilience of nationalist resentments directed against the French occupiers and German women who "colluded" with the "enemy." Similar resentments had been a major political dynamic during the 1920s "black horror" campaign against colonial French soldiers and their biracial German offspring.

The district health bureau's very significant involvement in the identification, racial classification, and biological "tracking" (via the *Sippentafeln*) of biracial "occupation children" sheds fresh light on the sizeable impact traditions of anti-black racism had on negative population policies during the Third Reich. At the same time, analysis of the role of the *Gesundheitsämter* in facilitating the 1937 sterilization campaign allows us to trace an insidious process by which public health officials and medical personnel increasingly turned into a type of "amateur anthropologists" who saw the ferreting-out of "racial aliens" (*Rassefremde*) as one of their supreme tasks. Dr. L. was not the only one at the health bureau who sought to emulate the work of race scientists like Eugen Fischer. Without the eager contributions of these local "racial detectives," the overall remarkably smooth implementation of Hitler's *Führer* order of April 1937 would not have been possible.

NOTES

Writing of this chapter was supported by a 2020–1 Presidential Arts and Humanities Program Research Fellowship, Indiana University—Bloomington. I am grateful to Jörg Pawelletz of Landeshauptarchiv Koblenz, who helped retrieve crucial denazification records. Brett Bowles of Indiana University—Bloomington generously facilitated initial correspondence with French archives. A number of colleagues offered thoughtful comments and suggestions on different versions of this chapter. Special thanks go to volume editor Stephanie Hilger, and to Donna Harsch, Emma Kuby, Emily Marker, and the participants in the October 28, 2022, History Department Research Seminar, Carnegie Mellon University.

1. The precise origin of the phrase, "schwarze Schmach," is somewhat unclear, partly due to the sheer volume of propagandistic materials published in a very compressed period of time.
2. I am grateful to Gisela Tascher for alerting me to the existence of this order. Hitler's order is mentioned, for example, in Arthur Gütt's circular, "Geheime Reichssache!," 21 April 1937, in Politisches Archiv des Auswärtigen Amts (PAAA) RZ 214/100683, p. 6–7.
3. In compliance with German privacy laws, I have anonymized the names of the doctors, victims, and victims' relatives.
4. The GzVeN defined nine (dubious) medical diagnoses: hereditary feeble-mindedness, schizophrenia, manic-depression, hereditary epilepsy, Huntington's chorea, hereditary blindness, hereditary deafness, hereditary malformations, and severe alcoholism.
5. Claude Hettier de Boislambert to Minister President Peter Altmeier and Minister of Justice Adolf Süsterhenn, 12 July 1948, in Ministère des Affaires Étrangères, Centre des Archives diplomatiques de La Courneuve (CAD-LC), Archives d'Occupation Française en Allemagne et Autriche, 1AJ/2577-327 (Affaire L. V.). Translations from the French and German are my own throughout this article, unless otherwise indicated.
6. Since this investigation focused primarily on evidence against Dr. L., the following discussion focuses on Dr. L., as well. Article II, Section 1. c. of Allied Control Council Law No. 10 of 20 December 1945 defined "*Crimes against Humanity*: Atrocities and offences, including but not limited to murder, extermination, enslavement, deportation, imprisonment, torture, rape, or other inhumane acts committed against any civilian population, or persecutions on political, racial or religious grounds whether or not in violation of the domestic laws of the country where perpetrated." Reprinted in George J. Annas and Michael A. Grodin, 318.
7. For the following, see the French translations of the two women's affidavits of 27 February 1948, in CAD-La Courneuve, ZFO Allemagne et Autriche, 1AJ/2577. The German original no longer exists.
8. French translation of A. H.'s statement of 27 February 1948 in CAD-La Courneuve, ZFO Allemagne et Autriche, 1AJ/2577.
9. The following is based on Frau R.'s statement of 15 March 1948 in CAD-La Courneuve, ZFO Allemagne et Autriche, 1AJ/2577.
10. For this and the following, see the minutes of the Mainz denazification tribunal of 17 June 1948, in Landeshauptarchiv Koblenz (LHAKo) Best. 856/134990.
11. For this and the following, see Dr. L.'s statement of 7 June 1947 in LHAKo Best. 856/134990.

12. Dr. L.'s letter to the public plaintiff at the Mainz denazification tribunal, 6 May 1948, in LHAKo Best. 856/134990.
13. Dr. L.'s letter to the public plaintiff at the Mainz denazification tribunal, 6 May 1948, in LHAKo Best. 856/134990.
14. For this and the following, see the report by the Mainz chief state prosecutor of 17 September 1948 in CAD-LC 1AJ/2577.
15. Walter Albath's letter to Dr. L. of 16 June 1937 in LHAKo Best. 856/134990.
16. Dr. L.'s letter to the public plaintiff (*öffentlicher Kläger*) of 10 October 1948, in LHAKo Best. 856/134990.
17. Dr. L.'s note of 10 May 1943 in Landesarchiv Speyer (LASp) Best. O49/374.
18. For this and the following, see Dr. L.'s report of 1 October 1944, in Landesarchiv Speyer (LASp) Best. O49 /374.
19. Report by the Mainz chief state prosecutor, 17 September 1948, in CAD-LC 1AJ/2577.
20. Hettier de Boislambert to the State Commissioner for Political Purification, 4 December 1948, in CAD-LC 1AJ/2577.
21. Frau H.'s re-fertilization surgery is documented in LASp O 49 Nr. 374.
22. A portion of K.'s application for restitution is preserved in LASp J 10 Nr. 5623.

WORKS CITED

Aitken, Robbie and Eve Rosenhaft. 2013. *Black Germany: The Making and Unmaking of a Diaspora Community, 1884–1960*. Cambridge: Cambridge University Press.

Annas, George J. and Michael A. Grodin, eds., 1992. *The Nazi Doctors and the Nuremberg Code: Human Rights in Human Experimentation*. New York/Oxford: Oxford University Press, 1992.

Bock, Gisela. 1986. *Zwangssterilisation im Nationalsozialismus: Studien zur Rassenpolitik und Frauenpolitik*. Opladen: Westdeutscher Verlag.

Campt, Tina M. 2004. *Other Germans: Black Germans and the Politics of Race, Gender, and Memory in the Third Reich*. Ann Arbor: University of Michigan Press.

Fischer, Eugen. 1913. *Die Rehobother Bastards und das Bastardisierungsproblem beim Menschen: Anthropologische und ethnographische Studien am Rehobother Bastardvolk in deutsch-Südwest-Afrika*. Jena: Gustav Fischer.

Forsbach, Ralf. 2015. "Die öffentliche Diskussion der NS-Medizinverbrechen in Deutschland seit 1945: Kollektivschuld, Vergangenheitsbewältigung, Moralismus." In *NS-Medizin und Öffentlichkeit: Formen der Aufarbeitung nach 1945*, edited by Stephan Brease und Dominik Groß, 97–132. Frankfurt am Main: Campus.

Freimüller, Tobias. 2001. "Mediziner: Operation Volkskörper." In *Karrieren im Zwielicht: Hitlers Eliten nach 1945*, edited by Norbert Frei, 13–69. Frankfurt am Main: Campus Verlag.

Hahn, Daphne. 2000. *Modernisierung und Biopolitik: Sterilisation und Schwangerschaftsabbruch in Deutschland nach 1945*. Frankfurt am Main: Campus.

Herzog, Dagmar. 2018. *Unlearning Eugenics: Sexuality, Reproduction, and Disability in Post-Nazi Europe*. Madison: University of Wisconsin Press.

Hohnholz, Rita. 2017. *Zwangssterilisationen in Wiesbaden von 1933 bis 1945*. Norderstedt: Books on Demand.

Klee, Ernst. 2003. *Das Personenlexikon zum Dritten Reich: Wer was was vor und nach 1945*. Frankfurt am Main: S. Fischer.

Kluchin, Rebecca. 2009. *Fit to Be Tied: Sterilization and Reproductive Rights in America, 1950–1980*. New Brunswick: Rutgers University Press.

Koller, Christian. 2001. *"Von Wilden aller Rassen niedergemetzelt:" Die Diskussion um die Verwendung von Kolonialtruppen in Europa zwischen Rassismus, Kolonial- und Militärpolitik (1914–1930)*. Stuttgart: Franz Steiner.

Labisch, Alfons and Florian Tennstedt. 1991. "Gesundheitsamt oder Amt für Volksgesundheit? Zur Entwicklung des öffentlichen Gesundheitsdiensts seit 1933." In *Medizin und Gesundheitspolitik in der NS-Zeit*, edited by Norbert Frei, 35–66. München: R. Oldenbourg Verlag.

Lösch, Niels C. 1997. *Rasse als Konstrukt: Leben und Werk Eugen Fischers*. Frankfurt am Main: Peter Lang.

Maß, Sandra. 2006. *Weiße Helden, schwarze Krieger: Zur Geschichte kolonialer Männlichkeit in Deutschland 1918–1964*. Kön: Böhlau Verlag.

Mitscherlich, Alexander and Fred Mielke. 1949. *Doctors of Infamy: The Story of the Nazi Medical Crimes*. New York: Henry Schuman.

Möhler, Rainer. 1992. *Entnazifizierung in Rheinland-Pfalz und im Saarland unter französischer Besatzung von 1945 bis 1952*. Mainz: Hase & Köhler Verlag.

Nelson, Keith L. 1970. "The 'Black Horror on the Rhine': Race as a Factor in Post-World War I Diplomacy." *Journal of Modern History* vol. 42: 606–627.

Pommerin, Reiner. 1979. *"Sterilisierung der Rheinlandbastarde": Das Schicksal einer farbigen deutschen Minderheit 1918–1937*. Düsseldorf: Droste.

Roos, Julia. 2023. "Constructing Racial Visibility: Biracial 'Occupation Children' in the Third Reich, 1933–37." *Holocaust and Genocide Studies*, 37, no. 1 (Spring): 2–24.

Roos, Julia. 2012. "Nationalism, Racism and Propaganda in Early Weimar Germany: Contradictions in the Campaign against the 'Black Horror on the Rhine.'" *German History* 30, no. 1 (March): 45–74.

Roos, Julia. 2009. "Women's Rights, Nationalist Anxiety, and the 'Moral' Agenda in the Early Weimar Republic: Revisiting the 'Black Horror' Campaign against France's African Occupation Troops." *Central European History* 42, no. 3 (September): 473–508.

Schmuhl, Hans-Walter. 2008. *The Kaiser Wilhelm Institute for Anthropology, Human Heredity, and Eugenics, 1927–1945: Crossing Boundaries*. Berlin: Springer.

Tascher, Gisela. 2016a. "Handeln auf Befehl des Führers: Die illegale und streng geheime Zwangssterilisationen der 'Rheinlandbastarde' von 1937 und die Strafverfolgung der ärztlichen Täter nach 1945." *Deutsches Ärzteblatt* 113, no. 10 (11 March 2016): 420–422.

Tascher, Gisela. 2016b. "Auf Befehl des Führers: Die Zwangssterilisierung der 'Rheinlandbastarde' und die Strafverfolgung der ärztlichen Täter." *Saargeschichte/n* 2: 7–14.

Tümmers, Henning. 2011. *Anerkennungskämpfe: Die Nachgeschichte der nationalsozialistischen Zwangssterilisationen in der Bundesrepublik*. Göttingen: Wallstein.

Vossen, Johannes. 2006. "Erfassen, Ermitteln, Untersuchen, Beurteilen: Die Rolle der Gesundheitsämter und ihrer Amtsärzte bei der Durchführung von Zwangssterilisationen im Nationalsozialismus." In *Lebensunwert-Zerstörte Leben: Zwangssterilisation und "Euthanasie,"* edited by Margret Hamm, 86–97. Frankfurt am Main: Verlag für akademische Schriften.

Weindling, Paul. 1989. *Health, Race and German Politics between National Unification and Nazism, 1870–1945*. Cambridge: Cambridge University Press.

Weindling, Paul. 2008. "Entschädigung der Sterilisierungs- und Euthanasie-Opfer nach 1945?" In *Tödliche Medizin im Nationalsozialimus: Von der Rassenhygiene zum Massenmord*, edited by Klaus-Dietmar Henke, 247–258. Köln: Böhlau.

Weiss, Sheila Faith. 2010. *The Nazi Symbiosis: Human Genetics and Politics in the Third Reich*. Chicago: University of Chicago Press.

Westermann, Stefanie. 2010. *Verschwiegenes Leid: Der Umgang mit Zwangssterilisationen in der Bundesrepublik Deutschland*. Köln: Böhlau Verlag.

Wigger, Iris. 2007. *"Die schwarze Schmach am Rhein": Rassistische Diskriminierung zwischen Geschlecht, Klasse, Nation und Rasse*. Münster: Westfälisches Dampfboot.

CHAPTER FIFTEEN

Tea, Race, and Ethnicity: Medical Knowledge of the Others in the German Lands, 1700–1830

HEIKKI LEMPA

In a book by Franz Anton May, titled *Medicinische Fastenpredigten* ["Medical Lent Sermons"], we find a claim that draws our attention. According to the author, the Germans were plagued by a "tea epidemic" ["Theeseuche"], a dangerous disease caused by the addiction to tea that caused "allzugrosen Flüßigkeit des Bluts" ["too great liquidity of blood"]. The consequences were grave: the people "ganz eigentlich schmelzen, niemals wieder gesund werden, und ganz erschöpft sterben" ["literally melt without ever recovering, and die completely exhausted"] and especially the women suffer from lost fertility (May 1793, 217–218). The author of the book, which included public lectures to the residents of the City of Mannheim, was a medical doctor and professor of midwifery at the University of Heidelberg. The introduction of the book was signed in the middle of the Revolutionary Wars, September 15, 1793. In January of the same year the French King had been decapitated and Marie Antoinette had heard her indictment. Tribal fervor was reaching its high pitch in the German lands. May's medical sermons added to the agitation, "um der Ansteckung der französischen Volksseuche vorzubeugen" ["to prevent the contamination of the French people's plague"] (May 1793, Vorbericht).[1] The plague was the French Revolution but the means of its proliferation were not only the weapons and political propaganda but also the pathologies of the German bodies and minds. The Revolution and its dangerous spread needed medical intervention. It is this medical intervention and especially its focus on such matters as tea that is in the center of this chapter. Why was tea so dangerous? What did this perceived danger mean? Tea was, I suggest, an important marker for the definition of the German body because this definition requested differentiation from the bodies of the others; for May tea was the vehicle that carried the contagion of the others into the Germanic realm—from near and afar.

Why tea and why tea in a history of the body? First, tea was a common beverage in the German lands in the eighteenth century. In East Frisia, it was a common, popular beverage in all social classes (Wassenberg 1991). Regional studies on German consumer culture indicate that tea was widely consumed in middling classes, urban elite, and nobility, although rural communities were generally excluded from this consumerism (North 2008, 68–70; Ogilvie 2015, 173–193). Second, tea allows a new approach in the history of the body. The methodological problems of the history of the body are well-known and well-debated. In 1991, the grand master of medical history, Roy Porter, wrote one of the first comprehensive reviews of the history of the body. He discerned three established fields of scholarship, body and mind, policing the body, and the study of sexuality and gender. The review ended with an agenda for future research. Porter saw no fewer than seven areas as trendsetters for scholarship: the body as human condition; the form of the body; the anatomy of the body; body, mind, and soul; sex and gender; the body and the body politic; the body, civilization, and its discontents (Porter 1991, 223–226). Twenty years later this agenda appears as visionary as having failed the test of time. Not only did Porter capture the range of themes that seemed to exhaust the topic at hand, but he also recognized the work that in German history became the paragon of the history of the body, Barbara Duden's magisterial work in the history of medicine, *The Woman Beneath the Skin*. And yet for a student of German history, Porter's review and agenda left something wanting. His focus was on Atlantic history—England, France, the United Sates—and he paid scant attention to the areas of body culture that in German history seemed most promising, such as sports, gymnastics, dancing, and the realm of topics that showed the closest political affiliation between the body and politics, eugenics, hygiene, and public education. All these topics had to wait. As Maren Lorenz noticed eight years later, it was not until the end of the 1990s that the real boom of the history of the body started in German history (Lorenz 2000, 10). Since then, an impressive amount of scholarship has been produced that has unearthed the meanings and socio-political underpinnings of human corporeality in German society from the Middle Ages into the late twentieth century. Yet the difficulties to find a nexus in the history of the body—something that we seem to have in the history of emotions, for instance—is obvious. Alys George's magnificent *The Naked Truth: Viennese Modernism and the Body* shows what it might take to cover the essential dimensions of what the body can be in a historical context. One must master not only different fields but different disciplines, such as film studies, literary studies, art history, social history, history of medicine, and history of dance (George 2020).

Yet the question remains: what brings these disciplinary approaches together, what makes the nexus of the history of the body? I do not pretend to have found an answer but there is something very appealing in the approach that the historian of medicine Pratik Chakrabarti has articulated. "The history of modern medicine," Chakrabarti argues, "cannot be narrated without the history of imperialism" (Chakrabarti 2014, ix). In the center of this new narrative are not the theories and the individual medical heroes but rather the new material forces that imposed themselves on the old forms of knowledge and practice. The discovery, classification, production, and global trade on *materia medica*, the pharmacopeia, medicinal herbs, were an important part of these forces (Chakrabarti 2014, 35). And tea was one of these medicinal herbs, in fact, a very important one.

In the early modern world, tea was not only a beverage but also a remedy, a commodity that served medicinal purposes as well as the indulgence of the wealthy and increasingly the middling classes and the poor. Erika Rappaport has recently shown how tea helped build empires, first the Chinese and then the British (Rappaport 2017). What is so appealing in tea for a history of the body and health humanities in general is that it is not only a metaphor, discourse, strategy or foil, but something material, something consumed by the body. It is this materiality and overall presence in everyday life that made tea a useful subject for what I call tribal talk. "Tribal talk" refers to the wide variety of ways of talking about groups and peoples that are considered to share a common origin, territory, climate, customs, and also bodies. The German term for "tribe" was "Stamm" but common were also terms "Nation" or simply "Deutsche" or "Teutsche," "Volk." In his German dictionary (1802) Johann Christoph Adelung defined "Stamm" as something that shared a common lineage (Adelung 1811, 278–279). Between 1700 and 1820 we see all these terms used as terms of distinction, as words of demarcation from others. Often, as we will see, the qualities of tea as remedy and beverage were described in tribal terms and thereby associated with the qualities of the bodies of these tribes. It is interesting that the term "Race" (in eighteenth-century German spelling) does not appear in the tribal talk on tea, although it was commonly used in philosophical and anthropological discourse after 1770. But was race, then, involved? Were the advocates, opponents, and consumers racial thinkers or, even more, were they racist? These are questions that are looming large in this chapter. "Race" and "tribe" were not accidental or external characteristics of tea but, as we will see, deeply embedded in its essence as a medicinal remedy. The change in these characteristics was also reflected in the change of medicine itself.

In scholarship, late-eighteenth century medicine, especially but not only in the German lands, has been identified as a field in crisis. The increasing awareness of a critical gap between theories of the body and the practices of healing amounted to a revival of the old Hippocratic medicine, which centered on practical cure, the art of healing (Broman 1996, 12, 140). At this juncture medical doctors turned to the public and the public turned to medicine. They gave rise to a strong public hygiene movement (*medicinische Polizey*) and they saw medical knowledge not only serving narrowly defined curative and therapeutic purposes but also applicable in such fields, as education, sports, and spa cures. Medical epistemes became public and, as in the case of May, an important part of political discourse (Lindemann 1996, 372; Loetz 1993, 74–78, 86). Recent scholarship has shown that the eighteenth-century crisis of medicine did not only mark a "return" of Hippocratic doctrines but also overlapped with the increasing import of medical epistemes outside of the European realm. Roberta Bivins has shown how for instance acupuncture and moxibustion—the fundamental ingredients of Ancient Chinese medicine—were received and critically discussed in eighteenth-century English medical literature (Bivins 2018, 339–347; Bivins 2007, 76–78). As Chakrabarti and especially Londa Schiebinger have shown, the transportation of medical epistemes was, however, not limited to these therapeutic practices. In fact, a much more successful transmission happened with *materia medica*, herbs and plants that reached the European realm from all directions of the globe, where the increasingly colonial occupation of the Dutch, Portuguese, Spaniards, British, and French had reached (Chakrabarti 2014, 20–35; Schiebinger 2017, 149–150). It is above all the *materia medica* that helped challenge and transform also those practices and ideas that medical doctors in the German lands were supporting. And tea was an important remedy. It serves as a case study in tracing the traveling of bodily epistemes into the Germanic world. In this chapter I will first take a look at the part of medical knowledge that May weaponized for Germanic identity: dietetics. I will then discuss how tea traveled to the German lands and was incorporated in dietetic therapeutics. Then follows a discussion of the introduction of (domestic) herbal teas as alternatives to the Chinese commodity. I will end the chapter by drawing some more general conclusions on the role of the bodies of the others in defining medical theories and practices in the German lands and the chemicalization of tea in the early nineteenth century.

As part of the Hippocratic Renaissance an old therapeutic practice, dietetics, gained in importance toward the end of the eighteenth century. In the classical medicine of the Hippocratic and Galenic tradition, which was canonized during the Middle Ages, health was understood as depending on the seven naturals, the six non-naturals, and the three contra-naturals. Although these categories overlapped at some important points, we can say that they roughly defined the scope of medical science. The seven naturals constituted physiology: elements (fire, air, water, earth), qualities (hot, cold, dry, moist), humors (blood, phlegm, yellow bile, black bile), members of the body, faculties, spirits (natural, vital, animal), and operations (hunger, digestion, retention, expulsion). The three contra-naturals defined pathology: Diseases, the causes of diseases, and the sequels of diseases. The six non-naturals made therapy and dietetics: Air, food and drink, motion and rest, sleep and waking, evacuations, and passions. The seven naturals were given by the constitution of the body; they were human nature and the basis of health. The pathological contra-naturals neither belonged to human nature nor contributed to its health but undermined it. Finally, the six non-naturals did not belong to human nature but still profoundly influenced its balance and health. In fact, the restoration of health was dependent on the balance of the non-natural with each other and the environment. Thus, dietetics emerged as a science and art of directing the contingencies of the human body and its environment. It is this dietetic theory that we find in May's *Medical Lent Sermons*. To make his argument May followed carefully the traditional breakdown of the six non-naturals but gave it a strong political reinterpretation: "Alles Gute ..., was der Staat und das Vaterland von der Würksamkeit seiner Bewohner erwarten kann, ist Resultat der Körper—und Geistes-Diätetik, Resultat einer gesunden körnigten Bevölkerung" ["All good ... that a state and fatherland can expect from the activities of its inhabitants, follows from the dietetics of the body and mind of a healthy and robust population"] (May 1793, 4). Dietetics was thereby a tool for an inhabitant (*Bewohner*) to make him- or herself useful for the state, a political tool of sorts. In the fifth lecture May came to warm drinks, as part of the second non-naturals, food, and drinks. Here, tea was one of the main targets of his critical comments.

There was a healing and healthy chemical compound in tea, argued May, but warmth destroyed its effect (May 1793, 210–214). In fact, tea was a striking example of how warm drinks made one's body droopy and weak, and therefore a person useless for the state (May 1793, 203–208). What we find here are rather typical complaints about civilizational degeneration of a people, similar to those the Swiss philosopher Jean-Jacques Rousseau had promoted in his early texts in the 1760s and then made widely popular in the German lands in the 1770s and 1780s by such educational reformers as Johann Bernhard Basedow, Joachim Heinrich Campe, and Christian Gotthilf Salzmann. But May's ethnocentric vitriol was something special. Tea, he accused, had entered the German lands because the cunning Dutch merchants managed to sell it as something exotic and appealing. "So ist es diesen erfinderischen Köpfen etwas sehr leichtes, den schlechtesten Thee in die Nachbarschaft wohlriechender Spezereien hinzulegen, und unsern leichtgläubigen Nasen etwas aufzubinden" ["It is therefore very easy for these inventive minds to place the worst tea next to flagrant spices and thereby lure our gullible noses"] (May 1793, 214). And yet, even for its original users, Chinese tea displayed negative symptoms, causing "Mademoisellen Chinesinnen bleiche Wangen, aufgedunsenes Fleisch, und hartes Fell" ["the Chinese lady her pale cheeks, puffed flesh, and hard skin"] (May 1793, 221). For May tea became a symptom of foreign invasion and un-Germanness.

How did tea become a target of accusations of degeneration and anti-Germanness? To answer this, let me now turn to the travel of tea from its origins in China into late eighteenth-century German teapots and *materia medica*. The first documented reports of tea stem from Southwestern China in the third century CE. From there it spread to the rest of China, Japan, Korea, and Southeast Asia as a remedy and stimulant. To Europeans it was introduced in the beginning of the seventeenth century by the Dutch who dominated the trade from the Far East (Rappaport 2017, 26–40). The consumption of tea as a luxury product spread quickly to other regions of Europe. In the German lands, tea consumption started around the mid-seventeenth century. The first treatises on tea in German were written in the 1680s. In the next twenty years, the number of studies increased rapidly. Tea became a topic of public discourse. By the end of the eighteenth century, dozens of books and pamphlets on tea, some in multiple editions, were published in the German lands. I have been able to locate a dozen treatises in German that explicitly discuss tea and dozens of books with substantive medical discussions on tea between 1682 and 1840. Not included were texts in Latin and journal articles and texts on tea trade only.

The question is not only the number of publications but also the locus of tea in the architecture of eighteenth-century medical knowledge. Two different genres should be discussed: dietetics and *materia medica.* As a medical remedy tea was made known by Dutch physicians, especially by Willem ten Rhijne and a host of others whose publications inundated the literary public in the 1680s and 1690s. One of the most influential texts was the work of the German medical doctor Engelbert Kaempfer who, after a lengthier stay in Persia, sailed in 1690 to Siam and then to Japan where he stayed two years and traveled around extensively with a Dutch delegation. Kaempfer interviewed people, medical doctors, officials and, above all, collected, described, and drew plants (Haberland 1996, 58–82). Kaempfer's work was important for botanical research (Gelder 2004, 211–225). Although he managed to publish some of the findings in his 1712 book *Amoenitatum exoticarum politico-physico-medicarum*, his most influential work, a detailed description of Japan, its political, social, and cultural life, remained unpublished until Hans Sloan, a famous British scientist and collector, acquired Kaempfer's manuscript from the author's estate and published it in English as *The History of Japan* in 1727. The book remained in several new editions and translations the standard presentation of Japan deeply well into the nineteenth century. The first German translations from Kaempfer's text were in the fourth volume of Jean-Baptiste du Halde's *Ausführliche Beschreibung des Chinesischen Reichs und der grossen Tartarey*, published in Rostock in 1749.

For us important is Kaempfer's description of Japanese and Chinese medicine. Along acupuncture and moxibustion, he pays special attention to tea. It was recognized as a stimulant and drink for socializing and travel, served in typical Japanese tearooms (Kaempfer 1749, 365). Kaempfer describes then in detail the symbolic and cultural meanings of tea, its botanical features, cultivation, and preparation (Kaempfer 1749, 467–478). Yet, he sees it as a remedy as well: "Ich glaube, daß in der ganzen Welt kein Gewächs ist, dessen man sich durch Aufgiessung des Wassers zum Getränk bedienet, das den Magen so wenig beschweret, so leicht paßiret, die niedergeschlagenen Lebensgeister erwecket, und das ganze Gemüth ermuntert, als der Japonische Thee" ["I believe that in the entire world there is no other plant that is served as a drink infused in water and that burdens the stomach so little, passes through so easily, awakes the depressed life spirits and enlivens the mind so well as the Japanese tea"] (Kaempfer 1749, 480). At the same time, Kaempfer warned, tea also had negative qualities. It did not go well with other remedies. The positive qualities, however, trumped the negative ones and Kaempfer saw in tea a remedy that "befördert ein langes Leben" ["promotes longevity"] (Kaempfer 1749, 482). In German medical literature of the mid-eighteenth century, Kaempfer's description of tea became one of the most cited. A long article on tea in the influential Zedler's lexicon praised tea as an exceptional stimulant and remedy for a large variety of diseases from gout to fevers (Zedler 1745, 537–538). In pharmacological literature—*materia medica*—tea was seen as an important remedy. For instance, Georg Heinrich Behr considered in his 1748 *Materia Medica* tea a wonderful universal medicine (Behr 1748, 112). Yet, some important authorities were more skeptical. A leading Dutch medical authority Hermann Boerhaave, for instance, did not list tea at all in his 1740 *De Materia Medica* and in his widely used and influential *Lectiones* considered tea even harmful because it thinned blood, as did all warm drinks. This hesitation was shared in dietetic literature. The leading authority of the Halle school of medicine, Friedrich Hofmann, saw in his early book on dietetics—the original Latin version was published in 1697—tea as a remedy that could be useful but not at all essential (Hoffmann 1744, 287–288). Samuel Schaarschmidt considered tea a good medicine when it was taken strong and for acute symptoms; as a permanent remedy it could only be taken mild—he considered it more a spice than a remedy—and then its remedial qualities remained weak (Schaarschmidt 1755, 619–624). This unenthusiastic interest was shared by Johann Gottlob Krüger who recommended tea mainly for older people (Krüger 1751, 302–305, 532–533). Another important authority in dietetics in the 1760s, Johann Friedrich Zückert recommended moderate use of tea and considered its remedial qualities weak (Zückert 1768, 97–98).

May inherited images of tea from both *materia medica* and dietetics. In both genres the initial euphoria, documented in Kaempfer and his contemporaries' texts, was cooling down.

In the latter half of the eighteenth century, tea was still an important, popular, widely known and recognized remedy, yet the faith in its remedial powers was eroding. At this juncture May felt comfortable shifting attention from tea's medical and botanic qualities to its civilizational and cultural meaning. Warm drinks—and tea was an important one—were harmful for the health and manners of the people. Tea originated from China and, May scoffed, "Es ist schon Unglück genug, daß die meisten Chineser dicke fette Schmeerbäuche haben. Nichts in der Welt begünstiget diesen unerträglichen Körperlast mehr, als warme Getränke" ["it is already unlucky enough that most Chinese have fat bellies. Nothing in the world causes more this unbearable bodily burden than warm drinks"] (May 1793, 208). For May, fatty bellies were not a result of the nature of the Chinese but rather their civilization. It was, however, the nature of the ancient Germans that made them the opposite of the Chinese: "Die einfachen Sitten, die Enthaltsamkeit der Urdeutschen kam gewiß größtentheils daher, weil sie die gekünstelten erhitzenden Getränke nicht kannten" ["The simple manners, the abstinence of the ancient Germans (*Urdeutschen*) resulted mainly from their ignorance of artificial hot drinks"] (May 1793, 246). The *Urdeutsche* were thereby superior because of the absence of the corrupting civilization, the simplicity of their nature in contrast to the complexity of the Chinese civilization. Tea expressed the pathologies of a civilization and civilizing.

Could we then say that May was a racist? Was he degrading the Chinese by degrading their favorite beverage and remedy? In the beginning of the eighteenth century, the term race had been introduced but rarely used. The famous French explorer and geographer Francois Bernier had in 1684 suggested the use of the external characteristics of the body to divide the peoples of the world into "Especes ou Races, qu'elle peut servir de juste fondement à une nouvelle division de la Terre" ["four or five human species or races whose differences are so notable that they can serve as a good foundation for a new division of the Earth"] (Bernier 1684, 148). By the mid-eighteenth century, the founders of natural history, Georges Buffon and Carl Linné, had adopted Bernier's concept though not always the terminology and classified the peoples of the world in groups that were determined by the climate. They considered the places, environments, weather conditions, and sun exposure the primary determinants of one's racial characteristics (Buffon 1752, 233–240; Linné 1773, 61–109). This climate theory of race dominated into the last quarter of the eighteenth century. Then important German and Dutch philosophers, medical doctors, and anthropologists started to cast doubts on the impact of climate. In 1775, Immanuel Kant argued—in a clear shift away from climate theory—that "Luft, Sonne und Nahrung können einen thierischen Körper in seinem Wachsthume modificiren, aber diese Veränderung nicht zugleich mit einer zeugenden Kraft versehen, die vermögend wäre, sich selbst auch ohne diese Ursache wieder hervorzubringen" ["air, sun, and nutrition can modify the growth of an animal body but this growth does not provide the power of procreation that would be capable of reproducing the body without the intervention of the original cause of growth"] (Kant 1912, 435). In the following fifteen years, German philosophers and anthropologists engaged the topic with increasing intensity. Dozens of articles and books were written on race or, as some authors called human variations and often following Kant's line of thinking. This was clearly the case with Friedrich Blumenbach, Peter Camper, and Samuel Sömmering, to name some of the most important and consequential racial theorists of the time. Much of this racial speculation was explorative, informed, and inspired by the rapidly expanding knowledge of the others, peoples outside of the European realm. There was a clear sense that the divisions were rather arbitrary and not absolutely grounded in real existing immutable facts. But the shift from climate theory to the hereditary theory of race was real.

And this reality started to gain a new kind of urgency in the 1780s. New explorations, such as James Cook's voyages to the Pacific, fed new information to the audience. For the German audience the explorations of James Cook became familiar through the detailed and philosophically grounded depictions of Georg Forster, a German-British explorer and ethnographer, who had accompanied with his father Cook's second exploration to the Pacific. The German version of Forster's book, *Reise um die Welt*, came out in two volumes 1778 and 1780. In 1786 Forster made an intervention in the race discussion. Unlike most of his fellow authors, Forster had met, discussed, and listened to the others that so many wanted to classify as races. Everything in living beings, argued Forster, is about nuances and although "eine Hauptform zu herrschen scheine, die in der reichsten Verschiedenheit wechselt" ["one main form seems to dominate, this form changes in multiple ways"] (Forster 1969, 85). Race was therefore less useful as a scientific category and virtually impossible to prove (Forster 1969, 88). In fact, its only utility was political. It helped justify slavery, claimed Forster, by depicting the enslaved as lower humans or even as separate species (Forster 1969, 96–101). A year earlier Johann Gottfried Herder had also raised doubts about the common use of the concept of race. "So haben einige z.B. vier oder fünf Abteilungen desselben, die ursprünglich nach Gegenden oder gar nach Farben gemacht waren, Racen zu nennen gewagt; ich sehe keine Ursache dieser Benennung" ["Some have had the audacity of calling races the four or five of its [human species] categories which originate from the regions or colors. I see no reason for this categorization"] (Herder 2002, 231). Instead of race the concept of people or folk was much more useful: "Denn jedes Volk ist Volk; es hat seine National-Bildung, wie seine Sprache; zwar hat der Himmelstrich über alle bald ein Gepräge, bald nur einen lindern Schleier gebreitet, der aber das ursprüngliche Stammgebilde der Nation nicht zerstöret" ["Because a people are a people; they have their national culture, their language. Although the sky has given one region a strong character and another only a thin veneer, the original tribal image (*Stammgebilde*) of a nation cannot be destroyed"] (Herder 2002, 231). And "folk" was also more useful in the new political situation that emerged as a result of the French Revolution. In 1792, the French Revolutionary wars had spread to German soil and German intellectuals were looking for concepts to rally the people in the German lands against the French. The political urgency was clearly on the side of "folk" and against "race." We see that in May's plea.

But there was another political urgency that had emerged before the French Revolution and was accentuated by its success. The anti-slavery movement took a radical step in 1787 with the founding of the Society for Effecting the Abolition of the Slave Trade in London. Forster's intervention was motivated by the discussions that led to this. Even more, it motivated another professor from the Hanoverian circle, Christoph Meiners who—a few years before May crafted his tirade against the French *Volksseuche*—drastically changed the understanding of what constituted the identity of a human group. Meiners, who in his earlier work from 1785, had argued that all humans are of the same species and thereby united in their origin, five years later started a campaign against this very principle and claimed that the equality of all humans was impossible and against all empirical evidence available (Meiners 1785, 17; Meiners 1790a, 387–388). Meiners's contribution to the rise and molding of a genuine racial theory is significant. Not only did he shift the emphasis from the climate and other external factors to such internal traits as lineage (*Abstammung*) and blood (*Blut*) but he also clearly argued for a racial hierarchy, for supremacy, "durch seinen Geist mehr als durch seinen Körper siegenden und beherrschenden Europäer zu beweisen, daß wenn auch die Neger, die Americaner, und andere diesen ähnliche Völker in aller Rücksicht weit unter ihm seyen" ["of the Europeans who win and dominate through their minds rather than their bodies" over the "Negros, Americans, and other similar people which in all respect are far below them"] (Meiners 1790a, 400–401). In the early 1790s his voice reached a feverish pitch in pointing out the inferiority not only of Blacks but also of East Asians and Native Americans (Meiners 1790b, 625–628; Meiners 1790c, 292).

Clearly May was not an advocate of the virulent racism of Meiners. His critique of the Chinese civilization was not that different from his remarks of the Dutch or French. Yet the (re)discovery of (domestic) herbal teas sheds the dispute in a different light. At the same time the medical doctors started to warn about the dangers of tea for the body and especially for the bodies of Germans, an alternative started to evolve: the replacement of Chinese tea with herbal teas. In fact, herbal teas appeared in German writings soon after the first promotions of Chinese tea were published. Friedrich Hoffmann, the Professor of Medicine at the newly founded University Halle and a leading medical authority in the German lands around 1700, advocated for herbal teas as a substitute for the Chinese original tea plant (Hoffmann 1705). Johann Heinrich Cohausen's *Neothea* (1716), a passionate promotion of herbal teas, went through three editions and a translation into Dutch. The dominance of Chinese tea had to be challenged with Dutch and German herbs, claimed Cohausen (Cohausen 1716, 4). In the seventeenth century, pharmacopeia had turned to foreign remedies so that "Es haben nunmehr die Englische Panace, der Italianische Milchzucker, der Venetianische Theriac, der Spanische Schnup-Toback, der Türckische Coffee, ihren Ruhm durch Teutschland sattsam verbreitet, fürnehmlich aber hat die Sinesische Thee unter den Erd—Gewächsen gleich dem Mond unter dem Gestirn, sich in Europa herfür gehoben" ["now there is the English cureall (*Panace*), Italian milk sugar, Venetian theriac, Spanish snuff, Turkish coffee which is well-known all over Germany. Above all it is the Chinese tea of all plants on the Earth, like the Moon among the stars, that has distinguished itself in Europe"] (Cohausen 1716, 2). Cohausen saw the remedies primarily as commodities that carried the label of their place of origin. These labels clearly indicated competition, competition in trade and influence that needed to be challenged with domestic herbs and plants, "welche in vielen Kranckheiten eben das, was die Thee, ja wohl noch mit besseren Nachdruck verrichten" ["which in many diseases do the same as tea and even with better results"] (Cohausen 1716, 6). Although Cohausen had a high respect for Chinese expertise in herbs, the challenge was clear (Cohausen 1716, 9). What then were the potential German alternatives for Chinese tea? Cohausen mentions several: rosemary, lavender, veronica, salvia, common hedge nettle, marjoram, and common agrimony (Cohausen 1716, 14). These herbs were, however, not only alternative and random substitutes but something that, for Cohausen, were "Einheimisch unserer Deutschen Natur mehr anständiges, reinigendes" ["domestic, more becoming and purifying for our German nature"] than the foreign ones (Cohausen 1716, 417). In the humoral medicine the nosology of diseases was not based on universal characteristics only but was always defined by the traits of the individual, by the constitution of the body, status, gender, location (climate) of the patient, and other idiosyncratic circumstances. Here, the location defined for Cohausen the "German nature" that required German remedies, as the climate theory of race would argue. We do not find any racial or tribal hierarchy in Cohausen's characterization. German bodies were not better or worse than the Chinese; they were only different.

After Cohausen's intervention, the idea of a domestic herbal tea went to hibernation. In the extensive literature on tea between 1750 and 1790, herbal tea does not get much attention. This changed after the French Revolution. A new physiological concept of the body moving beyond the traditional humoral medicine and its environmental conception of the body, launched by the Scottish medical doctor John Brown, was gaining traction in Germany. The body and its diseases, argued Brown and his German followers, were determined by two factors, irritability and sensitivity, and they were indigenous to the body and especially to its nervous system (Broman 1996, 132–135). What Cohausen had called "our nature" (*unsere Natur*) in 1716 (Cohausen 1716, 417) meant in the 1790s something that was not determined by the environment but indigenous and idiosyncratic to Germans' state of mind and neural system. The Romantics, among others, became keen believers in Brown and Brunonianism (Neubauer 1967, 367–382; Tsouyopoulos 1982). In the following decade the German tea authors dedicated more and more attention to the German substitutes for Chinese tea. Georg Piepenbring, for instance, saw in raspberry the best alternative because it was very common, had pleasant taste, and could grow anywhere (Piepenbring 1798, 55–58). Johann Rumpf was looking for a German gold mine with over seventeen domestic herbal substitutes for tea (Rumpf 1799, 56–60). In general, Rumpf was skeptical about the health benefits of Chinese tea because it enhanced the natural irritability and thereby set the body "in zu grosse Thätigkeit" ["in too great activity"] (Rumpf 1799, 53). Friedrich Langstedt agreed and suggested that "da aber die menschlichen Naturen ebenso verschieden als die Menschen selbst sind, so müssen ebenfalls die Wirkungen dieses Aufgusses verschieden seyn" ["because the human natures are as different as the humans themselves, so must be the effects of this [tea] infusion"] (Langstedt 1800, 37). The German body was simply different from the Chinese—and all the other ethnic bodies—and it needed its own domestic remedy, its own domestic tea: "So kann es nützlich seyn, alles mögliche Licht in dieser Hinsicht von dem Charakter eines Volks zu leiten, welches den Theeaufguß auf einander folgende Menschengeschlechter hindurch gebraucht hat" ["It can be therefore useful to derive all the possible understanding (*Licht*) from the character of a people that has used the tea infusion over many generations"] (Langstedt 1800, 66).

How should we understand May's and other medical authors' tribal talk on German and Chinese bodies in the 1790s? Clearly, they went beyond what was the traditional ethnic content of dietetic literature. They not only drew on the origins of tea in China but also associated tea with what they considered typical Chinese physiognomy and contrasted this with that of the Germans. And then they resorted to a peculiar German tea adjusted and tailormade to the German body. Thereby tea was not anymore, as an herbal tea, a global commodity as it had been for almost two hundred years but the very expression of the locality and domesticity of its consumer. Yet the main target of May's book was not China. It was France and the French Revolution. It was, however, not the French but the Dutch and the English who had specialized and made their mark as importers of tea. Tea, and especially traditional Chinese tea, functioned as a larger marker of civilization, a feature that connected all those peoples who had been corrupted and degenerated by the touch of civilization. Tea marked the body that was the opposite of the natural and strong German body. The bodies of others served and were weaponized for German identity formation but by doing so the German authors did not necessarily entertain fantasies of colonial conquests, as Susanne Zantop has argued (Zantop 1997, 43–65). For them, French could be as civilized or corrupted as Chinese. None of Meiners's racial and racist tirades found their ways to the minds and writings of German tea advocates. But clearly this was only waiting to happen. Yet it did not happen. In the first three decades of the nineteenth century, a new understanding of tea and its physiological impact emerged. And this understanding did not leave much space for tribal imagination.

The tribalization of tea, although long in the making, accelerated with the rising nationalistic rhetoric after the French Revolution. It changed the dietetic discourse that for so long had placed tea among other exotic remedies, such as coffee, cocoa, and tobacco. The dietetic discourse itself was interrupted when a series of new chemical discoveries were made in the 1820s. In 1820 Friedlieb Ferdinand Runge, a medical student from Berlin, published his discovery of a new compound that he named "Kaffebase" ["coffee base"]. By 1835 it was identified as an alkaloid making a major contribution to the emerging field of organic chemistry (Runge 1820, 147; Hudson 1992, 104–105). Runge had received the beans from Johann Wolfgang von Goethe, the preeminent German poet and author from Weimar, and set to extract with his new method the essence of coffee. Seven years later a French chemist, Alphone Oudry, managed to do the same with tea and extracted a compound that he called "Théine" ["thein"], a base that incorporated the essence of tea (Oudry 1827, 447–449). In 1838 a German chemist, Carl Jobst, could show that thein was identical with caffeine thereby setting the understanding of these stimulating beverages on a new chemical footing (Jobst 1838, 63–66). The great German chemist, Justus Liebig, made clear in his influential textbook, *Handbuch der organischen Chemie mit Rücksicht auf Pharmacie* (1843), that the essence of tea was not determined by soil and climate or any basic elements but by a host of compounds whose complicated structures a chemist had been able to decipher. An analysis of Chinese tea revealed "sulfuric acid, phosphoric acid, chloride, lime, potash, iron, silica" ["Schwefelsäure, Phosphorsäure, Chlor, Kalk, Kali, Eisen und Kieselerde"] (Liebig 1843, 643). The change of science happened with the shift in tea trade. In 1838 the first batch of Indian tea was shipped from Assam to London thereby launching the end of the Chinese monopoly in global tea trade. A new kind of chemistry and a new kind of capitalism started to transform tea from a dietetic remedy and remedial beverage into a "necessary luxury" and status symbol in England and elsewhere in Europe. At the same time the social and anthropological meaning of tea changed. In the nineteenth century, the differences between humans were established on the surfaces of the bodies, their colors, their gestalt, the shape of their body and especially in their civilizational levels. The humors and climates had been replaced by skins and skulls.

NOTE

1. All translations are mine, unless otherwise noted.

WORKS CITED

Adelung, Johann Christoph. 1811. *Grammatisch-kritisches Wörterbuch der Hochdeutschen Mundart: mit beständiger Vergleichung der übrigen Mundarten, besonders aber der Oberdeutschen*. Vol. 4. Wien: Bauer.

Behr, Georg Heinrich. 1748. *Zwey Bücher von der Materia Medica; oder, Vollständige Beschreibung aller und jeder Artzeney-Mittel: sampt beygefügter wohl-eingerichteter und höchst-nutzbarer Therapie*. Vol. 2. Strassburg: Johannes Beck.

Bernier, François. 1684. “Nouvelle division de la Terre, par les differenes Especes ou Races d’hommes qui l’habitant, envooyée par un fameux Voyager: À peu pré en ces terms.” *Journal des Sçavans*.

Bivins, Roberta. 2007. *Alternative Medicine: A History*. Oxford: Oxford University Press.

Bivins, Roberta. 2018. “Imagining Acupuncture: Images of the Early Westernization of Asian Medical Expertise.” In *Imagining Chinese Medicine*, edited by Vivienne Lo, Penelope Barrett, David Dear, Lu Di, Lois Reynolds, Dolly Yang, 339–347. Leiden: Brill.

Broman, Thomas S. 1996. *The Transformation of German Academic Medicine 1750–1820*. New York: Cambridge University Press.

Buffon, Georges Louis Le Clerc de. 1752. *Allgemeine Historie der Natur: nach allen ihren besondern Theilen abgehandelt; nebst einer Beschreibung der Naturalienkammer Sr. Maj. des Königs von Frankreich*. Mit einer Vorrede von Herrn Doctor Albert von Haller. Zweyter Theil. Hamburg/ Leipzig: Georg Christian Grund und Adam Heinrich Holle.

Chakrabarti, Pratik. 2014. *Medicine and Empire, 1600–1960*. New York: Palgrave MacMillan.

Cohausen, Joan Henrich. 1716. *Neothea: Oder Neu-angerichtete Medicinische Thee-Tafel Auff welcher Fürtreffliche so einfältig als künstlich zusammen gesetzte, theils aus einheimisch, theils ausländischen Kräutern und Gewächsen bestehende Kräuter-Thee. Denen Liebhabern der Gesundheit und landen Lebens auffgetragen und praesentiret werden*. Osnabrück: Michael Andreas Fuhrmann.

Forster, Georg. 1969. “Noch etwas über die Menschenraßen.” In *Werke in vier Bänden*, edited by Gerhard Steiner. 71–101. Vol. 2. *Kleine Schriften zur Naturgeschichte, Länder- und Völkerkunde: Ansichten von Niederrhein*. Frankfurt am Main: Insel.

Gelder, Roelof van. 2004 “Nec semper feriet quodcumque minabitur arcus – Engelbert Kaempfer as a Scientist in the Service of the Dutch East India Company.” In *Engelbert Kaempfer (1651–1716). Ein Gelehrtenleben zwischen Tradition und Innovation*, edited by Detlef Haberland, 211–225. Wiesbaden: Harrassowitz Verlag.

George, Alys X. 2020. *The Naked Truth: Viennese Modernism and the Body*. Chicago: The University of Chicago Press.

Haberland, Detlef. 1996. *Engelbert Kaempfer, 1651–1716. A Biography*. London: The British Library.

Herder, Johann Gottfried. 2002. *Werke*. Vol. III/1. *Ideen zur Philosophie der Geschichte der Menschheit*. Munich: Carl Hanser Verlag.

Hoffmann, Friedrich (Christoph Wilhelm Sattler). 1705. *Exercitatio physico-medica, de infusi veronicae efficacia praeferenda herba thee*. Halle: C.A. Zeitler.

Hoffmann, Friedrich. 1744. *Kurzgefaßte Diätetic oder hinlänglicher Unterricht, wie ein Mensch durch ordentliche Lebensart, auch wenige und wohlfeile Mittel sich lange Zeit gesund und beim Leben erhalten könne*. Jena: Gollner.

Hudson, John. 1992. *The History of Chemistry*. Houndmills: MacMillan.

Jobst, Carl. 1838. “Thein identisch mit Caffein.” *Annalen der Chemie* 25: 63–66.

Kaempfer, Engelbrecht. 1749. "Weiland berühmten Medici zu Lemgow, Beschreibung des Japonischen Reiches, nah seinem natürlichen, bürgerlichen und kirchlichen Zustande: Als eine Zugabe zur ausführlichen Beschreibung des Chinesischen Reiches." In Johann Baptista du Halde. *Ausführliche Beschreibung des Chinesischen Reichs und der grossen Tartarey*. Vierter und letzter Theil. Nebst Engelbrecht Kämpfers Beschreibung des Japonischen Reichs und einem Register über alle vier Theile. 1–537. Rostock: Koppe.
Kant, Immanuel. 1912. "Von den verschiedenen Racen der Menschen." In *Werke*. Vol. 2. *Vorkritische Schriften II, 1757–1777*, 427–443. Berlin: Georg Reimer.
Krüger, Johann Gottlob. 1751. *Diät oder Lebensordnung*. Halle im Magdeburgischen: Hemmerde.
Langstedt, Friedrich Ludwig. 1800. *Thee, Kaffee und Zucker in historischer, chemischer, diätetischer, ökonomischer und botanischer Hinsicht erwogen*. Nürnberg: Raspesche Buchhandlung.
Liebig, Justus. 1843. *Handbuch der Organischen Chemie: Mit Rücksicht auf Pharmacie*. Heidelberg: C.F. Winter.
Lindemann, Mary. 1996. *Health & Healing in Eighteenth-Century Germany*. Baltimore: Johns Hopkins University Press.
Linné, Carl von. 1773. *Vollständiges Natursystem: nach der zwölften lateinischen Ausgabe, und nach Anleitung des holländischen Houttuynischen Werks*. Vol. 1. Nürnberg: Gabriel Nicolaus Raspe.
Loetz, Franzisca. 1993. *Vom Kranken zum Patienten: "Medikalisierung" und medizinische Vergesellschaftung am Beispiel Badens 1750–1850*. Stuttgart: Franz Steiner.
Lorenz, Maren. 2000. *Leibhaftige Vergangenheit: Einführung in die Körpergeschichte*. Berlin: Edition Diskord.
May, Franz Anton. 1793. *Medicinische Fastenpredigten oder Vorlesungen über Körper und Seelen-Diätetik, zur Verbesserung der Gesundheit und Sitten*. Vol. 1. Mannheim: Schwan und Götz.
Meiners, Christoph. 1785. *Grundriss der Geschichte der Menschheit*. Lemgo: Meyer.
Meiners, Christoph. 1790a. "Ueber die Natur des Afrikanischen Neger, und die dabey abhangende Befreyung, oder Einschränkung der Schwarzen." *Göttingisches historisches Magazin* 6: 385–456.
Meiners, Christoph. 1790b. "Von den Varietäten und Abarten der Neger." *Göttingisches historisches Magazin* 6: 625–645.
Meiners, Christoph. 1790c. "Ueber die Natur der Völker im südlichen Asien, auf dem Ostindischen und Südsee-Inseln und in den Südländern." *Göttingisches historisches Magazin* 7: 258–310.
Neubauer, John. 1967. "Dr. John Brown (1735–1788) and Early German Romanticism." *Journal of the History of Ideas* 28, no. 3: 367–382.
North, Michael. 2008. "Material Delight and the Joy of Living." In *Cultural Consumption in the Age of Enlightenment in Germany*. Aldershot: Ashgate.
Ogilvie, Sheilagh. 2015. "Revolution des Fleißes: Leben und Wirtschaften im ländlichen Württemberg von 1650 bis 1800." In *Revolution des Fleißes, Revolution des Konsums? Leben und Wirtschaften im ländlichen Württemberg von 1650 bis 1800*, edited by Sigrid Hirbodian, Sheilagh Ogilvie and R. Johanna Regnath, 173–193. Ostfildern: Jan Thorbecke Verlag.
Oudry, Alphonse. 1827. "Note sur la *Théine*." *Nouvelle bibliothèque médicale* 1: 447–449.
Piepenbring, Georg Heinrich. 1798. *Teutscher Caffee und Thee, oder die zwey vorzüglichsten Mittel den ausländischen Caffee und Thee möglichst zu ersetzen*. Hannover: Ritschersche Buchhandlung.
Porter, Roy. 1991. "History of the Body." In *New Perspectives on Historical Writing*, edited by Peter Burke, 206–232. University Park: The Pennsylvania State University Press.
Rappaport, Erika. 2017. *A Thirst for Empire: How Tea Shaped the Modern World*. Princeton: Princeton University Press.
Rumpf, Johann Daniel Friedrich. 1799. *Deutschlands Goldgrube, oder durch welche inländischen Erzeugnisse kann der fremde Kaffee, Thee und Zucker möglichst ersetzt werden? Und was ist insbesondere von der Zuckerbereitung aus Runkelrüben und Ahornbäumen zu erwarten*. Berlin: Oehmigke.

Runge, Friedlieb Ferdinand. 1820. *Neueste phytochemische Entdeckungen zur Begründung einer wissenschaftlichen Phytochemie*. Berlin: Reimer.
Schaarschmidt, Samuel. 1755. *Diaetetik oder Lehre von der Lebensordnung für Gesunde und Kranke zur Erhaltung und Wiederherstellung der Gesundheit*. Berlin: Schützen.
Schiebinger, Londa L. 2017. *Secret Cures of Slaves: People, Plants, and Medicine in the Eighteenth-Century Atlantic World*. Stanford: Stanford University Press.
Tsouyopoulos, Nelly. 1982. *Andreas Röschlaub und die romantische Medizin: die philosophischen Grundlagen der modernen Medizin*. Stuttgart: G. Fischer.
Wassenberg, Karl. 1991. *Tee in Ostfriesland: Vom religiösen Wundertrank zum profanen Volksgetränk*. Bielefeld: Schuster.
Zantop, Susanne. 1997. *Colonial Fantasies: Conquest, Family, and Nation in Precolonial Germany, 1770–1870*. Durham: Duke University Press.
Zedler, Johann Heinrich. 1745. *Grosses vollständiges Universal-Lexicon Aller Wissenschafften und Künste*. Vol. 43. Halle: Zedler.
Zückert, Johann Friedrich. 1768. *Systematische Beschreibung aller Gesundbrunnen und Bäder Deutschlands*. Berlin: Rüdiger.

PART V

Gender

CHAPTER SIXTEEN

Suspicious Body Parts and Endangered Femininity: Western Medical Knowledge about Female Genitalia and Practices of Genital Cutting in the Early Modern Age

MARIACARLA GADEBUSCH BONDIO

A VERY SMALL PART OF THE PROBLEM?

In the debates about the one-sex/two-sex theories that were ignited around 2003, the external female genitals and the practices of clitoridectomy or nymphotomy play a rather minor role.[1] What explains this absence in the burgeoning field of observation, reflection, and intervention in early modern medicine, especially in anatomy and gynaecology? One explanation might lie in Thomas Laqueur's remarks on the clitoris. In defending his one-sex model, Laqueur defined the clitoris as "a very small part of the problem, if a problem at all, when the entire female genitalia were construed as a version of the male's" (in Park 1997, 187; Laqueur 1989, 113). Years earlier, in his reflections on the history of clitoridectomy, Laqueur concluded that "it is clear that clitorectomy was rejected in the West until the nineteenth century" (Laqueur 1989, 114). Another reason for the neglect of the pudenda may have been its seemingly marginal importance for the "new anatomy of sexual difference" that some critics of Laqueur's theory have convincingly advocated for (Stolberg 2003, 289). Early modern medical practitioners' approaches to the female genitalia are marked by the search for criteria that would allow them to differentiate between the sexes, especially in ambiguous cases. But these efforts are characterized by terminological and normative uncertainty and are very heterogeneous. As will be shown in what follows, the morphology and anatomy of the *pudenda*, as metamorphosing regions of the body, have proven stubbornly resistant to standardization. It is above all the clitoris in its disconcerting ambiguity that eludes easy determination of the binary gender order and—according to the thesis advanced here—is therefore of little help to historians seeking to shore up their two-sex theory.[2]

This article attempts to counteract this neglect and explores the following questions: What difficulties were associated with the exploration of these regions of the female body that were typically marked as shameful—i.e. both on living and deceased bodies—and how were they reflected upon? How did medical authors receive information about ritual clitoridectomy, genital cutting,[3] and infibulation and how did they relate these to supposedly preventive and therapeutic surgical procedures? These questions have prompted and guided the identification, analysis, and comparison of the sources presented here. Around the middle of the sixteenth century, physicians became increasingly interested in the physiological anatomy and morphology of women's external genitalia. Anatomical descriptions of the *pudenda* started to accumulate, becoming more detailed and, in some respects, more controversial. As early as 1997, in a seminal essay on the rediscovery of the clitoris in the early modern period, Katharine Park pointed out that anatomical descriptions of female genitalia are closely intertwined with descriptions of phenomena of ambiguous sexual attribution (hermaphroditism and tribadism) and with accounts of clitoridectomy (Park 1997, 183). The fact that some French physicians advocated clitoridectomy as a therapy for clitoral hypertrophy constitutes for Park "a striking sign" of the advancing sexual dimorphism in the medical discourse on biological sex (Park 1997, 183).[4]

Against this background, the positions of a group of physicians, especially anatomists and surgeons, deserve to be re-examined. The selection of authors and text passages emerges from internal cross-references: these authors entered into an ideational dialogue based on mutual reception because their opinions about the female genitalia did not always coincide. They offer a representative, if not exhaustive, picture of the state of knowledge about women's genitalia and the role they played in the search for criteria for the binary distinction between the sexes.

PUDENDA AND THE LIMITS OF MEDICAL INSPECTION

In the early modern period, women's pudenda were not only an unfamiliar and shameful domain for male physicians. As blood-rich, arousable, and swelling body parts, they differ substantially when inspected and observed on a living body as opposed to a corpse.[5] We learn, for example, from the Basel municipal physician Felix Platter[6] (1536–1614) how difficult it was for doctors to carefully observe, or even examine, these intimate regions of the female body. He reports on a female patient from a good family (*ex bona familiae femina*) with a growth "in the manner of a goose neck" in the genital area (*excrescentia instar colli anserini, in pudendo feminae*). At the upper part of the cleft of the pubis, "above the urethral orifice where the clitoris protrudes" (*supra meatum urinarium, ubi clithoris eminet*), an outgrowth in the "girth and length of a goose neck" had developed (*excrescentia quaedam enata, adeo excrevit, ut collum anserinum amplitudine et longitudine*). Whether this was an enlargement of the clitoris itself or of some other fleshy outgrowth, Platter could not distinguish, as the patient did not want to show him the problem area (*cum nollet hoc mihi ostendere*). She only allowed him to touch the surrounding region, which remained well covered. By palpating it, the doctor could see how to remove the excess flesh. As the patient did not allow excision, the surgeon tried to tie off the flesh formation with a thread soaked in arsenic. Due to great pain and a strong inflammatory reaction, the thread was removed immediately. The patient did not allow any further treatment. Because of the damage inflicted, but also for reasons of age—as Platter concludes his case report—the patient finally died, having meanwhile become a widow, at the age of about fifty.

This terse report, even though it does not reveal, for example, how long the patient lived with her problem after the treatment, provides important information about the discomfort of the respectable woman in showing the most intimate parts of her body to a doctor. She resolutely determines that the doctor may not see but only palpate the covered parts. She refuses excision, but undergoes the alternative and exceedingly painful procedure performed by the surgeon. The question that Platter could not answer during palpation, i.e. whether it was a clitoral hyperthrophy or a tumour that had grown at this site, remained unanswered even after the patient's death.

Although investigation and description of the morphology, size, and structure of the female genitalia were evidently carried out by some anatomists around 1550, it was a lengthy process, particularly among the living, for at least *three reasons*. *First and foremost*, for reasons of morality, inspection of the living remained a difficult undertaking for physicians. In the recorded case, Felix Platter did not perform a dissection after the patient's death. The reasons for this are not given. *Second*, the terminology for the pudenda was confusing because ancient and medical literature from late antiquity had several names for the clitoris and the labia.[7] This led to considerable misunderstandings when describing the female genitalia and the surgical interventions affecting them.[8] This made it difficult to transmit and receive previous observations and to study the area systematically. *Third*, for physiological-morphological reasons: though autoptic experience could be acquired from the corpse, it was soon found that these blood-rich and arousable body parts differed in a corpse and in a living woman. The question of whether a mere glance, palpation, or dissection of a corpse was necessary for the description and identification of a woman's genitals was discussed in differing ways. The physician and great collector of *observationes*, Johann Schenck von Grafenberg (1530–98),[9] stated that in cadaveric autopsy the clitoris was a small structure that was difficult to inspect.[10] It was different on the living body: here—according to Schenck—the "*muliebris virga*" was full of vital warmth and blood. Schenck specifies at this point that even where there was no abnormality (*etiam extra monstrosam constitutionem*) he could easily locate and identify this "female penis." The anatomists who were engaged in describing the pudenda around 1550 would first have to face these challenges in order to express and agree on the normal as well as divergent anatomy and function of the female genitalia.

THE "FEMALE PENIS" IN ANATOMICAL DESCRIPTIONS AND TRAVELOGUES

In medical historical research literature on early modern theories of the anatomy of the female genitalia and on the ritual and surgical practices of their modification, circumcision, and mutilation, the anatomist Andreas Vesal (1514–64) plays a peripheral role.[11] This despite the fact that he wrestled with this issue and gradually developed his own standpoint, partly through confrontation with other doctrines, as a comparison of the various editions of his anatomical work demonstrates. In the first edition of *De humani corporis fabrica libri septem* (1543), Vesal already devotes himself to these regions of the female corpse, but without mentioning the clitoris. Between the two editions of the treatise in 1543 and 1555, as well as the planned third edition,[12] there are considerable differences.[13] On closer comparative analysis of the passages, it is noticeable that there is a lack of consistency in the description of the individual structures: in one passage, for example, Vesal uses the Greek νύμφη (*nympha*) to designate two different structures. These are the *cuticulares carunculae*, i.e. the *labia minora*,[14] which vary individually in their dimensions, and the *tubercula*, i.e. the "remains of the hymen."[15] In the second edition (1555), he uses "myrtle berry," "hypoderis" (sic!), and "clitoris"[16] as further synonyms in addition to νύμφη. Taking his cue from ancient and late antique sources, Vesal describes the hypertrophy of the labia (*carunculae*)[17] and remarks that the enlargement was not only ugly and shameful for the woman, but was also considered a sign of shamelessness (*impudicitia*). The constant rubbing of the enlarged part against the clothing resulted in heightened libido. In Egypt—according to Vesal, who here refers to Aëtios of Amida[18]—it was the custom to excise the *carunculae* to avert this danger. In the second half of the 1550s, Vesal culled information from travelogues reporting practices of genital cutting in Ethiopia. In the handwritten commentary for the planned third edition[19] of *De humani corporis fabrica libri septem* as well as in *Anatomicarum Gabrielis Fallopii Observationum Examen*, there is evidence of his engagement with these sources. In the handwritten copy, after the remarks on excision practices among the Egyptians, Vesal added a note at the bottom of the page with reference to his own time[20]: among the "Scevani"[21] in Ethiopia, called by contemporaries "subjects of Presbyter John," i.e. the king of the Abyssinians, the practice of cutting newborn boys' and girls' genitalia was widespread "to this day." In boys the foreskin would be removed; in girls "these fleshy elevations" (*carnei isti processus*[22]). Vesal remarks that this particular custom was religious, although the other customs of these peoples were the same as the Christian ones. The kingdom of the legendary priest-king John, which Vesal equates with the region of the "Scevani" and Ethiopia,[23] is mentioned in various contemporary travelogues as a region in which, or in the vicinity of which, genital cutting was practiced.[24] This clarificatory addition by Vesal demonstrates how attentive he was to contemporary descriptions from travelers to north-east Africa. In the circulating travelogues, the information on circumcision or cutting practices was inconsistent, both in terms of ethnic groups and the anatomical structures of the women affected.[25] The painstaking search, documentation, and supplementation process that permeates Vesal's last anatomical writing attest to the anatomist's interest. Vesal's vigilant search for information may have been fueled by discussions in his field of anatomy. In 1559 and 1561, two anatomical treatises appeared in which a colleague of Vesal's, Realdo Colombo (*c.* 1516–59), and Vesal's student, Gabriele Falloppio (1523–62), vied with each other for primacy in describing the physiological anatomy of the *pudenda*—especially the seat of erotic arousal in women. Debates over correct designations, culminating in the creation of neologisms, and struggles over status of "first discoverer"[26] are closely connected in their writings.

Realdo Colombo, who correctly described the seat of female pleasure (*sedes delectationis mulierum*), speaks of the "*processus uteri*" when he talks of the clitoris. He also proposes *amor veneris* or *dulcedo* as names for this part of the body, which he claims to have "discovered," to this end deliberately avoiding the use of terms that have existed since antiquity.[27] He adopts the view of Galen of Pergamon, who had attributed a protective function to the smaller and larger "Nymphae."[28] Gabriele Falloppio's treatise appeared in 1561, only two years after Colombo's publication. Falloppio takes issue with the Greek and Arabic traditions. He also considers himself the first of his time to have rediscovered the clitoris. He nevertheless admits other contemporary anatomists may plausibly have addressed these questions without his own knowledge or that of the audience at his lectures. The basis of Falloppio's observations, as he himself points out, are previous dissections of these small and hidden structures (*Totum hoc pudendum, quia parvum est, et latitat*).[29] Falloppio sets out to thoroughly disclose the region neglected by anatomists: in the female pubis there would be a certain structure which Avicenna referred to as *virga* or *albathara*, Abulcasis as *tentigo*, and the Greeks as κλητορίς.[30] Falloppio characterises this structure in its blood-rich substance as analogous to the male member.[31] He does not comment further on the function of this female member. He confines himself to mentioning Albucasis' remarks on the consequences of clitoral hypertrophy, in which reference is made to the resulting tribadism (*quae* [*tentigo*] *solet aliquando ad tantum incrementum pervenire, ut mulieres hanc habentes coeant cum alijs, veluti si viri essent*).[32] Falloppio, like Colombo, makes no mention whatsoever of practices of genital cutting in other cultures.

Vesal's *Anatomicarum Gabrielis Fallopii Observationum Examen* appeared in 1564, only three years after Falloppio's anatomical work was printed and two years after his death.[33] The topic of the female genitalia continued to spark controversy. Even the question of their visibility or concealment was controversial. Vesal had declared as early as 1543 that "these regions are easily seen without cadaveric dissection, and need no description."[34] Falloppio, on the other hand, describes the *pudenda* as "small" and hidden in the upper part of the pubis in such a way that anatomical dissection was a prerequisite for autoptic access to these structures. Both anatomists were oblivious to the fact that the physiological anatomy of these blood-rich and swelling body parts needed to be explored in the living. Further points of contention hinged on the anatomical description, naming, and especially the normative ideas about the morphology, dimension, and physiology of the *pudenda*.[35] To the *labia minora*, which vary in size and which he continues to call *cuticulares carunculae*,[36] Vesal attributes the function of being undoubtedly created for pleasant rubbing, such as tickling, and to entice (*ad suauiorem indubie affrictum, ac ueluti titillationem, et illecebram procreatae*). In this context, Vesal adds a moralizing remark, comparing women from the northern regions with those from the southern regions. In the case of the "demure" women originating from the northern regions, the genitals are far smaller and only slightly prominent (*in septentrionalibus mulieribus, et pudicis, longè, quàm in caeteris, humiliores*). In this context, Vesal uses clitoris (*inter quae* κλιτορίς *etiam occurrit*)[37] as a synonym for the labia. Again, he points to the cutting practices of the Egyptians, who excised the labia of marriageable virgins. He adds information taken from travelogues, which can be found in his handwritten annotations: among the "Abdarites," also known as the "people of Presbyter John," genital cutting would take place "to this day" (*adhuc hodie*) among all little girls (*puellae*), just as among boys the *praeputium* was circumcized for religious reasons. Vesal explains the cutting by the fact that the sexual act is more difficult for the man because of the swelling of the labia as a result of constant friction due to rubbing against the clothing.[38] This is where Vesal launches his criticism of Falloppio's description of the clitoris: a pendulous structure (*penis*) that leads to an exaggerated sense of pleasure can—according to Vesal—only be found in hermaphrodites. In this, Vesal is not only criticizing Falloppio, but also doubts tradition by quoting Avicenna, who called it (sc. "penis") "albathara," and refers to the Greeks, who classified an enlarged "nympha" as a disease and excised it.[39] Nothing was more certain than that in women only the labia (*caruncula*e) were to be found at the outer rim of the vagina. Vesal could find no evidence at all of a "penis" or something very small, protruding from the bony region of the pubis, furnished with a few muscles, hidden under the skin and sensitive to arousal.[40] On the basis of his autopsy, he adamantly rejects the existence of a "female penis," i.e. a hypertrophic clitoris as an independent structure distinct from the labia. Thus, in his view, the cause of an exaggerated sense of pleasure can only be the enlargement of the *labia minora* that occurs in some women. Vesal does not pass judgement on the cutting of female genitals. In all published editions and in the planned third edition of his anatomical treatise, as well as in his discussion of Falloppio's theses, Vesal offers a matter-of-fact account of the religiously motivated, preventive practices of cutting to facilitate the sexual act, which were carried out from (late) antiquity until his own time. The painstakingly collected information from travelogues, which incorporated both legend and historical content, seems to have had an orientating function for anatomists in questions of the varying size and deviating morphology of these structures, which were perceived very differently in terms of their aesthetics.

SCHOLARLY VIGILANCE, EMPATHY, AND ISOLATED CRITICISM

The impact of this discussion can be found in gynaecological literature a good fifty years later. The Jewish city physician Rodrigo de Castro (1546–1627), who lived in Hamburg, wrote a treatise on women's medicine, *De universa mulierum medicina*, 1st ed. 1603, which would enjoy a long-lasting but highly selective reception.[41] In the theoretical part of his treatise, de

Castro deals with the anatomy of the female genitalia.[42] The description of the hymen leads him to describe existing uncertainties among anatomists, including forms of superstition.[43] He distances himself above all from the ideas common among the Arabs (*Arabes*) about the number and course of the blood vessels that supply the hymen. Autopsy shows that these are fantasies (*sunt imaginati*).[44] It is precisely such fantasies in combination with superstition (*tanta superstitio*) that de Castro sees as the cause of the spread of female infibulation in childhood. He condemns the practice on both ethical and medical grounds. He reports "that to this day in happy Arabia ... peoples are found—Arabs by origin, Mohamedans by faith—where the vulvas of their little daughters are sewn together. A small hole is left in the middle of them." He then continues with a factual description of the changes in the bodies of the girls concerned:

> The girls remain in this state until they are mature enough to be married to men. They are handed over to them closed and virtually sealed. Then the stitched labia [literally: the stitches and the wings of the uterus] are opened, which by this time have already grown together as if they had been formed this way by nature. [...]

Finally, de Castro describes the painful consequences of the procedure and emphasises that he gained this information from women:

> The more careful confirm that in those still inexperienced in sexual intercourse [virgins] the walls of the cervix are only semi-grown together and are thus closed and form a narrow neck there. During the first sexual act they are largely torn apart and, as it were, torn apart; therefore, as the women report, this [the first sexual act] is extremely painful; I am more than happy to agree with their opinions.
>
> (De Castro 1603a, 5f)[45]

De Castro does not name any written sources here.[46] We know, however, that in the 16th century, Cardinal Pietro Bembo (1470–1547) and the merchant and traveller Jan Huygen von Linschoten (1563–1611) reported infibulation practices in the Red Sea region and in India (Kingdom of Pegu).[47] Bembo's account suggests that the Portuguese, who traded extensively along the coasts of the Red Sea, brought information about these customs to Europe. It can be assumed that de Castro had heard oral reports about these practices when he was still living in Lisbon around 1588 and practiced, among other things, as a port physician.[48] De Castro does not confine himself to describing infibulation, which continues to be practiced today in some countries and regions.[49] He also describes the removal of the clitoris and the shortening or removal of the labia.[50] According to de Castro's understanding of medical tradition, *nymphotomia* is a synonym for clitoridectomy. He clearly distinguishes between the *nymphae* (pl.) and the *nympha* (s.) as a "muscular and membranous elevation (...) situated above the union of the wings of the pubis, where the orifice of the urethra appears."[51] This resolves the terminological ambiguity still present in Vesal. De Castro's accurate characterization of the individual structures of the female genitalia regards the labia majora as a skin-like addition or "*epiphysis*" (*cutacea quaedam* [...] ἐπὶ φυσις *sive additio*), which in its ornamental function corresponds to the male prepuce and forms a small outward elevation. On both sides of the inner parts, de Castro continues, there are two skin lobes that hang like a pair of lips (*carunculae* [...] *cuticulares instar geminae linguae propendulae*), to which the name *nymphae* (pl.) has been given and which are also called the "wings of the uterus" (*uteri alae*). De Castro compares the *labia minora, nymphae* (pl.) in their protective function—following Galen—with the *uvula*.[52] Where the labia unite, according to de Castro, they form a small hidden elevation like a small penis (*occultatus processus parvus; exiguus penis*), which ends in a glans and is covered by a foreskin (*praeputium*).[53] To this elevation, "which is also called the clitoris" (*cletoride* [*ita enim hunc processum vocant*]), de Castro attributes another function in addition to preventing the backflow of urine into the urethra and urinary bladder.[54] In this way, de Castro explicitly joins Realdo Colombo and his anatomical-physiological description of the clitoris.[55] Like Colombo, de Castro calls the clitoris a *processus*:

> In this [part of the body] an extraordinary excitement arises and for this reason it is considered the principal seat of women's sensation of pleasure during the act of love. In the same part of the body two elongated ligaments terminate; they are nerve-rich and hollow and originate at the sides of the uterus. Colombo latterly boasted that he had discovered it [the clitoris] as the main cause of women's greatest pleasure.
>
> (DeCastro 1603a, 6)[56]

De Castro sees hypertrophy as exceeding the natural measure and thus as aesthetically undesirable. In assessing the consequences, however, he takes an extremely tolerant stance:

> But that elevation sometimes exceeds the measure of nature, and grows to such greatness that it hangs over the uterus and leads to ugliness and shame, and, if it constantly rubs against the clothing, drives it to such desire that the women who are aroused by this [body] part cannot desist, throw themselves into love after the manner of men, and defile themselves by having sexual intercourse[57] alternately as *incubi* and as *succubi* [...].
>
> (DeCastro 1603a, 6)[58]

According to de Castro and other authors, the enlargement of the clitoris not only had aesthetic but also moral consequences: the abnormally developed and "ugly" part would cause an uncontrollable sensation of pleasure due to mechanical rubbing against the clothes.[59] The affected women would then lust like men and have both hetero- and homoerotic sexual intercourse. De Castro gives examples of the social effects of sexual desire that falls outside the norm. Following Amato Lusitano (1511–68) and based on his own experience from the time he lived in Lisbon, de Castro tells of two women who were denounced for homoerotic acts and had to endure a trial.[60] At this point, he mentions again the clitoridectomy practiced in Egypt, noting the ostensible preventative aim—to forestall socially condemned practices. De Castro is very frank in his criticism of this:

> Therefore it is customary among the Egyptians to cut out [this [sc. the clitoris]] in virgins; this [cutting] they consider necessary without distinction also in those membranous pieces of flesh [the *labia minora*] which are situated in front of the opening of the uterus; in my judgment, however, they err, because these [both] have a natural use, for they give great pleasure to women during sexual intercourse, and, as we have already said, protect the uterus against externalities.
>
> (DeCastro 1603a, 6)[61]

De Castro's precision in discussing interventions on the female genitalia and their consequences for the women concerned are exceptional in the medical literature of the early modern period.[62] The fact that he condemns them all equally is also remarkable. A comparison with Gerolamo Mercuriale (1530–1606) shows how similar observations could lead to divergent positions. Mercuriale, too, equated a hypertrophic clitoris with an aesthetic disfigurement (*deformitas*) that causes shame (*pudor*); de Castro uses the same term deformitas (*ugliness*) for this morphological conspicuousness and also emphasises the associated shame (*pudor*). But the two authors differ when it comes to the physiological-erotic consequences of this morphological deviation. For Mercuriale, the enlargement is in itself linked to increased erotic desire in the woman (*incredibile coitus desiderium*), which calls for surgical correction. De Castro describes the mechanical friction of the clothes on the enlarged part of the body and sees in this alone the cause of the increased excitability (*vestimentis jugiter attritus ad libidinem adeo irritat*), which then leads the affected person, who is in herself blameless, to engage in eruptive homoerotic behavior.

Three levels of argumentation formed the basis of de Castro's critical position: *First*, all body parts are considered functional and useful according to Galenic anatomical teleology. According to this, women's external genitalia by "nature" possess both a protective and erotic function, which alone justifies their existence. *Second*, de Castro refutes false anatomical ideas (hymen) and associated superstitious customs (infibulation). *Third*, the hypertrophy of female genitalia, which is regarded as deviating from the norm, is seen as the cause of the exaggerated homoerotic arousal of the women concerned (through mechanical friction); de Castro thus exculpates those affected. With these three arguments—usefulness/functionality of the female genitalia, errors of superstitious peoples, and desculpation of women with hyperthrophic genitalia—De Castro resolutely rejects supposedly preventative mutilating interventions. De Castro concludes that those who deny or ignore the anatomy, morphological variations, and natural functionality of women's intimate body parts are mistaken.

"UNCOMFORTABLE" BODY PARTS AND SELECTIVE TEXT RECEPTION

With the exception of de Castro's remarks, the controversies described have left their traces in anatomical[63] as well as in practice-related[64] and surgical texts.[65] To exemplify the selective treatment of this body of thought, the position of the anatomist and surgeon Marco

Aurelio Severino (1580–1656) should be mentioned in conclusion. In his work *De efficaci medicina libri* (1646), he advocates the propagation of nymphotomy as a surgical technique.[66] The difficulties of inspecting this region in the living and in the cadaver were known to Severino.[67] In addressing the question of whether to excise parts of the flesh that have grown too large against nature (*praeter naturae*) and have therefore become "useless, inconvenient and annoying" (*ociosa, incommoda, permolesta*), Severino falls back on the opinions of Falloppio and Vesal. Unlike Vesal, Falloppio had emphasized the natural state (*naturalis pars*) of the female genitals and had not mentioned corrective interventions at any point.[68] For Severino, Falloppio represents an isolated voice: the majority of physicians had followed Vesal (*sed aliquando plures sunt, qui Vesalio adhaeserint*) and advocated "nymphotomia."[69] With the phrase "Vesal rightly contradicted Falloppio," Severino introduces the section in which he talks of the hypertrophy common among women in southern regions, which he describes as a disease. Severino qualifies the excision procedures practiced by the Egyptians as "precaution" (*providentia*) and finally expresses the wish that contemporary surgeons engage more intensively with the procedure of nymphotomy.[70] One thing stands out when reading his impassioned plea: Roderigo de Castro is not mentioned anywhere. This omission is no accident.[71] Until the eighteenth century, authors of treatises discussing this complex of topics tended to draw on de Castro's work on gynaecology but ignored it in connection with "nymphotomia" and similar practices.[72]

Fifty years after de Castro's book on women's diseases was published, the English physician John Bulwer (1606–56) raised his criticisms. In his weighty work *Anthropometamorphosis* (1653), Bulwer succinctly but unequivocally condemned "female circumcision," which was common in Ethiopia, as a mistake.[73] Thomas Laqueur understood this testimony as *pars pro toto*, attesting to the supposed rejection of clitoridectomy "in the West" until the nineteenth century. The examples analyzed here show that in reality the vast majority of physicians read the reports on genital cutting, circumcision, and mutilation practices with cool curiosity and generally passed them on neutrally or even approvingly without medical or ethical justification or reservation. Against the prevailing acceptance of female genital cutting practices on the part of pre-modern physicians, De Castro and Bulwer stand out as rare exceptions.

The examination of the sources, which does not claim to be exhaustive and rather illustrates the need for further research, shows that de Castro's position was concealed and ignored for centuries. This may be interpreted as a sign of the prevailing uncertainties with which physicians had to wrestle in the process of exploring, uncovering, and standardizing the female genitalia. With the (re)discovery of the seat of female pleasure, the medical gaze turned to that which in women's nature grows "outwards," shows itself—or not—and varies greatly in shape and size. For the setting of normative boundaries and differences for biological sex correspondences, the measure (female/small vs. male/large) and the function (female/passive vs. male/active) become decisive. The unsettling idea that there was a *virga muliebris*—whether interpreted as a natural body part fluctuating in size, as a disease, a natural defect, or an ethnic trait—was apparently more easily accepted precisely because of the possibility of its surgical removal.

NOTES

This article is based on a previous study: Gadebusch Bondio/Förg (2022). In the present version, which has been abridged and given new emphases, findings are presented that were produced within the framework of the Collaborative Research Centre "Vigilance Cultures" (CRC/SFB 1369) funded by the German Research Foundation. A sub-project on pre-modern medical vigilance is led by the author in the CRC. Thanks are due to Kathatina-Luise Förg as former research assistant and co-author for the fruitful collaboration on the previous version. In the case of translations from Latin and Greek, the translator responsible is specified. I would also like to thank Karl Hughes without whose linguistic sensitivity and astute terminological-conceptual scrutiny this text would not exist in English.

1. For a critique of Laqueur's one-sex theory (Laqueur [1990]), the research by Michael Stolberg and Helen King is foundational. Stolberg (2003); King (2013). See also, with a focus on Rodrigo de Castro, Gadebusch Bondio/Förg (2020).
2. In her recent *longue durée* study, Camille Nurka critiques Katherine Park and interprets early modern medical discourses on clitoral hypertrophy in light of the clitoral/penile analogy—in Laqueur's sense. In the brief section on early modern authors (58–64), Nurka does not do justice to the complexity of the subject. For criticism of Park and "sympathetic explanation" of Laqueur, see Nurka (2019, 59f).
3. I am deliberately using a modern, "neutral" term here. In its vagueness, the collective term "genital cutting" includes the various practices of clitoridectomy, clitoris excision, labia excision, and infibulation. Genital cutting is limited to the procedure and does not refer to the consequences of cutting, or genital mutilation as such, for those involved.
4. "A striking sign of this general commitment to sexual binarism was the early modern French medical writers' promotion of clitoridectomy as a feasible remedy for clitoral hypertrophy and its inconvenients, not just in faraway Africa but in Europe itself" (Park 1997, 183).
5. On the medical preoccupation with the female genitals, the pathologically enlarged clitoris, and the medical treatment of the pudenda in the Middle Ages, cf. the overview in Green (2009, 97–102).
6. Platter (1614): In Extvberantia, p. 626: "Excrescentia instar colli anserini, in pudendo foeminae" ... "An clithoris sic adaucta fuerit, vel aliud sarcoma, non licuit, cum nollet hoc mihi ostendere, discernere; ex contactu tamen illius, quem non nisi locis vicinis bene tectis concedebat, carnem referre, cognoui."
7. On the terms derived from ancient sources that early modern authors either leave in Greek or adopt in Latin translation, see Gadebusch Bondio and Förg (2022).
8. Many early modern physicians preferred to leave designations of genitals in Greek letters. In doing so, they followed Celsus, who was of the opinion "that the designation of genitals in Greek was more acceptable than in Latin" because, on the one hand, Greek was, as it were, the specialist medical language and, on the other, it was held to be less unseemly than the Latin equivalents. Cf. von Staden (1991); Sauerteig (2005) Stamatu (2005); Fögen (2009, 79f. [citation on page 79] with note 34). Camille Nurka and Bernadette J. Brooten, among others, point out the terminological problems in the course of the tradition. Cf. Nurka (2019, 29–81); Brooten (2020, 192–201); here we also refer to our own paper in which we have carried out a terminological analysis Gadebusch Bondio/Förg 2022.
9. Schenck von Grafenberg (1600, 62)/(1596, 157): "Quod si non in omnibus mulieribus, si quidem venere potissimum exercitatas ad notionem hujus requirimus, secundum naturam constitutis, mentula illa in conspectum veniat, meminerint illi velim, id verius ob exiguitatem evenire, quo

minus cernatur, maxime si ex cadaveribus, ubi tam exilis hujusmodi particula ut plurimum conciderit inspectio petatur. In vivis vero cum omnia calore spiritu et sanguine turgent, etiam extra monstrosam constitutionem inventu faciliorem hanc muliebrem virgam judicaverim. Quae causa est, cur meam quoque observationem subijcere placuerit."

10. In the title of this chapter, Schenk already refers to the terms that circulate among ancient authors and contemporaries (mentula muliebris, columella, clitoris, nympha). Schenk, lib. IV. De genitalibus mulierum (1600, 59). On the history and terminology of the clitoris see: Di Marino/Lepidi (2014, 1–12, and 23–26).
11. In her view of an eroticized haptic and visual perception of the female genitalia by early modern anatomists, Bettina Mathes also refers to Andreas Vesal's abridged version of his anatomical treatise (*Epitome*). Vesal's remarks on the clitoris, however, go unmentioned. In his systematic, historical-ethnological monograph of 1986, Michel Erlich conducted a well-founded if compact "Parcours historique," listing the names and works of several anatomists and surgeons who reported on clitoridectomy or nymphotomy in the sixteenth and seventeenth centuries. Vesal is not mentioned. Erlich (1986, 49–55); likewise in Huebner (2009) and Johnsdotter (2012).
12. Vesal's handwritten notes on this were discovered in 2007. See Nutton (2012).
13. The processing of the information from the travelogues can be seen by comparing the texts: cf. Gadebusch Bondio/Förg Appendix, in which the relevant text passages are juxtaposed.
14. See here Garrison/Hast (2014, 1069 with note 39).
15. Vesal (1543): lib. V, cap. 15, p. 531f.: "Hic nanque perpetuò praeter laxos implexus cuticulares illas carunculas tuberculaque non aequaliter omnibus mulieribus propendula adipiscit, quae νυμφὼ Graeci vocant."
16. Vesal borrows at this point from the traditions of Rufus of Ephesus and Iulius Pollux; Vesal (1555): lib. V, cap. 15, p. 653: "Hîc namque perpetuò praeter laxos implexus, illas cuticulares carunculas non aequaliter omnibus mulieribus instar geminae linguae propendulas adipiscitur, quae Graecis νυμφὴ, μύρτον, ὑποδερίς [sic! et κλιτορίς uocantur."
17. Vesal (1543): lib. V, cap. 15, p. 536f.: "quod hae coriaceae quodammodo carunculae in nonnullis mulieribus ad tantam molem augeant, ut pudorem deformitatemque inducant, et multis nationibus quoque insignis impudicitiae argumento sint: imò à uestimentis iugiter attritae, ad libidinem irritant, et Veneris ardorem suscitant. Vnde etiam Aegyptijs praecipuè uisum est, ut anteaquam carunculae illae extuberent, tunc potissimùm amputentur, quum proximè uirgines nupturae sunt." Vesal (1555): lib. V, cap. XV, p. 653: "quòd illae carunculae nonnullis mulieribus ad tantam augeantur molem, ut pudorem deformitatemque inducant, et multis nationibus insignis quoque impudicitiae argumento sint: imò à uestimentis iugiter attritae, ad libidinem irritant. Vnde etiam Aegyptijs uisum est, ut anteaquam illae longiùs exerantur et propendeant, tunc potissimùm amputentur, quum proximè uirgines nupturae sunt."
18. Aëtios of Amida had described the consequences of the enlargement of the clitoris (which he called "nymph"/νύμφη) and the preventive removal of it among the Egyptians: Aët. XVI 103. See Blaschke (1998); Leven (2005).
19. Nutton (2012); Garrison/Hast (2014, 1078).
20. Nutton (2012, 429): "Quemadmodum hodie adhuc Sceuani Aetiopes {dicto} appellato nobis presbitero Janni < Abyssinorum regi > subditi, nuper natis puellis carneos istos processus religionis ipsorum iure haud secus prescindunt ac masculis praeputia auferunt, et si interim Christianae {alio} religioni in caeremoniis {alioquin} alias pleraque habeant communia." According to Vivian Nutton, this is one of the "most striking of such additions" Nutton (2012, 429).
21. According to Salvatore Tedeschi, the Scevani are inhabitants of the Ethiopian province of Shewa, whose (political) origins go back to the Middle Ages. Tedeschi (1985, 103).

22. The term *processus* (pl.) is newly introduced by Vesal and obviously refers to those structures which he has so far called *carunculae*.

23. Vesal probably borrowed from Paolo Giovio. Damião de Góis (1502–74) was the first to discuss the religiously motivated circumcision of girls, but he does not mention the "Scevani" in this context. Paolo Giovio (1483/6–1552), on the other hand, attributed this custom to the "Scevani" in Ethiopia in his work *Historiarum sui temporis*: Giovio (1550): lib. XVIII, p. 304. This led Nutton to assume that Giovio had been the reference source for Vesal. See Nutton (2012, 429–231).

24. In addition to Paolo Giovio, Francisco Álvares (*c.* 1465–1540), with his description *Legatio David Aethiopiae Regis* (1533) and *Verdadeira Informação das Terras do Preste João das Indias* (1544), or Giovanni Battista Ramusio (1485–1557), *Della descrittione dell'Africa et delle cose notabili che ivi sono* (1550), should be mentioned; on the latter see. Donattini (2016).

25. Cf. the remarks of the naturalist Pierre Belon (1517–64): According to him, the Copts in Ethiopia also circumcize women. Which structure exactly is removed is not entirely clear due to terminological contradictions. Belon (1588): lib. 3 cap. 28, p. 425f.: "Nous scauons aussi que les Cophtes Chrestiennes du pays de Prestre Iean en Ethiopie croyans en Iesus Christ, sont circoncises: car estant la loy telle que les femmes doiuent receuoir quelque impression de circoncision, ilz leur coupent les parties appellees en Grec Hymenea, en Latin Alae: car ilz les trouuent correspondantes au prepuce viril."

26. On the question of who is the first (re)discoverer of the clitoris, cf. Park (1997, 177f.); Stringer/Becker (2010, 132).

27. Colombo (1559): lib. XI, p. 243: "Processus igitur hi ab utero exorti prope id foramen, quod os matricis vocatur, extra abdomen exeunt; supra pubem ascendunt; desinunt autem in particulam quandam excelsam in vulvae apice circumvolutam supra id foramen, unde lotium exit. Et haec lector candidissimae illa, illa praecipue sedes est delectationis mulierum dum, venerem exercent [...] Hos igitur processus, atque eorundem usum cum nemo hactenus animadverterit; si nomina rebus à me inventis imponere licet, amor Veneris, vel dulcedo appelletur." In the terminological choice of Colombo, who spoke of *processus*, Laqueur saw an analogy with the penis: "[...] his nomenclature is decidedly odd and imprecise. His organ may be the clitoris but it is not the clitoris of modern anatomy" (Laqueur 1989, 104).

28. Colombo (1559, 242): "In cervicis uteri finibus vulvam versus nonnullae carunculae prominent, à quibus voluptas, ac delectio in coeundo non parum augetur. Sub hisce vulvae labellis duae adsunt à lateribus latae membranae Nymphae à veteribus dictae, quarum utilitas est, ut a pulvere, frigore, et aere uterum tueantur." Galen, De usu part. 15, 3: p. 344–346. See also Galen *On the anatomy of the uterus*: CMG V 2, 1, 2, 3, p. 36f.

29. Falloppio (1561) fol. 193r: "Anatomici verò nostri penitus neglexerunt, neque verbum quidem de ipsa faciunt." Cf. also fol. 193v: "Totum hoc pudendum, quia parvum est, et latitat in pinguiori pubis parte, ideò anatomicos etiam latuit, atque ita latuit, ut ego primus fuerim, qui superioribus annis idem patefecerim, et si qui alii da hac re locuti sunt, aut scripserunt, scias quòd ipsam aut à me, aut à meis auditoribus accepere, neque tamen obid rem ipſam bene norunt."

30. Ibid. fol. 192v–193r: "Sed haec levia, graviora, quae sequuntur sunt." Avicen. 3.lib. fen 21. "circa finem meminit cuiusdam partis in pudendo muliebri sitam, quam virgam vel albathara vocat." Hanc Albucasis lib. 2. cap. 71. "tentiginem appellat, quae solet aliquando ad tantum incrementum pervenire, ut mulieres hanc habentes coeant cum alijs, veluti si viri essent. Partem hanc graeci κλητορίδα vocarunt, unde verbum κλητορίζειν obscoenum diductum est."

31. Ibid.: "Particula haec eadem virili peni respondet, et ex duplici nervo constat intus spongioso, atque atriori crassiorique sanguine referto, uti in viris."

32. Ibid. fol. 192v–193r (see note 66).

33. See Nurka (2019, 60–62; 64f.) for a concise account based only on the first edition of 1543.
34. In the chapter on the uterus, at the point where Vesal comes to the external genitalia, he describes the skin, the hairiness and notes differences between older and younger women in terms of the size and consistency of the structures. Vesal [1543]: lib. 5, cap. XV, p. 536: "At quum haec citra mortuorum sectionem conspicua sint, enarratione neutiquam indigent: quemadmodum neque illi primi in pudendo implexus, et utrinque una prominens cuticularis caruncula, longa quidem, sed tenuis, et ex longa basi in mucronem desidens. Has νυμφὴ Graecis vocari innuimus, qui earum praecisionem […]." Likewise in Vesal (1555): lib. 5, cap. XV, p. 660: "At quum haec citra mortuorum sectionem sint obvia, quis omnium hoc Capite hactenus enarratorum sit usus, explicare modò conabimur."
35. Vesal (1564, 142f., esp. 143).
36. Ibid. p. 142: "In elatiore muliebris pudendi sede, quae anteriori pubis ossium regioni innititur, inter pudendi labra alasve duas lingularum fere in modum prominulas eminere scripsi cuticulares carunculas, quae non omnibus, vel eiusdem regionis mulieribus aequè sunt magnae ac procerae: uti etiam eidem quoque mulieri, ambae non pari semper modo eminent."
37. Vesal (1564, 142): "Quibus verò carunculae hae ad suaviorem indubie affrictum, ac veluti titillationem, et illecebram procreatae, et in septentrionalibus mulieribus, et pudicis, longè, quàm in caeteris, humiliores, et dimissae donentur nominibus (inter quae κλιτορίς etiam occurrit) […]."
38. Ibid.: "et qui apud Aegyptios iam nupturis virginibus (uti etiam omnibus puellis adhuc hodie apud Abdaritas seu vocati nobis Presbiteri Ioannis gentem, perinde ac masculorum praeputium, religionis ergo) praescindi soleant. Dein qui subinde vestium attritu veluti in tentiginem actae tumeant insurguntque, et interdum viro in venere molestius obsistunt magna ex parte, suo loco a me est descriptum."
39. Ibid. p. 143: "Existimo namque satis propendentem, et in tentiginem aliquando sese educentem in hermaphroditis (qui alioquin muliebria habuerunt perfectiora, et qui apud Aeginetam apertè describuntur) non semel mihi visum penem, et illum Auicennae albatharam, et Graecorum nimis excedentem et in morborum classe habitam nympham, mulieris cuipiam ita prouenisse, ut penis ille extra cutem non esset exortus, rudimentaque tantum quaedam pusillae mentulae haberet."
40. Ibid.: "Quaequum forte fortuna tibi inter secandum occurrit, illa huius tuae obseruationis causam dedit. Nihil namque certius est, quàm in omnibus mulieribus, in superiori pudendi sede, in qua à me descriptae, et adhuc in naturae metis comprehendendae eminent carunculae, penem, uel minimum haud reperiri, qui à pubis ossibus pronatus, et musculis aliquot praeditus, sub cute dictaue pudendi sede latitat, tentiginemque experitur, et illum innaturalem, quem fere ex Albucasi (qui aliàs de morbis hic loquitur) ipsi assignas vsum, praestat."
41. About De Castro see Gadebusch Bondio/Förg (2018). De Castro (1603a, 5ff).
42. See Gadebusch Bondio/Förg (2020). Borris (2004, 134–137).
43. De Castro compares the search for the hymen with that for the sectum transversum in the heart. The septum between the right and left ventricle had been postulated by Galen, but was not to be found in the cadaver dissections. The representatives of the "thick" consistency of the hymen, including Vesal, argue similarly, see Cunningham (1988); Manuli/Vegetti (1977).
44. De Castro (1603a, 5): "Arabes verò quinque venas ad cervicis uteris medium utrinque inferi tradiderunt, ac dextrarum venarum ora cum sinistris committi, ex hisque centonem ipsis appellatum atque adeò hymen efformari, quas tamen venas ex sanguine, qui in prima coitione profluit, potius, quàm ex sedula dissectione, cum ibi nullae reperiantur, procul dubio sunt imaginati."
45. De Castro (1603a, 5f.) (transl.: K.-. L. Förg/M. Gadebusch Bondio): "[…], tanta superstitione, ut adhuc reperiantur in felici Arabia nationes, non procul â regno preciosi Joannis, juxta BABEL MELEC urbem, natione Arabes, sectâ Mahumetani, apud quas filiolarum vulvae consuuntur,

medio relicto foramine, sicque quoad viris maturè conjungantur, dimittuntur, quibus eas obseratas et quasi sigillatas tradunt, ac tunc reserantur puncta et alae uteri, adeò jam cohaerentes ac si ita â natura fuissent fabricatae; [...] Diligentiores cervicis latera nondum venerem expertis duntaxat quasi conglutinata connivere, ac angustum ibi collum efficere affirmarunt, quae primus coitus magna ex parte divellit et quodammodo dilacerat, ideo, ut mulieres ferunt, acerrimus ille est, quorum ego sententiae libentius subscribo."

46. Paolo Giovio, whose reports on the "Scevani" and the kingdom of the priest-king John of Vesal, among others, were received (see note 57), does not mention infibulation.

47. Bembo (1552) lib. VI, p. 75v: "After these, other peoples left and entered the Red Sea, and many cities of black and good men and strong warriors came to them: who soon after their daughters were born, they took their nature into their hands; in such a way that the way to urinate is not impeded: and those who are grown, are married in such a way, that the first care of the husband is to cut the lips of the girl with an iron, so congealed and consolidated. So much is in honour with those barbarous men in taking wives, the certainty of their virginity." Van Linschoten (1599), ch. 17, p. 20: "Puellis infantibus quidam pudenda filo consuunt, ad usum naturae duntaxat relicto exiguo foramine, ita post sponsus membrum resecari suo arbitrio curat, unguento sive oleo ad medelam vulneri infuso." A linking of the "circumcision" practices of the "Mohamedans" with superstition is, however, used by the later author Jean de Thevenot (1633–67), s. Thevenot (1665), ch. 74, p. 497: "Les Mores sont Mahometans, mais ils ont quelques superstitions que les Turcs n'ont pas, car les Mores circoncisent leurs filles, leur coupant un petit morceau de ce qu'on appelle Nymphe, et ce sont des femmes qui sont cette circoncision de filles. Les Turcs ne sont point cela, ils circoncisent seulement les garcons."

48. De Castro (1614, 251). De Castro reports here how he examined and appraised slaves at the port of Lisbon and sailors in the course of embarkation (Spanish Armada, 1588).

49. The form described by de Castro corresponds to Type III of the WHO typology of female genital mutilation. See WHO (2008, 23–28). The term "Female Genital Mutilation" is the term favoured by the WHO but controversially discussed, which includes all variants of the irreversible procedure. See WHO (2008, 22); Nussbaum (1999, 118–219); Duivenbode/Padela (2019); Gillespie (2015). For geographical distribution, see WHO (2021). UNICEF (2016); Karim (1997). The number of women affected is currently around 200 million worldwide. In Germany, for example, around 2,000 women and girls are treated annually for the consequences of diagnosed genital mutilation. DÄ (04/12/2020).

50. The term *nymphotomia* goes back to Soranos of Ephesus. Cf. CMG IV, p. XX and 147 (Περὶ ὑπερμεγέθους νύμφης καὶ νυμφοτομίας); see Gadebusch Bondio/Förg (2022).

51. De Castro (1614, 7): "Ab his tamen nymphis differt alia pars nympha dicta, quia haec processus ille est musculosus, ac pelliculosus supra alarum pudendi commissuram situs, quo loco urinarius meatus existit, quam quidem particulam potius scindendam autores praecepisse arbitror, et hoc manuale opus nymphotomiam nominasse, non affectum ipsum ut Moschio perperam prodidit."

52. Galen, De usu part. 15, 3 p. 344–346, quotation p. 346. De Castro (1603a, 6): "[...] et est veluti cutacea quaedam hujus colli ἐπὶ φυσις sive additio, masculorum praeputio respondens; et ut praeputium ornamenti gratias existit in ambitu rimae seu oris genitalis, collibus seu monticulis protuberantibus, qui in partibus exterioribus crinibus in foeminis jam maturis ornantur; ab interioribus vero, carunculae illae cuticulares instar geminae linguae propendulae adnascuntur utrinque, quae Nymphae nomine donantur, quas uteri alas vocant, easdemque natura eo progenuisse creditum, ut uterum â pulvere, frigore, et alijs externis injurijs tutaretur; quale enim uva pharyngi propugnaculum est, tale utero nymphae [...]."

53. Ibid.: "[...] in cujus elatiori parte, ac pinguiori pubis loco, ubi hae carunculae conveniunt, juxta id foramen unde lotium exit, occultatum processum parvum efficiunt, exiguo peni, qualis est

cuniculi, admodum similem; substantia fungosa, nervosa, et sanguine plena: forma in glandem desinentem, parvo quoque praeputio obtectum, quem antea [cf. note 73] regressum urinae ad vesicae collum impedire diximus, quique alium praestet usum non contemnendum [...]."

54. Ibid. p. 5: In discussing the cervix, de Castro already addresses the clitoris en passant: "Juxta cervicem uteri in anteriori sua sede jam fermè supra pudendum vesicae collum ingreditur; per quod urina defertur, et Nympha fatiscente foras excernitur, (non enim ut Idiotae et mulierculae ipsae mingentes opinantur, per uteri cervicem lotium prodit) ibi cervicis portiuncula excrescit in ipsius cavitatem propendens, et postquam urinam cervicis uteri pars ferè extrema admittit, ipsius, alteriusve humoris regressum in collum vesicae impedit, illis processibus similis, qui regressum urinae â vesica ad urinarium meatum prohibent, hinc mulierum lotium occursante, impetuque collisa cletoride (ita enim hunc processum vocant) magis quàm virorum inter mingendum perstrepit."

55. In the second part of his gynaecological treatise, De universa mulierum medicina. Pars secunda, sive Praxis (Hamburg 1603b), de Castro repeats his terminological remarks and also lists the synonyms (p. 172): "Cuticularis illa Epiphysis, sive caruncula, supra alarum commissiorum sita, quam alibi descripsimus eiusque usus, quaeque Nympha dicitur sive clitoris, aliis colliculus, Hippocrati Columella, Avicennae Virga, vel Albatara virili peni respondens; [...]."

56. De Castro (1603a, 6) (transl.: M. Gadebusch Bondio): "In eo enim pruritus eximius efficitur, ideo praecipua sedes delectationis mulierum, dum venerem exercent, statuitur; In hanc etiam partem bina desinunt ligamenta oblonga, nervea cavaque, quae â matricis lateribus constituta praecipuam esse illius summae delectationis caussam invenisse se ex recentioribus gloriatur Columbus."

57. *Incubi* and *succubi* are, literally, those persons who "lie on" and "under" something (e.g. Van der Lugt [2001, 178–181]). An oversized clitoris leads the affected women to heterosexual as well as homosexual intercourse by "alternately lying on and under" their sexual partners.

58. De Castro (1603a, 6) (transl.: K.-L. Förg): "Verum processus ille aliquando naturae modum excedit, et ad tantam magnitudinem excrescit, ut extra uterum propendens deformitatem atque pudorem inducat, et vestimentis jugiter attritus ad libidinem adeo irritat, ut non desint, quae per hanc partem etiam erectae mulieres virorum instar in venerem ruant, et mutuis coitibus incubis, ac succubis sese polluant, [...]." See also De Castro (1603b, 172–174).

59. See Mercuriale (1601), lib. IV., cap. XIII, De nympha, et cauda, p. 192 ff.

60. De Castro (1603a, 6): "[...] quod de duabus Turcis Thessalonicensibus Amatus refert, et nos Vlisiponae ob simile foedissimum scelus aliquot mulieres publicè puniri vidimus, [...]." The case of the two Turkish women from Thessaloniki is described in detail by Lusitano; however, the latter does not report any punishment. Lusitano (1570): cent. VII, curat. 18, p. 59f.; Park (1997, 175–184); Lochrie (2005). On Lusitano, see von Engelhardt (2020).

61. De Castro (1603a, 6) (transl.: K.-L. Förg/M. Gadebusch Bondio): "Quamobrem Aegyptij in virginibus excidere consueverunt, quod quidam indistinctè faciendum esse putant in carunculis illis cuticularibus quae ante os uteri ad natae visuntur; qui tamen meo quidem judicio errant, quoniam illae suos habent â natura usus, nam et magnam foeminis in coitu delectationem pariunt, et uterum, uti diximus, ab externis tutantur."

62. De Castro's "clarity of vocabulary and style" is also emphasized by Santos Pinheiro in her analysis of the description of the uterus in *De universa mulierum medicina*. Rather cursorily, the author refers to de Castro's remarks on the hymen and clitoris, in which he included "controversial practices of his time," but in principle adhered to Vesal as his main source: Santos Pinheiro's statement (2021, 309) that "Castro also makes use of some Vesalian comments on social or religious practices and shows his clear approval of the moralistic tone of Vesalius' text," however, does not apply to the remarks on excision or infibulation.

63. Thomas Bartholin may be mentioned here as an example. His composition of sources in reproducing the anatomical knowledge of women's genitalia is remarkable. Bartholin (1651): cap. XXXII, p. 182f.: "De pudendo muliebri externo in genere." On excision practices he positions himself favourably: p. 188f.: "[...] nam aliquando una ala, aliquando utraque, et rarius in virginibus quam mulieribus adeo excrescunt, praesertim cum digitis frequenter attrahuntur, aut alias, humores affluunt; ut ob impedimenta, quae sequuntur, excisione opus sit."

64. The medical case collections (*Observationes*) are among the texts relevant to practice. See: Schenck von Grafenberg (1596): obs. LXXXIX. "Mentula Muliebris, Hippocrati Κίων, id est, columella, alijs Clethoris, quibusdam Nympha dicta: recens ex veterum scriptis et neotericorum observatione inventa et descripta." p. 149–157; obs. XCII. "Clethoris seu mentula muliebris Matronae cuidam ad eam deformitatem excrevit, ut collum anserinum, crassitie et longitudine, aequaret." p. 160f.; obs. XCIII. "Mentualae muliebris ubi ad deformem magnitudinem excreverit: velut et Cercosis ex veterum praescripto praesectio." p. 161f.; See also Platter (1614), lib. III, In Deformatione Observationes, p. 550f.: "Hermaphroditus putatus, quia scrotum illius pudendum muliebre nonnihil repraesentabat." and also the case of a distinguished lady, already mentioned above (p. 626), with an excrescentia in the region of the pudenda, which cannot be closely looked at or palpated by Coiter.

65. Operations to reduce hyperthropic female genitalia were already described in detail by Paré; see also Fabrizio da Acquapendente (1666, 277). In "De Hermaphroditis" he describes, after Paul, the nymphotomia practiced by the Egyptians. Da Acquapendente's description of the operation is also adopted by Johannes Schultes (1595–1645). Schultes (1666, 102): "De [...] clitoridis inutiliter auctae abbreviatione [...]" With reference to the 43rd plate and the illustrations contained therein, the instrument used by Fabrizio da Acquapendente to extract polyps is used to remove the clitoris.

66. Severino (1646): cap. XCIII, De Nymphotomia, p. 119f.

67. See ibid. p. 120, where the difficulties in the living (*partim verecundia non licere*) and the restrictions in cadaveric dissection are mentioned (*in mortuis vero abolitas et cassas has partes ut vix vestigia manserint, adstruuntur*).

68. Ibid.: "Convenerunt isti omnes in exscindenda re non inutili solum et ociosa, sed incommoda et permolesta; ita scilicet alienum et praeter naturae modum incrementum illud carnis aestimarunt. Contraria sententia *Gabrielis est Fallopii obseru. anatom.* non qui de amputando aliquid decreverit, sed qui naturalem hanc partem et sexui faemineo communem arbitratus fuerit; [...]." Ibid.: "[arbitratus fuerit]; dissentiente tamen ac repugnante *Andreâ Vesalio, qui in Examine observ. Falloppii, anat.* contendit aut monstrum aut morbum hunc esse."

69. Severino (1646, 120): "sed aliquanto plures sunt, qui Vesalio adhaeserint; è quibus est Hieron. Mercurialis, l.4.de morb. mul. cap. 13. et hunc imitatus sequutusque suppresso nomine autoris Ioannes Schenckius indicato iam loco." North of the Alps—Severino specifies—Volker Coiter (1534–76) had represented Falloppio's position. Coiter (1573, 10): "Virga muliebris, à piae memoriae praeceptore meo Fallopio ex antiquorum Arabum scriptis eruta, virorum peni similis, sed multò minor, et magis occultata, à Sorano et Ruffo κλητορίς, ab Arab: albathar, ab albucasi (sic!) tentigo dicitur: habet suam glandem et praeputium virili proportione respondens: lingua samior: νυμφή."—This passage is also quoted by Schenck von Grafenberg (1596, 153). In the Suda, there is a reference in the lemma Νύμφαι that this is a Samian term for the clitoris: "[...] Σάμιοι γὰρ τὸ ἀνὰ μέσον τῶν γυναικείων αἰδοίων νύμφη καλοῦσι. [...]." In the lemma Νύμφη there is the reference to the passage just mentioned: "[...] Νύμφη γὰρ καλοῦσι καὶ τὸ ἀνὰ μέσον τῶν γυναικείων αἰδοίων, ὡς προσεγράφη."

70. Severino (1646, 120): "Mirum autem non tractatam hanc tractationem à nostris neotericis qui libros operationum Chirurgicarum reliquêre." A detailed description of *nymphotomia* can be found in the surgical work of Falloppio's well-known successor, Girolamo Fabrizio da Acquapendente (1533–1619). Fabrizio da Acquapendente (1666, 276f).

71. Thomas Bartholin also mentions contemporary infibulation practices half a century after de Castro. However, he does not seem to have used de Castro's remarks as a model for this report. Bartholin 1651, lib. I, cap. 31, p. 180: "Si ex petulantia ruperint virgines digito vel alio instrumento. Hinc quidam populi in recens natis foemellis vulvas consuunt, interea spatium exiguum pro egressu urinae relinquentes; nec aperiunt usque ac tempus nuptiarum: tum vero sponsus aperiri curat, ut certo virginem habeat."

72. See e.g. Schurig (1729a) sect. II, cap. II, De nymphis, §9 Nymphotomia (p. 140–142), §10 Circumcisio feminarum (p. 142f.); ders. (1729b): sect. III, cap. IIX, De virginitatis custodia, §1 Per vulvae consutionem (p. 366–368); Osiander (1795, 69–72). On the reception of de Castro's work on women's health, see Gadebusch Bondio/Förg (2020).

73. John Bulwer is known, among other things, for his defence of the rights of the deaf to education and to the recognition of sign language (*Philocopus: or, the Deafe and Dumbe Man Friend* of 1648). Bulwer (1653, 380f.): "In *Ethiopia*, especially in the Dominions of *Prester John*, they Circumcise women. These *Abassines* have added errour upon errour, and sin upon sin, for they cause their Females to be circumcised, whom they call Cophles. A thing which was never practised in Moses Law, neither was there ever found any expresse Commandement to do it; I know not where the Noselesse Moores learned it, for they cut their Females, although they be of marriage estate, taking away a certaine Apophosis, or excrescence of musculous skin that descendeth from the superiour part of the Matrix, which some call *Nympha*, or *Hymenea*, one growing on either side, even so far as the Orifice of the neck of the Bladder, which serve the erection to coition. Many women both here and elsewhere have caused themselves to be cut, as being over-great, and exceeding Nature, but not for any matter of Religion. In all which places it is done by cutting that part which answereth the Prepuce or Foreskin in a man." Bulwer quotes Belon and Giovio here (cf. notes 59 and 57).

WORKS CITED

Primary Sources

Aëtios von Amida. 1542. *Medizinische Bücher.*

Aetii medici graeci contractae ex veteribus medicinae tetrabiblos [...]. Basel: Froben.

Avicenna. 1555. *Liber canonis, de medicinis cordialibus, et cantica, iam olim quidem a Gerardo Carmonensi ex arabico sermone in latinum conuersa.* Venedig: Giunta.

Bartholin, Thomas. 1651. *Anatomia reformata.* Brittenburg: Franciscus Hackius.

Belon, Pierre. 1588. *Les Observations de plusieurs singularitez et choses memorables, trouvees en Grece, Asie, Iudée, Egypte, Arabie, et autres pays estranges.* Paris: Hierosme de Marnef, & la Veuve Guillaume Cavellat, au mont S. Hilaire, à l'enseigne du Pelican. M.

Bembo, Pietro. 1552. *Della Historia Vinitiana [...] libri XII.* Venedig: Scotto.

Bulwer, John. 1653. *Anthropometamorphosis: man transform'd: or, The artificiall changling, historically presented, in the mad and cruell gallantry, foolish bravery, ridiculous beauty, filthy finenesse, and loathsome loveliness of most nations, fashioning and altering their bodies from the mould intended by nature; with figures of those transformations.* London: William Hunt.

Coiter, Volker. 1573. *Externarum et internarum principalium humani corporis partium tabulae.* Nürnberg: Dietrich Gerlach.

Colombo, Realdo. 1559. *De re anatomica libri XV.* Venedig: Bevilacqua.

De Castro, Rodrigo. 1603a. *De universa mulierum medicina, novo et antehac a nemine tentato ordine opus absolutissimum. Et Studiosis omnibus utile, Medicis verò pernecessarium. Pars prima Theorica.* Hamburg: Froben.

De Castro, Rodrigo. 1603b. *De universa mulierum medicina: Pars secunda, sive Praxis*. Hamburg: Froben.
De Castro, Rodrigo. 1614. *Medicus-politicus: Sive de officiis medico-politicis tractatus*. Hamburg: Froben.
De Thevenot, Jean. 1665. *Relation d'un voyage fait au Levant*. Paris: Thomas Iolly.
Fabrizio da Acquapendente, Girolamo. 1666. *Opera Chirurgica*. Padua: Matthei de Cadornis.
Falloppio, Gabriele. 1561. *Observationes anatomicae*. Venice: Marcus Antonius Ulmus.
Galen. *De usu partium*.
Galeni. 1909. *De usu partium libri XVII*, edited by Georg Helmreich. Vol. 2. Leipzig: B.G. Teubner.
Galen. *De uteri dissectione*.
Galen. 1971. *Über die Anatomie der Gebärmutter [Galeni: De uteri dissectione.]*, edited, translated and commented on by Diethard Nickel. (= Corpus Medicorum Graecorum V 2,1) Berlin: Akademie Verlag.
Giovio, Paolo. 1550. *Historiarum sui temporis*. Vol. 1. Florence: L. Torrentini.
Linschoten, Jan Huygen. 1599. *Navigatio Ac Itinerarium [...] In Orientalem Sive Lusitanorum Indiam*. Den Haag: Ægidium Elsevirum.
Lusitano, Amato. 1570. *Cvrationvm Medicinalivm Centuria Septima. Thessalonicae curationes, [...] varia multiplicique doctrina referta*. Lyon: Gulielmus Rovilius.
Mercuriale, Girolamo. 1601. *De morbis mulieribus praelectiones*. Venice: Giunta.
Osiander, Friedrich Benjamin. 1795. *Denkwürdigkeiten für die Heilkunde und Geburtshülfe*. Vol. 2. Göttingen: Vandenhoeck-Ruprechtischer Verlag.
Paré, Ambroise. 1973. *Des monstres et prodiges*, edited by Jean Céard. Geneva: Droz.
Platter, Felix. 1614. *Observationum [...] libri tres*. Basel: Ludwig König.
Schenck von Grafenberg, Johann. 1596. *Observationvm medicarvm [...], liber quartvs, de partibvs genitalibus utriusque sexus [...]*. Freiburg im Breisgau: Martin Böckler.
Schurig, Martin.1729a. *Muliebria historico-medica, hoc est partium genitalium muliebrium consideratio physico-medico-forensis [...]*. Dresden, Leipzig: Hekel.
Schurig, Martin. 1729b. *Parthenologia historico-medica, hoc est, virginitatis consideratio [...]*. Dresden, Leipzig: Hekel.
Schultes, Johannes. 1666. *Armamentarium Chirurgicum bipartitum [...]*. Frankfurt: Johann Görlin.
Severino, Marco Aurelio. 1646. *De efficacy medicina libri III. [...]*. Frankfurt: Johannes Beyer.
Vesal, Andreas. 1543. *De humani corporis fabrica*. Basel: Oporinus.
Vesal, Andreas. 1555. *De humani corporis fabrica*. Basel: Oporinus.
Vesal, Andreas. 1564. *Anatomicarum Gabrielis Fallopii Observationum Examen*. Venice: Franciscus de Franciscis.
Vesal, Andreas. 2014. *The Fabric of the Human Body. An Annotated Translation of the 1543 and 1555 Editions of "De Humani Corporis Fabrica Libri Septem,"* edited by Garrison, Daniel H. and Malcolm H. Hast. Basel: Karger.

Secondary Literature

Blaschke, Andreas. 1998. *Beschneidung: Zeugnisse der Bibel und verwandter Texte*. Tübingen, Basel: Francke.
Borris, Kenneth, ed. 2004. *Same-Sex: Desire in the English Renaissance. A Sourcebook of Texts, 1470–1650*. London/New York: Routledge.
Brooten, Bernadette J. 2020. *Liebe zwischen Frauen: Weibliche Homoerotik in hellenistisch-römischer Zeit und im frühen Christentum*, translated into German by Gerlinde Baumann. Berlin: LIT Verlag.
Cunningham, A. 1988. "William Harvey: The Discovery of the Circulation of the Blood." In *Man Masters Nature: Twenty-Five Centuries of Science*, edited by Roy Porter, 65–76. New York: George Braziller.

Deutsches Ärzteblatt. 2020. Immer mehr Fälle von Genitalverstümmelung in Deutschland. Hamburg 14/12/2020. (https://www.aerzteblatt.de/nachrichten/sw/Genitalverst%FCmmelung?s=&p=1&n=1&nid=119322).

Di Marino, Vincent and Hubert Lepidi. 2014. *Anatomic Study of the Clitoris and the Bulbo-Clitoral Organ*. Heidelberg/Dordrecht/London/New York: Springer.

Donattini, Massimo, Ramusio, Giovanni Battista. 2016. *Dizionario Biografico degli Italiani* 86. (https://www.treccani.it/enciclopedia/giovanni-battista-ramusio_%28Dizionario-Biografico%29/).

Duivenbode, Rosie and Aasim I. Padela. 2019. "Female Genital Cutting (FGC) and the Cultural Boundaries of Medical Practice." *The American Journal of Bioethics* 19, no. 3: 3–6.

Erlich, Michel. 1986. *La Femme blessée: Essai sur les mutilations sexuelles féminines*. Paris: L'Harmattan.

Fögen, Thorsten. 2009. *Wissen, Kommunikation und Selbstdarstellung: Zur Struktur und Charakteristik römischer Fachtexte der frühen Kaiserzeit*. München: C.H. Beck.

Gadebusch Bondio, Mariacarla and Manuel Förg. 2020. "*De mulierum morbis* – Frühneuzeitliche Beiträge zu einer geschlechterspezifischen Medizin." In *Natur – Geschlecht – Politik: Denkmuster und Repräsentationsformen vom Alten Testament bis in die Neuzeit*, edited by Andreas Höfele and Beate Kellner, 217–244. München: Brill/Wilhelm Fink.

Gadebusch Bondio, Mariacarla and Katharina Luise Förg. 2022. "Erkundungen des Fremden: Über ‚korrigierende' Eingriffe an den weiblichen *pudenda* in der vormodernen Medizin." *Medizinhistorisches Journal* 57, no. 1: 2–35.

Gillespie, Gannon. 2015. "FGC? FGM? Female circumcision? Why Language Matters in Helping Communities Abandon Harmful Practices." Tostan International (03/02/2015). (https://www.tostan.org/fgc-fgm-female-circumcision-why-language-matters-helping-communities-abandon-harmful-practices/.)

Green, Monica H. 2009. *Making Women's Medicine Masculine: The Rise of Male Authority in Pre-Modern Gynaecology*. Oxford: Oxford University Press.

Huebner, Sabine. 2009. "Female Circumcision as a Rite de Passage in Egypt – Continuity through the Millennia?" *Journal of Egyptian History* 2: 149–171.

Johnsdotter, Sara. 2012. "Projected Cultural Histories of the Cutting of Female Genitalia: A Poor Reflection as in a Mirror." *History and Anthropology* 23, no. 1: 91–114.

Karim, Mahmoud. 1997. *Female Genital Mutilation: Historical, Social, Religious and Legal Aspects*. Cairo: Ain Shams University.

King, Helen. 2013. *The One Sex Body on Trial: The Classical and Early Modern Evidence*. Farnham: Routledge.

Knight, Mary. 2001. "Curing Cut or Ritual Mutilation? Some Remarks on the Practice of Female and Male Circumcision in Graeco-Roman Egypt." *Isis* 92, no. 2: 317–338.

Kölling, Anna. 2008. *Weibliche Genitalverstümmelung im Diskurs: Exemplarische Analysen zu Erscheinungsformen, Begründungsmustern und Bekämpfungsstrategien*. Berlin: LIT.

Laqueur, Thomas. 1989."Amor Veneris, vel Dulcedo Appeletur." In *Fragments for a History of the Human Body*.Vol. 3, edited by Michael Feher, 91–131. New York: Zone.

Laqueur, Thomas. 1990. *Making Sex: Body and Gender from Greeks to Freud*. Cambridge: Harvard University Press.

Leven, Karl-Heinz. 2005. "Beschneidung." In *Antike Medizin: Ein Lexikon*, edited by Karl-Heinz Leven, 145. München: C.H. Beck.

Lochrie, Karma. 2005. *Heterosyncrasies: Female Sexuality When Normal Wasn't*. Minneapolis: University of Minnesota Press.

Manuli, Paola and Mario Vegetti. 1977. *Cuore, sangue e cervello: Biologia e antropologia nel pensiero antico*. Mailand: Petite Plaisance.

Mathes, Bettina. 2003. "As Long as a Swan's Neck? The Significance of the 'Enlarged' Clitoris for Early Modern Anatomy." In *Sensible Flesh: On Touch in Early Modern Culture*, edited by Elizabeth D. Harvey, 103–124. Philadelphia: University of Pennsylvania Press.

Nurka, Camille. 2019. *Female Genital Cosmetic Surgery: Deviance, Desire and the Pursuit of Perfection*. Cham: Palgrave Macmillan.

Nussbaum, Martha C. 1999. *Sex and Social Justice*. Oxford: Oxford University Press.

Nutton, Vivian. 2012. "Vesalius Revised: His Annotations to the 1555 *Fabrica*." *Medical History* 56, no. 4: 415–443.

Park, Katharine. 1997. "The Rediscovery of the Clitoris: French Medicine and the Tribade 1570–1620." In *The Body in Parts: Fantasies of Corporeality in Early Modern Europe*, edited by David Hillman, and Carla Mazzio, 171–193. New York/London: Routledge.

Santos Pinheiro, Cristina. 2021. "From Flesh to Text: The Chapters on the Uterus and Its Parts in Roderigo de Castro's *De universa mulierum medicina*." *Ágora: Estudios Clássicos em Debate* 23, no. 1: 293–317.

Sauerteig, Lutz. 2005. "Klitoris." In *Antike Medizin: Ein Lexikon*, edited by Karl-Heinz Leven, 504. München: C.H. Beck.

Stolberg, Michael. 2003. "A Woman Down to Her Bones: The Anatomy of Sexual Difference in the Sixteenth and Early Seventeenth Centuries." *Isis* 94, no. 2: 274–299.

Stamatu, Marion. 2005. "Geschlechtsorgane." In *Antike Medizin: Ein Lexikon*, edited by Karl-Heinz Leven, 343–345. Munich: C.H. Beck.

Stringer, Mark D. and Ines Becker. 2010. "Colombo and the Clitoris." *European Journal of Obstetrics and Gynecology and Reproductive Biology* 151, no 2: 130–133.

Tedeschi Salvatore. 1985. "Paolo Giovio e la Conoscenza dell'Etiopia nel Rinascimento." In *Atti del Convegno Paolo Giovio: Il Rinascimento e la Memoria. Como 3–5 guigno 1983*, 93–116. Como: Società storica comense.

United Nations Children's Fund (UNICEF): Female Genital Mutilation/Cutting: A Global Concern. New York 2016. (https://www.unicef.org/media/files/FGMC_2016_brochure_final_UNICEF_SPREAD.pdf).

Van der Lugt, Maaike. 2001. "The *Incubus* in Scholastic Debate: Medicine, Theology and Popular Belief." In *Religion and Medicine in the Middle Ages*, edited by Peter Biller and Joseph Ziegler, 175–200. Woodbridge: York Medieval Press.

Von Engelhardt, Dietrich. 2020. "Amato Lusitano (1511–1568): Leben und Werk eines verfolgten Botanikers und Arztes auf der Flucht von Portugal ins Osmanische Reich." In *Menschennatur in Zeiten des Umbruchs: Das Ideal des politischen Arztes in der frühen Neuzeit*, edited by Mariacarla Gadebusch Bondio, Christian Kaiser, and Manuel Förg, 115–139. Berlin: De Gruyter Oldenbourg.

Von Staden, Heinrich. 1991. "Apud nos foediora verba: Celsus' Reluctant Construction of the Female Body." In *Le latin médical: La constitution d´un langage scientifique*, edited by G. Sabbah, 271–296. Saint Étienne: Publications de l'Université de Saint-Etienne.

World Health Organization. 2008. Eliminating Female Genital Mutilation: An Interagency Statement - UNAIDS, UNDP, UNECA, UNESCO, UNFPA, UNHCHR, UNHCR, UNICEF, UNIFEM, WHO. (https://apps.who.int/iris/bitstream/handle/10665/43839/9789241596442_eng.pdf?sequence=1&isAllowed=y).

World Health Organization. 2021. Prevalence of Female Genital Mutilation. (https://www.who.int/reproductivehealth/topics/fgm/prevalence/en/).

CHAPTER SEVENTEEN

Establishing a New Order? Queer Performativity, Embodied Precarity, and the Pathologization of the Transgressive Body in *Melusine* (1456) and *Fortunatus* (1509)

BENJAMIN R. DAVIS

From *Landesordnungen* to *Kleiderordnungen* to *Kirchenordnungen* to regulations on court life and the like, the idea of *Ordnung* was important to maintaining and enforcing the seemingly inseparable and indistinguishable triad of religious, political, and social order in the early modern era (Dingel and Kohnle, 2014). While *gute Ordnung* was intended to maintain a stable society in a pragmatic manner rooted in Christian doctrine, it is clear both in the literary imaginary and the historical record that such strict control of social order was challenged if not outright rejected in lived experience. Natalie Zemon Davis (1975, 131) shows us how women could use their perceived inherent disorderliness to their advantage to invert the social-sexual order in times of festivals and beyond in an effort not to reaffirm the standard of social order, but rather to undermine it and to create a wider set of behavioral options for women in the early modern era. Scientific discourse, too, suggested that socio-sexual order was a fluid concept, despite its attempts to confirm perceived male dominance. Thomas

Laqueur, critiques of his theory notwithstanding (see, for example, Park, 1997; Cislo, 2010), argues that "at least two genders correspond to but one sex, where the boundaries between male and female are of degree and not kind, and where the reproductive organs are but one sign among many of the body's place in a cosmic and cultural order that transcends biology" (1992, 25). Indeed, this was an attempt by scientists to confirm the male and the masculine as the perfect, fully expressed human form, but inversions and perversions of "perfection" challenged that very notion. Todd Reeser (2006), for example, argues that understandings of hegemonic masculinity in the early modern period are dependent on "scapegoats of nonmasculinity" (20) who are marked in terms of absence or excess. Despite such attempts to render manifestations of gender variance as "scraps of dominant masculinity in order that male masculinity may appear to be the real thing" (Halberstam 1998, 1), their mockery of dominant modes of masculinity, marked in terms of moderation and nonperformativity, encourages us to probe those very foundations of what upheld gender-based power in the early modern era. If we consider masculinities in the plural, then indeed we must question what mode was the "original." But these challenges to hegemonic order extend to and are pervasive in the literary landscape as well. In this article I will focus on two textual examples, *Melusine* (1456) and *Fortunatus* (1509) which present challenges to *gute Ordnung*, by serving as examples where wealth and social power are acquired through strange manners in the absence of *Land und Leut*.[1] Traditional means of wealth accumulation are called into question and the texts attempt to promote new conceptions of generational wealth in the early modern era (Rohrman 1975; Classen 2000; Classen 2015). Building on these arguments, I suggest that the texts transgress established order in a queer manner, whereby precarious bodies acquire value, but not without a cost. The transgressive bodies of the titular figures become pathologized in an attempt to reverse the non-normative values these bodies represent.

To understand the applicability of queer theory to early modern texts, an explanation of my usage of "queer" is in order. Building on Carla Freccero's (2006) and José Esteban Muñoz's work (1999, 2009), I am using "queer" as a flexible position of resistance to social and sexual binaries; a position that in its indeterminacy and resistance of rigidity configures change and imagines other ways of being in the world. Indeed, following Sarah Ahmed, "[t]he queer orientation might not simply be directed toward the 'same sex,' but would be seen as not following the straight line" (2006, 7). My usage does not intend to examine same-sex desire in these texts, but rather posits that these *Prosaromane* refuse to follow the dominant straight line of "*gute Ordnung*" as the superior and default mode of being in the early modern world and that they do so through breaking down and calling into question the binaries of sex and gender in order to imagine something new. Indeed, according to Muñoz, "[q]ueerness is essentially about the rejection of the here and now and an insistence on potentiality or concrete possibility for another world" (2009, 1). In these texts other worlds are created where money and power stem from magical and supernatural sources closely tied to sexual transgressions (Wailes 1986; Williams 1991), indeed, advancing on these arguments, transgressions of the queer, corporeal type. But how does one conceive of queer ways of being in the early modern literary world as liberating when at the end "*gute Ordnung*" is seemingly restored through the pathologization of such transgressions? The key, as Muñoz points out, is to look beyond the here and now and to orient toward a future potential: "Unlike a possibility, a thing that simply might happen, a potentiality is a certain mode of nonbeing that is eminent, a thing that is present but not actually existing in the present tense" (2009, 9). While order is seemingly restored in our texts, the potential to disrupt it is present, even if not fully articulated or actualized. This potential creates narrative ruptures and poses a threat to the established order such that the body, as a sign of this potential, becomes the exact space that is marked in its nonconformity. Consequently, these transgressive bodies risk being viewed as a failure.

Yet queer potential can be connected to acts of failure or loss in a seemingly contradictory, productive manner. Jack Halberstam's *The Queer Art of Failure* (2011) argues that while normative ways of being in the world are often associated with success, interrogating acts of failure, which have often been considered unproductive, can provide insights into new ways of being in the world, of community building, and of knowledge creation. Halberstam states: "The queer art of failure turns on the impossible, the improbable, the unlikely, and the unremarkable. It quietly loses, and in losing it imagines other goals for life, for love, for art, and for being" (2011, 88). In short, under certain circumstances, where challenges to social and sexual binaries are present, failure can be read as a means of queer productivity, or as another way to establish queer potential, despite efforts to render such potential as invisible or devalued. Connecting failure to queerness allows us, according to Halberstam: "[to] recognize failure as a way of refusing to acquiesce to dominant logics of power and discipline and as a form of critique. As a practice, failure recognizes that alternatives are embedded already in the dominant and that power is never total or consistent; indeed, failure can exploit the unpredictability of ideology and its indeterminate qualities" (2011, 88). The connection of narratives of success to normative power structures invites us to interrogate those always-already present alternatives—the queer "losers" lurking on the margins and questioning established "truths."

In our *Prosaromanen, Melusine* (1456) and *Fortunatus* (1509), one way the queer art of failure, and queerness more general, emerges is by the introduction of magical elements in the texts. Through the presence of magic, social and moral binaries collapse to the point that characters find themselves in a space of productive liminality that is connected to queer sexual and bodily economies. As such we can view failure in the early modern world not merely by way of negative example (which could be assumed by the return to apparent normativity in the works) but rather also on the basis of the *productive potential* it might engender. We have to ask ourselves, quoting Halberstam: "What happens when failure is productively linked to ... gender variance and different formulations of the temporality of success?" (2011, 92). Indeed, what happens when queer failure becomes associated with nonconformativity and critique in a way that works with, against, and on dominant ideology in order to transform and create (Muñoz 1999)?

MELUSINE

Thüring von Ringoltingen's 1456 *Melusine,* which depicts the founding of the noble house of Lusignan, demonstrates what occurs when *gute Ordnung* is abandoned. Chaos seemingly ensues, monstrous and grotesque elements enter the scene, and social and sexual transgressions occur. All of these consequences suggest we examine the intersection of the magical and the natural and the human and the monstrous as a space where queer potential and possibility can be realized, building upon how Scholz Williams characterizes magic in the early modern era: "Magie steht für Wissen, Forschen, für das Eindringen in die Geheimhisse des Universums; und Magie steht für Macht über die Natur, über den Menschen, über die Geister" ["Magic represents knowledge, discovery, penetration into the secrets of the universe; and magic represents power over nature, over people, over spirits"] (1991, 81–82).[2] Indeed, Melusine and Reymund create a magical world that abandons traditional understanding of lineage and heritage—a concept that was key to upholding social order at the time.

The connection between transgression, sex, and magic is important in *Melusine*, but Reymund's acts of transgression are quite peculiar in their relationship to queer failure and potential. Reymund's failures initially correspond to gender variance that leads to prosperity and a re-configuration of social order as determined by Melusine. As Scholz Williams states "[Melusine] hat nichts Geringeres zum Ziel, als die dynastische Bräuche und die vassalische Ordnung im Lande des Grafen von Poitiers grundsätzlich zu verändern" ["Melusine has no other goal than to fundamentally change the dynastic customs and the vassalistic order in the Count of Poitiers' lands"] (1991, 93). This new order is maintained through magic, the marriage contract, and Melusine's performance of female masculinity. When Reymund voids the marriage contract through his visual betrayal of Melusine, he becomes astutely aware of the queerness upon which this new order depends. Reymund is initially able to overcome the distress brought on by this awareness, but it ultimately proves too much as he exposes both himself and Melusine to the world.

Reymund's first transgression, accidentally killing his uncle on the hunt, occurs quite early in the text. This act leaves him in a vulnerable position where he sacrifices his current societal position in an attempt to atone for his sin—he is no position to return to his family and laments his transgression, continuing to wander awry, leading to his first encounter with Melusine. Distraught and in a state of shock, Reymund spots Melusine, an apparently beautiful woman of noble heritage and stature, near the magical space of a well. Reymund finds himself trapped in the borderlands, somewhere between life and death: "Da Reymund die Edle schöne Jungfrauwe ersahe, da erschracke er, und wusste nicht, ob er lebendig oder todt was, oder ob das ein Gespenst oder ein Frauw was" ["Reymund became terrified as he laid eyes on the noble and beautiful maiden, and he did not know if he was living or dead, or if it was a ghost or a woman"] (11). The state of confusion brought about by committing the cardinal sin of killing his family member renders Reymund weak of mind. Indeed, unable to return home and mourn the death of his uncle out of fear that he would be accused, Reymund finds himself without a home, on the boundary of order and disorder, where his queer potential can be realized and where "the time is out of joint."[3] Melusine takes advantage of Reymund's disposition and offers him riches and power beyond his expectations if he marries her: "Reymund, ich weiss deine noht und klage, und das ungefell, das dir zu dieser stund an deinem Herren unnd Vettern widerfahren ist … unnd wenn du meiner Lehr wilt folgen unnd nachkommen, so sol dir Gut, Ehr, Glücks unnd Gelts nimmermehr gebresten …" ["Reymund, I am aware of your distress and lamentation, and the current misfortune that befell you regarding your lord and cousin. But if you follow and comply with my teachings, you will never want for land, honor, happiness, and money"] (12). Melusine offers Reymund an escape (and herself as well if you recall her own past), however, only under the condition that he marries her and remains obedient to her will. Her offer of marriage comes with an important stipulation: he is not allowed to look for her on Saturdays at the risk of losing the prosperity that she promises him: "Reymund, ist es sach, dass du mir nicht leistet oder heltest, das du mir gelobet unnd geschworen hast, so solt du mich warlich verlieren, und mich nimmermehr gesehen, und es wirdt darnach deinen Kindern und Erben fast missgehen ..." ["Reymund, it is settled, that if you do not carry out and hold true to what you have sworn, you will truly lose me, and never see me again, and matters will turn bad for your children and heirs"] (14). With these words Melusine creates a marriage contract that is based on bodily control and control of the gaze.[4] This contract is created and determined solely by Melusine, suggesting that here, on the edge of the magical and natural space, social power structures are inverted. Indeed, now, as throughout their marriage, Melusine plays an active role while Reymund assumes a passive role.

In such an arrangement the noble house is founded and the union is prosperous and (re) productive. Indeed their children travel across the world from East to West to expand the noble house. But all is not as orderly as it seems as the text hints that something is strange and queer within the marriage in regard to bodily integrity and visibility. All but two of their children have a certain bodily deformation to them. Uta Störmer-Caysa states: "Melusines Kinder tragen beide Naturen in sich, und man sieht es ihnen—anders als Melusine—allzeit an. Anna Mühlherr hat das auf die schöne Formel gebracht, die Familie sei 'gezeichnet' und 'ausgezeichnet' zugliech" ["Melusine's children carry both natures in them, and it is always visible, as opposed to Melusine. Anna Mühlherr formulated it nicely: the family is marked and distinguished at the same time"] (1999, 245). The process of marking the children shows the sign of the mother and her supernatural qualities being passed on through to her children, highlighting her dual nature. While Melusine is able to hide her own bodily disorderliness, the hybrid nature of her and Reymund's created world is projected and marked onto the bodies of their sons: "Doch was [ihr erster Sohns] Angesicht nicht schön, sondern einer seltzamen form unnd gestalt, denn er war gar Kurtz und breyt, und flach under den Augen ..." ["But still her first son's face was not fair, rather it was of a peculiar form and shape, it was very short and wide and flat under the eyes"] (31). Others are also portrayed with a marked body, be it through a red marking on the face, one eye being placed slightly above the other, having only one eye, one elongated tooth, and the like.[5] The text is quite clear to note that their bodies, aside from the faces, are for the most part quite unremarkable (31–34). Thus, the text suggests that these sons represent a sort of hybrid identity—albeit a different one than that of Melusine. Unlike their mother, the sons are forced to confront their othered bodies at every moment which comments further on the inverted order in the text. While the passive Reymund believes himself to be in marital bliss, his anxieties are presented to him directly, that is on the faces of his sons. The hybrid nature of the family as human and mythical, masculine and feminine continues to be engendered in terms of the body when Melusine's truth is revealed to him and a rigid separation ensues.

The prosperity born out of failure and loss and contingent on control of the body does not, however, last forever. Reymund is convinced by the Graf vom Forst, a skeptic of Melusine and the reconfigured order, that his wife might be committing acts of adultery on Saturdays. Reymund loses control of his emotions and becomes pale and enraged; he decides to examine the situation:

> er machet mit sinem Schwerdt ein Loch durch die Thür ... Reymundt sahe durch das Loch hineyn und sahe, dass sein Weib im Bad nacket sass, sie war oberhalb dem nabel ein schön Weiblich Bild, und von Leib und Angesicht gantz schön aber von dem Nabel hinab war sie ein grosser langer und ungehewer Wurmschwantz ...
>
> (70–71)

> [He made a hole through the door with his sword ... Reymund looked in through the hole and saw his wife sitting naked in the bath. She was the picture of a beautiful woman from navel up, her body and face truly beautiful, but below the navel she had a large, long, monstrous serpent tail ...]

The scene is marked in voyeuristic terms with the emphasis on the gaze as Melusine's othered body is put on display. Despite being an enraged, jealous husband, Reymund nevertheless hides his body from Melusine's sight when he peeps through the hole to discover her secret. This incident proves to be a key turning point in Reymund's understanding of his Self (Classen 2004), an understanding, though, that is engendered in queer bodily anxieties. With the secret revealed, Reymund reacts astoundingly: "Reymundt, da er nun diese greußliche und gar frembde Geschöpff an seinem Gemahel sahe, da ward er gar sehr bekümmert, und von allem seinem Gemüt betrübet, unnd erschracke sehr von diesem Gesicht, und stund also vor forcht in grosen sorgen, das im der schweiss vor angst außgienge ..." ["Reymund, having seen his wife in this ghastly and completely foreign form, became very distressed and deeply saddened all over. He was terrified by this image, and stood in such fear and great worry, that sweat poured out of him"] (72). Reymund's frightened disposition is the result of confronting the fragmented body. Describing the theoretical implications of such bodies with the example of Medusa, Lennard J. Davis (1995, 132) argues that

> [s]he is the necessary counter in the dialectic of beauty and ugliness, desire and repulsion, wholeness and fragmentation. This intersection [of a normal and disabled body] is marked by the power of the visual. The "normal" person sees the disabled person and is turned to stone, in some sense, by the visual interaction. In this moment, the normal person suddenly fees self-conscious, rigid, unable to look but equally drawn to look. The visual field becomes problematic, dangerous, treacherous ... [the disabled body] provides a caution about the body as a construct held together willfully, always threatening to become its individual parts.

Reymund, in essence, turns to stone when gazing at Melusine's body as the means of his new found prosperity is revealed; feelings of bliss change to fear and anxiety and manifest in the loss of control of his own bodily functions. The visualization of Melusine's bodily transformations had previously been under strict control through the marriage contract, but now that Reymund subverts this contract, her body becomes the space where his own anxieties are projected, where his subjecthood is both constituted and threatened (Huot 2003, 412). Indeed, with her plan to hide her bodily fragmentation foiled, the body becomes a further site of pathologization, blamed for all misfortune, and the visual representation of disorder.

Immediately following this voyeuristic act, Reymund begins to panic. His failures have up to this point been engendered, and hidden, in terms of productive non-normativity. Yet now his failures are revealed to him through the sight of Melusine's visibly fragmented, queer body and this revelation emphasizes his own non-normativity, so tightly bound to Melusine, before proving detrimental. He laments:

> Und vor leyd und jammer zog er sich auß, und legt sich an ein Bett, unnd weynet bitterlich, unnd sprach: "Ach Melusina, sol ich dich verlieren, so wil ich doch durch die Wüste fahren, unnd mich gantz und gar von der Welt thun, und ein Einsidel oder Münch werden, und mich der Welt nichts annemmen." Solche klage triebe er den gantzen Tag und die lange nacht ohn aufhören ...
>
> (73)
>
> [In his suffering and misery, he undressed and laid down in bed, crying bitterly, and spoke: "Oh Melusine, if I were to lose you, I would travel through the desert, turn away from the world, and become a hermit or monk, and accept nothing else from this world." Such lamentations continued the whole day and long night, without end ...]

The male body is not merely desexualized by the reference to a monastic and reclusive life, but also related to a sense of passivity. Reymund strips his body and remains lying in bed, crying and lamenting in this marked sexualized space, which was previously so fruitful. The relationship between his desexualized desires and sexualized passive body is striking in the narrator's description:

> In dem so kompt Melusina, unnd entschloß mit einem Schlüssel die Kammer, und gienge hineyn zu Reymunden, und schloss hinder ihr wider zu, und zog sich gar nackendt auß, und leget sich also wieder zu ihm an sein Bett, unnd küsset und umbfieng ihn gar tugendtlich, sie befande auch wol, dass er sehr kalt, unnd vor leyd und unmut ungesundt wordern war, denn er war gar verkehrt.
>
> (73–74)
>
> [And so Melusine came and unlocked the room with a key and went inside to Reymund, locking the door behind her. She undressed fully naked and laid down with Reymund in his bed. She kissed and embraced him virtuously and discovered that he was very cold and sick from distress and unhappiness. He was completely amiss.]

Melusine shows not only control of bodies but also of space, as she marches into the room and plays the active, healer role in this sexualized scene. Ahmed reminds us that:

> Bodies take the shape of norms that are repeated over time and with force. Through repeating some gestures and not others, or through being oriented in some directions and not others, bodies become contorted: they get twisted into shapes that enable some action *only in so far as they restrict the capacity for other kinds of action.*
>
> (2006, 91)

Up to this point, Melusine's control over Reymund's body enables him prosper in their created world, but this means giving up the old world completely, which, it turns out, he is unable to do. Melusine mentions nothing of the scene of exposure although she knows that he has seen her dual body and turns her attention to bringing Reymund back to their world created out of queer potential as her fragmented, grotesque, female body demonstrates more control than the perceived complete body.

The attempt to reconcile their world is unsuccessful. Reymund betrays her after discovering that one of his sons, Goffroy, has burned down the cloister where one of his other sons, Freymund, was living. Goffroy's reasoning is the supposed feminization of his brother in the cloister which drives him to burn it down and kill all of the monks therein (80–81). Reymund blames this heinous act on Melusine's monstrosity and reveals her secret to all. Melusine, however, does not leave quietly. Just as Melusine had control at the beginning of the text with the creation of the marriage contract, so too does she at the end of it all. She flips the script, stating: "Du schendlicher ehrloser Schalk und Bösewicht, aller untreuw voll, Du meineydiger und falscher Ritter, wie hast du mir gehalten, wie hast du so lästerlich unnd schendtlich dein Gelübd, Ehr und Lob ubersehen" ["You disgraceful and dishonorable rogue and wretch, full of disloyalty, you perjurious and false knight! Oh, how you treated me, how you so blasphemously and disgracefully lost sight of your vow, honor, and accolade!"] (87). Reymund's failure again comes to the fore as he is also chided for breaking the contract which produced prosperity. Again, it is Reymund's incompleteness and fragmentation that is being emphasized und juxtaposed against Melusine's visibly fragmented torso. This fragmentation had been the source of their queer order, in which Reymund is unable to continue. Melusine not only brings Reymund's fragmented nature to the forefront, but also foretells the downfall of Reymund's fortunes in her farewell speech. Perhaps the most telling of her predictions is that Reymund will have to kill one of their sons in order to remain prosperous, at least for a while (88). Her absence, in effect, requires a sacrifice of the masculine, here a son, which once again underlies the inversion of gender roles in the *Prosaroman* and the precarious potentiality of their queer world. Melusine departs in a spectacle-like fashion which forces the entire community to confront their bodily—be it the social or material—anxieties. The narrator describes her departure: "Melusine die schoß durch den Lufft schnelle, unnd umbfuhre das Schloß dreymahl, unnd ließ zu jedem mahl einen grossen schrey, gar zumahl erbärmlichen, unnd schoß also durch den Lufft hin schnell, dass von stundt darncach alles Volck noch niemandt sie mehr gesehen mochten." ["Melusine shot quickly through the air and circled the castle three times and each time she let out an enormous, particularly wretched scream, and bolted through the air quickly, that from that moment on, no one would ever see her again"] (92). By revealing her serpent body to the entire population and encircling her territory one final time, Melusine again presents herself as superior, although she ultimately leaves the story. The spectacle in this instance serves to remind the entire community of Reymund's betrayal and at the same time confronts them with the visible sign of the Other. While the queer world crumbles, the text, in its representation of the body and gender, points to both the precarity of power and the queer possibility transgressions engender, particularly when connected to the magical realm.

FORTUNATUS

While queer potential is connected to sexual and bodily economies in *Melusine, Fortunatus* connects it more markedly to the rising money economy and bourgeois consciousness (Rohrmann 1975; Moser 1999; Classen 2000). Even if larger socioeconomic shifts take center stage in the tale, the text still connects such developments to bodily control and the binary of success/failure. Halberstam reminds us that capitalism always has its winners and losers: "Failure goes hand in hand with capitalism ... [it] requires that everyone live in a system that equates success with profit and links failure to the inability to accumulate wealth" (2011, 88). Failure becomes "a hidden history of pessimism, a history moreover that lies quietly behind every story of success" (88). Beyond the central role of money in the text, *Fortunatus* challenges acceptable means of productivity and forces us to question what happens when productivity emerges from perceived failure queerly tied to gender variance and (bodily) loss.

Fortunatus tells the life story of the titular character as he abandons his family home, travels the known and unknown world, experiences wealth and loss, and is aided by magical elements on his journeys. Fortunatus leaves his parents in Cyprus to ease the burden on his family after his father squanders their wealth. He enters the service of the Count of Flanders where he wins his favor and excels in all courtly matters—in short, he finds himself comfortable and content with tradition. However, Fortunatus' fellow servants become jealous and attempt to craft a plan to encourage him to leave. Rupert, a fellow servant, claims that if Fortunatus stays with the count, he will be castrated which shocks and frightens Fortunatus:

> Fortunatus sprach/ "wer solliches beger/so wölle got das es ym widerfar/ich will nicht Darvon hören sagen/unnd der mir die wal gäb/ob ich mir ließ außschneiden/das ich künig zu Fracnckreich wär/oder unverschnitten müßt bettlen gan/und ain nacht nit ligen/so bedörfft ich kaynes radts noch darauff mich zu bedencken. Ich wolt ee bettlen gan ..."
>
> (17)

> [Fortunatus spoke: "Whoever desires that, may God let it befall them! I do not want to hear any of that, and if I were given the choice to be castrated and become the King of France or to be a beggar while still intact, I would not need to consider any advice. I would become a beggar ..."]

For Fortunatus the threat to his masculinity is clearly more pressing than living a comfortable life connected to loss and stagnation, and he determines to leave the court. Fortunatus' mobility brings the focus of the text to a non-traditional economic order where power and security are connected to a sexual economy of potency. Wailes comments: "The metaphorical linkage of sexual and financial potency through the imagery of scrotum and purse was part of the literary culture of the late Middle Ages, with a marked presence in the narrative of eastern Bavaria during the fifteenth and sixteenth centuries" (1986, 11). Indeed, it is Fortunatus' body that plays a central role in his negotiations of a burgeoning economic mobility.

Having determined to leave the count, and the associated comforts, Fortunatus lands in London where he squanders all of his money on prostitutes and other vices: "alles [was] verthon mit schönen frawen/und die schönen frawen tailten es mit den buoben/tailten es so lang und vie byß doch Fortunato noch sinen gesellen kain gelt im sechel belayb …" ["Everything was wasted on beautiful women, who shared it with their knaves, to the point that neither Fortunatus nor his companions had any more money in their sacks"] (23). Fortunatus once again faces an attack on his *seckel.* He leaves Flanders out of fear of stagnation, loss, and impotency, but falls victim to his very potency in London where it is evident that he fails to navigate the money economy. While we could view these failures in terms of a negative example, the ensuing episodes indicate ways in which failure can be both positive and productive. After leaving London, Fortunatus finds himself in a predicament. While lost and starving in a forest, he is attacked by a bear that he ultimately kills before drinking its blood: "Mit erschrockem hertzen stig er herab/unnd nam seinen tegen/und stach yn in den beren/legt seinen mund auf die wunden und sauget das warm bluot in sich/das ym ein wenig krafft gab/und gedacht ym/'het ich yetzund ain feür/ich wölt mich des hungers wol erweren'" ["He climbed down with a frightened heart and took out his dagger and stabbed it into the bear. He put his mouth on the wound and drank the warm blood, which gave him a bit of strength, and he thought, 'If I had a fire, I could also sate my hunger'"] (44–45). Just as Reymund finds himself in a state of shock after his failure, so too does Fortunatus. Both instances are also uniquely connected to animality and a dissolving sense of social order. But, as Mara Wade (2016) has pointed out, the scene references a Germanic ritual where drinking bear's blood is a testament of masculinity, thus an attempt to restore order. Yet it is here on the margins of society where not only magic is present, but also where gender variance and queer elements of the text push the boundaries of the normative.

The similarities between the tales of Reymund and Fortunatus continue as Fortunatus forges a new path back into the social world with the help of magic and a mysterious female figure. Lady Fortuna offers him the choice among six virtues: wisdom, wealth, strength, health, beauty, or long life. Fortunatus selects wealth: "Allso bedachte er sich nit lang und sprach/'so beger ich reichtumb/das ich alweg gelts gnuog hab'/tzu stund zoch sy herfür ainen sechel und gab den Fortunato …" ["He did not ponder it too long and said, 'I desire wealth, then, so that I will always have enough money.' At that moment she pulled forth a sack and gave it to Fortunatus"] (46). Fortunatus does not hesitate at all, his choice of wealth seems to follow natural impulse as opposed to rational ideals. The *seckel* that Fortuna provides him is a double signifier of power, both sexual and economic. Fortuna bestows upon him all that he has lost (in London) or fears losing (in Flanders). As such the magical source emphasizes his past and potential future failures and points to a fluid understanding of social power and gender, in that it is connected to a female allegorical figure with the ability to provide a key signifier of masculinity. Fortunatus' sexual and social power, however, does not come without conditions:

> "Du solt auff den tag feyeren/uff den tag kain eelich werk volbringen/unnd auff den tag alle jar in wölchem land du seyest/frag haben/wo ain armer man ain tochter hab die manber sey ir gern ainen man gäbe unnd es vor armuot nit vermag/die soltu eerlich klaiden ihren vater und muoter und sy begaben und erfreüwen mit vierhundert stuck goldes des selben lands werschafft ..."
>
> (47)
>
> ["On this day you should celebrate, abstain from sex, and wherever you find yourself, search for a poor man with a marriageable daughter who would like to provide her with a husband, but is too poor to do so. You should clothe her honorably and delight both the daughter and parents with four hundred pieces of gold in the currency of their land ..."]

Fortuna insists that Fortunatus abstain from sexual activity at least one day throughout the year and to provide a dowry for a poor woman. Once again control of the body, in *Fortunatus* more temporary, reminds him yearly of the source of his (re)productivity. As such the economy of social and sexual power in Fortunatus' new subjectivity toward the world is both masculine (in its signification) and feminine (in its source and control), indeed both queer and born out of failure.

But this new subjectivity does not go unquestioned. Traditional notions of order, power, and wealth attempt to reestablish themselves in a scene where Fortunatus attempts to purchase some horses with his new found wealth. Consequences of transgressing order ensue, as Fortunatus outbids a noble lord. In doing so, Fortunatus exposes himself as a fraud: he has no material goods, nor servants, yet he contests the wishes of the lord. Fortunatus' transgression against social order does not go unnoticed nor unpunished. The lord claims that the money Fortunatus found belongs to him since it was "found" on his land and wishes to punish Fortunatus: "Der graff sprach/'mir ligt nicht daran das du es nit gewißset hast/has du nit gehört? Wer nit waißt der soll fragen/unnd kurtz richt dich darnach/heüt nym ich dir als dein guot und morgen das leben.'" ["The count spoke, 'It does not matter to me if you did not know, didn't you hear? Whoever does not know should ask. Simply put, prepare yourself: today I will take your goods and tomorrow your life'"] (51). With his life threatened, Fortunatus begs for forgiveness and is released. He only dares to use the sack again at a far distance from the count.

Fortunatus becomes more moderate and careful with the use of his sack until, on his travels through the West, Fortunatus' queer potential is figuratively attacked. One innkeeper is a thief and decides to steal Fortunatus' money. He sneaks into Fortunatus' room at night and cuts off his seckel. Fortunatus responds with anguish:

> Doch so was der schreck so groß gewesen, das er so bald nitt wider zů seiner farb noch stercke kommen mocht vnd blib also den tag still ligen. Lüpoldus wolt yn trösten vnd

> sprach: O herr, gehabt üch nit so übel. wir haben noch schöne roß, silberin ketten, guldin ring vnd andere klainat vnd so wir nit gelt haben, wöllen wir eüch mit der hilff gotes auch wol haim helffen ... Fortunatus redett gar onmechtigklich vnd sprach: wer das gůt verlürt, der verlürt die vernunfft. Weißhait wär zuerwölen für reichtumb, stercke, gesunthait, schöne, langes leben, das mag man kaim stelen vnd darmit swig er.
>
> (68)
>
> [But his shock was so intense, that he could not regain his color nor strength, and he remained bedridden the entire day. Leopold wanted to comfort him and spoke, "Oh Sir, do not perceive matters so horribly. We still have our fair horses, silver chains, golden rings, and other jewels. Even though we do not have money, with the help of God, we will get you home" ... Fortunatus spoke faintly, "He who loses his possessions, loses his reason. I should have chosen wisdom instead of riches, strength, health, beauty, or long life, for no one can steal it." With that, he fell silent.]

The *seckel* provides Fortunatus with his new precarious identity and without it (or its secret exposed) he becomes weak and pale. He regrets choosing wealth and this incident brings about a moment of self-realization that exposes the unstable potential of Fortunatus' power.

With his queer potential exposed, Fortunatus eventually returns to Cyprus where he loses his mentor and becomes a father of two children. In Cyprus Fortunatus lives rationally and moderately, having established an orderly home with his new money. Although he builds many structures with his wealth, he is careful to hide its source. It would seem then that Fortunatus begins an orderly lifestyle after his years of disorderly adventure. But, having lived twelve years of this moderate lifestyle, Fortunatus decides to once again travel after finding out that his wife will bear no more children. Deborah Prager (2014, 110) relates his wish to travel again to a desiring sense of self: "The hat in *Fortunatus* thus represents the notion that even when needs are fulfilled, there remains a desire for more, and that wish for more can only find its mode of expression in fantasy" (2014, 110). The desire for more is connected to a desire to push boundaries of the natural and fantastical and the known and unknown as he travels to the East, where he cleverly steals the magical hat from the Sultan before returning home to an ailing wife. Despite being comfortable at the boundaries of the normative, Fortunatus laments his choice of wealth, and therewith the queer identity it bestowed upon him, and warns his children of the potential dangers of those items as he is on his deathbed.

CONCLUSION

Fortunatus' regret and resignation at the end could suggest that he is a negative example. Indeed, just as Reymund regrets his life with Melusine at the end, herself betrayed and destined to her serpent form, both texts seem to argue against non-normativity. Yet reading against the grain shows us that failure is marked in terms of queerness, in a transient, liminal space where boundaries between masculinity and femininity, the natural and supernatural, monstrosity and humanness, and the productive and non-productive are blurry, at best. Furthermore, the texts complicate our understanding of masculinity in a queer manner: Melusine's female masculinity is the backbone of the noble house and Fortunatus' denial of economic order and social stability lands him in precarious situations. Indeed, viewing the early modern through a queer lens forces us to, at the very least, question hegemonic systems in the then and there and the here and now. It is this indeterminacy that emphasizes the potential potency of queer world-making projects, in particular in the face of a strict hegemonical social order that is imposed by multiple regulatory apparatuses. In Halberstam's words: "There is something powerful in being wrong, in losing, in failing, and all of our failures combined might just be enough, if we practice them well, to bring down the winner" (2011, 120).

NOTES

1. *Fortunatus*, edited by Hans-Gert Roloff (Ditzingen: Reclam, 1996) and Thüring von Ringoltingen, *Melusine*, edited by Hans-Gert Roloff (Ditzingen: Reclam, 1991). All citations are to these editions and are made parenthetically within the text.
2. All translations from the German are my own, unless otherwise indicated.
3. For further discussion of queer spectrality, mourning, and loss, see Freccero, especially 70 ff.
4. On the central role of contracts in *Melusine* and other early modern texts, see Williams and Schwarz (2003). For a queer phenomenological reading of Melusine's and Reymund's relationship regarding normative constructions of happiness, see Pfleger (2017).
5. For a more complete depiction of the marked bodies of the children, see pages 31–4 in the text or Strömer-Caysa (1999).

WORKS CITED

Ahmed, Sara. 2006. *Queer Phenomenology*. Durham: Duke University Press.
Cislo, Amy Eisen. 2010. *Paracelsus's Theory of Embodiment: Conception and Gestation in Early Modern Europe*. London: Pickering & Chatto.
Classen, Albrecht. 2000. "The Role of Money in Mideaval and Late-Medieval German Literature." *Neuphilologische Mitteilungen* 101, no. 3: 415–428.
Classen, Albrecht. "Love and Fear of the Foreign: Thüring von Ringoltingen's *Melusine* (1456): A Xenological Analysis." 2004. *Daphnis* 33, no. 1–2: 97–122.
Classen, Albrecht. "Family and Kinship in Early Modern German Prose Novels: Thüring von Ringoltingen's Melusine and the Anonymous Fortunatus." 2015. *Orbis Litterarum* 70, no. 5: 353–379.
Davis, Lennard J. 1995. *Enforcing Normalcy: Disability, Deafness, and the Body*. London and New York: Verso.
Dingel, Irene and Kohnle, Armin, eds. 2014. *Gute Ordnung. Ordnungsmodelle und Ordnungsvorstellungen in der Reformationszeit*. Leipzig: Evangelische Verlagsanstalt.
Fortunatus. 1996. Edited by Hans-Gert Roloff. Ditzingen: Reclam.
Freccero, Carla. 2006. *Queer/Early/Modern*. Durham: Duke University Press.
Halberstam, Jack. 1998. *Female Masculinity*. Durham: Duke University Press.
Halberstam, Jack. 2011. *The Queer Art of Failure*. Durham: Duke University Press.

Huot, Sylvia. 2003. "Dangerous Embodiments: Froissart's *Harton* and Jean d'Arras's *Melusine*." *Speculum* 78, no. 2: 400–420.

Laqueur, Thomas. 1992. *Making Sex: Body and Gender from the Greeks to Freud*. Cambridge: Harvard University Press.

Moser, Marc. 1999. "Adel und Bürgertum in *Fortunatus*, Einleitung." In *Etudes médiévales*, edited by Danielle Buschinger, 367–373. Amiens: Presses de l'UFR Clerc, Univ. Picardie.

Muñoz, José Esteban. 1999. *Disidentifications: Queers of Color and the Performance of Politics*. Minneapolis: University of Minnesota Press.

Muñoz, José Esteban. 2009. *Cruising Utopia: The Then and There of Queer Futurity*. New York: New York University Press.

Park, Katharine. 1997. "The Rediscovery of the Clitoris: French Medicine and the Tribade, 1570-1620." In *The Body in Parts: Fantasies of Corporeality in Early Modern Europe*, edited by Carla Mazzio and David Hillman, 171–193. New York: Routledge.

Pfleger, Simone. 2017. "The Promise of (Un)happiness in Thüring von Ringoltingen's *Melusine*." In *Melusine's Footprint: Tracing the Legacy of a Mediaeval Myth*, edited by Misty Urban, Deva F. Kemmis, and Melissa Ridley Elmes, 208–221. Leiden: Brill.

Prager, Debra. 2014. *Orienting the Self: The German Literary Encounter with the Eastern Other*. Rochester, NY: Boydell & Brewer.

Reeser, Todd. 2006. *Moderating Masculinity in Early Modern Culture*. Chapel Hill: University of North Carolina Press.

Ringoltingen, Thüring von. 1991. *Melusine*. Edited by Hans-Gert Roloff. Ditzingen: Reclam.

Rohrmann, P. 1975. "The Central Role of Money in the Chapbook *Fortumatus*." *Neophilologus* 59: 262–272.

Scholz Williams, Gerhild. 1991. "Frühmoderne Transgressionen: Sex und Magie in der Melusine und bei Paracelsus." *Daphnis* 20, no. 1: 81–100.

Scholz Williams, Gerhild and Schwarz, Alexander. 2003. *Existentielle Vergeblichkeit: Verträge in der Mélusine, im Eulenspiegel und im Dr. Faustus*. Berlin: E. Schmidt.

Störmer-Caysa, Uta. 1999. "Melusines Kinder bei Thüring von Ringoltingen." *Beiträge zur Geschichte der deutschen Sprache und Literatur* 121, no. 2: 239–262.

Wade, Mara. 2016. "Geld, Geschlecht und gute Ordnung im frühdeutschen Roman *Fortunatus*." In *Eigennutz und "gute Ordnung" Ökonomisierungen der Welt im 17. Jahrhundert*, edited by Sandra Richter and Guillaume Garner, 207–224 and 581–582. Wiesbaden: Harrassowitz.

Wailes, Stephen L. 1986. "Potency in *Fortunatus*." *The German Quarterly* 59, no. 1: 5–18.

Zemon-Davis, Natalie. 1975. *Society and Culture in Early Modern France: Eight Essays*. Stanford: Stanford University Press.

CHAPTER EIGHTEEN

Making Intersex Identity ILLegible: Oskar Panizza's "Ein skandalöser Fall"

JOELA JACOBS AND BASTIAN LASSE*

As of 2018 in Germany and 2019 in Austria, parents can register the sex of their newborns as *divers* to indicate intersex identity instead of male or female. They also have the option of leaving the entry empty altogether (as of 2013 in Germany). This new sex designation appears on all official documentation and has become a required category, for instance, in job listings, making these countries the first in Europe and some of a few worldwide to recognize intersex individuals in such a way. Intersex and trans organizations have flagged the requirement for medical evidence to achieve such legal recognition as a potentially traumatic re-pathologization, but a new law that would enable self-identification (*Selbstbestimmungsgesetz*) is now under discussion in Germany. Despite open questions and valid criticisms about aspects of the process, the successful legal struggle for a positive recognition of intersex identity has overall raised broader awareness about the ubiquity of gender check boxes in everyday life and the rampant medical ramifications of not fitting the available options.

While it might seem surprising that the legal recognition of identities beyond the male/female binary would begin with intersex persons, the long medical history of and insistence on intersex bodies as material evidence perhaps explains the relative ease of acknowledging them in language and law. Accordingly, historians of sexuality like Michel Foucault and

* The collaboration for this article emerged in the context of a lecture series on the anniversary of Oskar Panizza's death in 2021 (see panizza.arizona.edu). Our writing is based on many conversations that reinforced the value of collaborative work in the humanities to us.

gender theorists such as Judith Butler have engaged with the Western history of intersex identity, previously called "hermaphroditism," as a designation that predates many other conceptualizations of sex, gender, and also sexual orientation.[1] While early sexology coined terminology such as "homosexuality" for criminalized behavior in the second half of the nineteenth century, Prussian law contained a so-called *Zwitterparagraph* already in 1794, which determined for almost a century that intersex individuals could choose their place in the gender binary when coming of age. Whether protected by law or not, the decision was nonetheless mostly determined by physicians, such as in the case of the arguably most famous historical intersex individual, the French Herculine or Abel Barbin (1838–68), whose memoirs were published by Foucault in 1978 and discussed at length by Butler and many others. As the only known autobiographical record of an intersex person from early nineteenth-century Europe (see Dreger 1998, 23) and one of few available before the 1990s, Barbin's memoir "has become a touchstone in contemporary queer, trans, and intersex scholarship" (Malatino 2019, 39). The text and its afterlife have just as much to offer to health humanities research that is invested in giving visibility and a voice to pathologized individuals of the past and present.

Foucault appended a French translation of a little-known literary adaptation of Barbin's life by German author Oskar Panizza (1853–1921) to the memoirs of the headline-making historical figure. The trained physician Panizza was an ardent critic of psychiatry in his writing and died disenfranchised in a mental institution. He likely read about Barbin in Tardieu's *Question médico-légale de l'identité* while he lived in France in 1881.[2] Published in his 1893 short story collection *Visionen*, Panizza's narrative fictionalizes and partly alters the circumstances surrounding the historical change of Barbin's sex designation from female to male in 1860. Called "Ein skandalöser Fall" (literally "A Scandalous Case," or in the English translation of the French rendering, "A Scandal at the Convent"), the story is situated at a Catholic boarding school for the upper-class teenage daughters of France, where two pupils—Henriette and Alexina—develop a close relationship, until the discovery of its sexual nature prompts medical and religious authorities to intervene.[3] An examination outs the latter as intersex, and in the biggest deviation from the historical original, the text hints that the former has become pregnant. Panizza's story is one of the author's many censored texts about individuals in conflict with biopolitical norms that are enforced by church, state, and society, and—as this article shows—underpinned by medical science and discursive strategies.[4]

The characters in the story represent these regulatory mechanisms, beginning with Monsieur l'Abbé and Madame la Supérieure, who supervise the convent school. Among the many girls attending class is the Supérieure's niece, 17-year-old Henriette, who is described as a spoiled and charming troublemaker. She has befriended 18-year-old Alexina, who is an intellectual prodigy and a charity case on her way to becoming a teacher. Alexina Besnard is modeled on the historical Herculine Barbin, who was called Alexina, became a teacher, and was forced to live as a man after the discovery of their intersex identity in the wake of several relationships with pupils. The character disposition and physical appearance of all protagonists, including the fictionalized Alexina, are described in great detail not only by the narrator of Panizza's story, but also by various other figures, such as the schoolgirls, the villagers, and ultimately the examining doctor. The following sections analyze these discursive constructions of deviation from the norms of sex, gender, and sexuality, which cannot result in life as an intersex individual, according to nineteenth-century realities, but only lead to the enforced attempt to fit one of the sides of the binary (see Reis 2021, 59)—a biopolitical enactment that made the historical Barbin take their own life.

This article argues that the Abbé, the schoolgirls, and the people of the surrounding village, the doctor, and the narrator make Alexina ILLegible with their descriptions: Initially, this means that the more Alexina is discussed, the less we actually know about Alexina. The intersecting attempts to render Alexina legible or comprehensible by fitting their identity into known contexts—from mythology to medicine—teach us something about the characters who draw on them, but not Alexina. In a second step, this illegibility is pathologizing, as Alexina's body and mind are inscribed with an ill(ness) through the repeated description of deviations from the expectations of science and society. Alexina is marked as not fitting these norms on the three levels of sexuality, gender, and sex, which this article will use as its structuring principles. Panizza's narrative exposes that the many overlapping approaches to determining Alexina's identity from the outside are grounded in each character's self-conception and the norms governing their own sex, gender, or sexuality. Ultimately, the Abbé, the girls, the people of the village, and the physician try to fit Alexina into existing categories that constrict everyone's identity. Therefore, these attempts do not only make Alexina ILLegible, but also obscure the other characters in the story, so that the reader is left with aberrant types rather than fully developed individuals.

SEXUALIZING ALEXINA

Monsieur l'Abbé is introduced as a person who samples books with gusto. His daily habits, in fact, parallel reading and consumption. Described as an overweight "Schlecker" (Panizza 2020, 87) ["gormandizer"] (Panizza 2010, 156), he consumes theological treatises "als Frühstückscigarre" (Panizza 2020, 94) [literally "as breakfast cigar"]. Since the notion of a Catholic priest and a sensual consumer are not meant to go together, the narrator points to the Abbé's "sublime Natur" (Panizza 2020, 88, see also 94). Sublimation, understood as a "culturally promoted processing of frustrated instinctual desires" (Goebel 2012, 7), was famously theorized by Sigmund Freud as a diversion of the "normal sexual aim" (Freud 1981, 149) onto other sexual objectives. In the case of the Abbé, these prohibited, displaced erotic desires attach themselves not only to his books, but also to the "case" in question. When he learns that Alexina and Henriette have been found in bed together, he turns to his library to investigate what he considers a "case of the greatest scientific and moral-theological significance" (Panizza 2010, 179):

> Dieser hatte inzwischen das *Dictionnaire ecclésiastique* hervorgezogen und unter dem Titel "Sappho" gesucht; und als er hier nicht fand, was er wollte, suchte er unter "Lesbos"; und als ihm dies auch nicht genügte, holte er den Artikel "Tribade". Diesen nahm er mit auf's Tigerfell, und blieb über ihn wohl eine halbe Stunde –
>
> (Panizza 2020, 104)

[He had meanwhile pulled out his Ecclesiastical Dictionary and was reading the entry under "Sappho." When he did not find what he was looking for, he went on to "Lesbos" and, still unfulfilled, he found the article on "Tribadism." This he took with him to his tiger skin and pored over it for a good half-hour.]

(Panizza 2010, 172)

The nineteenth century proliferated the many "fictions of Sappho" (Andreadis 2014, 26) in such a way that "Sappho," "Lesbos," and "Tribadism" became synonymous with sexual encounters between women. The Abbé's awareness of this tradition immediately awakens his sublimated interests, and the suggestive scene on the tiger rug ends in a dash (left out in the translation) that entails the potential omission of an emission. Just as the famous Kleistian dash in the "Marquise von O…." stands for a sexual act, this ambiguous narrative moment raises questions about whether the supposedly abstinent Abbé pleasures himself on the rug. While the narrative leaves purposefully unclear (i.e., illegible) whether more than just the Abbé's desire for knowledge was satisfied on the tiger rug, his lengthy engagement with the details of the encounter confirms that he takes pleasure in his pursuit either way. The notion of such undefined solitary pleasure while reading up on Sappho emphasizes the ill associated with this moment, since the nineteenth century thought homosexuality and masturbation to be causally related. Both were considered amoral (even for those who had not declared their celibacy) and same-sex relations were illegal in most jurisdictions (Laqueur, *Solitary Sex*). The suggestion of a masturbatory scene therefore sexualizes and pathologizes the Abbé, just as he does with his two pupils.

As the Abbé continues to read Alexina and Henriette through the lens of sexuality to make sense of their "case," he interrogates the head teacher about the bounds of typical behavior among women. His many questions betray a fixation on touch and touching:

"Ob selbe [Berührungen] sinnlicher Natur seien?" […] "Kämen Ineinanderschlingungen und Umarmungen bei solchen Zusammenschlafungen vor?" […] "Ob es gewöhnlich sei, daß Mädchen sich gegenseitig unter die Röcke langten?" […] "Ob ein directes Berühren der Körpertheile der Andern dabei beabsichtigt sei?"

(Panizza 2020, 113–114)

["Is such contact sensual in nature?" […] "In such cases, would they embrace and intertwine their limbs?" […] "Is it fairly common for girls to put a hand under each other's skirts?" […] "Does this lead to their touching each other?"]

(Panizza 2010, 180–181)

In his obsessive attempt to distinguish the boundaries between friendships and sexual relationships, the Abbé's focus on predominantly tactile and corporeal aspects takes on a voyeuristic level of curiosity about details (a curiosity that the earlier dash stoked but not rewarded by refusing to provide any details of the scene on the tiger rug). Once again, the text suggests that the answers might be at least as important for the Abbé's moral-theological pursuits as they are for fueling his sexual imagination and—whether as second-hand knowledge or his own touch—pleasurable. The Abbé's sublimated sexuality determines how he reads the "case" of Alexina and Henriette, and it does not occur to him to question Alexina's sex or gender (who remains "la Maitresse" for him throughout the text), as he only focuses on sexuality as a physical act between bodies—the very thing that his profession denies.

Temptations of the flesh are therefore serious moral-theological problems to him, and he wonders whether the girls' relationship is a "teuflische, sinnliche Anreizung" (Panizza 2020, 115) ["diabolic sensuality," or more literally "a diabolic incitement or temptation"] (Panizza 2010, 181). Once the medical examination makes clear that Alexina does not bear the mark of the devil, his erotic fascination ends. Even while Alexina and Henriette provide fodder for his fantasies, he pathologizes their same-sex desire in his religious worldview, and when the impact of the devil is ruled out, only sin, or the illness of religious deviation, remains: "war aber der Teufel nicht im Spiel, dann hatten offenbar Henriette und la Maitresse ein frevelhaftes, sündig-gottloses Spiel mit einander getrieben" (Panizza 2020, 129) ["If [...] the devil was not involved at all, then Henriette and the Schoolmistress had evidently been playing a most heinous, sinful game with one another"] (Panizza 2010, 195). The paradoxical perspective of the Abbé, which would render Alexina's and Henriette's behavior acceptable only if the devil were involved, makes clear just how much taboo and desire are entangled in the Abbé's subconscious. His "sublimated nature," i.e., his own sexual desire, determines this initial interpretation of the "case," while Alexina's identity remains illegible, both unreadable and pathologized, because of the sexualization and subsequent demonization.

GENDERING ALEXINA

Alexina and Henriette were discovered in bed by the other schoolgirls, who do not accuse them of sexual transgressions but are more concerned with (in)appropriate behavior for young women. Since sexual innocence in both theory and practice is part of these gendered expectations, the schoolgirls both perform and collectively reinforce the contemporary norms for female behavior about which the Abbé had inquired. While they accuse Henriette and Alexina of inappropriate looks, touches, and kisses, the pupils predominantly describe what they perceive as Alexina's deviations from expected feminine appearance and behavior, such as reluctance to bathe with or urinate in front of other girls, ill-fitting underwear, a walk that is not girly, and hairy legs "wie der Teufel" (Panizza 2020, 107) ["like the Devil"] (Panizza 2010, 174). One of the girls concludes, "sie glaube überhaupt nicht, daß Alexina ein Mädchen sei; sie sei viel zu gescheidt [...]; sie glaube Alexina sei ein böser Geist in Mädchengestalt" (Panizza 2020, 108) ["She did not think that Alexina was a girl at all; she was much too smart [...]. She felt sure that Alexina was an evil spirit in the semblance of a girl"] (Panizza 2010, 174). While the girls question whether Alexina is one of them on the basis of a slew of gender stereotypes, they do not say explicitly that she behaves like a man. Instead, they call Alexina and Henriette "*le diable et sa fiancée!*" (Panizza 2020, 111) ["The Devil and his bride!"] (Panizza 2010, 177), demonizing and—perhaps accidentally—rendering Alexina grammatically masculine in the process.[5] Since Alexina is perceived as the stronger of the two, both physically and mentally, the focus is increasingly on this character alone.

As the young women turn Alexina into the devil to align the perceived deviations with their worldview, the narrator objectifies and massifies the girls' bodies by describing them as a material collective that is, among metaphors such as a flood, storm, and lava stream, called a "Bienenschwarm" (Panizza 2020, 97) ["bee swarm"] (Panizza 2010, 165) in the text. The convent and indeed the entire narrative are abuzz with sounds like "summen [...] Klirren [...] und ein Stumpen, Drücken, Gilfen, Kichern und Pst! Rufen" (Panizza 2020, 98) ["humming [...] rattling [...] and stamping, pressing, giggling and shushing sounds"] (Panizza 2010, 166). The soundscape escalates into a frenzy, depicting the girls on the brink of—clearly gendered—mass hysteria: "die Schaar der auf's Höchste erregten und vor Neugier fiebernden Mädchen [...] fuhr[...] wie von einer plötzlichen Panik ergriffen, kreischend und Abscheu ausdrückend [...] vor Alexina, zurück" (Panizza 2020, 109–110) ["the [...] young chatterboxes, feverish with excitement and curiosity [...] drew back from the two sinners violently, as if in a sudden panic, screaming and showing their disgust"] (Panizza 2010, 176). Their description as a collective that is made of noisy bodies has rendered any individual young woman illegible, and the expectations for gendered behavior fall apart. Rather than controlling their emotions and not speaking out of turn, the religiously fueled hysterics leave nothing but a stereotype of overly strictly monitored girls whose emotions emerge in pathologized excess that is only one step away from violence.

Violence comes more explicitly into play with the mass of the villagers, who take up the girls' religious ideas once they hear about the "case" and demand that Alexina be exorcized. When a local forester confirms the sexual nature of the relationship, saying that he saw the two in a compromising position in the forest, the townspeople materialize into a threatening mob: "vor dem Kloster ständen mehrere hundert Leute, mit Mistgabeln und Aexten, die die Faust gegen das Gebäude ballten, Verwünschungen ausstießen, und fortwährend riefen, der Teufel sei im Kloster" (Panizza 2020, 123) ["a crowd of several hundred people had gathered at the gate, armed with pitchforks and axes, shaking their fists at the cloister, cursing aloud and insisting that the Devil was being harbored in the convent"] (Panizza 2010, 189). This stereotypical pitchfork-wielding crowd is convinced that "ein Incubus, oder der Teufel selbst, habe die schöne Henriette [...] vergewaltigt" (Panizza 2020, 123–124) ["an incubus—unless it was the Devil himself—had raped [...] the lovely Henriette"] (Panizza 2010, 190). The text highlights the dangerously volatile powers of masses of bodies, whose discourse makes Alexina a diabolic aggressor by insistence alone. At this point of impending loss of control over the situation, the Abbé calls a doctor, to find "die bekannten Male und Zeichen von Teufels-Besessenheit an ihrem Körper" (Panizza 2020, 124) ["the well-known marks and stigmata of diabolic possession [...] on the girl's body"] (Panizza 2010, 191). Unlike the Abbé, whose own sexual desires enabled him to picture a consensual relationship between Alexina and Henriette, the villagers and the schoolgirls can only interpret the observed behavior through a lens of religious transgression. Despite their hysterical imaginings, none of them seem to think that Alexina's sex is not female, which shows how pervasively the gender binary continues to shape Alexina's perceived appearance as a woman.

SEXING ALEXINA

The doctor, who is meant to settle the "case" of Alexina as much as cure the spreading hysteria and end the superstitious siege, is a young man with top academic credentials. As a representative of science, he is perceived as threatening by the Abbé, who introduces an opposition between science and religion: "Ja, glauben denn diese neuen Aerzte, sie können die Welt ohne Geistlichkeit in Ordnung bringen?" (Panizza 2020, 129) ["Did these young doctors imagine they could keep the world in order without any help from the clergy?"] (Panizza 2010, 194). The order of things will indeed be shaken up by this figure, as his medical report does not engage with religious interpretations and instead reassigns Alexina's sex, making both patient and physician illegible in the process.

Though the doctor was asked to the convent for a big revelation, the final determination of the "case" happens in private, with an examination behind almost closed doors. The narratorial voice recounts what the sole witness—la Supérieure—hears, but we will learn only later, from the report with which the story ends, what the clinical gaze of the physician saw. In contrast to the report that makes Alexina's body appear in supposedly plain sight, the narrator's description foregrounds the removal of all lighting: "Das Licht wird gerückt, so daß die Helle jetzt ganz aus der Thürspalte verschwindet" (Panizza 2020, 127) ["The lamp was moved so that all the light was gone from the minimal opening of the door"] (Panizza 2010, 193). As other commentators have noted, the examination scene is notoriously suggestive:[6]

> eine Aufforderung; dann ziehen und schleifen von ausgezogenen Gewändern; Pause, neue Aufforderung; Entgegnung; wiederholte Aufforderung in festerem Ton! ein Seufzen; dann wieder Ausziehen und Rutschgeräusche; strumpfiges Aufstampfen auf dem Boden; erst einmal; dann noch einmal; dann noch ein Rutschgeräusch; und jetzt ein weiches, schilfriges Gleiten; wie Epidermis auf Epidermis; und begleitet von zustimmenden *Ah, c'est cela; c'est cela, oui* des Arztes. Längere Pause. Dann wieder ein Commando; man hört die knerzenden Bewegungen eines Bettgestells und das knistrige Hingleiten auf eine Matraze; ein ruhiges Commando; ein stärkeres Commando; dringende, unwillige Aufforderung; seufzendes Wimmern von der andern Seite; *Ah, vous me faitez mal, Monsieur*; rief auf einmal Alexina laut und wie explosiv; dumpfe Entgegnung des Arztes, dessen unterbrochenes Athmen auf schwieriges, intensives Arbeiten hinwies. Nunmehr ausgiebiges Schluchzen ohne Unterlaß von Seite Alexina's, ohne stärkere Schmerzensrufe, aber mit unstillbarem Weinen, hingebend, machtlos, verzweifelnd, sich gänzlich überlassend; die Stimme des Arztes nunmehr weich und bedauernd, ohne plötzliche Commandorufe. Der Culminationspunkt schien überschritten.
>
> (Panizza 2020, 127)[7]

> [A directive was given, followed by the sounds of garments being slipped off. There was a pause, followed by another order and a reply. The order was repeated more firmly; a sigh, and the sounds of more clothing being pulled off, sounds of slipping, of someone stamping on the door in stockinged feet, once, then again, and again; another sliding sound, and

> then a soft, slippery gliding, like skin on skin, accompanied by an encouraging: "Yes, that's it, that's it, fine," from the doctor. A long pause, then another order; the bed creaking, then the sound of a body slipping onto a mattress; a quiet request, repeated more firmly, followed by an urgent, impatient command. The response was a sigh and whimper, "Ah, you're hurting me, Monsieur." Then Alexina suddenly cried out, loudly and explosively. There was an indistinct reply from the doctor, whose uneven breathing suggested that he was concentrating hard, meeting with difficulty. Alexina sobbed without restraint, not crying out with pain, but weeping in total self-abandonment, powerless, despairing. The doctor's voice became gentle, compassionate, without further commands. The worst seemed to be over.]
>
> (Panizza 2010, 193, more literally, the last sentence says, "the culmination point was transgressed")

The word "directive" (*Aufforderung* or *Commando*) appears seven times in this passage, which emphasizes that Alexina is resisting the various steps of the procedure and not consenting. By describing only what can be heard, the scene seems to avoid the pitfalls of voyeurism, while bringing the violence and terror of this non-consensual physical examination to the fore. Except for two utterances, the exact directives and Alexina's replies are not spelled out. Alexina's cry of pain that parallels the one intelligible sentence "you're hurting me" stands out against a seemingly endless parataxis of speech acts. Read in conjunction with the doctor's report, this scream presumably marks the moment of digital penetration. According to current law, penetration without consent constitutes rape, and the heavy breathing of the physician along with the unstoppable sobbing of Alexina and the final sentence about the passed "climax" (*Culminationspunkt*), which the report reveals to be an ejaculation by Alexina, strongly support this interpretation. The medical procedure is as invasive and traumatic as rape, but what happens exactly behind the door remains nonetheless illegible. Similar to the suggestive dash that omitted the details of the Abbé's acts on the tiger rug but underscored his sublimated sexual desire by association, the suggested rape highlights the violence of this unwanted moment, which is only the beginning of a series of pathologizing decisions that force Alexina to live as a man. The illegibility of the situation expands to the figure of the physician through his report, which consists of a letter addressed to the Abbé. Opening in French, the salutations state the doctor's name as "Adolph Duval" (Panizza 2020, 131). However, the closing lines—written in German, just like the rest of the letter—use the German spelling "Adolf Duval" (Panizza 2020, 133) suggesting that Adolph/Adolf himself has an ambiguous identity. Moreover, the etymological proximity of "Duval" to the old high German *tiuval* (Totzke 2015, 294–295) picks up on the persistent invocation of the devil throughout the text. Adolph/Adolf Duval's dual and potentially diabolical identity makes him illegible, while he purports to reveal Alexina's "true sex" (Foucault 2010, vii), or one unambiguous identity, with his medical methods and distinctly scientific language:

> Somit ist Alexina Besnard ein *Zwitter*; und, da derselbe während der Untersuchung [...] auch eine unwillkürliche *ejaculatio seminalis* hatte, deren Bestand unter dem Mikroscop

> das deutliche Vorhandensein normaler, beweglicher Spermatozoen ergab, so muß Alexina als *männlicher Zwitter* angesprochen werden; somit ist Alexina ein *Mann* und zwar ein zeugungsfähiger Mann.
>
> (Panizza 2020, 133)

> [Such being the case, Alexina Besnard is a hermaphrodite and, inasmuch as he had, in the course of the examination, [...] an involuntary emission of semen, which proved under the microscope to contain normal, mobile spermatozoa, Alexina must be regarded as a male hermaphrodite. Alexina is, in fact, a *man*, and indeed a man capable of procreation.]
>
> (Panizza 2010, 199)

The report's language provides a false sense of clarity. The word *somit* (ergo) is repeated twice in the original, evoking flawless causality. The scientific prose style accounts for supposedly "objective" and therefore authoritative observations that have led to a seemingly indubitable result. However, the letter of the ambiguous physician that was meant to deliver an unambiguous verdict report that Alexina is both intersex and male. The ambivalent physical traits at the core of the decision are interpreted retroactively in one particular way due to the emission of semen. It is therefore not the body that determines Alexina's sex but the doctor, who takes reproductive ability to be more important than his patient's gender expression and does not ask Alexina for their opinion. Even though the designation as male usually comes with societal power, Alexina remains utterly powerless. Since the nineteenth century strove to align gender, sex, and sexuality in the "business of creating women and men" (Reis 2021, 70), the seemingly clear doctor's report ultimately keeps Alexina's body illegible.

A NARRATIVE OF ILLEGIBILITY

While we have so far mostly focused on the ways the narrator works with omissions, such as the dash obscuring what the Abbé did on the tiger rug and the door that leaves the examination scene invisible, there are also voyeuristic moments of seeing, in which the narrator inserts themselves into the narrative. These instances of deixis place the narrator seemingly in the plot, although nobody responds to this presence. In all of these examples, the narrator is trying to observe or look at something more closely, which then becomes illegible. The first time this happens, the narrator looks over the Abbé's shoulder, while the latter is reading: "Wir können nicht erkennen, welches Capitel Monsieur aus Liguori las, wie sehr wir auch über seine Schulter gebeugt uns den Text zu entziffern bemühen" (Panizza 2020, 94) ["Which chapter Monsieur was reading in Liguori, we cannot tell, no matter how hard we try, leaning over his shoulder, to decipher the text"] (Panizza 2010, 162). Unable to decipher what is on the page, this moment marks literal illegibility, while at the same time potentially including the reader in the formulation of a "we." Deixis draws the narrator's omniscience into doubt and renders illegible whether the voice is actually part of the diegesis as a character or not.[8]

The voyeuristic nature of these deictic insertions becomes particularly clear when the narrator visits the girls' dormitory and describes what "one saw." Just like with Alexina, the more "one" is looking, the less one seems to see clearly:

> In dem ganzen Schlafsaal sah man jetzt nur weiße Lichter und Flächen; chamoisgelbe Arme und Nacken; blendendweiße Röckchen und Hemdstücke; und manchmal glitzernde Punkte von aufgesperrten Mündern; und ein Schliefen, Rutschen, Anziehe- und Auskleide-Geräusch, ein Knipsen der Strumpfbänder, ein Schlappen, Wischen und Wenden ging durch den Saal.
>
> (Panizza 2020, 96)

> [The whole dormitory was now a vision of white lights and surfaces, the skintones of bare arms and necks amid the gleaming white of petticoats and camisoles, and sometimes pearly glimmerings between open lips. There were sounds of slippings and slidings, of clothing being pulled off and on, the snapping of garters, the flapping of slippers, the swishing of washcloths.]
>
> (Panizza 2010, 164)

The body parts and intimate objects become blurry, as they are listed in unconnected sequence in the original.[9] Without clearly establishing the relationship between individual bodies and objects, the girls—once again—turn into a material mass. The voyeuristic moment of seeing young girls' bodies lets loose the imagination and introduces a suggestive, erotic element that becomes disturbing due to the age of the observed and the absence or impossibility of consent. At the same time, since the body parts blur, "one" is not seeing anything, and despite the description of a detailed observation, the passage almost also becomes an omission. Seeing turns into its opposite, just as the earlier moment of reading over the shoulder rendered the text illegible. As the Abbé did with the help of his library and the doctor through his report, the narrator and the narrative as a whole attempt to read bodies to make sense of them, but they grow increasingly illegible—and both narrator and readers become implicated in the process.

MEET ALEXINA

Mererid Puw Davies and Sonu Shamdasani recently analyzed the interrelations of health and humanity in documents such as the WHO Charter and came to the conclusion that "[m]edicine has come to define the human" (2020, 5). As Jones et al. (2017) describe, the hegemony of medicine in discourses about what is human is precisely what stifled the shift in vocabulary from medical to health humanities. Panizza's story shows that the human is lost whenever it becomes an object of classification, medical or otherwise. Every figure's attempt to read Alexina—be it through the lens of gender, sex, or sexuality—renders the individual human at the center of the story illegible, and the narrative shows how the characters are themselves implicated in the discourses they are drawing on, thus casting doubt on whether the norms they uphold actually exist outside of theoretical discourse. Yet Alexina gets their own voice in Panizza's narrative, too, and we therefore invite you to finally meet Alexina. Concluding our article by examining how the narrative features Alexina's perspective will recenter the human, but it will not resolve Alexina's identity. Alexina's voice can be heard in dialogue with the Abbé and in letters to Henriette—instances that create a seemingly unmediated presence. Through these letters, Panizza paints a picture of a strong-willed, very articulate individual, who is deeply in love with their companion's body and mind, sees nothing wrong with their relationship, and can hold their own in defending it. In their letters, Alexina sounds like this:

> Weißt Du, daß Du in meine Hände gegeben, wie Wachs dem Bildner? Daß Du das unglückliche Mädchen Alexina lieben mußt [...] Und willst Dich in die bestialischen Arme eines Mannes werfen [...]? Bin nicht ich Dein Mann!? [...] Und was wir verbrochen haben, Berührungen, und unerlaubte Küsse, und Umarmungen und Ergießungen, und was wir im Geheimen thaten, ist an und für sich nichts, ist nicht das Eigentliche, was wir wollten, war nur symbolisch gemeint, weil wir es durch Worte nicht ausdrücken konnten [...] Deine Liebe zu mir, Henriette, das ist für mich Alles.
>
> (Panizza 2020, 118–119)

> [Don't you know that you have been given into my hands, like wax in the hands of a sculptor? That you must love the unhappy Alexina [...] Do you intend to throw yourself into the bestial arms of a man [...]? Aren't I your husband? [...] The wrong we have done, touching each other, those forbidden kisses and embraces and effusions, and the things we did in secret, all that doesn't matter in itself; it's not what this is really all about. It's only symbolic of what we could not express in words [...] Your love for me, Henriette, is all that matters to me.]
>
> (Panizza 2010, 184–186)

Without perceiving any conflict between sex/gender designations, Panizza's Alexina self-identifies both as a "girl" and as Henriette's "husband" or "man" in their writing. The letters also make clear that the prohibited sexual intimacy of the couple is a physical expression of their love and inner connection, of the things that they "could not express in words." These "symbolic" actions contrast with what is expected of them by society, and the image of "throwing oneself into the bestial arms of a man" instead of Alexina's conveys not just jealousy but also disgust of potential heterosexual encounters, along with a fear of what the future might hold. By giving Alexina a voice, Panizza lets Alexina emerge as a human and a full-fledged character with fears and desires, confidence and vulnerability in the narrative.

Yet the doctor's examination challenges Alexina's confident self-conception and, in a rare occurrence, the text briefly presents Alexina's inner monologue:

> Was war denn dann mit ihr so besonderes los? Diese Kleinigkeit, über die Henriette so oft gelacht?—Aber es mußte doch etwas sein! Denn woher der schreckliche Schmerz?
>
> (Panizza 2020, 131)

> [So what was all the fuss about, where she was concerned? Was it that little thing that made Henriette laugh every time? If it wasn't that, then why the terrible painfulness there?]
>
> (Panizza 2010, 196)

Here, the text breaks with the distance of the usual third-person perspective, creating a brief moment for the reader to share Alexina's confusion and concern, which show Alexina as vulnerable, though not weak. The passage suggests that Alexina does not know "what is going on" either, but rather than being illegible to themselves, Alexina is just Alexina.

As Panizza's narrative navigates the balance between familiarizing the reader with an individual and exposing the dehumanizing tendencies of an "authoritative" reading of a body, it resonates with the challenges of today's discourse in the health humanities. In particular, when it comes to bodies that are understood as deviating from a perceived norm, certain voyeuristic impulses of storytelling can do as much harm as enforced medical diagnostics or biopolitics. Yet storytelling can also expose the discourses at work in reinforcing normativity, and it can be an empowering tool of self-determination. There is hope that the new *Selbstbestimmungsgesetz* in Germany can present such an opportunity to give a voice to intersex individuals and ultimately every gender identity out there, beyond select countries.

NOTES

1. For current terminology debates, see Rubin (2017, 141–152) and Malatino (2019, 71–99).
2. For a detailed account of Panizza's life, see Bauer (1984 and 2019).
3. The spelling of the title has been inconsistent since its first publication in Panizza (1893), as the table of contents lists "Ein scandalöser Fall," while the heading of the text itself reads "Ein skandalöser Fall." Both spellings are common in scholarship and new editions, but this text follows Panizza (2020) by spelling the title with a "k."
4. For more information about these aspects of Panizza's short prose, see, e.g., Jacobs (2015a and b). For a discussion of this particular text, see Totzke (2015), Bachmann (2016), and Ketterl (2016 and 2017).
5. Small portions of dialogue appear in French in the German original, but the English translation does not retain this strategy of reminding readers of the story's setting.
6. See Ketterl (2016, 108–111) and Totzke (2015, 293–294).
7. As Matthias Lorenz observes in his review of Panizza (2020), this quote does not follow Panizza (1893), where it says "Epidermus auf Epidermis" (171) (see Lorenz 2022, 686).
8. For a discussion of the narrative situation as omniscient or extradiegetic/heterodiegetic, see Bachmann (2016, 207) and Ketterl (2016, 106).
9. The translation takes some liberties that obscure the passive voice and list-like quality of the original. Literally, the passage says, "In the whole dormitory, one now saw only white lights and surfaces; sheep-skin-yellow arms and necks; blinding-white little skirts and shirt pieces; and sometimes glittering points of gaping mouths; and a slipping, sliding, dressing and undressing sound, snapping of garters, a shuffling, wiping, and turning went through the room."

WORKS CITED

Andreadis, Harriette. 2014. "The Sappho Tradition." In *The Cambridge History of Gay and Lesbian Literature*, edited by E. L. McCallum and Mikko Tuhkanen, 15–33. Cambridge: Cambridge University Press.

Bachmann, Magdalena Maria. 2016. "Der Psychiater als Literat – der Literat als 'Psichopat' – der 'Psichopat' als Psychiater: Zu den Fallgeschichten des Falls Oskar Panizza. Mit einem Seitenblick auf Foucaults *Hermaphrodismus*." In *Fallgeschichte(n) als Narrativ zwischen Literatur und Wissen*, edited by Martina King and Thomas Wegmann, 195–223. Innsbruck: Innsbruck University Press.

Bauer, Michael. 1984. *Oskar Panizza: Ein literarisches Porträt*. Munich: Hanser.

Bauer, Michael. 2019. *Oskar Panizza: Eine Biographie*. Munich: Allitera.

Butler, Judith. 2007. *Gender Trouble: Feminism and the Subversion of Identity*. New York: Routledge.

Davies, Mererid Puw and Sonu Shamdasani. 2020. "Medical In/Humanities: The Human and the Humane in the German-Speaking World: An Introduction." In *Medical Humanity and Inhumanity in the German-Speaking World*, edited by Mererid Puw Davies and Sonu Shamdasani, 1–12. London: UCL Press.

Dreger, Alice Domurat. 2000. *Hermaphrodites and the Medical Invention of Sex*. Cambridge: Harvard University Press.

Foucault, Michel. 2010. "Introduction." In *Herculine Barbin: Being the Recently Discovered Memoirs of a Nineteenth-Century French Hermaphrodite*, edited by Michel Foucault, xii–xvii. New York: Vintage Books.

Freud, Sigmund. 1981. *The Standard Edition of The Complete Psychological Works of Sigmund Freud. Volume VII: A Case of Hysteria, Three Essays on Sexuality and Other Works*. Translated by James Strachey. London: The Hogarth Press.

Goebel, Eckhart. 2012. *Beyond Discontent: "Sublimation" from Goethe to Lacan*. Translated by James C. Wagner. New York: Continuum.

Jacobs, Joela. 2015a. "Assimilating Aliens: Imagining National Identity in Oskar Panizza's *Operated Jew* and Salomo Friedlaender's *Operated Goy*." In *Alien Imaginations: Science Fiction and Tales of Transnationalism*, edited by Ulrike Küchler, Silja Mähl, and Graeme Stout, 57–71. New York: Bloomsbury Academic.

Jacobs, Joela. 2015b. "'Verbrechen wider die Natur': Oskar Panizza's First Encounter with Censorship." In *Protest and Reform in the German Literature and Art of Modernity, 1871–1918*, edited by Godela Weiss-Sussex and Charlotte Woodford, 125–138. Munich: Iudicium.

Jones, Therese, Michael Blackie, Rebecca Garden, and Delese Wear. 2017. "The Almost Right Word: The Move from Medical to Health Humanities." *Academic Medicine* 92, no. 7 (July): 932–935.

Ketterl, Anja. 2016. "Von Hegemonie und Unentscheidbarkeit: Oskar Panizzas *Ein scandalöser Fall*." *Aussiger Beiträge* 10: 99–114.

Ketterl, Anja. 2017. "Skandalöses Erzählen: Panizza – Bernhard – Walser." PhD Diss., University of Maryland. ProQuest (10285032).

Laqueur, Thomas W. 2003. *Solitary Sex: A Cultural History of Masturbation*. New York: Zone Books.

Lorenz, Matthias. 2022. "Peter Staengle, Günther Emig (Hrsg.). Oskar Panizza: Werke. Verlag Günther Emigs Literatur-Betrieb, Niederstetten 2019 ff., 10 Bde." Review of "Oskar Panizza: Werke," ed. by Peter Staengle and Günther Emig. *Zeitschrift für Germanistik* XXXII, no. 3: 683–687.

Malatino, Hil. 2019. *Queer Embodiment: Monstrosity, Medical Violence, and Intersex Experience*. Lincoln: University of Nebraska Press.

Panizza, Oskar. 1893. "Ein scandalöser Fall." In *Visionen: Skizzen und Erzählungen*, 112–181. Leipzig: Wilhelm Friedrich.

Panizza, Oskar. 2010. "A Scandal at the Convent." In: *Herculine Barbin: Being the Recently Discovered Memoirs of a Nineteenth-Century French Hermaphrodite*, edited by Michel Foucault, 155–199. New York: Vintage Books.

Panizza, Oskar. 2020. “Ein skandalöser Fall.“ In *Visionen: Skizzen und Erzählungen*, edited by Peter Staengle and Günther Emig, 86–134. Niederstetten: Günther Emigs Literatur-Betrieb.

Reis, Elizabeth. 2021. *Bodies in Doubt: An American History of Intersex*. Baltimore: Johns Hopkins University Press.

Rubin, David. 2017. *Intersex Matters: Biomedical Embodiment, Gender Regulation, and Transnational Activism*. Albany: State University of New York Press.

Totzke, Ariane. 2015. “Schwindsüchtige Erlöser, psychotische Pfaffen und der Fall ‘Barbin’.” In *Religion und Literatur im 20. und 21. Jahrhundert: Motive, Sprechweisen, Medien*, edited by Tim Lörke and Robert Walter-Jochum, 277–295. Göttingen: Vandenhoek & Ruprecht.

CHAPTER NINETEEN

Reading as a Trans-Corporeal Act

NECIA CHRONISTER

What role does our body play when we read? To be sure, our eyes, ears, or fingers receive and perceive the words, depending on how we read. We sit, stand, or recline, comfortably or not; maybe we pace. Is that the extent of our body's role when we read? Scholars working in a number of research areas such as disability studies, gender studies, and queer studies have long investigated the tensions between the fleshy material body and the social constructions that it challenges. Those working with affect theory are linking reading and the body through emotions and feeling. Yet scholarship on embodied reading still typically assumes a one-way relationship between the fictional world and the body. We may get tension in the pits of our stomachs, hold our breath, or get sexually excited by what we read. In this paradigm, the bodies of readers react to representation and are not typically considered to have an active role in the construction of the fictional world itself. But what if bodies do have an active role in the construction of fictional worlds? What if we can interpret the world of fiction precisely because we are embodied, and what if our bodies' reactions to texts, be they affective, emotional, and/or sexual, are evidence of our bodies' contributions to literary worlds? Might our bodies be more central to the reading experience than previously thought?

In 2015, I participated in a brilliantly designed seminar at the annual conference of the German Studies Association titled "New Feminist and Queer Approaches to German Studies." This group of some twenty scholars discussed theoretical works by Stacy Alaimo, Karen Barad, Rosi Braidotti, Judith Butler, Elizabeth Grosz, Donna Haraway, Susan Hekman, and Eve Sedgwick, among others, theorists who champion a reconsideration of the relationship between the world of discourse and the world of materiality. Most notably Alaimo, Barad, Braidotti, and Hekman call for an understanding of the material world as infusing, and infused by, the intellectual one. They argue for the agency of matter, its discursive ability, and thereby they relativize human intellect, situating it among an array of agencies operating in the world.

These are thrilling ideas, but they also created an impasse for our seminar participants, most of whom were literary scholars. How do we reconcile the world of materiality with the fictional worlds we construct in our minds as we read? The theorists we discussed in this seminar insist that matter and its agencies, its situatedness, and its complex impacts on human experiences are real and not to be understood metaphorically. How, then, do we employ these theories when working in the world of literature, a world that necessarily deals in metaphor and linguistic construction? This discussion prompted me to build on my previous work on the linguistic construction of gender in fiction, this time reconsidering our material facticity, our embodiment, as part of the endeavor of reading. Here, I present the theoretical underpinnings of the two articles that I wrote attempting to answer the following two questions: (1) how can we understand fiction as infused with materiality? and (2) how might our own bodily materiality be affected, perhaps even altered, by our interaction with fiction?[1]

I take as a starting point the notion of a porous humanness, such that the discursive world of literature and the material world of the body enter and impact one another. It is important to note that when speaking about bodies, we must recognize just how variable and situated a person's experience is. Alaimo frames this situatedness as exposure—to climates, landscapes, discourses:

> Exposure, then, is terribly uneven, across such simultaneously social and material categories as class, race, and the disparities between the global north and global south. [...] it is crucial to point out that ideological and discursive categories position bodies differently and have material effects. For feminists, LGBTQ people, people of color, persons with disabilities, and others, thinking through how corporeal processes, desires, orientations, and harms are in accordance with or divergent from social categories, norms, and discourses is a necessary epistemological and political process.
>
> (Alaimo 2016, 184)

Ability, age, culture, education, gender identity, physical environment, race, sexual identity, upbringing, and innumerable other factors impact how we experience our embodied relationship with the environment and the world of discourse. I want to take this moment to acknowledge this situatedness and point out that there are inherent limits to theorizing embodied reading based on my own interpretation of theorists, my literary analysis, and limited findings in the neurosciences, which I present below. This essay is meant to be a contribution to thinking beyond the apparent mind-body split when we read, but it can be only that. My hope is that my ideas can be complicated, fleshed out (as it were), and nuanced by those who inhabit positionalities different from my own.

READING, THE INDEXICAL TRACE, AND THE AGENTIC FICTIONAL BODY

In the last two decades, new material feminisms have emerged from the natural sciences that are reconceiving what matter is and what kinds of agency it may have. As Braidotti explains, "a new brand of 'materialism' is current in our scientific practices, which reinstates the vital, self-organizing capacities of what was previously seen as inert matter. As a result, the dualistic mode of thinking supported by social constructivism is no longer sufficient [...]" (Braidotti 2011, 16). These material feminisms are reconsidering the kinds of agency operative in the material world, what relationship those agencies have to human cultures, and what that means for feminism. This new direction in philosophical and scientific reasoning thus prompts questions about the relationship between the material world and human consciousness that literary studies, and feminist literary studies in particular, should be prepared to address. As Braidotti writes, the objective of new material feminisms is to understand "the embodied and embedded material structure of what we commonly call thinking. It is a materialism of the flesh that unifies mind and body in a new approach that blurs all boundaries" (Braidotti 2011, 2). The question of body materiality is of particular importance to feminism; scholars such as Alaimo, Barad, Braidotti, Grosz, Hekman, and others investigate how we can bring the body back into the discussion of feminism without losing what we gained with postmodernism. That is, how do we think about the material body as something that is not comprehensible only as a product of discourse without falling into the traps of essentialism that dominated understanding of the material body previously?

The questions brought up within material feminist discourse pose a unique challenge to literary scholars, who necessarily work in the world of language and metaphor. Can we think about an imagined diegetic world in the same way we think about material reality? Can fictional bodies be anything other than symbolic, metaphoric, or figurative? Can they be understood as material at all? The long-entrenched assumption is that language and the body, though related, stand in opposition to one another. Language is conceptual, a system of arbitrary signs, and therefore not material. The material body, on the other hand, belongs to the world of things and is to be interpreted through language. I contend, however, that we can understand the material bases of fiction when we recognize that the material bodies of the reader and author stand at the interstices of the material world and the linguistically constructed one. To explain what I mean, I will first expand my theoretical framework, demonstrating how indexical traces of material reality exist in fiction, so that our embodied experiences of material reality as readers, authors, and scholars are integral to the construction of fictional worlds. Then, because the question of agency as conceived of outside of human subjectivity is central to material feminisms, I will discuss the kind of agency that a fictional body may exhibit.

In order to reconceive of the role that the material body plays in the construction of literary worlds, we must first think about the nature of literary representation as distinct from other kinds of artistic representation. This is necessary, because differing modes of representation are understood to fall in line with the distinction between the material and language. Images, for example, are presumed to be more in line with the material because they appear to reproduce what they represent, whereby fictional worlds are considered to be solely linguistic constructions. In fact, in his treatise on photography, *Camera Lucida*, Roland Barthes argues that the indexicality of the photographed subject is the defining characteristic of photography as an art form and the primary distinction between photography and language:

> Photography's Referent is not the same as the referent of other systems of representation. I call 'photographic referent' not the *optionally* real thing to which an image or a sign refers but the *necessarily* real thing which has been placed before the lens, without which there would be no photograph. [...] Discourse combines signs which have referents, of course, but these referents can be and are most often "chimeras."
>
> (Barthes 1981, 76)

The index, the material trace left on the representation by the thing represented, in this case the blockage of light, is thus the distinctive characteristic of photography and what distinguishes it from discourse. Discourse can only indirectly refer to its subject, whereas the photograph relies on the physical presence of its subject before the lens for its very existence.[2]

Barthes's assumption, of course, is that discourse does not exhibit indexicality. I would like to problematize this assumption by creating a caveat for fictional literature. I propose that fictional bodies in literature do contain indexical traces of real, lived bodies and are not solely the indirect referents of discourse. I propose that bodies we encounter in literature are more immediate and materially real to us than those offered in the visual media because our own material bodies are imprinted on and leave traces on those fictional bodies. Literature is unique in its representation because unlike any other medium, it requires the active imagination of the reader in the construction of the diegetic world. One of the major contributions of reader response theory was to establish the role of the reader in this process of construction, and I expand upon that premise to show how the reader is involved in the construction of characters' fictional bodies specifically. When a narrator communicates information about a text's characters, the reader completes the act of constructing bodies by imagining their contours, postures, and gestures. A character's body is thus dependent upon both the narrator's speech—the use of nouns, pronouns, and adjectives—and the reader's expectations. Reading literature, and thus constructing fictional bodies, is always an act of collaboration between the author and the reader, and the indexes of our own materiality are evident in the metamorphic characteristic of fictional bodies. Each body takes shape differently according to the particular reader-author constellation, because each reader will construct a different body in their reading of the same literary piece. As a reader, my own embodied experiences inform the way I contribute to the construction of bodies in literature; those bodies exhibit traces of my materiality. Just as importantly, our bodies have long-lasting effects on the fictional world. The gestures and contours with which we endow fictional characters when we read will remain with them in our future imaginings of them. We thus leave traces of our own physicality on them. The fictional body's characteristics are determined by the material, embodied experience of both the author and reader. The fictional body is thus both material and relational, never only discursive or symbolic.

Barad provides us another way to think about this collaboration. In her work that reinterprets quantum physicist Niels Boehr's theories of materialization, she describes the inseparability of the observer, the thing observed, and the apparatus in scientific practices. An apparatus, according to Barad, is a specific configuration (a "phenomenon" as she calls it) of observer and observed, assembled in such a way that certain factors become controlled or eliminated so that underlying relationships can become apparent. She writes: "any measurement of 'position' using this apparatus cannot be attributed to some abstract independently existing 'object' but rather is a property of the phenomenon—the inseparability of 'observed object' and 'agencies of observation'" (Barad 2008, 132). The scientific observer or team constructs the apparatus, and thus their position necessarily affects and effects what is observed. Therefore, the basic unit of understanding anything, any object, anything observable, is not the distinct entity, but rather the configuration.

For readers, authors, literary critics, and scholars, the text is our apparatus. Language is stylized and metaphor employed to control certain elements so that underlying relationships can come to light. The author is not solely capable of assembling the apparatus; the presence of a reader is also required to decipher the underlying relationships brought to light by the author's work. Any paratextual discourse on the literary text, be it from critics, scholars, marketing, et cetera, necessarily contributes to the perpetual reconstruction of the fictional world. No one interacting with the text stands outside its apparatus, and as Barad writes, no apparatus is distinct and separate from other apparatuses: "Apparatuses are open-ended practices. [...] any particular apparatus is always in the process of intra-acting with other apparatuses" (Barad 2008, 134). The apparatus of the author and reader interacts with the apparatuses of the literary critic and scholar, the marketing of the book, et cetera.

The worlds of fiction and the material world necessarily leave imprints on one another. What is more, this involvement is intensely material. Both the author and the reader, who are the main agents in the collaborative process, are embodied entities, and thus their own embodied experiences must necessarily inform the way in which they imagine, construct, and shape bodies in fiction. The bodies of authors and readers are part of the makeup of the apparatus; they stand at the interstices of the real world and the fictional one. To refer back to Barthes, if the indexical referent must be present in order for the photograph to take place at all, then at the very least, the embodied author and reader must also be present in order for the fictional world of literature to take shape.

If the fictional body is interpellated via the author's word and the reader's imagination and carries traces of the materiality of both those people, another conceptual problem arises for a material feminist reading of the body in literature. One of the most important tenets of material feminisms is that the body, the material world, the non-human, and even the human-made inorganic are not inert, but rather, have their own agency beyond what we can understand and control. As Barad writes, "To restrict power's productivity to the limited domain of the 'social,' for example, or to figure matter as merely an end product rather than an active factor in further materializations, is to cheat matter out of the fullness of its capacity" (Barad 2008, 128). Theorizing agency outside the realm of the social, the field of human power, has been one of the central challenges of material feminisms. Focusing on the human body, Alaimo and Hekman contend that we must understand its materiality "as itself an active, sometimes recalcitrant force" (Alaimo and Hekman 2008, 4), and both Braidotti and Barad speak of nature's self-organizing and self-differentiating tendencies that have little need for human logics or interventions. By reconceptualizing nature, the material world, and even the inorganic as having their own agency and processes, rather than as inert matter at our disposal, these theorists re-think the relationship between mind and matter and flatten the hierarchy between human consciousness and other forms of agency operating in the material world.[3]

The fictional body cannot be considered a material entity that operates separately from human consciousness, but it does belong to the realm of the human-made inorganic. For the fictional body, agency might be understood as the willful resistance to control by those who construct it. Bodies in literature act in ways we cannot wholly control, and this emerges from the slippages that necessarily arise in the collaborative process between reader and author and which exhibit themselves in the text as ellipses. Ellipsis is one of the intrinsic features of discourse that allow interpretation to be possible. While the author has control over the fictional body to the extent that they can describe certain features and make it act in certain ways, they can never describe a body completely or account for the actions of the body in the ellipses of the fictional text. Likewise, the reader cannot predict what the fictional body will do, even though they are necessarily employed to complete the body's construction. A body in fiction thus has its own agency because even though it is imbued with our materiality and experiences as readers and writers, it exceeds them at the same time, defying our expectations and resisting being fully controlled through representation. Material feminists draw on terms such as "transformation," "metamorphosis," and "process" to describe the kinds of agency in the material world that evade human logic and control, and these are precisely the kinds of agency that fictional bodies also possess. Bodies in literature are unpredictable and metamorphose in any number of ways. They have agency because they can willfully evade our control and because they have the power to foreground the processes—social, material, and historical—that debunk a conventional concept of an essential body. Because of literature's ability to create a space for the free play of the symbolic, material, discursive, and relational, it can be an excellent site for rethinking the material body, its agency, its processes, and its place in fictional worlds.

READING AS TRANS-CORPOREAL

If our experience of embodiment is what allows us to imagine fictional bodies at all, then our bodies must be understood as primary to the reading experience. Reading, considered this way, is both discursive and material, a border crossing between bodies, fictional, and real, as we co-construct the bodies we encounter in fiction. I want to go a step further now and maintain that the effect might be reciprocal, that these fictional bodies might also make their way into our materiality and leave their traces there. Here, I depart again from the conventionally held notion that what happens in literature happens only in the mind, that reading is a kind of "simulation" (see for Oatley 2012, 426). In this part of my essay, I take a cue from Alaimo and Barad and ask the following: what if what happens in literature happens to us not only in an intellectual sense, but in another, more physical sense as well? What if our bodily materiality is changed by the reading process?

In her entry in *The Posthuman Glossary*, Stacy Alaimo states that trans-corporeality as a concept "means that all creatures, as embodied beings, are intermeshed with the dynamic, material world, which crosses through them, transforms them, and is transformed by them" (Alaimo 2018, 435). With this statement, Alaimo puts forth two priorities for thinking about our situatedness. First, as embodied beings, we are always influenced and even transformed by external materialities. A case in point is that we must eat: "Perhaps the most palpable example of trans-corporeality is that of food, whereby plants or animals become the substance of the human" (Alaimo 2008, 253).[4] Toxins similarly make the permeable and interdependent nature of the material and social worlds evident:

> the traffic in toxins reveals the interconnections among various movements, such as environmental health, occupational health, labor, environmental justice, popular epidemiology, environmentalism, ecological medicine, disability rights, green living, antiglobalization, consumer rights, and children's health and welfare. The traffic in toxins may render it nearly impossible for humans to imagine that our own well-being is disconnected from that of the rest of the planet.
>
> (Alaimo 2010, 18)

As the examples of food and toxins illustrate, the human body is never an autonomous, static, or stable entity because it constantly interacts with its physical and discursive environments.

The second priority that Alaimo posits for considering embodiment is that the material world is dynamic. The material world does not merely comprise the raw materials with which we build our lives, but rather, is agentic in its own right. Certain natural agencies evade human reasoning and exist independently of human utility, although we interact with them, knowingly or not, on a regular basis. In pointing this out, Alaimo counters notions of human exceptionalism by relativizing human subjectivity among a variety of other kinds of logic in the natural world. Here the influence of Barad is recognizable, who theorizes materiality and discourse as an entanglement. For Barad, the agency of matter is evidenced by our ability to perceive it. The self-organizing tendency of matter, as matter differentiates itself from other matter, is a performance of iteration, a form of discourse (see Barad 2007).

By foregrounding the material existence of embodied beings, Alaimo and Barad battle the millennia-long held notion in Western thought that human subjectivity is separate from and elevated above the material world. Not only is the human body enmeshed within its physical environment, our physical existence a "fleshy permeability" (Alaimo 2016, 78) through which air, water, microscopic organisms, food, and other substances pass, but, as she is keen to point out, our subjectivity is part of this entanglement. For Alaimo, the material and social worlds are infused with one another, so that, as she writes, the "'body' and 'nature' are comprised of the same material, which has been constituted, simultaneously, by the forces of evolution, natural and human history, political inequities, cultural contestations, biological and chemical processes, and other factors too numerous to list" (Alaimo 2008, 257).

In my own literary analysis of work by Antje Rávic Strubel, Jenny Erpenbeck, and Juli Zeh, I have developed close readings to foreground the entanglement of the body, subjectivity, community, governance, capitalism, the environment, toxicity, and other human bodies thematized in their works. In Strubel's novel *Kältere Schichten der Luft* (2007), the main character's fleshy materiality is altered through the interpellation of a second gender that emerges from within her/him. This interpellation requires a particular constellation—the third person narrator, a second character in the text, and the reader's imagination—and thus the body is shown to be discursive and relational in addition to material (Chronister 2015). In Erpenbeck's *Geschichte vom alten Kind* (1999), the main character's physical awkwardness and her body's ability to metamorphose challenge the reader to imagine it, making our active participation as co-constructors of the body all the more apparent. We draw on our own experiences of physical awkwardness to imagine her body, unwittingly yet still cruelly burdening the protagonist with our own difficult experiences of embodiment (Chronister 2018). In Zeh's *Corpus Delicti* (2009) and *Unterleuten* (2016), characters ingest toxins, poison one another, and manipulate their physical environments in order to send discursive messages to one another and assert resistance to power. Bodies ingest aspects of the environment and, reciprocally, expel body materiality outward for others to ingest (Chronister 2023). In all four of these literary texts, discourse and materiality are entangled. The body is the porous flesh through which the personal and the social flow, which, in terms that bring us back to Alaimo and Barad, highlights the duality of materiality and discourse. The boundaries that differentiate the fictional from the real also become porous, as the reader's body becomes the materiality out of which fictional bodies are built. The question remains whether the fictional characters' materiality is similarly expelled outwards for us to ingest as readers, that is, whether reading can truly be considered trans-corporeal in nature.

Recent studies in the cognitive sciences may support an understanding of reading as trans-corporeal, such that the reader's body not only contributes to, but is also impacted by, the reading experience. In such studies, brain scanning techniques using functional Magnetic Resonance Imaging (fMRI) and single pulse Transcranial Magnetic Stimulation (TMS) have shown how reading both activates areas of the brain associated with the performance of specific motor skills and stimulates electrical activity in the nervous system and muscle groups outside of the brain. For example, in an oft-cited study from 2009, a team of researchers led by Nicole Speer demonstrated through fMRI that areas of the brain associated with specific motor skills are activated when the reader reads a passage in which a character is undertaking an analogous action in the text. When a character pulls a lamp cord, the region of the reader's brain responsible for grasping is activated, which means that we comprehend the representation of a person pulling a lamp cord in narrative through the same mechanisms of the brain that we use to actually pull a lamp cord (Speer et al. 2009). Some scholars call this neurological ability to interpret the linguistic representation of activities by utilizing the same brain functioning as performing them "embodied semantics" (see, for example, Aziz-Zadeh and Damasio 2008, 35). According to this theory, our comprehension of action concepts is primarily embodied. A number of other studies have had similar findings (see, for example, Aziz-Zadeh and Damasio 2008; Aziz-Zadeh et al. 2006; Glenbert et al. 2008; Jacobs and Willems 2018). These studies make the case that when we read, we may step into someone else's shoes metaphorically, but also in a much more physical sense as well (as put by Jacobs and Willems 2018, 154). Of course, these studies are small with controlled groups of norm-conforming bodies. More work is warranted among populations with more diverse experiences of embodiment.

Other studies have suggested, furthermore, that embodiment is central to the interpretation of more abstract functions of language and literature than just the representation of actions, such as metaphor and even narrative structure. George Lakoff and Mark Johnson's now classic work *Metaphors We Live By* (1980) offers a deep study into the ways in which the use of metaphors in our speech and thought shapes the way in which we conceptualize and navigate our immediate physical environments and social world. According to Lakoff and Johnson, the body is primary to the make-up of these metaphors:

> [Orientational metaphors] have to do with spatial orientation: up-down, in-out, front-back, on-off, deep-shallow, central-peripheral. These spatial orientations arise from the fact that we have bodies of the sort we have and that they function as they do in our physical environment. Orientation metaphors give a concept a spatial orientation; for example, HAPPY is UP. The fact that the concept HAPPY is oriented UP leads to English expressions like "I'm feeling up today." Such metaphorical orientations are not arbitrary. They have a basis in our physical and cultural experience.
>
> (Lakoff and Johnson 1980, 14)

Not only do metaphors derived from physical experience help us navigate our physical and social worlds, but they are also key to our interpretation and creation of narrative. The basic metaphor of the container (we conceptualize an inside and outside of our bodies; therefore, we conceptualize space and the material world in the same way) leads us to think about story in terms of its "content." Similarly, the metaphor of the journey leads us to expect certain norms in narrative structure, such as a beginning, middle, and end. Even if these elements are out of order or missing, we perceive them as such (Lakoff and Johnson 1980, 92–96; see also Glenberg 2008, 906).[5] Finally, our embodiment is key to our aesthetic experience:

> From the experientialist perspective, metaphor is a matter of imaginative rationality. It permits an understanding of one kind of experience in terms of another, creating coherence by virtue of imposing gestalts that are structured by natural dimensions of experience. [...] And conceptual structure is not merely a matter of the intellect—it involves all the natural dimensions of our experience, including aspects of our sense experience: color, shape, texture, sound, etc.
>
> (Lakoff and Johnson 1980, 235)

Indeed, a study conducted by Lisa Aziz-Zadeh and Antonio Damasio found neurological evidence for the embodied knowledge required to understand metaphor. The first time a test subject encountered an expression like "grasping the situation," the same sensory-motor areas were activated that are used for actually grasping something. They found, however, that once sayings like "grasp the situation," "bite the bullet," or "kick the bucket" become standard to the test subject, they no longer utilize the same neural networks, meaning that the brain has since organized this language differently (Aziz-Zadeh and Damasio 2008). Such metaphorical language requires first embodied knowledge for interpretation before it can be organized intellectually.

These studies make a strong case that reading is trans-corporeal in nature, that reading literature—indeed interpreting language more generally—is a full-body physical endeavor. They challenge the notion of a mind-body split in powerful ways. Yet the question remains whether these trans-corporeal moments make a lasting impact on our materiality. There is some evidence that they do, particularly when we consider the brain itself as material. A 2013 study by Gregory S. Berns et al. set out with the following premise: "It seems plausible that if something as simple as a book can leave the impression that one's life has been changed, then perhaps it is powerful enough to cause changes in brain function and structure" (Berns et al. 2013, 590). While previous studies had shown changes in the functional connectivity of certain brain regions while reading, it was unknown how long those changes might last. The participants in this study were assigned a novel to read over nine days and given regular fMRI scans before, during, and after the study to determine connectivity change. While some new connections in the brain associated with reading comprehension eroded rapidly after the completion of the novel, "[l]ong-term changes in connectivity, which persisted for several days after the reading, were observed in bilateral somatosensory cortex, suggesting a potential mechanism for 'embodied semantics'" (Berns et al. 2013, 590). The reading experience had, indeed, a longer-term effect on the brain. The evidence is still scant, but further studies might explore whether reading impacts the materiality of our nervous and muscular systems in lasting ways.

The work done in the cognitive sciences on embodied reading comprehension builds upon studies that show how important embodiment is to language comprehension more generally (Speer et al. 2009, 997; Pulvermüller 2005; Buccino et al. 2005; Glenberg et al. 2008, 912). To be sure, language comprehension is a full-body endeavor, and reading is one of many language-based activities that requires embodied knowledge. Watching films, television, or theater; listening to speech; and observing others, for example, all require embodied experience for the organization of information and interpretation of events. Yet reading fiction, as I argued above, is particularly intimate. Unlike in visual representation or observation, we actively construct the bodies that we read, crawling into their skins and constituting and altering their makeup. We are the food, the toxin, that infuses and alters these bodies, and perhaps they are doing the same for us, to us, creating new pathways in our brains and activating our nervous systems and muscle groups. Maybe, then, the physicality of reading that has been explored in areas like affect studies—the tension we get in the pit of the stomach, the abatement of breath, the sexual excitement—is not merely a response to what we are reading, but rather, our bodies' active involvement in the construction of the meaning. Our bodies are providing our imaginations with conceptual information, as those fictional bodies summon our nervous and motor responses, leaving their marks on our brains. The infusion of bodies, fictional with real and real with fictional, is mutual. The reading experience is trans-corporeal in nature.

NOTES

1. This essay is developed from two articles previously published: Necia Chronister. 2018. "Conceiving of a Realfictional Body: Material Feminisms and Jenny Erpenbeck's *Geschichte vom alten Kind* (1999)." *German Quarterly* 91, no. 2; and Necia Chronister. 2023. "Beyond the Simulation: Reading, Trans-Corporeality, and Juli Zeh." *German Studies Review* 46, no. 2.
2. Of course, Barthes is speaking here of celluloid photography, which requires the presence of the object depicted before the lens. While digital photography does not rely on the index to the same extent, viewer expectations established with celluloid photography persist. We continue to assume some indexical relationship between the object represented and the digital photograph even with the most manipulated of images.
3. Material feminists are taking cue here from environmental feminists, who have long contended that we must relinquish the anthropocentric and patriarchal notion that we have mastery over nature.
4. Here, Alaimo references Gatens (1996).
5. Here, I extrapolate from Lakoff and Johnson's discussion of argumentation.

WORKS CITED

Alaimo, Stacy. 2010. *Bodily Natures: Science, Environment, and the Material Self*. Bloomington: Indiana University Press.

Alaimo, Stacy. 2016. *Exposed: Environmental Politics and Pleasures in Posthuman Times*. Minneapolis: University of Minnesota Press.

Alaimo, Stacy. 2008. "Trans-corporeal Feminisms and the Ethical Space of Nature." In *Material Feminisms*, edited by Stacy Alaimo and Susan Hekman, 237–264. Bloomsbury: Indiana University Press.

Alaimo, Stacy. 2018. "Trans-corporeality." In *The Posthuman Glossary*, edited by Rosi Braidotti and Maria Hlavajova, 435–438. London: Bloomsbury.

Alaimo, Stacy and Susan Hekman. 2008. "Introduction: Emerging Models of Materiality in Feminist Theory." In *Material Feminisms*, edited by Stacy Alaimo and Susan Hekman, 1–19. Bloomington: Indiana University Press.

Aziz-Zadehab, Lisa and Antonio Damasio. 2008. "Embodied Semantics for Actions: Findings from Functional Brain Imaging." *Journal of Physiology – Paris* 102: 35–39. doi:10.1016/j.jphysparis.2008.03.012

Aziz-Zadeh, Lisa, Stephen M. Wilson, Giacomo Rizzolatti, and Marco Iacoboni. 2006. "Congruent Embodied Representations for Visually Presented Actions and Linguistic Phrases Describing Actions." *Current Biology* 16 (Sept): 1818–1823. doi:10.1016/j.cub.2006.07.060

Barad, Karen. 2007. *Meeting the Universe Halfway: Quantum Physics and the Entanglement of Matter and Meaning*. Durham: Duke University Press.

Barad, Karen. 2008. "Posthumanist Performativity: Toward an Understanding of How Matter Comes to Matter." In *Material Feminisms*, edited by Stacy Alaimo and Susan Hekman, 120–154. Bloomington: Indiana University Press.

Barthes, Roland. 1981. *Camera Lucida: Reflections on Photography*. Translated by Richard Howard. New York: Hill and Wang.

Berns, Gregory S., Kristina Blaine, Michael J. Prietula, and Brandon E. Pye. 2013. "Short- and Long-Term Effects of a Novel on Connectivity in the Brain." *Brain Connectivity* 3, no. 6 (Dec): 590–600. doi:10.1089/brain.2013.0166

Braidotti, Rosi. 2011. *Nomadic Theory: The Portable Rosi Braidotti*. New York: Columbia University Press.

Buccino, G., L. Riggio, G. Melli, F. Binkofski, V. Gallese, and G. Rizzolatti. 2005. "Listening to Action-Related Sentences Modulates the Activity of the Motor System: A Combined TMS and Behavioral Study." *Cognitive Brain Research* 24 (Aug): 355–363. doi:10.1016/j.cogbrainres.2005.02.020

Chronister, Necia. 2023. "Beyond the Simulation: Reading, Trans-Corporeality, and Juli Zeh." *German Studies Review* 46, no. 2 (Spring): 227–245.

Chronister, Necia. 2018. "Conceiving of a Realfictional Body: Material Feminisms and Jenny Erpenbeck's *Geschichte vom alten Kind*." *The German Quarterly* 91, no. 2 (Spring): 123–137.

Chronister, Necia. 2015. "Language-Bodies: Interpellation and Gender Transition in Judith Hermann's 'Sonja' and Antje Rávic Strubel's *Kältere Schichten der Luft*." In *German Women's Writing in the 21st Century*, edited by Hester Baer and Alexandra Merley Hill, 18–36. Rochester: Camden House.

Erpenbeck, Jenny. 1999. *Geschichte vom alten Kind*. Frankfurt: Eichborn, 1999.

Gatens, Moira. 1996. *Imaginary Bodies: Ethics, Power and Corporeality*. New York: Routledge.

Glenberg, Arthur M., Marc Sato, Luigi Cattaneo, Lucia Riggio, Daniele Palumbo, and Giovanni Buccino. 2008. "Processing Abstract Language Modulates Motor System Activity." *The Quarterly Journal of Experimental Psychology* 61 (June): 905–919. doi:10.1080/17470210701625550

Jacobs, Arthur M. and Roel M. Willems. 2018. "The Fictive Brain: Neurocognitive Correlates of Engagement in Literature." *Review of General Psychology* 22, no. 2 (June): 147–60. doi:10.1037/gpr0000106

Lakoff, George and Mark Johnson. 1980. *Metaphors We Live By*. Chicago: University of Chicago Press.

Oatley, Keith. 2012. "The Cognitive Science of Fiction." *WIREs Cognitive Science* 3 (July/Aug): 425–430. doi:10.1002/wcs.1185

Pulvermüller, Friedemann. 2005. "Brain Mechanisms Linking Language and Action." *Perspectives* 6 (July): 576–582. doi:10.1038/nrn1706

Speer, Nicole K., Jeremy R. Reynolds, Khena M. Swallow, and Jeffrey M. Zacks. 2009. "Reading Stories Activates Neural Representations of Visual and Motor Experiences." *Psychological Science* 20 (Aug): 989–999. doi:10.1111/j.1467-9280.2009.02397.x

Strubel, Antje Rávic. 2007. *Kältere Schichten der Luft*. Frankfurt am Main: S. Fischer Verlag.

Zeh, Juli. 2009. *Corpus Delicti. Ein Prozess*. Frankfurt am Main: Schöffling Verlag.

Zeh, Juli. 2016. *Unterleuten*. Munich: Luchterhand.

PART VI

Trauma

CHAPTER TWENTY

Death by Despair: Destroying Health in Schiller's *Die Räuber*

ELEOMA BODAMMER

INTRODUCTION

Lack of attention to the emotion despair in published research on Schiller's first play *Die Räuber* (1781) means that its importance as a central theme which unites all plot strands has not been fully explored. In the play, Schiller conceptualizes a pathology of despair as a condition of the spirit that makes the body ill and explores the idea that despair can be immorally exploited and weaponized as a destructive emotion. He uses his villain Franz Moor as a mouthpiece for medical, religious, and philosophical ideas about how emotions, in particular despair, affect the body, soul, health, and wellbeing, and to test their effects. Moor explains that he is like a doctor in reverse, "wie der gescheide Arzt, (nur umgekehrt.)" (Schiller 1988, 2: 53) ["like a skilled doctor—only the other way about"] (Schiller 1979, 56), meaning that he wants to make his victims ill or assist their deaths, but not cure them. The theme of despair is key to Franz Moor's plan to use an emotional weapon to destroy his father and brother, and it contributes to his own mental breakdown and suicide, in the form of religious despair. Schiller not only explores the possibility of controlling the contexts that create despair, but in relation to the other main characters, he also demonstrates that despair has different causes that lead to a renunciation of life and to death. For example, despair drives Karl Moor to join the band of robbers, abandon his love for Amalia, and all hope of reuniting with his father; despair eventually kills Old Moor when he discovers that his son Karl is the captain of the band of murderous robbers; despair becomes a prerequisite for joining the band of robbers, which is evident when Karl Moor tells the recruit Kosinsky that he should only join the robbers if he has abandoned all hope and reached the point of despair; despair drives Amalia to demand to be killed when she is confronted with the truth about Karl Moor's crimes at the end of the play and the prospect of a future without joy or love. In effect, despair is the context for Schiller's presentation of suffering in this tragedy.

In his preface to *Die Räuber*, Schiller argues that he has reconfigured tragic figures so that they have villainous traits and makes a case for it being possible for the viewer to feel pity or sympathy for the suffering villain or criminal. He defends his villains as not being completely evil and states that he regards a completely evil character as not morally suitable for the stage. There is an apparent contradiction here, because it is difficult to find any redeeming characteristic in his villain Franz Moor. I propose, however, that if we examine the idea of despair and relate it to Schiller's later essay *Über den Grund des Vergnügens an tragischen Gegenständen* (1792) (Of the Cause of the Pleasure We Derive from Tragic Objects) (1992, vol. 8), it is possible to argue that Franz Moor's capacity for despair shortly before his death serves as evidence of an acceptance of moral law and his suffering evokes some sympathy in the spectator or reader. Schiller has therefore not contradicted himself, and Franz Moor is not a completely evil villain. This is made possible by employing despair as a mechanism for self-judgment and atonement, as evidence of a guilty conscience and a moral compass, and for invoking suffering in order to produce sympathy in the viewer or reader.

DEFINITIONS OF "VERZWEIFLUNG"

In theological and philosophical contexts and historical dictionaries, "Verzweiflung" is generally associated with a loss of hope, a profound sadness, and a state of personal crisis that overwhelms the individual who becomes unable to resolve the problem through action. The person suffering from despair often perceives suicide as the only solution to the suffering experienced. In religious contexts, "Zweifel" (doubt) is a component of the German word for despair, "Ver-*zweifl*-ung," (despair) and acknowledges the role that doubt plays in undermining the despairing person's hope of a resolution to the crisis (Ohly 1995, 177; Ruprecht 1959, 80). In scholastic thinking, theological or religious despair comes to be regarded as a sin, because it derives from the belief that comfort cannot be found in God's grace, mercy, or compassion. Religious despair arises from doubts about one's own salvation and is apparent in the inability to repent or show remorse for the sins committed (Ohly 1995, 183). It is not regarded as a justified reason for avoiding confession (Ruprecht 1959, 80). In St Augustine's teachings in Sermon 71 on Matthew 12:32 and Luke 12:8–12, despair in its religious context is understood as blasphemy against the Holy Spirit and as an unpardonable sin that leads to eternal damnation if death comes before remorse (Ohly 1995, 177; Ruprecht 1959, 12). For St Augustine, it was still possible for a person in a state of despair to have their sins forgiven and achieve the salvation of the soul, but only in cases where the individual felt remorse before death (Ohly 1995, 183–184). St Augustine understands blasphemy as the "unrepentant heart that resists the forgiveness of sins." Since St Augustine, sinful despair has been referred to as a form of sinful sadness that derives from the fear that the sins committed are so serious that God will not forgive them (Ruprecht 1959, 12; Jacob 1966, 154; Ohly 1995, 177–216). Despair is therefore a threshold and potential point of no return, and in its religious form, it can be the point at which the salvation of the soul and God's forgiveness are no longer possible.

In eighteenth- and early-nineteenth-century German dictionaries "Verzweiflung" in general is defined as a condition of the spirit or soul that affects the mind, body, and senses dramatically and negatively. According to J. G. Krünitz's *Oeconomische Encyclopädie* (1773–1858) [Economic Encyclopedia], a person in the state of despair is inconsolable and in a state of mental confusion; they cannot judge rationally or determine right from wrong; they can be driven to the point of madness; the consequences of despair are suicide and death. Krünitz's definition describes the physical effect of despair as producing unnatural convulsive gestures that emphasize a loss of control over the body, such as wringing hands, grinding teeth, and rolling eyes. The despairing person's behavior appears strange; they cannot find peace or rest; their speech is incoherent and is expressed in wild bursts; they curse and swear (Krünitz). For Krünitz, despair also interacts with other emotions and physical states, such as extreme pain and fear. This definition of despair conceptualizes it as an irrational state and encodes despair with a specific set of gestures that indicate a physical and mental loss of control.

The Grimms' dictionary considers "Verzweiflung" first and foremost as the highest form of spiritual pain and a state of hopelessness, the threshold beyond which there is nothing except the abyss, self-abandonment, or the deed that rescues the person. The Grimms foreground the experience of religious despair as one of the seven deadly sins. As a sin against hope, religious despair is defined as a sin against faith and is therefore an insult that God will not forgive. Drawing on Matthew 12:31, the Grimms state that all human sins and blasphemy will be forgiven, except for those spoken against the Holy Spirit, such as religious despair. They refer to Judas as the prototypical figure of religious despair. In their second definition, despair is defined as the most effective weapon that the devil can use in his battle for the human soul. In their worldly definition, it is the feeling of helplessness when not being able to find a way out of an internal crisis or external predicament. For the Grimms, despair is a state of extreme sadness that arises from impending misfortune and pairs with pain and fear.

In his general remarks on aesthetic reflective judgments in the *Critique of the Power of Judgment* (1790), Kant defines despair as an affect, as relating to "tumultuous and unpremeditated" feelings, whereas passions are "sustained and considered," "belong to the faculty of desire," and render choice difficult or impossible (2000, 154; 1974, 198–199). Kant classes despair as aesthetically sublime when it takes the form of rage rather than despondency (154).[1] Like anger, he regards it as one of the courageous affects "which arouses the consciousness of our powers to overcome any resistance (animi strenui)" (154–155). Similar to Kant, Schiller connects despair to the sublime. In *Die Räuber*, despair, in combination with the suffering individual and their realignment with moral law, creates the conditions for the aesthetically sublime, as Schiller notes in his essay *Über den Grund des Vergnügens* (1992, 8: 244).

The prototypical figures of religious despair in the Bible are Judas, Cain, and Saul (Ohly 1995, 190); in German literature, they are Hartmann von Aue's Gregorius and Wolfram von Eschenbach's Parzival (Ohly 1995, 177). Susan Snyder points out that despair as a religious crisis of belief in salvation is a significant feature of English Renaissance literature and from the mid-sixteenth century "despair episodes have a [...] place in the prodigal son dramas" (1965, 18), becoming a central theme of late sixteenth- and seventeenth-century plays in

England. Snyder cites works by Donne, Bunyan, and Marlowe's *Doctor Faustus* as examples. Considering that Schiller's original title for *Die Räuber* was the prodigal son (*Der verlorene Sohn*) (Koc 1986, 94), and that the topos of despair was usually employed in literature as a warning against despairing (Snyder 1965, 25), Schiller's play should be viewed as part of the canon of dramas of despair.

The concept of despair in eighteenth-century Germany has been an under-researched field of study until Katja Kauer's very recent book *Verzweiflung im 18. Jahrhundert: Eine Diskursgeschichte* [*Despair in the Eighteenth Century: A Discourse Analysis*], which argues that there was a re-coding or new shift in the meaning of "Verzweiflung" in the eighteenth century in Germany, from a purely negative emotion that inhibits action, to a positive emotion experienced by the active and rational individual (2022, 7). Kauer finds the roots of the idea that a rational person is not defenseless against "Verzweiflung" in the religious movement of pietism when it becomes possible to overcome it through a practice of self-optimizing (10–11). Despair is also centered in Lutheranism as a way of engaging with God whilst working on establishing a foundation for faith (11). In philosophy, Kauer pinpoints Kant's *Critique of Pure Reason* (1781) as an important milestone in transforming the idea of a despairing and doubting person into an independent thinker, capable of action (12). Kauer concludes that the modern definition of "Verzweiflung" has origins in epistemology rather than "Affektlehren" [theories of affects] (11).

In a very brief discussion of *Die Räuber*, Kauer positions Schiller's literary treatment of despair in this play between the positive and negative trends and decides that the characters are provoked into action by despair, but that this leads to negative actions and outcomes (2022, 184–185). She argues that despair fuels Karl Moor's courage and Franz Moor's malice, and leads to direct action in the former and indirect in the latter (Kauer 184). Kauer's conclusion is that Karl Moor overcomes his despair but that this is not a positive reconfiguration of the meaning of despair because it does not translate into "an edifying end" ("ein erbauliches Ende") (185). She states: "Die tatkräftige Überwindung seiner Verzweiflung kostet Karl die bürgerliche Existenz und seine soziale Akzeptanz" (185) ["In actively overcoming his despair, Karl loses his civic existence and his social acceptance"] (my translation). However, in my view, if we understand his surrender to the authorities as a renunciation of life, and since this act poses no hope of a future but certain death, this decision is therefore not a surmounting of despair but giving in to it. Ultimately, the characters' despair in this play is founded on the complete loss of hope and joy, which in fact none of them can overcome.

SCHILLER'S MEDICAL IDEAS: HOW THE SOUL AFFECTS THE BODY

While the origins of Schiller's early concept of despair are partly philosophical, they are also partly medical: they are present in his medical dissertation, *Versuch über den Zusammenhang der thierischen Natur des Menschen mit seiner geistigen* (1992, vol. 8) (*Essay on the Connection between the Animal and Spiritual Nature of Man*), which he submitted in 1780 to the Military Academy at the Karlsschule in Stuttgart in order to complete his medical training. This dissertation examines how the soul interacts with the body and how intense passions, including despair, psychosomatically affect physical health (Dewhurst and Reeves 1978, 253). Here, he sets out the philosophical and medical thinking that Franz Moor draws on when presenting his mechanistic worldview at the beginning of Act 2 Scene 1, as he devises a plan to undermine his father's health by using the spirit as an instrument with which to destroy the body, "den Körper vom Geist aus zu verderben" (Schiller 1988, 2: 54) ["to destroy the body through the soul"] (Schiller 1979, 56). Moor's intention is to employ emotions to harm the lifeforce of the body. This amounts to weaponizing emotions for the destruction of the sweet, peaceful union between the soul and the body, "diese süße friedliche Eintracht der Seele mit ihrem Leibe stören" (Schiller 1988, 2: 54) ["to disturb the sweet peace and harmony of body and soul"] (Schiller 1979, 57). His aim is not to heal but do the opposite of a doctor, to shorten and end his father's life (Schiller 1988, 2: 53). Arguing that "der überladene Geist drückt sein Gehäuse zu Boden" (2: 53) ["the overburdened spirit weighs down its vehicle"] (Schiller 1979, 56), Franz Moor understands the body as functioning like a machine that chimes in accordance with the mood of the spirit (Neubauer 1982, 277). In Act 2 Scene 1, he states: "Philosophen und Mediziner lehren mich, wie treffend die Stimmungen des Geists mit den Bewegungen der Maschine zusammen lauten" (Schiller 1988, 2: 53) ["Doctors and philosophers have taught me how finely the motions of the mind are attuned to those of the machine that houses it"] (Schiller 1979, 56). Franz Moor acknowledges that health and life are at the mercy of the passions, "Leidenschaften mißhandeln die Lebenskraft" (Schiller 1988, 2: 53) ["passions disturb the vital force"] (Schiller 1979, 56) and that mechanical dissonances in the body are accompanied by what he calls gouty emotions.

Paragraph 14 of Schiller's medical dissertation has the subtitle "Geistiger Schmerz untergräbt das Wohl der Maschine" (Schiller 1992, 8: 144) ["Mental anguish undermines the health of the human machine"] (Dewhurst and Reeves 1978, 271) and here Schiller explains that mental anguish is caused by unpleasant emotions, such as anger or fear, which produce mental convulsions, "Konvulsionen des Denkorgans" (Schiller 1992, 8: 144) ["convulsions of the thought organ"] (Dewhurst and Reeves 1978, 272) and affect the nervous system. He observes that this state of mental anguish is accompanied by physical symptoms, such as irregular and fast heartbeats, forcing blood into the lungs and a failing pulse (Schiller 1992, 8: 144). Such convulsions, Schiller argues in paragraph 14, "bringen die Kräfte des Lebens in jene Mißstimmung, die seinen Flor zernichtet, und alle Aktionen der Maschine aus dem Gleichgewicht bringt" (144) ["bringing the vital spirits into such discord that health is destroyed and all bodily functions are upset"] (Dewhurst and Reeves 1978, 272). He concludes this paragraph with the general statement that when the soul is in the most extreme state of suffering, it is also in the most extreme state of physical illness, "der Zustand des größten Seelenschmerzens ist zugleich der Zustand der größten körperlichen Krankheit" (Schiller 1992, 8: 144) ["the state of greatest mental anguish is also that of the greatest physical sickness"] (Dewhurst and Reeves 1978, 272).

In paragraph 15 of the dissertation, Schiller gives examples of the negative impact of "deep, chronic pain in the soul" [my translation], "[t]iefe chronische Seelenschmerzen" (Schiller 1992, 8: 144) on physical health when it is accompanied by excessive mental activity caused by emotions. He explains that the emotions anger and indignation gnaw at the foundations of the body, dry out the juices of life, and cause the body to waste away, leading to a deathly pallor and sunken eyes. The emotions despair (Verzweiflung), fear (Furcht), disquiet (Unruh), and a guilty conscience (Gewissensangst) are described as having no less of an impact than the highest fever (Schiller 1992, 8: 144–145). In Act 2 Scene 1, when considering with which emotion to torture his father, Franz Moor lists most of the emotions Schiller refers to in paragraph 15 of the dissertation and discusses their effects: these are "Zorn," (anger) "Sorge," (carking care) "Gram," (sorrow) "Furcht," (fear) "Schreck," (terror) "Jammer," (grief) and "Reue" (repentance) (Schiller 1988, 2: 54; Schiller 1979, 57). Moor settles on "Verzweiflung" as the emotional weapon he wants to use against his father, giving the reason that it leaves no trace of the dissector's knife and no wound or evidence of poison (2: 55). Franz Moor's plot to kill his father therefore tests the theory that there is a direct link between mental and physical states (i.e., that the state of the soul affects the state of the body).

While Franz Moor clearly draws on the philosophical and medical ideas that Schiller presented in his medical dissertation, the opposite is also the case. In paragraph 15 of the dissertation, Schiller refers directly to Franz Moor as a fictional case that supports his medical theory that emotions undermine the health of the body. To preserve his anonymity, Schiller disguises this reference to his as-yet unpublished play as an English tragedy by the fictitious author Krake, called *Life of Moor*, thus implying that the German extract he is citing is a translation from an English original (Schiller 1992, 8: 145). Schiller includes in paragraph 15 a shortened quotation from Act 5 Scene 1 of *Die Räuber* with a comment on Franz Moor's state of mind and physical symptoms when he is talking to his servant about his apocalyptic dreams (145). Schiller describes him as pale, breathless, and breaking out into a cold sweat because of the crimes he has committed; he is plagued by nightmares and visions of future trials, and he struggles to order the sensations and rationalize the horrors of his imagination (145).[2] In this quotation from Act 5 Scene 1 in the dissertation, the servant tells Franz Moor that he looks deathly pale and is stammering with fear.[3] Moor says that he has a fever and that an illness is the cause of his bad dreams and symptoms, and then he faints (146). Since despair is the cause of these physical symptoms, Schiller's explanation can be regarded as a pathology of despair. Schiller establishes that the dreams have set dark ideas into motion which have shut down his organ of thought and produced a pain that has undermined his soul and the nervous system (146). He argues that such shaking and convulsing are responses to planning and committing evil deeds and that these symptoms resemble patients in feverish states (145). He concludes that vices and emotions, such as anger, envy, and hatred, when experienced constantly, destroy health and happiness, which should therefore serve as a deterrent (147).

ACT 1 SCENE 1: "VERZWEIFLUNG" AS AN EMOTIONAL WEAPON

The opening scene and the motto indicate that health is central to *Die Räuber*. The Hippocratic motto[4] placed before the dramatis personae notes that what medicine does not heal, iron, or in other words the operative knife heals, and what iron does not heal, fire heals. But the play is not about healing, at least not until we reach the end, when Karl Moor symbolically returns to the fold and "heals" the disrupted order of things, saying: "Aber noch blieb mir etwas übrig, womit ich die beleidigte Gesetze versöhnen, und die mißhandelte Ordnung wiederum heilen kann" (Schiller 1988, 2: 160) ["But still something remains that can reconcile me to the laws against which I have offended, and heal the order which I have violated"] (Schiller 1979, 159–160, my addition).

The play is about destroying health. In Act 1 Scene 1, Franz Moor feigns concern about his father's health and introduces the idea that words and emotions can have a detrimental effect on the health of the body; they can cause suffering, shorten life, and kill. In this scene, it quickly becomes clear that Franz Moor is practicing an insincere ethics of care by pretending he wants to preserve his father's health and prevent the harm that the upsetting news about his brother Karl could cause. Franz Moor recommends postponing reading out a letter, which unbeknown to his father, he has forged and which he alleges is from an informant and contains distressing news about Karl's scandalous behavior in Leipzig. Playing the role of the concerned, caring, and compassionate son, Franz begins the pretense with a kind of "trigger warning" by first asking his father for reassurance that he is physically fit enough to hear the content of the letter because of a potentially traumatizing reaction. Franz announces that avoiding the news would be the safest option if his father is even the slightest bit unwell: "Wenn ihr krank seid – nur die leiseste Ahndung habt es zu werden, so laßt mich – ich will zu gelegnerer Zeit zu euch reden, *halb vor sich*. Diese Zeitung ist nicht für einen zerbrechlichen Körper" (Schiller 1988, 2: 20) ["If you are not well – if you have the slightest suspicion that you are not well, then let me – I will tell you at some more appropriate moment. [*Half aside*] This is no news for a delicate constitution"] (Schiller 1979, 25). Even before the news has been conveyed, the recommendation to delay disclosing the content because of its potential to harm is already having a negative effect on his father's wellbeing. The trigger warning reinforces the idea that the words in the letter will cause emotional and physical pain and as a result Old Moor starts thinking about Karl's wild antics as undermining his emotional resilience, saying: "O Karl! Karl! wüßtest du wie deine Aufführung das Vaterherz foltert!" (Schiller 1988, 2: 20) ["Oh, Karl, Karl! If only you knew how your wild ways torture your old father's heart"] (Schiller 1979, 25–26).

While Franz Moor promotes the view in this scene that written and spoken words are a stimulus for emotional harm, his father puts forward the opposite position, that they can also reduce distress and potentially have a rejuvenating effect. Old Moor acknowledges this by saying that good news would add ten years to his life and turn him into a younger man, whereas bad news would bring him closer to the grave (Schiller 1988, 2: 20–21). Opting to hear everything, Old Moor continues with the medical metaphor by referring to these attempts to prevent an intense physical and emotional reaction as unnecessarily providing crutches: "Alles, alles—mein Sohn, du ersparst mir die Krücke" (2: 21) ["Everything, everything – my son, you will spare me the need for crutches"] (Schiller 1979, 26). Old Moor's decision to be exposed to the deleterious news is motivated by a desire for access to the truth, which, of course, is a misperception because the letter has been written by Franz Moor. Franz Moor's deception is not discovered because, under the pretense of a duty of care, he does not allow his father to read the fake letter. Franz Moor explains to his father that he is already intervening by censoring the letter and reading out the less distressing content. When he reads out a section that describes the likely reaction to the news that the fictional correspondent expects Old Moor to have, he is priming his father further to believe that the words will cause harm. In the letter, the correspondent imagines Old Moor to be deathly pale and reeling in his chair on receiving the news, and Franz Moor reinforces this by claiming that his father's reaction matches this description. Quoting the informant's words in the forged letter, Franz Moor says "'mir ists, als säh ich schon deinen alten, frommen Vater Totenbleich'" (Schiller 1988, 2: 21) ["'it is as if I could see your good old father, deathly pale already'"] (Schiller 1979, 26). Comparing his father's appearance to the description in the letter, Franz Moor falsely declares that he can see the effect of the distress in his father's deathly pallor: "Jesus Maria! ihr seids, eh ihr noch das mindeste wisset?" (Schiller 1988, 2: 21) ["Dear God! and so you are, already, before you have heard anything at all?"] (Schiller 1979, 26). When reading out a list of his brother's scandalous acts, Franz Moor stops mid-sentence and declares that he will not continue to read the letter, because he will never murder his father with his lips. On the one hand, this context of Franz Moor's performance of a duty of care is a pretext for destroying the letter on the false grounds of protecting his father and, on the other, it also protects Franz Moor from being discovered, since it destroys the evidence of the forgery.

The opening scene consequently sets up the idea that words can be used to torture and destroy the health of the soul and the body. It also presents an idea that we find in twenty-first-century debates about trigger warnings, that they can induce the very psychological trauma that they are trying to avoid and protect the individual from. Franz Moor writes the letters to his father and brother with the specific intention of provoking affective states. This comes close to what the critic Ramzi Fawaz calls a pedagogical model of "affective curation" that deliberately "centralizes the value of intentionally eliciting, or 'triggering,' uncomfortable affective responses (...) in order to develop new strategies for retuning, rerouting, or altogether altering (...) sense perceptions of the world" (2016, 760). Franz Moor's warnings that signpost potential harm and pre-empt damaging reactions are a performance of care for the psychological wellbeing of his father, but later his curation of triggering materials extends to other props, such as the fake bloodied dagger that falsely proves to Old Moor and Amalia that despair has driven Karl to his death in battle (Schiller 1988, 2: 62–69).

The critic Richard Koc suggests that Franz Moor chooses this "self-destructive feeling of 'Verzweiflung'" as an emotional weapon to use against his father, because it is the same emotion that his father repeatedly tells him he should not inflict on his brother Karl (Koc 1986, 93). Indeed, Act 1 Scene 1 ends with Old Moor repeatedly asking Franz not to bring his brother to the point of despair when he communicates their father's disavowal to Karl in a letter that Old Moor asks Franz to compose for him. Old Moor asserts: "Schreib ihm daß ich tausend blutige Tränen, tausend schlaflose Nächte—Aber bring meinen Sohn nicht zur Verzweiflung! (...) Schreib ihm daß die Väterliche Brust—Ich sage dir bring meinen Sohn nicht zur Verzweiflung" (Schiller 1988, 2: 27) ["Tell him that a thousand tears of blood— tell him that a thousand sleepless nights—But do not drive my son to despair. (...) Tell him that his father's bosom—I tell you, do not drive my son to despair"] (Schiller 1979, 32). Franz Moor's decision to weaponize despair is informed by medical knowledge and an understanding of how the body reacts to it and the kinds of acts it causes.

ACT 1 SCENE 2: THE BODY AND SOUL AND THE METAPHOR FOR LEADERSHIP

Act 1 Scene 2 continues with the idea that words shock and produce a range of symptoms that can give the appearance of death. In this scene Karl Moor receives a letter from his brother that falsely declares that his father has disowned him and that there is no hope of mercy unless he lives on bread and water in his father's dungeons, a fate that eventually befalls Old Moor later in the play. The robber Grimm describes Karl Moor as leaving the group as pale as a corpse after reading the letter (Schiller 1988, 2: 38), which echoes the first scene of the play and the fictional informant's fabricated expectation that Old Moor will respond by becoming "[t]otenbleich" (2: 21) ["deathly pale"] (Schiller 1979, 26). This scene reinforces the idea that "Trauerpost," ["a letter announcing a death"] (my translation), a term that Schiller uses in his own review of *Die Räuber* (the "Selbstrezension"), affects health negatively (Schiller 1988, 2: 294).

Furthermore, the healthy relationship between the body and the soul is the source of the metaphor that is used in the robbers' leadership discussion. Shortly before returning to the robbers, after Karl Moor has read his brother's letter, which has had the desired effect of triggering despair, the robber Roller refers to Karl Moor as the soul in relation to the robbers' body. He says: "Ohne den Moor sind wir Leib ohne Seele" (Schiller 1988, 2: 43) ["Without Moor we're a body without a soul"] (Schiller 1979, 47). When choosing a captain, the robbers are not looking for an enlightened and political mind to lead them, which is what Spiegelberg wants to represent, but are instead in search of a soul that breathes life and passion into the "body" of the group. Karl Moor demonstrates his capacity to do this when he becomes emotionally animated by despair in his response to the letter from his brother. His decision to become the captain of the robbers is preceded by the wild convulsive gestures of despair associated with this emotion, and as Karl S. Guthke rightly argues, Karl Moor's actions have an emotional cause, and not just an idealistic one; his decisions are not entirely free will choices but are determined by passionate responses (2005: 50). The shock of the letter causes a tumultuous reaction, and his body moves wildly as he paces up and down the room. His language descends into comparisons between human beings and exotic wild animals, whilst he condemns human treachery and his brother's and father's betrayals. As the soul to the robbers' body, Karl Moor's leadership represents the element that can be affected by emotions, despair, and conscience. Furthermore, if the robbers are aligned with the concept of the body and Karl Moor represents the soul of the band of robbers, despair will also disturb the harmony of the robbers' union, which connects this metaphor to Franz Moor's comments on soul-body interactions. The "health" and viability of the group depends on the favorable influence of the soul on the body.

ACT 2 SCENE 2: "VERZWEIFLUNG" AND THE LOSS OF HOPE

Despair and the loss of hope are noted as the reasons why Karl Moor chooses to die in battle in Herrmann's fabricated account of Karl Moor's death, which Herrmann relates to Amalia and Old Moor, at Franz Moor's instigation. As part of Franz Moor's plot to undermine the health of his father, he persuades Herrmann to explain to Old Moor that his rejection caused his son Karl to lose hope and motivated him to become a soldier and desire to die as a hero on the battlefield. Herrmann talks of Karl Moor's loss of hope: "Er sprach viel von seinem alten Vater (...) und von vereitelten Hoffnungen" (Schiller 1988, 2: 62) ["He talked much of his old father (...) and of disappointed hopes"] (Schiller 2006a, n.p.); he went to battle "da er auf der Welt nichts mehr zu hoffen hatte" (Schiller 1988, 2: 62) ["and as he had nothing left to hope for in this world"] (Schiller 1979, 65). Herrmann then continues his false report, saying that Karl Moor wanted his father to know that his curse caused his despair and sent him into battle to die: "Sag ihm sein Fluch hätte mich gejagt in Kampf und Tod, ich sei gefallen in Verzweiflung!" (Schiller 1988, 2: 63) ["Tell him it was his curse that drove me into battle, war and death, tell him I am fallen in despair!"] (Schiller 1979, 66). In a theatrical performance of a duty of care, Franz pretends to become angry that Herrmann is trying to hasten Old Moor's death with the news of his brother's death, again pretending to shield him from the effects of the news. With a question that supports his theory that words and emotions can harm, Franz deceives his father again by feigning concern about his health and pretending to criticize Herrmann: "Bist du hierher kommen unserem Vater den Todesstoß zu geben?" (Schiller 1988, 2: 63) ["Have you come here to deal our father his death-blow?"] (Schiller 1979, 66). Franz Moor reveals here that despair can be caused by creating a particular set of circumstances that lead to a loss of hope and a desire for death. He also insinuates in this question that being responsible for creating the conditions for despair has the potential to cause despair in the person who has caused despair in others.

ACT 3 SCENE 2: "VERZWEIFLUNG" AS THE FOUNDATION FOR THE ROBBERS' ALLIANCE

Despair is central to Schiller's characterization of Karl Moor, whom he describes in the "Selbstrezension" (1782) ["Self-Review"] as "der zur Verzweiflung gehetzte Abenteurer" (Schiller 1988, 2: 294) ["the adventurer hounded by despair"] (my translation). Here, Schiller specifies that despair is the driving force behind Karl Moor's decision to lead the robbers as their captain. In his review of his play, Schiller writes of the effect of Old Moor's rejection on Karl Moor: "Karl, durch diesen Schritt zur Verzweiflung gebracht, verwickelt sich mit seinen Gefährten in ein Räuberkomplott, wird ihr Anführer, und führt sie in Böhmische Wälder" (2: 293) ["Karl, driven to despair by this act, becomes embroiled in a robbers' complot with his companions, becomes their leader and leads them into the Bohemian Forest"] (my translation). Despair also becomes a prerequisite for becoming a member of the band of robbers. This is evident in Act 3 Scene 2, when Karl Moor explains to the new recruit Kosinsky that joining them involves first knowing the depth of the abyss into which he is about to jump. Moor advises Kosinsky to consider any remaining element of joy or hope that he may still have, "eine einzige Freude" or "ein Funken von Hoffnung" (2: 103) ["one single joy" or "one single spark of hope"] (Schiller 1979, 103), that could save him, thus revealing that Karl Moor's concept of despair relates to the absence of hope and joy. What leads Kosinsky to the robbers is the impossibility of hope, which becomes evident when he recounts what has happened to him, saying, "die Hoffnungen meines Lebens hab ich müssen sehen in den Grund sinken" (Schiller 1988, 2: 101) ["I [...] have seen my life's hopes sink beneath the ocean"] (Schiller 1979, 101). Without a foundation in hope, his despair prompts him to act, and he first becomes a soldier to suppress the torturing memory of the loss of hope because, he says, the alternative would have been madness (Schiller 1988, 2: 101). While despair is on the one hand an absence of the hope of ending the crisis and is self-destructive, on the other hand it also creates a context for violence directed at others. Kosinsky's motivation to accept a violent life as a robber is presented here as a distraction from the experience of despair and a means of finding a way to live with it. After hearing Kosinsky's account of his despair over losing his Amalia, who chose to save his life by becoming the prince's mistress, Karl Moor is galvanized into seeking out his own Amalia. With the exclamation, "Aber bei der Hoffnung des Himmels!" (2: 105) ["But by every hope of heaven!"] (Schiller 1979, 106), Moor considers that he has perhaps not lost all grounds for hope and returns to Amalia.

Act 3 Scene 2 is a key scene for explaining the ways in which despair is challenged by hope and that when there is no hope of a way out of the state of despair, there is only space for actions so heinous that they suppress rather than overcome the state of despair. It also locates the experience of despair in relation to time as not future-oriented but present-centric. Schiller constructs an idea of despair in this scene that aligns itself with Anthony J. Steinbock's definition in his article on the phenomenology of despair, which states that "despair is oriented to the present" (2007, 449) and finds no connection to a future or resolution in the past. Steinbock argues that despair imprisons the individual in the present.

ACT 5 SCENE 1: RELIGIOUS DESPAIR

Franz Moor experiences a physical and mental loss of control throughout his final scene in Act 5 Scene 1: he faints, is pale, has a fever, slurs his speech, is in a state of confusion, is shaking, has memory loss, paces up and down, falls into a chair and convulses with terrifying movements. These symptoms correspond to Krünitz's definition of how despair presents in physical symptoms.[5] Franz Moor attributes the cause of his symptoms, however, to an illness that is affecting the brain and causing his nightmares that focus on how he will be judged on Judgment Day. Nevertheless, the religious nature of these dreams motivates him to call on Pastor Moser to interrogate him about the existence of God, the immortality soul, the prospect of salvation, and the consequences of committing unpardonable sins against the Holy Spirit. Moor defends his materialist and atheist position by rejecting the idea of God and the soul, and by reducing the human being to merely the body or matter whose spirit and thoughts end when life ends. Moser, on the other hand, paints a picture of an all-knowing, judging God who does not need to defend His existence. In this theodicy debate, Moser admits the existence of both good and evil in the world as evidence of God's greatness, which acknowledges that the existence of evil is compatible with the existence of God. Moser finds that human tyranny does not undermine God's greatness. Of God he says: "Er ist eben so groß in deinen Tyranneien, als irgend in einem Lächeln der siegenden Tugend" (Schiller 1988, 2: 145) ["For His greatness is as surely seen in your tyrannies, as in any smile of triumphant virtue"] (Schiller 1979, 144). In response to Franz Moor's explanation that the existence of the mind and the spirit end when life ends, and to Moor's disbelief in the immortal soul or eternal life, Moser exclaims: "Das ist die Philosophie eurer Verzweiflung" (2: 145) ["That is your philosophy of despair"] (Schiller 1979, 145). Moser argues that the fact that Franz Moor's heart is beating with anxious dread against his ribs is evidence that he is lying to himself and suggests he believes that there are consequences for his actions in relation to his soul, i.e., the physical symptoms indicate a conscience and concern for the salvation of his soul.

Despair is also presented in this scene as a state that can be experienced after death, in the hereafter, when Moser gives an account of the suffering that Moor has inflicted on others and warns him that those who have suffered in life will triumph in eternity, but those who have triumphed in life will be condemned to eternal, never-ending despair. When the discussion moves on to unpardonable sins, despair is not included amongst these, but instead fratricide and patricide.

THE CAPACITY FOR "VERZWEIFLUNG" AS A REDEEMING CHARACTERISTIC

In the preface to the play, Schiller defends his decision to depict vices, despicable acts, and villainous characters as didactically necessary to promote virtue and discourage vice (Schiller 1988, 2: 15). Unwilling to fully condemn his immoral characters, he refers to his approach as characterizing whole humans. He explains that the strong points of the evilest characters relate to the spirit more than the heart (2: 17). Schiller asserts that everyone, even the wickedest person, is made in the image of God and suggests that the greater villain has the shorter path to righteousness than the lesser villain (2: 17). He explains that his villains are never completely evil, giving the reason that a completely evil human being should not be the subject of art: "Auch ist ein Mensch, der ganz Bosheit ist, schlechterdings kein Gegenstand der Kunst, und äußert eine zurückstoßende Kraft, statt daß er die Aufmerksamkeit der Leser fesseln sollte" (2: 18) ["Besides this, a man who is so utterly depraved as to be without a single redeeming point is no meet subject for art, and would disgust rather than excite the interest of the reader"] (Schiller 2006a, n.p.).

Although Schiller makes it clear in the preface that he did not intend his villains to be understood as entirely evil, it is difficult to establish which strong, positive, or redeeming characteristics Franz Moor could possibly have. The critic Alan Menhennet, for example, acknowledges that Franz Moor should be regarded "a monster of heroic proportions" (1973, 163), whilst also recognizing that, like his brother Karl, he is part of the central theme of "'the sublime criminal,' the intertwining of the abominable and the admirable" (160), but Menhennet is not specific about any non-villainous or admirable characteristics that Franz Moor has. Lesley Sharpe comments that in the first version of the play, Franz Moor's "only moral impulse is the terror and panic he feels at the approach of retribution" (2005, 126), which suggests that the experience of the feelings that precede his suicide are evidence of a moral core.[6]

In the "Selbstrezension" ["Self-Review"] of 1792, Schiller expands on the idea of villains being both human and sublime and proposes that sublime criminals produce sympathy and admiration, alongside "die Empfindung des Abscheus" (Schiller 1988, 2: 296) ["the feeling of disgust" (my translation). While he recognizes that in Franz Moor he has created "dieses Monstrum" (2: 300) ["this monster"] (my translation) and "die ganze menschliche Natur in der Person eines Teufels" (2: 301) ["the whole of human nature in the figure of a devil"] (my translation), he nevertheless writes that it is not his evil actions nor despicable philosophy ("die abscheuliche Philosophie") (2: 301) that we should be outraged about, but the ease with which he is able to act in this manner. Most importantly, Schiller mentions that Franz Moor's humanity and capacity for despair are characteristics that allow the spectator to sympathize with him. Schiller explains: "seine Verzweiflung fängt an, uns mit seiner Abscheulichkeit zu versöhnen" (2: 303) ["his despair helps us to reconcile with his detestableness"] (my translation). He points to Franz Moor's humanity as his redeeming quality, which is identifiable in the cowardice that prevents him from committing murder by his own hand (2: 302) and in his human suffering and feelings of torment before he takes his own life because he is terrified of the prospect of eternal damnation. Schiller asserts that he suffers as a human: "Endlich in der unglücklichen Katastrophe seiner Intrige, wo er menschlich leidet?" (2: 303) ["Ultimately, in the unfortunate catastrophe of his intrigue, he suffers as a human?"] (my translation).

The intention to evoke "Mitleid" ("pity") as a reaction to suffering is central to Schiller's early concept of tragedy in his essay *Über die tragische Kunst* (*On the Tragic Art*) (1792). In his interpretation of Aristotelian catharsis, the spectator achieves what he calls "Rührung" (Schiller 1992, 8: 274) ("emotion" or "stirring"), which is the mixed feeling of suffering ("Leiden") and pleasure ("Lust") when watching suffering (8: 239). Schiller specifies that only the suffering of moral beings comparable to us can evoke pity ("Mitleid") (8: 273) and that this can be caused by the circumstances (8: 259). The person suffering can only be a tragic subject and evoke pity in the viewer if they (the tragic subject) align themselves with moral law ("Sittlichkeit") (Schiller 1988, 8: 273). He elaborates on the tragic subject further in his essay *Über den Grund des Vergnügens* (*Of the Cause of the Pleasure* by stating that the suffering of the criminal is not less tragically pleasing than the suffering of a virtuous person, and that this is a morally inappropriate subject matter for tragedy if there is no return to the moral law. Schiller proposes then that the suffering criminal realigns with the moral law via remorse, self-damnation, and in the state of despair. He states:

> Reue, Selbstverdammung, selbst in ihrem höchsten Grad, in der Verzweiflung, sind moralisch erhaben, weil sie nimmermehr empfunden werden könnten, wenn nicht tief in der Brust des Verbrechers ein unbestechliches Gefühl für Recht und Unrecht wachte, und seine Aussprüche selbst gegen das feurigste Interesse der Selbstliebe geltend machte.
>
> (Schiller 1992, 8: 244)

> [Repentance, [self-damnation,] even despair, have nobleness morally, and can only exist if an incorruptible sense of justice exists at the bottom of the criminal heart, and if conscience maintains its ground against self-love.]
>
> (Schiller 2006b, n.p., my addition)

If the capacity to feel despair is a sign that a person has not abandoned moral law, then Schiller is presenting the case here that not only Karl but also Franz Moor has redeeming characteristics. Franz Moor's suffering reaches the point of self-condemnation and his despair becomes the indicator of an internal judge and conscience that he cannot suppress. Schiller states in this essay:

> Reue und Verzweiflung über ein begangenes Verbrechen zeigen uns die Macht des Sittengesetzes nur später, nicht schwächer;
>
> (Schiller 1992, 8: 245)

> [Repentance and despair at past crimes show us the power of moral law, only later and not weaker;]
>
> (my translation)

If despair is evidence that the moral law has not been abandoned, Schiller is supporting the notion that Franz Moor's suffering and suicide produce pity and catharsis in the viewer, and that this provides an answer to the question of Franz Moor's redeeming quality, i.e., there is an indication of his humanity and acknowledgment of the moral law. Schiller intends for both Karl and Franz Moor's suffering to produce pity or sympathy in the viewer, and therefore both to be considered as morally sublime villains.

CONCLUSION

With his first play *Die Räuber*, Schiller offers the Sturm und Drang movement a tragedy about the impact of despair on human health. Drawing on his early medical studies at the Karlsschule in Stuttgart, which had an interdisciplinary focus on philosophy and medicine, he examines in the play how the spirit or soul interacts with the body. He conceptualizes a medical view of despair as a condition of the spirit that makes the body ill and builds dramatic tension around the testing of the theory that the health of the body can be undermined and destroyed by despair, which sets the individual on a pathway of suffering that ends in death. Despair produces physical reactions in the body that not only resemble illness and death but are also part of the process of the deterioration of health and dying.

Exploring the cause-and-effect link between the soul and the body, Schiller constructs a plot around the different ways in which despair can be induced in an individual: for example, by using his villain Franz Moor as a doctor in reverse whose aim is not to heal but to shorten life by bringing others to the point of despair. The characters in the play suffer and are driven to despair for different reasons, giving Schiller the opportunity to illustrate that the loss of love, hope, purpose in the world, and religious skepticism all lead to despair; in fact, despair unites all plot strands in the play.

Schiller shows how chance circumstances and deliberate influence over an individual's understanding of their circumstances create contexts for the experience of despair. Tragic events can be generated when contexts and actions are misrepresented, and perceptions manipulated. The actions that arise from despair relate to violence directed at oneself and others, thus providing a context for suffering and the viewer's experience of pity. The pathway from despair to death operates in a similar way to tragic fate, as an unstoppable and necessary life-ending force. When fully invoked, despair does not allow for hope, optimism, or improvement, it instead drives the individual to renounce the self, body, kinship, relationships, and life.

Schiller states in his preface to the play that the portrayal of a complete villain is inappropriate for the stage, but critics have struggled to find any redeeming characteristic in Franz Moor. In his essay *Über den Grund des Vergnügens* (*Of the Cause of the Pleasure*) Schiller reflected further on despair, stating that the criminal's ability to feel remorse and condemn himself, even in a state of despair, is an example of the morally sublime and evidence that he has not rejected moral law. Since Schiller regards despair, remorse, and self-condemnation as indicators of an incorruptible moral core, we can understand Franz Moor's capacity for despair as his redeeming characteristic because his apocalyptic dreams indicate the surfacing of suppressed guilt that is subconscious remorse. While the tragic outcome of the play depends on Franz Moor's successful employment of despair to produce suffering and his use of despair as an emotional weapon to destroy health and life, it is nevertheless also relevant to his own demise, when religious despair appears to contribute to his suicide. If Franz Moor genuinely experiences religious despair, which his physical reactions seem to indicate, then this is evidence that he is not an entirely villainous villain and that he acknowledges moral law, thus providing the redeeming characteristic that Schiller posits is essential for his evil characters.

Ultimately, in *Die Räuber*, Schiller demonstrates that despair is pernicious and produces tragedy if the characters are morally worthy and the events are preventable. In centering despair and examining its hold over the soul and body, Schiller reveals that whoever has the power to produce this emotion in others can torture them, disrupt the order of things, and cause tragic events.

NOTES

1. In the original German: "die Verzweiflung (nämlich die entrüstete, nicht aber die verzagte)" (Kant 1974, 199).
2. The wording in paragraph 15 of the dissertation is: "Der von Freveln schwer gedrückte Moor, der sonst spitzfindig genug war, die Empfindungen der Menschlichkeit durch Skelettisierung der Begriffe in nichts aufzulösen, springt eben izt bleich, atemlos, den kalten Schweiß auf seiner Stirne, aus einem schrecklichen Traum auf" (Schiller 1992, 8: 145) ["Moor, who had previously been cunning enough to annihilate humanitarian feelings by reducing logic to a bare skeleton,

is now so heavily burdened by crimes that he starts up from a nightmare, pale, breathless, with his brow bathed in cold sweat"] (Dewhurst and Reeves 1978, 272). This echoes the comment on this passage in the preface to *Die Räuber*: "Es löst in Franzen all die verworrenen Schauer des Gewissens in ohnmächtige Abstraktionen auf, skelettisiert die richtende Empfindung, und scherzt die ernsthafte Stimme der Religion hinweg" (Schiller 1988, 2: 16) ["In Francis it resolves all the confused terrors of conscience into wild abstractions, destroys virtuous sentiments by dissecting them, and holds up the earnest voice of religion to mockery and scorn"] (Schiller 2006a, n.p.).

3. The deathly paleness is similar to the reactions of Old Moor in Act 1 Scene 1 (Schiller 1988, 2: 21) and Karl Moor in Act 1 Scene 2 (2: 38).
4. "Quae medicamenta non sanant, *ferrum* / sanat, quae ferrum non sanat, *ignis* sanat" (Schiller 1988, 2: 12) ["What drugs cure not, *iron* will cure; / what iron cures not, *fire* will cure"] (Schiller 1979, 22).
5. His physical state resembles Krünitz's definition of a person in a state of despair: "Er ringt die Hände, er knirscht wohl auch mit den Zähnen, verdreht die Augen, hat nirgends Ruhe und Rast, er stößt wilde, unzusammenhängende Reden aus, wenn nicht gar Verwünschungen und Flüche" ["He wrings his hands, he even grinds his teeth, rolls his eyes, finds no peace or rest, he launches into wild, incoherent speeches, or even imprecations and curses"] (my translation).
6. Sharpe also notes that Franz Moor's immorality posed problems of decorum for actors of the time and that the later *Trauerspiel* version of the play was less problematic because Franz Moor "asserts some moral feeling" by not plotting to kill his brother (2005, 126).

WORKS CITED

Augustine. *The Works of Saint Augustine*. 1991. Electronic Edition. Volume III.

Dewhurst, Kenneth, and Nigel Reeves. 1978. *Friedrich Schiller: Medicine, Psychology and Literature*. Oxford: Sandford Publications.

Fawaz, Ramzi. 2016. "How to Make a Queer Scene, or Notes toward a Practice of Affective Curation." *Feminist Studies* 42, no. 3: 757–768.

Grimm, Jacob and Wilhelm Grimm. *Deutsches Wörterbuch*, available online: https://woerterbuchnetz.de/?sigle=DWB&lemid=V06856#0 (accessed 14 February 2021).

Guthke, Karl Siegfried. 2005. *Schillers Dramen: Idealismus und Skepsis*. Tübingen: Stauffenburg Verlag.

Guthrie, John. 1999. "Schiller's Early Styles: Language and Gesture in *Die Räuber*." *The Modern Language Review* 94, no. 2: 438–459.

Guyer, Paul. 2012. "The German Sublime after Kant." In *The Sublime: From Antiquity to the Present*, edited by Timothy M. Costelloe, 102–117. Cambridge: Cambridge University Press.

Jacob, Günter. 1966. *Kirche auf Wegen der Erneuerung: Gesammelte Aufsätze aus drei Jahrzehnten*. Göttingen: Vandenhoeck & Ruprecht.

Kant, Immanuel. 1974. *Kritik der Urteilskraft*, edited by Wilhelm Weischedel. Frankfurt am Main: Suhrkamp.

Kant, Immanuel. 2000. *Critique of the Power of Judgment*, edited by Paul Guyer and translated by Paul Guyer. Cambridge: Cambridge University Press.

Kauer, Katja. 2022. *Verzweiflung im 18. Jahrhundert: Eine Diskursgeschichte*. Würzburg: Königshausen & Neumann.

Koc, Richard. 1986. "Fathers and Sons: Ambivalence Doubled in Schiller's *Räuber*." *The Germanic Review* 61, no. 3: 91–104.

Krünitz, Johann Georg. *Oeconomische Encyclopädie (1773–1858)*, available online: http://www.kruenitz1.uni-trier.de/ (accessed 23 May 2022).

Menhennet, Alan. 1973. *Order and Freedom: Literature and Society in Germany from 1720 to 1805*. London: Weidenfeld & Nicolson.

Neubauer, John. 1982. "The Freedom of the Machine: On Mechanism, Materialism, and the Young Schiller." *Eighteenth-Century Studies* 15, no. 3: 275–290.

Ohly, Friedrich. 1995. "Desperatio und Praesumptio. Zur theologischen Verzweiflung und Vermessenheit (1978)." In *Ausgewählte und neue Schriften zur Literaturgeschichte und zur Bedeutungsforschung*, edited by Uwe Ruberg and Dietmar Peil, 177–216. Stuttgart/Leipzig: Hirzel.

Ruprecht, Dietrich. 1959. *Tristitia: Wortschatz und Vorstellung in den althochdeutschen Sprachdenkmälern*. Göttingen: Vandenhoeck & Ruprecht.

Schiller, Friedrich. 1979. *The Robbers and Wallenstein*. Translated by F. J. Lamport. London: Penguin Books.

Schiller, Friedrich. 2006a. *The Robbers: A Tragedy*. Produced by David Widger, available online: https://www.gutenberg.org/files/6782/6782-h/6782-h.htm#link2H_4_0001 (accessed 14 December 2022).

Schiller, Friedrich. 2006b. *Of the Cause of the Pleasure We Derive from Tragic Objects*. Produced by David Widger, available online: https://www.gutenberg.org/files/6798/6798-h/6798-h.htm#link2H_4_0047 (accessed 14 December 2022).

Schiller, Friedrich. 2006c. *On the Tragic Art*. Produced by David Widger, available online: https://www.gutenberg.org/files/6798/6798-h/6798-h.htm#link2H_4_0046 (accessed 14 December 2022).

Schiller, Friedrich. 1988. *Werke und Briefe in zwölf Bänden*, vol. 2, *Dramen I*, edited by Gerhard Kluge. Frankfurt am Main: Deutscher Klassiker Verlag.

Schiller, Friedrich. 1992. *Werke und Briefe in zwölf Bänden*, vol. 8, *Theoretische Schriften*, edited by Rolf-Peter Janz, Hans Richard Brittnacher, Gerd Kleiner, and Fabian Störmer. Frankfurt am Main: Deutscher Klassiker Verlag.

Sharpe, Lesley. 2005. "Schiller and the Mannheim National Theatre." *The Modern Language Review*, 100, no. 1: 121–137.

Snyder, Susan. 1965. "The Left Hand of God: Despair in Medieval and Renaissance Tradition." *Studies in the Renaissance* 12: 18–59.

Steinbock, Anthony. J. 2007. "The Phenomenology of Despair." *International Journal of Philosophical Studies* 15, no. 3: 435–451.

CHAPTER TWENTY-ONE

The Bodies Kept the Score: Two Case Studies on Health and Violence after the Great War

ALLISON SCHMIDT

Each individual of the millions involved in the First World War and its aftermath had a personal experience, and, to quote the writer Nadezhda Teffi, each was "the axis" to their story (Teffi 2016, 3). This article presents two archive-based case studies of people who dealt with health issues following 1918.[1] The first narrative concerns Anna Soukopp, an Austrian Red Cross nurse who treated typhus in Ukraine; the second, Alfred Barta, a veteran who suffered from morphine addiction during the tumultuous early years of the Weimar Republic. Both stories include a twist—the subject had an encounter or alleged connection with political violence that defined the embattled atmosphere of the postwar years. Scholars have argued that the First World War left "legacies of violence," especially in postwar Central and Eastern Europe; not everything was in equilibrium after the Treaty of Versailles, as much as civilians and politicians wished for peace (Böhler et al. 2014). This article emphasizes the entanglement of that violence with lingering, destabilizing health issues, whether it was typhus that continued to spread through Eastern battlefronts or veterans' struggles with morphine addiction. In some ways, Soukopp's and Barta's experiences were unique in the general postwar setting. Most German veterans did not develop morphine addiction. Most Austrian professional nurses did not volunteer for Red Cross missions and then find themselves captured by the Bolsheviks. Still, they had the "shared experience" of "enormous changes and tensions in almost all spheres of life" (Pudłocki and Ruszała 2021, 1), including struggles with health.

AN AUSTRIAN NURSE IN THE RUSSIAN CIVIL WAR

Dietrich Neufeld, a Mennonite teacher and writer who lived in Ukraine during the Russian Civil War (*c.* 1918–22), described the setting as a "verzauberten Labyrinth des tollen Totentanzes" ["bewitched labyrinth of the great dance of death"] (Neufeld 1921, 3).[2] Millions of people suffered from violence, starvation, and disease. Millions were uprooted as refugees, soldiers, prisoners of war, or civilian internees. Each regime change brought different rulers and different expectations of political allegiance, with partisans operating in the wings (Engelstein 2018, 214). Yet, as historians have recently questioned, how did these power struggles precisely affect individual subalterns in Ukraine? How did everyday people exact agency in an age of warring ideologies and mass death and destruction (Velychenko 2021, 9; Betlii 2019, 937)?

A witness statement by Anna Soukopp, an Austrian nurse who had been part of a Red Cross commission to treat typhus in Ukraine, provides an example of a civilian who tried to navigate the complexity and confusion of regime changes, ideologies, and egos. Originally recorded on September 25, 1920, in the Office of Prisoners of War and Civilian Internees in Vienna, her testimony was forwarded to German authorities (and thus found in the *Bundesarchiv*) presumably because she mentioned an Austrian Communist under warrant for arrest in Germany. Though caught within larger forces such as epidemics and ideological warfare, Soukopp comes across as savvy, resourceful, and understandably self-protective. Her testimony defies the stereotype of the nurse as the self-sacrificing angel in the field, solely a witness for the pain of soldiers. A growing subset of historiography has focused on the trauma experienced by nurses during the First World War. The autobiographical texts of nurses who served Austria-Hungary, Christa Hämmerle argues, contain "trauma as a consequence of their attempts to cope with violence and horror" (Hämmerle 2014, 90). This shock extended to the victors, as well. Bridget E. Keown established that British and Irish nurses expressed their own physical and psychological war injuries in personal writings (Keown 2021, 29–30).

Soukopp's testimony on the typhus epidemic and the Russian Civil War similarly illustrates a nurse's difficulties and fight for self-preservation. She begins by recounting how she was recruited:

> Ich war als Berufspflegerin im Wiener allgemeinen Krankenhaus in günstiger Stellung, als ich mich im August bzw. September 1919 unglückseligerweise vom Stabsarzt Dr. Nowak bereden liess, mich der ersten ukrainischen Seuchenabwehrkommission anzuschliessen.
>
> [I was in a favorable position as a vocational nurse at the Vienna General Hospital when, in August 1919, or rather September 1919, I was ill-fatedly persuaded by medical officer Dr. Nowak to join the first commission to fight epidemics in Ukraine.] (Soukopp testimony)

Her recollection has a common trope of war survivors—disillusionment had replaced initial optimism. She never explains exactly why she agreed to join the commission. Perhaps the prospect of an income, patriotism, humanitarianism, the search for adventure, or a mixture of motives drove her. Whatever the reason, she certainly expresses regret. The twenty-seven-year-old signed a contract, which also contained a travel visa from the Austrian Red Cross and from the Ukrainian embassy in Vienna. Though mentioned as short details, both of these institutions reflected recent major changes that shaped Soukopp's experience. The Red Cross-organized commissions and field hospitals of the First World War "provided women a rare opportunity to witness combat and thereby enter a traditionally male domain" (Little 2014). The Ukrainian consulate and its required visa were also fairly new. Ukraine had declared independence from the Russian Empire after the 1917 Revolution. Dr. Yaroslav Okunevsky, a former medical officer in the Austro-Hungarian military-turned proponent of the Ukrainian republic, had blessed the contract with his signature. On September 15, 1919, Anna departed Vienna via train with three doctors, ten nurses, four disinfectors, and a Swiss entourage, presumably for diplomatic reasons, that left the commission at an unnamed city on the Dniester river.

Earlier in 1919, delegates of the International Committee of the Red Cross (ICRC) had met to organize responses to the typhus epidemic in Eastern and Southeastern Europe. Humanitarian organizations such as the ICRC rose to deal with issues such as shellshocked veterans, stateless refugees, and "widespread famines and epidemics" (Cabanes 2014, 5). Health conditions were especially dire for the population in Ukraine. Years of blockades, violence, and lack of resources and medical personnel had depleted and demoralized people, and the International Red Cross "was the only important foreign organization that realized Ukraine's human crisis and was prepared to send aid" (Velychenko 2021, 10). In order to garner international support, the organization portrayed its intervention as a preventive measure to stop the disease from spreading to the West. The Western Front of the First World War, though crawling with lice, had not had the exposure to the bacterium and had thus avoided the typhus epidemic. Various national Red Cross organizations became involved. The looming epidemic "reunited the countries of the former Austro-Hungarian Empire in a joint action of defense," which explains the presence of Austrian Red Cross personnel in Western Ukraine ("Grave Typhus" 1919, 1134). The health commissions also served as a nationalistic tool for Germany and Austria as they tried to regain their "medical prestige" after the war (Weindling 2000, 141). The commissions faced a gargantuan task. Anywhere from 2 to 3 million people died from typhus during the Russian Civil War (Patterson 1993, 361). The disease spread as soldiers moved to different battle points (and quartered with civilians) and refugees fled their homes. Due to pillaging and disruption of trade routes, people often did not have the hygienic items to curb the lice-born disease (Neufeld 1921, 56). In June 1919, the Austrian Red Cross planned to send "eighty typhus-immune personnel" with medical supplies to Ukraine (Weindling 2000, 142).

Soukopp's group, which departed from Vienna in September 1919, did not seem to have that immunity upon arrival. The entire Austrian Red Cross commission in Ukraine suffered from dysentery and typhus fever. Soukopp believed she was the first member to successfully return home. Dr. Nowak, who had recruited her, "hat sich im Fleckfieberdelierium die Adern geöffnet und ist gestorben" ["in a delirium from typhus fever, opened his veins and died"] (Soukopp). Her description reflects others' experience with the disease. High temperatures caused the infected to lose control of their senses, and, thus, they felt like they had lost control of their body (Neufeld 1921, 65). Furthermore, the group was constantly robbed (herself three times) and worked in appalling conditions. Soukopp started in a field hospital in Vinnytsia and then moved to Tiraspol, where she was able to obtain a wage, albeit a low one. She eventually reached the port city of Odessa on the Black Sea from where she hoped to travel home. Authorities had organized a transport from Odessa to the Mediterranean harbor of Trieste for Austrian prisoners of war and civil internees (Formanek). Soukopp's testimony on this time in Ukraine matches the apocalyptic descriptions given by journalists, doctors, and officials on all sides of the war. According to a Bolshevik report on the Novomoskovsk district, four out of eighteen doctors and five out of sixty-five medics died in 1919 (Velychenko, 2021, 69).

When Soukopp left Vienna in September 1919, the former Russian Empire (which included Ukraine) was in the midst of a Civil War, brought on after the Bolshevik Revolution. The former Central Powers, such as Austria, and the Allies, such as the United States, supported the White Guard (e.g., pro-tsarists, Social Democrats, and a mix of others determined to stop the Bolsheviks). At that point, it seemed that the White Guard was winning against the Red Army (i.e., the Bolsheviks and their conscripts) and had pushed them out of Ukraine. The Red Army had come to symbolize for many people torture and terror. That did not mean, however, that the White Army or partisan groups treated people in occupied territory well, as Soukopp and her companions experienced. Soldiers robbed and abused peasants and carried out pogroms on Jews. The war turned in fall 1919, and by February 1920, the Red Army had made gains and marched into Odessa, disrupting Anna's evacuation (Mawdsley 2005, 194).

With the immediate possibility of return delayed, Anna applied to work as a nurse in a local hospital but was instead sent by the Bolsheviks to serve on the Polish front. The newly emerged nation-state of Poland had gone to war with the Bolsheviks over borderland territories. Anna asserts that if she had said no, she would have been labelled as "konterrevolutionär" ["counter-revolutionary"] (Soukopp). Her fears were warranted. Before their retreat from Ukraine in Summer 1919, the Red Army had carried out mass executions of "bourgeois" people or sent them to labor camps (Werth 2008, n.p.). Soukopp emphasizes that the Bolsheviks sent her to the Polish front even though she was technically an invalid from a wounded leg in 1915 (she had likely been a nurse at the front). After the three weeks at the Polish front, Soukopp traveled to Moscow "und von da nach Hamburg unter den abenteuerlichsten Verhältnissen, teils bettelnd teils schwarzfahrend unter falschen Papieren" ["from there to Hamburg under the most adventurous circumstances, partly begging, partly traveling illegally with false papers"] (Soukopp). Moscow was a transfer point for a number of prisoners of war and internees, who could, through international negotiations, return home. Having taken a route through the port city of Hamburg, Soukopp was designated for transport to Vienna. However, bad luck struck again. In a conversation with two other internees, she remarked that she thought circumstances in Vienna were better than in Russia. Karl Toman, a former Austrian prisoner of war who had adopted the Communist agenda and become an Internationalist, overheard her comment, arrested her as a "*Konterrevolutionär*," and took her back to Moscow.

The Internationalists, or former prisoners of war who adopted Bolshevik ideology, became fervent proponents of the cause in Western Europe. Roland Starch argues that they could be considered "the direct forerunners to Comintern," the organization that attempted to spread Communism worldwide (Starch 2009, 48). After the 1917 Revolution, in line with Communist ideology, the Soviets declared the 2.3 million prisoners of war as equal in status to its citizens, with the expectation that the prisoners of war would work and devour a heavy dose of Bolshevik propaganda. The Soviets hoped that the more sympathetic prisoners would then spread Communism once they returned to their home countries. The Internationalists were put in charge of the prisoner of war camps, where, according to famous Swedish Red Cross nurse Elsa Brändström, they attempted to pressure prisoners into Bolshevism through humiliation, starvation, and mistreatment. Brändström also claimed that the Internationalists interned their fellow prisoners who had not sworn allegiance to the Communist organization the Third International and thus eliminated the freedom the Soviets had initially promised (Brändström 1922, 110).[3] Soukopp's forced return to Moscow supports this claim. Brändström viewed the interest of these former Austro-Hungarian prisoners of war in the Bolshevik cause with skepticism. She thought that, while a few were true believers, most of the small number who joined were looking to improve their means of living. The true believers, according to Brändström, were educated men who had lost their senses during capture and now "ihre idealistischen Theories mit wahrem Fanatismus verfochten" ["advocated for their ideals with real fanaticism"] (Brändström 1922, 110).

Soukopp's statement that Russian Communists treated her better than Austrian or Hungarian Communists reflects Brändström's description of the "converted" former prisoners of war. Whereas the Internationalists volunteered for their roles, the Red Army conscripted its soldiers, which meant varying degrees of commitment to the cause (Gilley 2014). In the rest of her witness statement, Soukopp does not explain how she eventually returned to Vienna but names Austrian and Hungarian Internationalists whom she encountered. She lambasts them for their treatment of Austro-Hungarian prisoners of war and details their travel strategies:

> Tomann[4] und einige andere Kommunisten sind unter falschen Namen, mit wechselnder Barttracht als angebliche [Kriegsgefangenen] fort auf dem Wege zwischen Wien und Moskau. Tomann soll von den deutschen Behörden steckbrieflich verfolgt werden, dennoch gelingt es ihm in den Gefangenentransporten durchzukommen.
>
> [Toman and other Communists, with the aid of false names and changing beard styles, constantly travel between Moscow and Vienna disguised as alleged prisoners of war making their return. Tomann is under warrant for arrest by German authorities. Nevertheless, he manages to get through in prisoner transports.]

Not only did authorities in the newly founded Austrian Republic and Weimar Republic concern themselves with the repatriation of civilians, but they also feared the spread of undesirable political ideas through former internees. German and Austrian authorities had well-founded reasons to believe that former Austro-Hungarian prisoners of war-turned Soviets could eventually wield more power. One such former prisoner, Béla Kun, had led the Hungarian Soviet Republic. While that regime was only in place from March to August 1919, it signaled that the spread of Bolshevism to the newly formed nation-states was a possibility.

Soukopp's witness statement ends with her denunciation of the Internationalists. We do not know why she gave the witness statement and whether it was voluntary or involuntary. She might have felt the need to clarify why she at one point worked for the Bolsheviks. Former prisoners of war had a tenuous relationship with their home countries after they returned and were often viewed with skepticism for their contact with the Soviets (Moritz, n.d.). Perhaps she wanted to avenge herself against the Austrian Communists who had delayed her return. Or she wanted people to hear what happened to her and her Red Cross associates who had left for Ukraine in 1919. Or, like many people who have been through traumatic experiences, vocalizing the experiences helped her process them.[5] She was, at any rate, a survivor with a story to tell.

A VETERAN'S STRUGGLE WITH MORPHINE ADDICTION

In the popular German television series *Babylon Berlin* (2017–present), detective Gereon Rath secretly uses morphine to calm his shellshock from the First World War. The series has (re)drawn attention to the plight of veterans who became dependent on the effective yet highly addictive painkiller during the war and into the Weimar Republic. Scholars of German medical history have focused on rehabilitation from physical injuries (Perry 2014) or shellshock (Lerner 2003) that resulted from the First World War. Yet the real-life stories of individual veterans who developed and navigated drug dependency still remain largely hidden. A 1923 police report located in the Saxon State Archives provides an opportunity to examine an actual case of a veteran dealing with morphine addiction. This document was included among reports from April to August 1923 entitled "Police Exchange of Messages about Political Events." Thus, instead of delving into the history of addiction and drugs as a category of analysis in itself, this case study contextualizes an individual's addiction in a time and place of heavy political discord.

A number of studies have delved into the historical use of drugs to deal with war and war trauma, in general. These studies are usually top-down histories of drug enforcement laws and the discourse of psychologists, scientists, and physicians of the era (Kamieński 2016; Lewy 2017). Historiography has largely overlooked cases of everyday people who dealt with morphine addiction, possibly because a relatively small percentage of people developed an addiction in the battlefield or shortly thereafter, even if numbers were noticeably higher from the pre-war era. Given the personal nature of addiction, historical studies on the Weimar Republic usually cite public figures with well-known issues such as the Nazi leader Hermann Göring or the writer Hans Fallada who published a treatise on the drug. Clinical psychiatric studies of the era describe anonymous individual veteran cases and focus on the patient's medical history and subsequent treatment (Horst 1920; Hogrefe 1924; Dansauer and Rieth 1931). The case of Alfred Barta came to police attention and made one of these veterans visible.

On the afternoon of May 12, 1923, Alfred Barta, a Czechoslovak citizen who lived in Germany, was accused of panhandling on a train from Prague to Dresden. When interrogated by German authorities at the border station of Bodenbach (*Podmokly* in Czech), Barta made an astounding claim: disguised as an invalid, he planned to shoot the "Deutschenfeind" ["enemy of Germans"] Ferdinand Foch when the official visited Prague in the next few days (Barta quoted in May 28, 1923 report). The young man's assassination threat echoed a postwar pattern of targeting political leaders. According to certain factions, these leaders had humiliated the German nation through postwar concessions and agreements. Victims included German Foreign Minister Walther Rathenau, gunned down by right-wing extremists after the Treaty of Rapallo in 1922. Foch had been a French marshal and later commander of the Allied forces and had dictated the terms of the 1918 armistice. That included the return of Alsace-Lorraine from Germany to France. Barta's emphasis on avenging "Germanness" parroted right-wing nationalist rhetoric of the time. It is unclear whether Barta actually subscribed to those politics, or whether, as he claimed later on, he was just telling the police what he thought they wanted to hear. His veteran status plays into the historiographical stereotype of the disgruntled ex-soldier seeking to avenge the betrayed homeland, though newer scholarship stresses that most veterans did not engage in political violence (Gerwarth 2016, 12). Both officials present told Barta that his declared plan was not only inexcusable, but also would probably damage Germany's reputation. While a police report would obviously attempt to paint the officials in the best legal light, there was general disapproval amongst German citizens of these assassinations (Storer 2013, 52). Upon their response, Barta seemed to doubt his plan but contended that he had an oath to fulfill to another person.

Due to pain management for a severe wound from the war, Barta had developed an addiction to morphine, which seemed in part to explain his erratic behavior. He had both the drug and syringes on his person. At this time in Germany, people could legally consume morphine, though possession without a doctor's or pharmacist's prescription was illegal (Lewy 2017, 130). The reports do not say whether Barta had a prescription. Łukasz Kamieński highlights the historical use of drugs in warfare, especially as stimulants in battle and depressants or opiates afterward (2016, xvii). Soldiers were often given morphine during the war for psychological and physical pain, and veterans had access to the drug in the following years. Without a doubt, morphine saved lives and provided relief from temporary and chronic pain. Yet growing accessibility, widespread usage in the war, and persistent health problems had their effect. A perfect storm of circumstances increased the visibility of morphine-addicted veterans such as Barta in the Weimar Republic.

Germany had ties to morphine from the drug's inception at the beginning of the nineteenth century (Stephens 2022, 390). The young pharmacist Friedrich Sertürner derived the alkaloid from opium, which resulted in a purer, more measurable narcotic. The Merck company began manufacturing the drug in the 1830s (Lewy 2017, 69), and German pharmacological production dominated the market. Morphine's export to the United States and its use during the US Civil War garnered morphine addiction the label of the "soldiers' disease" (Kamieński 2016, 89). In Germany the association of soldiers with morphine addiction stemmed from the Wars of Unification (1864–70) (Lewy 2017, 70). Drug laws carried over from the *Kaiserreich* into the early Weimar Republic. Scientists and medical doctors knew of dependency but how to treat it, was (and still is) debated. However, during the 1920s, growing concern of veterans becoming addicted to morphine led to more laws and ordinances in Germany (Lewy 2017, 136). Popular rhetoric and scientific literature referred to people who developed an addiction to the drug as *Morphinisten* (morphinists). The Saxon police reports never label Barta as such, and thus, in a sociolinguistic sense, do not define him as an addict.

The police statements emphasize Barta's frayed nerves and the officers' carefulness not to upset him. They refer to him as a "schwerkranken" ["seriously ill"] man "der sich nur mittelst Morphiums künstlich über Wasser hält" ["who keeps his head above water artificially by means of morphine"] (May 12, 1923 report). The gendarme told an officer named Hermsdorf to accompany Barta on a train back to Dresden and then hand him over to the Dresden police for *Schutzhaft*, "protective custody" (May 12, 1923 report). However, things went awry en route. On the train, Barta wanted to inject morphine but Hermsdorf dissuaded him. A distraught Barta began to cry and believed himself betrayed by the officers and destined for jail. Fearing Barta's delicate state, Hermsdorf had planned to tell him of the arrest first at the Dresden train station. The officer said he was now off duty and was merely accompanying Barta because he himself had to take the train home as usual. Hermsdorf's white lie became a problem when Barta wanted to stop in the town of Schandau to buy cigarettes and send his parents a telegram. The officer kept an eye on him while Barta ordered and paid for the telegram. Once Barta had stepped away, Hermsdorf told the telegraphist to defer sending the message until the train reached Dresden to avoid any third-party interference. Meanwhile, Barta announced he was leaving the waiting room and then did so while Hermsdorf showed the telegraphist his police identification. Though only a few seconds behind, Hermsdorf could not find Barta outside the waiting room or on the train. He then scouted the local ship and ferry in case Barta had made his escape via the Elbe River. He sent alerts to the nearest villages and towns. Hermsdorf returned to Bodenbach at 8 a.m. the next morning, without Barta, after allegedly searching for him the whole night.

Police immediately sought out Barta's contacts in Dresden for clues to his whereabouts and intentions. Though a Czechoslovak citizen, Barta had actually been born in Dresden and seemingly had spent most his life there. However, the German state only recognized *jus sanguinis* citizenship through parents, not *jus soli*, or being born on German soil. Barta's parents had probably emigrated to Saxony from the Austrian Empire, as many people had during the *Kaiserreich*, and their original home town was now in Czechoslovakia. While pressures of national allegiance and citizenship increased after the First World War, many Bohemians still lived and/or worked in Saxony during the Weimar Republic and traveled back and forth across the border (Murdock 2010, 112). According to Barta's former landlady in Dresden, he had relinquished his apartment two weeks prior and had been often away on business trips. Barta's parents, bicycle salesman Gustav and his wife Helene (née Grünberger), worried about their son, whom they claimed not to have seen for three to four weeks. They believed the assassination threat to be "unsinniges Gerede" ["nonsensical talk"] and that his morphine consumption had completely made him unaware of what he was doing or saying (May 15, 1923 report). He had already been to a sanatorium twice for treatment. Barta had been in a romantic relationship with Fanny Lange (née Gruner), a slightly older widow who also lived in Dresden. On the evening of Sunday, May 12, she told someone that she was leaving for about a month and was herself unsure of the destination, perhaps to her parents in Klingenberg, perhaps to another small town. Police doubted, however, that she and Barta would hide at her parents, who disapproved of the relationship. Saxon police circulated a wanted notice for the veteran around the province.

Almost two weeks later, police found Barta and Lange in a pension named "Villa Helene," located in the district of Pötzscha in the small village of Wehlen (May 28, 1923 report). It lies on the bank of the Elbe near the picturesque area known as Saxon Switzerland. Barta explained his behavior on the 12. He claimed that he had been en route from Prague to Dresden with papers in order to marry Lange. A fellow passenger on the train, an employee of the German consulate in Prague (thus, possibly someone familiar with Barta), informed train personnel that Barta had been begging for money. Though Barta denied the accusation, he admitted that, two weeks prior, he had asked people on the train for money to finance his ticket home. Barta claimed that he escaped from Hermsdorf's custody in Schandau because he felt that the officer was really on duty and would turn him over to the police in Dresden. After his escape, Barta wandered through the night to the town of Pötzschau, where earlier he had booked two rooms to vacation with Lange, marry her, and go through morphine withdrawal.

Regarding the assassination threat, the Barta claimed that, due to the agitation caused by having his passport taken away in Bodenbach, he had taken a dose of morphine and lost control of his senses. He then reasoned that the German officials would think his plan a boon to Germany (they told him it would not) and that they would then return his passport to him (they did not). Police concluded that the assassination threat was hollow and that Barta, through his illness and addiction, "für seine unvernünftigen Handlungen auch nicht voll verantwortlich gemacht werden zu können" ["could not be made fully accountable for his unreasonable behaviors"] (May 28, 1923 report). He had sustained serious injuries during the war, lost interest in work, and lost control of his life. A thorough search of Lange's apartment in Dresden, where Barta kept his belongings, produced no evidence of a gun or political conspiracy to commit the assassination.

Police questioned his multiple border crossings (via notations in his passport) and how he was able to afford weeks in a hotel. Barta denied he had been smuggling, except twice when he sold two perfume bottles and then two pieces of soap at the Bodenbach train station. He asserted that he had unsuccessfully looked for work in Czechoslovakia as a technician or draftsman. Out of pity, the factory owners gave him donations in crowns, which, were much more valuable than the inflating Mark. He stated that he lived off these donations—from what the police deemed "Betteltouren" ["beggar's tours"]—and his "Kriegsinvalidenrente" ["war disability pension"] (May 28, 1923 report). Lange claimed to not know anything about Barta's smuggling and that she lived off her pension as a teacher's widow. The police voiced doubt that she could afford the vacation hotel on her income. She agreed and replied that she had sold some of her deceased husband's clothes. Police still suspected that Barta and Lange engaged in smuggling, or some other type of illegal business, though a thorough search of their hotel rooms and Lange's apartment in Dresden produced no evidence. The police returned to Barta the 1,000 Mark that he had paid for his telegram before Hermsdorf had intervened. However, they did not return his passport because of two forgeries, including the etching of a date to extend a visa.

The police reports show broader political-economic tensions facing Germany in the early 1920s, such as smuggling and a spree of political assassinations. Inflation of the Mark especially made smuggling over the Saxon-Czechoslovakian border an appealing, if illegal, method to subsidize income. This marks the end of the 1923 police report on Alfred Barta, though more documentation appeared in a 1934 collection of reports by the League of Nations, the international organization that, among its many goals, attempted to stop trafficking across borders. He was listed as one of a number of people who had smuggled morphine and cocaine from Czechoslovakia into Germany from 1931 to 1932 (*League of Nations* 1934, 26–27). Like the fictional Rath, Barta was wrapped in the fallout of drugs and war.

CONCLUSION

Both of the case studies in this article provide a subaltern perspective to the aftermath of the First World War, which changed individual lives as much as the power systems they lived within. An analysis of a police report takes the historical literature beyond scientific or legal discourse and contextualizes the case of a veteran dealing with morphine addiction. The testimony of an Austrian nurse adds a civilian perspective to the epidemics and fighting in Ukraine. Public health concerns were irrevocably entangled with war and trauma, and both stories address an iteration of political violence from the left and right. Literature on these postwar years, especially in East-Central Europe, has been growing in wake of centennial anniversaries of treaties and treatises. Digitization of sources has made searching for individuals in records easier, though these detailed stories were randomly discovered in archival holdings. Because these stories are often hidden under broad subjects and timeframes, it is important to make them visible in order to (re)construct the totality of the whole.

NOTES

1. Thank you to the Staatsbibliothek zu Berlin, Bundesarchiv Berlin-Lichterfelde, Hauptstaatsarchiv Dresden, and Österreichisches Staatsarchiv—Archiv der Republik. On-site research was made possible through the German Historical Institute in DC and Munich Centre for Global History. I received helpful feedback at the 2019 Association for Slavic, East European, and Eurasian Studies and 2020 German Studies Association conferences. Lastly, thank you to Stephanie Hilger for assembling and editing this collection.
2. All translations are mine unless otherwise stated.
3. In the German version, her name is spelled "Else" due to phonetics.
4. The source spells Toman's name with two "n"s.
5. As Margaret R. Higonnet observes in her introduction to her 2001 edition of two nurse autobiographies, sometimes "writing to expose wounds … is surely a first step toward healing wounds" (xxxi). Borden, Mary and Ellen Newbold La Motte. 2001. *Nurses at the Front: Writing the Wounds of the Great War*, edited by Margaret R. Higonnet. Boston: Northeastern University Press.

WORKS CITED

Archival Sources

Dr. Franz Formanek: Direktiven für Heimbeförderungen der Kriegsgefangenen von 1919. AT-OeStA/KA FA AOK KgfFürsorge 3862. Österreichisches Staatsarchiv, Kriegsarchiv.
Testimony of Anna Soukopp (copy). 25 September 1920. R 1501/118375, Bd. 4, S. 99. Bundesarchiv, Berlin-Lichterfelde.
Testimony of Anna Soukopp (original). 25 September 1920. OeStA/AdR, KGF 1920, Rubrik 13-9/94. Österreichisches Staatsarchiv, Archiv der Republik.
Report from the Sächsische Grenzgendarmerie-Kommissariat Bodenbach to the Polizeipräsidium in Dresden. 12 and 13 May 1923. Ministerium des Innern (MdI) 11097 Teil 2: 199–200. Sächsisches Staatsarchiv, Dresden (StAD).
Report by the Über-Kriminal-Kommissar. 15 May 1923. MdI 11097 Teil 2: 201–202. StAD.
Report by the Über-Kriminal-Kommissar. 28 May 1923. Later forwarded from the Dresden
Polizeipräsidium to the Saxon Ministry of the Interior. MdI 11097 Teil 2: 204–208. StAD.

Printed Primary Sources

Brändström, Else. 1922. *Unter Kriegsgefangenen in Rußland und Sibirien 1914–1920*. Hannover: F.E. Haag, Melle.
Dansauer, Friedrich and Adolf Rieth. 1931. *Über Morphinismus bei Kriegsbeschädigten: nach amtlichen Unterlagen*. Berlin: Hobbing.
"Grave Typhus Situation in Central Europe." 1919. *Public Health Reports* 34, no. 21 (May 23): 1134.
Hogrefe, Heinrich. 1924. "Über Entziehungskuren bei Morphinismus." Med. Diss., Kiel.
Horst, Oskar. 1920. *Die Zunahme des Morphinismus während des Krieges*. Kiel: Schmidt & Klaunig.
League of Nations Advisory Committee on Traffic in Opium and Other Dangerous Drugs: Summary of Illicit Transactions and Seizures Reported to the Secretariat of the League of Nations Between July 1st and September 30th, 1934.
Neufeld, Dietrich. 1921. *Ein Tagebuch aus dem Reiche des Totentanzes*. Emden: M. Wilkens.
Teffi.2016. *Memories: From Moscow to the Black Sea*. Translated by Robert and Elizabeth Chandler, Anne Marie Jackson, and Irina Steinberg. New York: New York Review Books.

Secondary Sources

Betlii, Olena. 2019. "Revolution through the Lens of Ordinary Life in Kyiv." *Slavic Review* 78 (4): 935–941.
Böhler, Jochen, Wlodzimierz Borodziej, and Joachim von Puttkamer, eds. *Legacies of Violence: Eastern Europe's First World War*. 2014. München: Oldenbourg Verlag.
Borden, Mary and Ellen Newbold La Motte. 2001. *Nurses at the Front: Writing the Wounds of the Great War*, edited by Margaret R. Higonnet. Boston: Northeastern University Press.
Cabanes, Bruno. 2014. *The Great War and the Origins of Humanitarianism, 1918–1924*. Cambridge: Cambridge University Press.
Engelstein, Laura. 2018. *Russia in Flames: War, Revolution, Civil War, 1914–1921*. New York: Oxford University Press.
Gerwarth, Robert. 2016. *The Vanquished: Why the First World War Failed to End*. Allen Lane.
Gilley, Christopher. 2014. "Red Army." In *1914–1918-online: International Encyclopedia of the First World War*, edited by Ute Daniel, Peter Gatrell, Oliver Janz, Heather Jones, Jennifer Keene, Alan Kramer, and Bill Nasson, issued by Freie Universität Berlin, Berlin. https://encyclopedia.1914-1918-online.net/pdf/1914-1918-Online-red_army-2014-10-08.pdf.

Hämmerle, Christa. 2014. "'Mentally Broken, Physically a Wreck …': Violence in War Accounts of Nurses in Austro-Hungarian Service." In *Gender and the First World War*, edited by Christa Hämmerle, Oswald Überegger, and Birgitta Bader Zaar, 89–107. New York: Palgrave McMillan.

Kamieński, Łukasz. 2016. *Shooting Up: A History of Drugs and War*. New York: Oxford University Press.

Keown, Bridget E. 2021. "'A Perfect Hell of a Night which We Can Never Forget': Narratives of Trauma in the Private Writings of British and Irish Nurses in the First World War." In *Languages of Trauma: History, Memory, and Media*, edited by Peter Leese, Jason Crouthamel, and Julia Barbara Köhne, 29–45. Toronto: University of Toronto Press.

Lerner, Paul. 2003. *Hysterical Men: War, Psychiatry, and the Politics of Trauma in Germany, 1890–1920*. Ithaca: Cornell University Press.

Lewy, Jonathan. 2017. *Drugs in Germany and the United States, 1819–1945: The Birth of Two Addictions*. Baden-Baden: Nomos Verlagsgesellschaft.

Little, Branden. 2014. "State Civil Society and Relief Organizations for War." In *1914–1918-Online: International Encyclopedia of the First World War*, edited by Ute Daniel, Peter Gatrell, Oliver Janz, Heather Jones, Jennifer Keene, Alan Kramer, and Bill Nasson, issued by Freie Universität Berlin. http:ss//encyclopedia.1914-1918-online.net/article/state_civil_society_and_relief_organizations_for_war.

Mawdsley, Evan. 2005. *The Russian Civil War*. New York: Pegasus Books.

Moritz, Verena. "'Rücktransport' aus der Gefangenschaft." Accessed July 25, 2022. https://ww1.habsburger.net/de/kapitel/ruecktransport-aus-der-gefangenschaft.

Murdock, Caitlin. 2010. *Changing Places: Society, Culture, and Territory in the Saxon-Bohemian Borderlands, 1870–1946*. Ann Arbor: University of Michigan Press.

Patterson, K. David. 1993. "Typhus and Its Control in Russia, 1870–1940." *Medical History* 37 (4): 361–81.

Perry, Heather R. 2014. *Recycling the Disabled: Army, Medicine, and Modernity in WWI Germany*. Manchester University Press.

Pudłocki, Tomasz and Kamil Ruszała. 2021. "The War That Never Ended: East-Central Europe After 1918." In *Postwar Continuity and New Challenges in Central Europe, 1918–1923: The War That Never Ended*, edited by Tomasz Pudłocki and Kamil Ruszała, 1–6. New York: Routledge.

Starch, Roland. 2009. "Die KPÖ und Komintern." Magister der Philosophie, Universität Wien.

Stephens, Robert P. 2022. "Germany's Role in the Modern Global Drug Economy." In *The Oxford Handbook of Global Drug History*, edited by Paul Gootenberg, 389–407. New York: Oxford University Press.

Storer, Colin. 2013. *A Short History of the Weimar Republic*. New York: I.B. Taurus.

Velychenko, Stephen. 2021. *Life and Death in Revolutionary Ukraine: Living Conditions, Violence, and Demographic Catastrophe, 1917–1923*. Montreal: McGill-Queen's University Press.

Weindling, Paul Julian. 2000. *Epidemics and Genocide in Eastern Europe, 1890–1945*. New York: Oxford University Press.

Werth, Nicolas. "Crimes and Mass Violence of the Russian Civil Wars (1918–1921)," *SciencesPo*. Last modified March 21, 2008. https://www.sciencespo.fr/mass-violence-war-massacre-resistance/en/document/crimes-and-mass-violence-russian-civil-wars-1918-1921#title6.

CHAPTER TWENTY-TWO

Refracting War Violence: Psychiatric Discourse in the Soviet Occupation Zone and the Early East German State

ANKE PINKERT

Throughout the twentieth century, the history of studying psychological trauma, and particularly trauma related to human atrocities, such as war and captivity, has alternated between periods of active inquiry and forgetting. In the years after the Second World War, the memories of earlier discussions of war trauma appeared to be lost in Germany and other national and transnational postwar contexts. Little public and medical interest existed in the psychological conditions of returning soldiers and the civilian population, let alone camp survivors (Leys 2000, 5; Herman 1997, 7–33).[1] Instead, German psychiatrists reinvested in traditional hereditary and organic models of mental illness that eclipsed the relationship between historical and psychological experience. In 1945 and the following years, psychiatrists observed a relatively low number of psychogenic (experience-conditioned) disorders among the German population (Schwarz 1950, 291; Müller-Hegemann 1973, 128). (According to the *Diagnostic and Statistical Manual of Mental Disorders* [DSM-IV, 1994], psychogenic illnesses result from mental stressors, where symptoms manifest in the patient without biologically identifiable causes.) This notion of absent psychological responses to the war and the collapse of the Third Reich was reproduced in the 1960s by the West German psychoanalysts Alexander and Margarete Mitscherlich in their seminal book *The Inability to Mourn: Principles of Collective Behavior*. Despite its importance for a critical assessment of Germany's past two decades after the war, the book obscured the experience and traumatic consequences of the all-pervasive, multi-layered violence among the German postwar population (Geyer 1997, 17n35, Pinkert 2008, 1–18; Parkinson 2015, 113–146). Here, the authors contended that the Germans had avoided what should have been a psychological reaction to war destruction, mass death, and defeat, namely a massive fall into depression (Mitscherlich and Mitscherlich 1967, 37, 40). This argument helped foster the idea that Germans survived the Second World War without experiencing considerable psychological harm. More than fifty years needed to pass until the German experience of the Allied bombings, for example, belatedly recurred in public discourse in the 1990s. This delay further reinforced the assumption that obstinacy and resilience had prevented the German postwar population from collapsing at the end of the Second World War. However, since notions of psychological harm largely depend on the historical practices and social contexts that provide it with meaning (Foucault 1954; Hacking 1996),[2] this article examines how German psychiatric discourse in the immediate postwar years contributed significantly to the seeming absence of psychological disorders related to the war. Seen from this perspective, Germans experienced the immediate postwar years not only as an inescapable state of emergency, which, as one East German psychiatrist put it, essentially absorbed the psychic drives responsible for the formation of psychic symptoms, but the psychiatric discourse itself reproduced this traumatic numbing that in many respects became the primary characteristic of the postwar period (Müller-Hegemann 1973, 128; Geyer 1997, 17).

While other historical accounts have focused on the continuities and transformations of the psychiatric profession in West Germany after the end of the Second World War (Cocks 1994), this study turns to psychiatric practices and discourse that emerged in the Soviet Occupation Zone and early years of the East German state. My discussion is primarily based on an archive assembled by research reports, eye-witness accounts, and narrative case histories, published in public health-oriented and medical journals between 1945 and the early nineteen fifties. These case records may be unconventional documents—their mediated, often fragmentary, and summarized nature could raise doubts regarding their validity as sources for historical research. Therefore, extracting any "authentic" voice of patients from these files may easily be a misguided effort. And yet, these case histories aid my argument that Germans were more impaired by the effects of the war than contemporary memory culture tends to acknowledge. After all, to draw on Ana Antic's insight, case files contain a multiplicity of voices and narratives, which allows for "viewpoints of patients to enter into an (unequal) competition with the dominant psychiatric tone" (Antic 2016, 27).

Shortly after the war, *Das Deutsche Gesundheitswesen,* commissioned by the Central Health Administration of the Soviet Occupation Zone, became the designated professional publication venue of the Society of Psychiatry and Neurology, which was constituted in 1947 through order 124 of the Soviet Military Administration. In 1949, the society founded its journal, *Psychiatrie, Neurologie, Medizinische Psychologie*, which served as the single professional journal for the various psychiatric disciplines in the German Democratic Republic (GDR). Relevant medical publications in the Western zones at the time included *Medizinische Klinik* (Munich) and *Der Nervenarzt* (Berlin-New York). Although, immediately after the war, the journals published in the Eastern and Western zones remained little influenced by the politics of the respective occupational forces (Schagen 1999, 168), socio-psychiatric discussions, and especially those related to the psychological disorders of the war returnee, began increasingly to diverge. The official ideological commitment to antifascist renewal in the Soviet Occupation Zone resulted in an "active and future-oriented health politics" ["aktive, vorausschauende Gesundheitspolitik"] (Radetzky 1946) that relied on a psychiatric discourse that by and large sidestepped the significance of war experience in the etiology of psychological trauma. By 1950, the psychiatric profession in the Eastern sector widely replaced psychogenic approaches, according to which symptoms were caused by the experience of external realities, with physiological concepts imported from Soviet psychology.

(DIS)CONTINUITIES ACROSS 1945

Following the end of the Second World War, German psychiatrists, psychotherapists, and psychoanalysts aimed at re-establishing their profession, thereby avoiding any critical assessment of their "missed resistance" to the Nazi regime (Cocks 1994). Recent research shows the extent to which psychiatrists were involved in the Nazi eugenics program. Dagmar Herzog argues that the Nazi mass murder of "the disabled" served as an overt reference point in the debates of the 1960s and 1970s over abortion rights in Western European Nations (Herzog 2018, 9; Friedländer 1995; Roelcke 2008). After 1945, however, only a few psychiatric practitioners were prosecuted for their roles in the involuntary sterilization and killing of "the mentally disabled." Moreover, in some cases, they were absolved of any responsibility when German courts ruled that doctors had acted in the belief that the program was legally constituted (Cocks 1994, 315n12, 315n13; Seidel and Werner 1991, 14; Bock 1986, 237–238). In July 1933, a few months after Hitler had come to power, the Higher Court passed the so-called sterilization law, which introduced compulsory sterilization for persons suffering from various mental and physical disorders and defined the groups to be excluded from the national community. Starting in 1939 (based on the so-called "T-4-Aktion"),[3] the systematic and secret calculated murder of "the disabled," including the mentally ill suffering from schizophrenia, hereditary epilepsy, manic-depressive psychosis, progressive paralysis, congenital feeble-mindedness or certain neurological illnesses, was implemented.[4] The disabled were initially killed by injection, shooting, and carbon monoxide on-site at various psychiatric institutions. From 1941 onward were gassed in so-called operational killing centers that proved to be the "testing ground" for the Nazi genocide. Although the reputation of the psychiatric profession had suffered considerably due to its involvement with the destructive racial policy of the Nazis, the demand for medical expertise to rebuild a devastated society led to a significant carryover of medical personnel from the Third Reich into postwar Germany. Obscuring these institutional and personal continuities between postwar Germany and the Nazi era and in line with the "zero-hour" rhetoric at the time, psychiatrists in the Soviet Occupation Zone constructed their position after the collapse of Nazi Germany in terms of a complete break that dramatically separated the Third Reich from postwar Germany.

As W. Lindenberg put it in the inaugural issue of the journal *Psychiatrie, Neurologie und Medizinische Psychologie* in 1949:

> Als 1945 die Gewaltherrschaft der Nazis zusammenbrach, standen wir auf dem Gebiete der psychiatrischen Fürsorge vor einem Nichts. Von den 150,000 Betten, die wir in Deutschland vor 1933 in rund 393 Anstalten für Geisteskranke hatten, waren nach dem Zusammenbruch nur noch knapp 30,000 mit Geisteskranken belegt. Die durch Morde schwer belasteten Ärzte und Pfleger flohen aus den Anstalten und überliessen die noch nicht euthanasierten Patienten ihrem eigenen Schicksal.
>
> [When Nazi tyranny collapsed in 1945, we were left with nothing in the field of psychiatric care. Of the 150,000 beds, we had in around 393 institutions for the mentally ill in Germany before 1933, only just under 30,000 were still occupied after the collapse. The doctors and nurses, who were heavily burdened by the murders, fled the institutions and left the patients who had not yet been euthanized to their fate.]
>
> (Lindenberg 1949, 4)[5]

It is against the background of approximately 250,000 psychiatric patients eradicated during the Third Reich (a number listed by medical articles at the time) that psychiatrists in the Soviet Occupation Zone viewed the increasing number of people admitted to mental institutions after 1945 as a sign of progress.[6]

However, at least in the short run, the desire to compensate for the outcome of Nazi eugenics also hampered the potential democratization and reform of psychiatric care in general and the recognition of war trauma and its lasting effects in particular.[7] Instead of critically re-examining psychiatric practices and theories, psychiatrists were invested mainly in rebuilding the old institutions. Still far from implementing modern clinical practices, these asylum-style institutions centered on the confinement and care of patients suffering from illnesses labeled hereditary, incurable, or endogenic. At the time, this referred to psychoses, including schizophrenia, paranoia, and forms of epilepsy, illnesses with a strong constitutional basis generally seen as irreversible and affecting the personality. With little room for psychotherapeutic interventions, psychiatrists commonly treated these illnesses with somatic therapies, such as electroshock, insulin coma, continuous water bed, or hot packs, which, in many cases, immobilized and shut down the patients rather than integrating and rehabilitating them (Weisse and Uhle 1990; Gross 1996, 28–31). According to the memoirs of Friedrich Rudolf Gross, an East German psychiatrist, the outdated asylums were only slowly, and in most cases belatedly, transformed into modern psychiatric clinics (Gross 1996, 17–27). This process continued to be caught up in traditional notions of psychiatric institutions, where the mentally ill who appeared to pose a public danger had to be confined and monitored. How much such notions informed both the general population and medical practitioners was pointed out by those few doctors who insisted that even psychotic illnesses could be approached with more open and flexible forms of psychotherapy (Nobbe 1948, 15–19). Despite the dominance of psychiatric approaches to mental illness throughout the nineteen-forties, an institutional structure and professional discourse concerned with curable psychological suffering emerged in the Soviet Occupation Zone. By and large, however, these psychotherapeutically oriented practices seemed to exist in a historical vacuum. They were largely oblivious to the psychological impact of war, defeat, and reconstruction on the German population.

The institutional reestablishment of psychotherapy in the Soviet Occupation Zone took place quickly, given that the Hermann Göring Institute, "The Reich Institute for Psychological Research and Psychotherapy," was reduced to rubble in the final days of the war. According to the historian Geoffrey Cocks, on May 15, 1945, Harald Schultz-Hencke, a psychotherapist formerly affiliated with the Göring Institute, reported that the Russians were actively interested in psychotherapy (Cocks 1997, 357; Cocks 1990, 321). And indeed, only a few weeks after the end of the war, Schultz-Hencke and Werner Kemper, who emerged as the leading organizers of psychotherapy in Berlin, were able to establish "an outpatient clinic in the ruins of the city to care for patients from the Göring Institute and to treat new patients emerging from the rubble of the war" (Cocks 1997, 357). In late November, 1946, eighty-five psychiatrists, neurologists, and psychotherapists from East Berlin gathered at a meeting in the house of the Central Administration. The same year, "the Versicherungsanstalt Berlin agreed to underwrite the treatment of psychoanalysis and psychotherapy performed by medical and nonmedical practitioners within what was now officially named the Central Institute for Psychogenic Illnesses [...] The original permission for the clinic to function as an official entity was given by Ferdinand Sauerbruch, who had been placed in charge of Berlin's health administration by the Russians" (Cocks 1997, 357). In 1947, the Central Institute became the outpatient clinic for the newly founded Institute for Psychotherapy. Notably, in 1948, the first "Research Meeting of Psychiatrists and Neurologists" from throughout Germany took place in the Soviet Occupation Zone. In 1949, Schultz-Hencke was granted a teaching position at Humboldt University in the Russian sector of Berlin. In the same year, he and Kemper joined the editorial board of *Psychiatry, Neurologie und Medizinische Psychologie* published under the head editorship of Alexander Mette (Weimar) by Hirzel, in the eastern German city of Leipzig.

Yet even as the Russians seemed to have expressed interest in making psychological counseling services available in the shattered city of Berlin, Schultz-Hencke's and Kemper's accounts indicate that they construed their role in rebuilding a "mental hygiene" system in postwar Germany in terms of a pioneering, even conspiratorial project. According to them, these efforts were carried out under significant emotional and financial hardship by an isolated group of closely linked collaborators who needed to appeal to disinterested, if not openly hostile, public offices and administrations (Kemper 1949). The inclusion of psychotherapeutic theories and practices in mainstream psychiatry was hampered by the elitist reputation of psychoanalysis (here called depth psychology) *and* a great deal of professional competition among psychiatrists, neurologists, and neo-analytically trained psychotherapists. They all attempted to gain a foothold in a health service system that, after the war, was stressed to the limits and focused its primary efforts on medical supplies, hygienic prophylaxis, and the control of bacterial epidemics (Konitzer 1946; Radetzky 1946; Beyer 1946; Reinisch 2013, 220–254). During those years Schultz-Hencke, Kemper, and other leading psychotherapists and psychoanalysts struggled to have neurotic disorders recognized as an essential mental health concern. They underlined the urgency of the matter by describing the existing neurotic illnesses analogous to the widely spread bacterial and venereal diseases as a mass epidemic. According to them, 500,000 cases of depression, anxiety-neurosis, and what was then called neurasthenic disorder—a combination of anxiety, restlessness, obsession, and localized organic disorders—were already registered in Germany and required immediate therapeutic as well as administrative attention. Harking back to the German tradition of socialized medicine that had prospered during the Weimar era, they challenged the dominant notion of psychoanalysis as a bourgeois luxury primarily construed for treating rich women (Schultz-Hencke 1946, 251; Kemper 1949, 49; Derbolowsky and Lindenberg 1949, 58). Instead, they continued to insist on a shorter neo-psychoanalytical psychotherapy that would be able to provide services to a wide range of the population, including all classes, both genders and adults as well as children. The need to position themselves in a broader socio-medical context points as much to the resistance, even rejection that psychotherapeutic practitioners ultimately faced from communist officials as it does to the willingness of the psychotherapists and psychoanalysts previously trained at the Göring Institute to accommodate the new political and economic system in the Soviet Occupation Zone.

Schultz-Henke and Kemper were highly invested in emphasizing neurotic suffering as a pressing health concern among the German population. By extension, they aimed to delineate psychotherapy as an independent field interrelated with rather than subsumed by the discipline of psychiatry. Their concept of hereditary neurotic illness, however, tended to deflect attention from those external conditions which could have lent psychotherapeutic theories and practices legitimacy and urgency in postwar Germany: the experience of loss, mass death, and violence caused by the war (Kemper 1949; Schultz-Hencke 1949; Besold 1949, 374). This avoidance is most notable where psychotherapists insisted that the increasing number of neurotic illnesses needed to be recognized *despite* the postwar crisis rather than seeing the diffuse symptoms of depression and anxiety intimately linked with it. Attesting to the gradual divergence between psychological illness and the external conditions of war since the 1920s, this argument is part of a more extensive dialectical history of the twentieth century in which the study of psychological trauma shifted in and out of focus.

ECHOES OF THE FIRST WORLD WAR

Throughout the 1930s and especially the1940s, legal, psychiatric, and ideological strategies had helped corrode the linkage between war and traumatic suffering (Küchenhoff and Warsitz 1991, 48; Cocks 1997, 305–329). The First World War had given rise to the perception that traumatic war neurosis occurred as a mass epidemic. The successful treatment of shell-shocked soldiers through psychotherapeutic methods convinced some psychiatrists, including Freud, to challenge the hitherto prevailing efforts to attribute the cause of the disorder to organic lesions of the nervous system brought about by the mechanical force of explosions (Freud 1961, 10–11; Micale 2008). Sigmund Freud followed the French clinical neurologist Jean-Martin Charcot and others in relating traumatic hysteria or shell shock observed in soldiers (exposed and unexposed to war combat) to psychological rather than anatomic-physiological changes. In the context of the massive waves of disability claims in the decade following the First World War, health administrators increasingly conflated the mental debilitations of the former soldiers with an unwillingness to re-enter civilian life (Lerner 2009; Micale and Lerner 2001; Cohen 2001). Although psychotherapeutic services continued to exist into the Third Reich, the Second World War and the uncompromising Nazi demands of allegiance and performance fostered an environment of punishment in which "difficult" soldiers were either simply sent back to the front or risked being labeled abnormal (Cocks 1997, 319). According to Joachim Küchenhoff and Peter Warsitz, by the end of the Second World War, the only way the contingency between war violence and mental suffering continued to exist was through conscious efforts to reject any such relationship in the first place (Küchenhoff and Warsitz 1991, 48). Indeed, even though, by the end of 1944, the estimated number of classical "war neurotics" in all branches of the German Army was around 100,000 (Shephard 2001, 311), the psychiatric discourse had eclipsed the relationship between warfare and psychological stress to the point that the term "war neurosis" itself appeared obsolete.

Questions fiercely debated after the First World War, such as whether or not psychological illness is triggered or caused by war, the nature of trauma, the cathartic-abreactive cure, and processes of remembering, remained largely untouched in the years following the Second World War. The publications and discussions in postwar psychiatric and socio-medical journals show that wherever psychological trauma is about to come into view, the different neurological, psychiatric, and psychotherapeutic disciplines deployed their discipline-specific conceptions to undermine the notion that people could be deeply penetrated and lastingly affected by the intense experience-conditioned impact of war violence. In other words, psychological distress was continuously resituated in relation to the body, nerves, organs, brain, muscle tissue, and the vasomotoric system. The more intangible traumatic effects of war violence, mass death, and historical collapse became less apparent in these organic reconstructions.

The shift away from the external conditions of war within the psychiatric discipline up to the end of the Second World War tied into an official public sphere in the Soviet Occupation Zone where the atrocities committed by the Germans (together with the enormous destruction, economic problems, epidemics, and malnutrition) inevitably prevented a closer look at war suffering experienced by the Germans themselves. In 1946, the journal *Deutsches Gesundheitswesen*, published by the German Central Administration of Health in the Soviet Zone, began immediately to sketch out the discursive and legal limits within which psychological war suffering was to be understood (Kröber 1946). Clearly outlining the practitioner's task in assessing the war damage to the nervous system, the publication vehemently rejected any relationship between the conditions of war and so-called "nervous disturbances"—at the time, a general term for the ailments of tremblers, mutes, physically paralyzed as well as more diffuse symptoms, such as headaches, fatigue, depressed moods, lack of concentration, irritability, and fits of anger. Arguing that these symptoms are either conditioned by constitutional factors or, in many cases, without any basis, faked and the product of wishful thinking, *Das Deutsche Gesundheitswesen* urged the general practitioner to decline all applications for monetary compensation. Here, the medical journal revived the longstanding dispute of whether people with traumatic symptoms are genuinely suffering or malingering, whether or not they are entitled to care and financial support or deserving of contempt and public neglect. Physicians were told that the First World War had already shown that the external conditions of war do not generate real mental illnesses. The repeated reminder that the general practitioner served as a trustee of public money, together with the insistence that doctors should not be all too easily fooled by the soldiers' stories of hardship during the war and that diffuse nervous symptoms rarely developed in response to extraordinary physical and mental duress (Kröber 1946, 348–351), all played into larger discursive and fiscal efforts to contain war-related psychological damage. Any potential breakdown of the German population, and especially of the returning soldiers, was foreclosed by the notion that the doctor's rejection of compensation would itself function as a therapeutic measure. This measure was to foster the productivity and resilience necessary to jump-start postwar reconstruction.

There was one early exception to this bureaucratic approach to Germany's economic and psychological maladies: those who suffered traumatic brain injuries—presumably around 20,000 in the Soviet Occupation Zone—were given a special status in the broader group of the physically disabled, which also included amputees, the blind, and the hearing impaired. The brain-injured were, thus, transformed into *the* most tangible reminder of war violence (Lindenberg 1948; Lindenberg 1947a).[8] Evidently, the pre-First World War anatomic-physiological notion of trauma as a surgical wound was the one relatively stable concept in which former soldiers' psychic debilitation and rehabilitation could be legitimized. The subsequent efforts to reintegrate the brain-injured into postwar society were buttressed by social-psychiatric institutional spaces that sprung up on the local scale. This network included special care units in psychiatric clinics or general hospitals (such as in Berlin-Spandau for patients in Brandenburg and Mecklenburg and Bernburg for patients in Sachsen-Anhalt), counseling offices for the brain-injured and their relatives (Dresden), as well as compensatory regulations, a series of professional conferences, and public informational campaigns. The idea of a universally recognizable sign—a round yellow badge with three black dots and the label "brain injured" ("Hirnverletzter")—also recirculated, turning war-wounded former soldiers into a publicly visible group of casualties, if not victims (Lindenberg 1948, 145). In the medical vocabulary of the time, the personality of these men who had experienced traumatic brain injuries had radically altered: they developed neurological symptoms of aphasia, spasms, epilepsy, and paralysis; their speech appeared blurred, their cadence flattened, their general motoric system was slowed down, and their sex drive seemed to have weakened. Notably, these symptoms were accompanied by physical deformities and idiosyncrasies, such as missing eyes, scars, and limp facial muscles, and, as it recurs over and over again in the case studies presented in medical journals in both the East and the West, many of the brain-injured had completely withdrawn from any social life. Reportedly, they often "starrte[n] ins Leere" ["stared into space"], "erkenne[n] auch Bekannte nicht" ["no longer recognized acquaintances"], and exhibited "weiches, leises Lächeln, stille Traurigkeit" ["a soft, quiet smile and silent sadness"] that amounted to a general mental disposition described as "versandend" ["severely abstracted"] (Lindenberg 1947a, 225; Busemann 1948, 120, 122; Busemann 1947). According to these records, the wounded men had turned into ghosts.

The social implications of such severe dejection did not elude the key professional actors who led the socio-psychiatric reorganization in the Soviet Occupation Zone. Because of these fundamental changes in their personality, the brain-injured constantly faced conflicts, blame, and shame at home and in public. Even in those private spaces where soldiers were still considered heroes, they complained that no one wanted to know the real truth about war combat (Herman 1997, 8). In post-1945 Germany, men returning from the war were no longer idealized members of society. They had not only been dislodged from their stabilizing role as head of household in the private sphere but also represented the shameful investment in a horrific extermination war that the German people had supported. Although among those men who participated in the Second World War, the brain-injured were the only group construed as legitimate victims, the recurring appeal not to mistake them for the insane and not to admit them to mental institutions intimates that the notion of the war-damaged soldier continued to tap into the deepest anxieties and biases among the postwar population (Lindenberg 1948). These anxieties were also widely negotiated by early DEFA films (Pinkert 2008, 19–72).[9]

At the same time, the first signs of a return to a more modern medical discourse were established in the Soviet Occupation Zone. In 1948, *Das Deutsche Gesundheitswesen* set out to confront the presumably still widespread pre-enlightenment assumptions about psychic suffering as madness with a socio-medical explanation (Kröber 1948, 227–230). Now three years after the war's end, the journal recommended taking the psychological complaints of citizens as seriously as traditional concerns with the body. The general practitioners were asked to allow patients to share their problems and concerns and provide some form of counseling with light sedatives as a temporary treatment for chronic irritation and physiological overdrive. Medical professionals were licensed to address the diffuse nervous symptoms observed among the exhausted and underfed postwar population. The conventional perception of soldiers' suffering as manipulated performances of pension neurotics was primarily maintained.

Reportedly, the public perceived those often displaced and homeless men who appeared brain-damaged as "lethargic idiots," wandering lunatics, or even criminal psychopaths (Lindenberg 1948, 145–147; Lindenberg 1947a, Lindenberg 1947b). It is worth noting that interest in the repetitive intrusion of traumatic flashbacks and nightmares into the survivor's life, which had been relevant for Freud's and Abram Kardiner's discussion of combat neurosis, had vanished from postwar medical discourse after 1945 (Freud 1961, 11; Kardiner and Spiegel 1947, 201). Among all case studies of patients classified as brain-injured soldiers that appeared in the psychiatric journals in the second half of the forties, only one (in the West) refers to a patient's occasional recurrence of past memories. A report by Adolf Busemann published in *Der Nervenarzt* in 1948 states:

> Ju. [Joh], Schreinergeselle von 30 Jahren, dessen Verwundung 4 Monate zurückliegt, [....] *gibt zu*, [m]anchmal kämen die Erinnerungen an Tage, da es so *schwer war, was er durchgemacht habe*. Er "sieht noch das Mündungsfeuer der Pistole" bei seiner Verwundung. "Das Schlimmste war, wie ich im Feldlazarett lag, *ich konnte nicht sprechen, nicht [...] [verstummt]*. Da dacht ich, du bist ein armer Mensch dein Lebtag, *wärst du lieber draussen geblieben.*"
>
> (my emphasis)

> [A 30-year-old patient, a carpenter wounded 4 months ago, *admits* that sometimes the memories of the days *when he had to endure such difficulty* resurfaced. He still sees "the muzzle flashes of the weapon" when he got injured. "The worst happened when I was at the mobile army hospital, *and I could not talk [. . .] [pauses]*. Then I told myself, you are an unlucky man; if *I could have only stayed outside*."]
>
> (Busemann 1948, 124)

Astonishingly, this is one of the rare archival sources in the journals where the subjective, first-person voice of the brain-injured patient is reproduced. We should note that the physician renders the patient's recall of his intrusive war experiences in the trenches as an "admission." This gives not only a sense of the relation between trust and power in the doctor-patient relationship, which delineates the contours of "scientific" knowledge, but the first-person narrative also registers a particular tension, if not public taboo, regarding the ambiguous psychic hauntings of the Second World War and the former soldiers' precarious survival. Most importantly, this discursive space is rife with silences on multiple temporal scales. While the first-person patient account alludes to a diffuse sense of self-pity ("'you are an unlucky man'"), an unspoken, privately held historical regret about participation in combat and mass destruction is also implied ("'if I could have only stayed outside'"). Again, the sporadic nature of such subjective narrative forms entering the psychiatric discourse in these journals cannot be overemphasized.

If immediately after the end of the war, anxieties concerning the widespread emergence of psychological suffering went hand in hand with the reinforced circulation of traditional ideas about "malingerers" that reached back to the First World War, then, in subsequent years, psychiatrists began to wonder why no mass epidemics of experience-conditioned illnesses had occurred among the postwar German population. This seemed especially puzzling given the enormous physical and mental strains the population had endured (Kröber 1948). The seeming absence of massive psychic reactions similar to those after the First World War, especially of "hysterics" and "tremblers," gave rise to the overall understanding that Nazism, the Second World War, and its aftermath had revealed the human brain, nerve system, and psyche to be much more adaptable to any strain and disruption than previously assumed (Schwarz 1950, 291; Henssge 1949, 133; Bonhoeffer 1947). Paradoxically, in the postwar era, this assumption helped sustain a valorization of hardiness, endurance, and compliance that had already been cultivated under National Socialism and supported conventional notions of masculinity. All these different factors—the insistence on endogenic models of explanation, the reproduction of an ideological link between dignity and endurance, the all-pervasive public and even medical stigmatization of reactive psychic illness to war and postwar experience, as well as privately and publicly enforced ethics of health and work as the only remaining source for a livable future—might have been the historically contingent forces that helped confine war trauma to the private sphere (Schwarz 1950, 290) and the most inner recesses of the body.

THE SILENT PSYCHIC WORK OF WAR

It was, however, also in the margins of psychiatric discussions more generally invested in debating the relations between body/mind, organ/psyche, endogenic and exogenic explanations that war suffering translated the "private" effects of violence and historical rupture into public representations. If most medical practitioners understood the absent psychic symptoms as a sign of the extreme adaptability of the human psyche, some interlocutors stated the problem differently. The psychiatrist E. Henssge (based in Dresden) suggested in 1949: "Should we not rather conceive it as abnormal when people exposed to great psychic impact ('seelische Erschütterungen') do not develop intense reactions?" (Henssge 1949, 133). With some distance from the immediate crisis of 1945, the seeming absence of psychogenic disorder in postwar Germany itself came more clearly into view as a pathological symptom of psychic failure:

> Die durch Hunger und Not, durch die chronifizierte Damoklessituation und durch eine schicksalsmässig empfundene Ausweichunmöglichkeit hervorgerufene Hypodynamie nahm den Menschen die Kraft und Energie zu gestaltungsbedürftiger Darstellung psychogener Inszenierung, liess aber, zumal soziale Verlockerungen fehlten und individuelle Differenzierungen ihren Reizwert verloren zu haben schienen, das psychische Versagen in die Tiefenperson bis zur vegetativen Atonie absinken. Steudner wies unlängst darauf hin, dass sich die psychogenen Reaktionen jetzt viel eher unter dem "stilleren" Bild einer Organneurose verbergen, also wohl nicht geringer geworden, sondern nur anders gefärbt sind. *Man könnte vielleicht sagen, aus der aktiven Flucht in die Krankheit wurde die passive Krankheit der Flucht.*
>
> (my emphasis)
>
> [Starvation, deprivation, an environment of chronic danger, and the feeling of utter hopelessness produced hypodynamia in members of the population. This hypodynamia consumed all the energy and drive necessary to have psychogenic symptoms. Moreover, social incentives and individual differentiation no longer acted as stimulating forces. All these factors allowed psychic degeneration to sink into the depth of a people's personality ("Tiefenperson") to the point of vegetative atony. Recently, Steuder pointed out that current psychogenic reactions are concealed in "less dramatic" symptoms of an organ neurosis; thus, psychogenic reactions have not abated but produce different symptoms. *One could say that the active flight into the illness has been transformed into the passive illness of flight.*]
>
> (Schwarz 1950, 291)

To put it into more contemporary terms, what is implied here is a startling recognition that more people develop acute posttraumatic stress symptoms after the threat has safely passed rather than in the face of continuing danger. The sense of hopelessness and immobility (together with the notion of "vegetative atony," an increasing limpness of muscle tissue) described here resonates with an observation by the historian Reinhart Koselleck who has argued that the experience of wholesale death in the Second World War sat like a "congealed lava mass" in all survivors (Geyer 1997, 18). In 1946, an eye witness account captured this state of psychic paralysis, if not traumatic dissociation, among the German postwar population in metaphoric fashion:

> Trümmer- und Schuttberge machten die Strassen unkenntlich oder versperrten sie. Durch die Wohnungen drangen Zug, Kälte, und Regen: Fenster und Türen waren zersplittert. Die unter den Trümmern verendeten Menschenleichen und Tierkadaver bekamen eine gefährliche Rattenplage. Küchenreste und verdorbene Lebensmittel dienten unzähligen Insekten als Brutstätte. [...] Es war ein abnormaler Zustand, eine grauenerregende Verdrossenheit des ganzen Mileus. In ihm vegetierten durch Elend und Not, Angst und Affektstupor jeder Initiative unfähige, in Lethargie verfallene, völlig deklassierte Geschöpfe, die weder Lust noch Freude empfanden, so dass jede normale Beeinflussbarkeit fehlte.
>
> [Mountains of rubble and ruin made streets completely unrecognizable or impassable. Windows and doors were shattered and broken; apartments were drafty, cold, and wet. The human and animal corpses decomposing under the rubble were the cause of a life-threatening plague of rats. Piles of kitchen waste and rotting food were breeding grounds for countless insects. [...] it was a catastrophic situation; an entire milieu was engulfed in a horrifying degradation. Completely destitute creatures languished in this environment of deprivation, misery, fear, and affect-stupor. Sunk in passive resignation, they were incapable of taking any initiative or feeling any desire or joy; normal suggestibility was lacking.]
>
> (Beyer 1946, 641)

In other words, symptoms manifesting the experience of war and mass death did not vanish after the Second World War (Becher). Instead, to draw on the historian Michael Geyer, they found more silent or intimate articulations, often localized in particular organs, especially the stomach (and we can add the skin, muscles, and nerves); they were directed inward through "a restriction of the sensorium, everywhere accompanied by an inability of communication bordering on speechlessness" (Geyer 1997, 18). Under immediate postwar conditions where a person's life was reduced to the goal of survival, psychological constriction or numbing became an essential mode of adaptation. This altered state of consciousness—identified by Judith Lewis Herman as one of the cardinal symptoms of psychological trauma, in addition to hyperarousal and intrusion—combines a feeling of indifference, emotional detachment, and profound passivity in which the person relinquishes all initiative and struggle (Herman 1997, 42–43). As the above account of the situation in destroyed German cities at the end of the war indicates, this narrowing of psychological capacities was in many ways all-consuming, applying to nearly every area of life, including activities, thoughts, memories, and emotions.

In the aftermath of the Second World War, death and violence continued to permeate all aspects of the everyday lives of ordinary people in Germany and Eastern Europe. The only comprehensive study on psychogenic illnesses in the postwar period, published in *Psychiatrie, Neurologie, and Medizinische Psychologie* in 1949, reveals the more specific articulations of psychic reactions to war violence (Henssge 1949; Schulte 1948). Based on 1200 cases of patients living in Dresden between 1945 and 1946, the study exposes what the writer W. G. Sebald in the late 1990s described as the lasting effects of a shameful taboo in Germany's postwar public. During a new moment of reckoning with the Second World War in the aftermath of Germany's unification, Sebald's essay "Luftkrieg und Literatur" (On the Natural History of Destruction) spurred the widespread recirculation of narratives about the destruction and deaths caused by the Allied bombings among the German civilian population. Given the damage and death the Germans had inflicted on others during the Second World War, a social context was lacking in the postwar period that would have made it possible to translate the traumatic events of the air war bombings into public narratives. In the 1990s, this led to the widely acknowledged claim that the Germans' experience of the air war had receded into collective forgetting and needed to be recovered through literature, historiography, and personal accounts (Sebald 1999; Sebald 2003; Friedrich 2002). It surprises in retrospect how lastingly the collective experience of German war death became erased in the official realm, especially in the East, if we consider just how palpably the experience was recorded in medical records shortly after the war. For instance, the psychological study of people in the 1940s who had survived the air raids of Dresden provides detailed descriptions of the psychosomatic effects caused by war loss and destruction:

> Kurt St., 63, totalausgebombt, Frau beim Luftangriff verloren. Vorher nie seelische Störungen. Elfriede Z., 43, Periode seit 18 Monaten weggeblieben, totalausgebombt, früher nie seelisch krank, bewohnt ein Zimmer, wo sie auch kocht und schläft. Klagen: Schlaflosigkeit, Juckreiz an Kopf und Nacken, Müdigkeit, Brustschmerzen, traurige Stimmung, Antriebs- und Lustlosigkeit [...] Martha M., 49, 1944 Mann verloren, am 13. 2. 45 ausgebombt, wollte sich nach dem Angriff mit Veronal vergiften, wurde daran gehindert [....] Elfriede K., 30, totalausgebombt, am 13. 2. 45 Mann vermisst, Periode seitdem weggeblieben [....] Elizabth H., 39, totalausgebombt, nach dem Angriff laut Angabe 9 Wochen steif gewesen. Subjektiv: Geschlechtsteil wie abgestorben, taubes Gefühl in den Fingerspitzen, Lustlosigkeit [....] Elizabeth Sch., 53, totalgeschädigt, Mann verloren, Sohn gefallen. Subjektiv: Schwindelanfälle, Herzklopfen, innere Unruhe, Angstzustände. Objektiv: rote Hautschrift [....] Margarete Th., 63, totalausgebombt, früher Schneiderin [...] nie depressive [...] trauriger und ängstlicher Gesichtsausdruck, glaubt sterben zu müssen [...] Wegen drohender Selbstmordgefahr kam sie in das Krankenhaus Löbauer Strasse [...] Der Ehemann, 64 Jahre [...] sieht keinen Ausweg mehr, hat das Leben satt, hat an nichts Freude, kann nicht schlafen, leidet an Angstzuständen und hat in letzter Zeit Selbstmordgedanken [....].
>
> [Kurt St, 63, bombed out of his home, lost his wife in an air raid, son killed in action, no mental disorders before [....] Elfriede Z., 43. No period in last 18 months, bombed out of her home, previously no mental illness. Complaints: sleeplessness, itching on head and neck, fatigue, chest pains, sad moods, listlessness [....] Martha M., 49, lost her husband

> in 1944, bombed out on February 13, 1945, wanted to poison herself with Veronal, was deterred [. ...] Elfriede K., 30, bombed out, husband missing since February 13, 1945, no periods since then [....] Elisabeth H., 39, bombed out, reports she was stiff for nine weeks after an air raid. Subjective: sex organ appears dead, numbness in fingertips, listlessness [....] Elisabeth Sch, 53, house totally destroyed, lost husband, son killed in action. Subjective: fits of dizziness, heart palpitations, restlessness, anxiety attacks. Objective: red marks on skin [....] Margarete Th., 63, totally bombed out, used to work as a seamstress, never depressive before [...] sad and fearful facial expressions, thinks she has to die [...] suicidal, and admitted to hospital [...] her husband, 64, [...] sees no way out. Is sick of life without joy, unable to sleep, suffers from anxiety attacks, recent suicidal thoughts [. ...].]
>
> (Henssge 1949, 135–136)

Here, the complex symptoms of insomnia and anxiety, as well as the lack of affect, severe sexual inhibitions, hopelessness, and suicidal preoccupations, signal a tenacious state of depression that results from staggering psychological losses (Herman, 94–95). Rather than the more active modes of mourning and sorrow, the patients display persistent signs of numbness that constrict their emotional capacities. One woman who had lived through the bombing of Dresden laconically stated: "'Ich lebe wie in einer anderen Welt, man ist zu Stein geworden.'" ("'I live as if I am in a different world; one has turned into stone'") (Henssge 1949, 135). We need to probe further why the narrative and perceptual frameworks by which the experience of Elfriede Z. could have become legible in the larger public realm did not exist in the aftermath of the Second World War and the following decades. The French-Bulgarian cultural critic and psychoanalyst Julia Kristeva suggests that the horrific and painful sights of death in the Second World War have damaged our systems of perception and representation (Kristeva 1989, 233). In the specific context of early postwar Germany, a diffuse sense of shame and guilt among the population prevented the emergence of a viable public sphere in which the individual and collective experience of mass death and destruction could be addressed (Geyer 1997, 19). The lack of public articulation in the immediate postwar years reinforced a sense of dissociation and numbness among the survivors of the war. This numbness represents, at the same time, "the achievement of defense and the failure of defense, the success of protection and the breaching of the protective shield" associated with traumatic stress today (Leys 2000, 35).

The contributions in the health and medical journals of the Soviet Occupation Zone forestalled a notion of a more permeable affective-psychic space that is susceptible to contingent biographical and historical relations. If, for Freud, traumatic memory was "inherently unstable or mutable owing to the role of unconscious motives that confer meaning on it" (Leys 2000, 20), psychiatric discourse after the Second World War continued to follow a tradition that reduced the effects of traumatic impact to quasi-objective bodily phenomena. Centering on the relationship between psychological trauma and neuro-somatic symptoms, studies juxtaposed case histories related and unrelated to the conditions of war in a way that continued disregarding the historical specificity of wartime experience (Schwarz 1950, 293–295). Whether victims of war combat or a work-related accident, whether victims of family loss caused by war killings or a fear-inducing encounter with an animal, all these patients were viewed as casualties of an external trauma that triggered changes in their vasomotor system in ways that tended to eliminate the issue of historical and moral meaning.

COLD-WAR REALIGNMENTS

In the Soviet Zone and early German Democratic Republic (GDR), the ritualized commemorations dedicated to the official (communist) victims of fascism left little room for representing the experience of Germans who had lost relatives, were severely wounded, imprisoned, bombed out, or displaced. In contrast, the politics of memory in the early Federal Republic of Germany (FRG) was openly defined by conflating German wartime suffering with victimization. This was particularly apparent in the public construction of the German prisoner of war returning from Soviet internment, to which psychiatric discussions in the West contributed significantly. While the East German psychiatric journal seems to have published only one abbreviated study of psychic disorders among German prisoners of war in North Africa, various medical studies appeared in professional journals in the Western zones. Here, psychiatrists used the concept of "dystrophy" to describe the somewhat diffuse physiological and psychological effects of starvation and maltreatment experienced by many prisoners of war in Soviet camps. In addition, the concept of "returnee depression" ("Heimkehrerdepression") served to make sense of the various psychic and psychosomatic symptoms developed by returnees who, upon their reentry into German postwar society, experienced a profound sense of geographical, social, and psychological dislocation. Amid mass mobility, entire populations were pulled into new conflicts as national boundaries were redrawn. Hundreds of thousands of dispersed military units, POWs, re-settlers, refugees, and camp survivors of all countries were stumbling across Europe. Medical case studies published by *Der Nervenarzt* open a "window" into a postwar Germany traversed by thousands of displaced physically and mentally injured men who had returned from imprisonment in Soviet camps. Two should be cited here:

> Zweiter Fall, H. Sche., 30. Aufnahme am 11. November 1946. Angaben der Mutter: [...] Zwei Jahre Militärdienst bei der Infantrie. Von 1941–43 Lokomotivführer. 1943 wurde Sche. wieder zum Militär eingezogen und kam 1944 nach Russland, wo er im Frühjahr 1945 in Kriegsgefangenschaft geriet. Arbeitet in der Nähe Moskaus in einem Steinbruch. Bekam nach seinen Angaben nur Wassersuppe zu essen und wurde viel geschlagen. Im Juni 1946 wegen Fieber und Durchfall aus der Gefangenschaft entlassen. Auf dem Transport verschlechterte sich sein Gesundheitszustand, so dass er ins Krankenhaus Erfurt eingeliefert wurde. Von dort im Sammeltransport über die Zonengrenze gebracht, kam er sofort in ein Krankenhaus. Ref. hat ihren Sohn am 16. Oktober das erste mal wieder gesehen. Sie meinte er habe einen scheuen und ängstlichen Blick bekommen. Die schwerere Wesensveränderung bemerkte die Mutter zunächst nicht. [...]

Dritter Fall, P. Rö., 34, [...] Am 9. Mai 1945 kam er in der Tschechei in russische Kriegsgefangenschaft. Er wurde von Breslau nach Stalino befördert und arbeitete auf Kolchosen und beim Häuserbau. Er war während seiner Gefangenschaft längere Zeit "dystrophiekrank." Ödeme will er nie an sich beobachtet haben. Im November 1947 wurde er aus russicher Kriegsgefangenschaft entlassen, von November 1947 bis Februar 1948 war er bei seiner Schwester in Thüringen. Dort wurde er dadurch auffällig, dass er in dranghafter Unruhe fast täglich eine Strecke von 10 km von Stotterheim und Erfurt hin und her zurücklegte und sich durch diese sinnlosen Märsche die Füsse völlig wund lief. Er musste in ein Krankenhaus eingewiesen werden, verschwand von dort aber eines Tages in die amerikanische Zone, ohne eine weitere Nachricht zu hinterlassen. Er kam mit Sammeltransport über Eisenach nach Bebra [...] Von hier aus wurde er in ein Lazarett verlegt und wegen psychischer Auffälligkeiten in unsere Klinik eingewiesen.

[A second case, H. Sche., 30, admitted on November 11, 1946 [...] Stated by the mother: [...] Two years of military service in the infantry, locomotive driver between 1941 and 1943. 1943 again drafted into the military, got to Russia in 1944, and became a prisoner of war in the spring of 1945. He worked near Moscow in a quarry. He said he was only fed water soup and was regularly beaten. He was released from prison in June 1946 due to fever and diarrhea. His health worsened during the transport; he needed to be admitted to a hospital in Erfurt. From there, he was taken by mass transport across the borders into the Western zones and immediately admitted to a hospital there. The mother saw her son for the first time again on October 16. She said he now had a shy and anxious look on his face. She did not immediately notice the severe changes in his personality. [...]

A third case, P. Rö, 34 [...] on May 9, 1945, became a prisoner of war in a Russian camp in the Tschechei. He was transported from Breslau to Stalino, where he worked on a collective farm and in construction. During his internment for a prolonged time, he suffered from dystrophy. He claims he never saw edemas on his body. In November 1947, he was released from Soviet internment, and from November 1947 until February 1948, he stayed with his sister in Thuringia. There he became conspicuous since he displayed urgent restlessness almost daily and walked 10 km back and forth between Erfurt and Stotterheim. Through these senseless marches, he got severe sores on his feet. He had to be admitted to a hospital, from which one day he ran away to get to the American zone without leaving a note. He came from Eisenach to Bebra in a mass transport [...] From there, he was transferred to a military hospital and admitted to our clinic due to noticeable psychic problems.

(Schmitz 1949, 305–309)

A closer reading of these narrative files could provide further insights into the complex positioning of former POWs returning from Soviet camps to a split-up postwar Germany, grappling with defeat and its repercussions (Goltermann, 2014). Suffice it to say, due to the common belief that dystrophy and returnee depression would not result in long-term psychological damage, most former prisoners of war returning to Germany did not receive any thorough neurological and psychiatric examination. Psychiatrists nevertheless hoped that these concepts would help identify and perhaps prevent suicidal pursuits among a postwar male population, profoundly diminished, as one psychiatrist put it, of substance, roots, affect, courage, and any vitality. Patients often articulated this depressed state as anxiety concerning their sexuality and masculinity (Schulte, 1953, 417–448). The ubiquitous concern with sexual dysfunction across multiple medical studies in the early postwar years reveals a larger anxiety about reproducing a depleted, war-torn society. Paying attention to these feelings of diminished self-worth, especially in the sexual realm, among returnees from Soviet internment, early postwar psychiatric discourse in the West helped register the historical and personal changes experienced by many former Wehrmacht soldiers as a fundamental rupture in their lives (Schulte 1953, 417):

> [...] die tiefgreifende Erschütterung der Selbstwertgefühle, das elementare Erlebnis der Leistungs- und Seinsinsuffizienz gerade auch auf sexuellem Gebiet. Dadurch ist der dystrophisch Geschädigte vorzeitig in die biologisch gefährliche Situation versetzt, die sonst Greisen mit dem Anheben ihrer sexuellen Insuffizienz verhängnisvoll werden kann.
>
> [[...] men experienced a significant blow ("Erschütterung") to their sense of self-worth, especially regarding their sexual performance. Due to these conditions, the person incapacitated by dystrophy finds himself prematurely within a biologically dangerous state that only older men experience when their sexual insufficiency increases.]
>
> (Schulte 1953, 419)

At the same time, however, historians Svenja Goltermann, Frank Biess, and Robert Möller have pointed to the oversight of multiple historical conditions. By linking the physical and psychological troubles of former prisoners of war to their maltreatment in the Soviet camps, the psychiatric studies overlooked that the etiology of these symptoms might have been related to the even earlier experience of participating in a war of mass destruction whose goals included the extermination of European Jewry and the subordination of "inferior races" in Eastern Europe and the Soviet Union (Möller 2001, 108, 179; Goltermann 2001, 344; Biess 2009, 70–94; Ulrich 1992, 182–183).

In that sense, the concept of dystrophy ostensibly caused by capture and Communist atrocities enabled a displacement of guilt onto the Soviets that was sustained more generally by a public sphere in the West centered on German war suffering. Needless to say, this strategy could not gain much currency in the East, where the public narrative of a new beginning revolved around the antifascist education and transformation received by POWs at training schools in the Soviet Union and the atonement of former Wehrmacht soldiers performed through the particular hardship endured in Soviet internment (Naimark, 42–43; Biess, 126–152; "Wer is der Angeklagte"). Bruno Lewin's study of three thousand prisoners of war held in British camps in Egypt between 1941 and 1947, which was published by *Psychiatrie, Neurologie, and Medizinische Psychologie* in 1950, is as close as it gets to constituting discursive spaces in the East German public realm for a discussion of the so-called "barbed-wire sickness" ("Stacheldrahtkrankeit") brought on by capture and deprivation that dominated the West German politics of memory throughout the 1950s. The circulation of the concept also harked back to the First World War. Lewin's focus on POWs who suffered from nervous-depressive disorder (insomnia, nightmares, lack of appetite, weight loss) and psychosomatic symptoms (ulcers, etc.) discloses a sense of impaired masculinity that the political and cultural discourse in the early GDR shored up with exemplary notions of antifascist male subjectivity. Suggesting, however, that psychological reactions to the war were least likely to occur among "Anti-Nazis," the study supported the dominant idea that antifascist transformation was a matter of collective mental health (Lewin 1949; Vischer 1918).

Political contexts played a significant role in producing or containing pathologies in the postwar era. In many ways, the psychiatric profession and studies in the Soviet Occupation Zone and the early GDR contributed to the apparent absence of traumatic responses to war violence among the German population. The psychiatric discourse thereby helped sustain the exclusion of the experience of death and destruction from public representation. In contrast, I have argued elsewhere, the cinematic culture in the Soviet Occupation Zone produced, albeit often inadvertently, an elegiac public memory in the immediate aftermath of Nazi Germany and the Holocaust, where wartime suffering was registered in the margins of the visible field. At the same time, Jennifer Kapczynski has shown how postwar German culture wrestled with specters of fascist constructions of health and illness, reproducing to a certain extent the biopolitical rhetoric of the Nazis (Kapczynski 2008). Although some socio-medical and psychiatric publications pointed to notable symptoms among the German population and thus supplied a viable language for recognizing psychic ailments, the overall conceptual shift from psychodynamic to biological approaches, together with a renewed focus on the asylum-style confinement of the endogenically mentally ill, stifled a modern understanding of transient mental dispositions affected by historical experience in the early GDR.

In 1950, the increasing ideological resistance to the viability of psychogenic illnesses under the political and social conditions of socialism culminated in the first massive public denouncement of depth-psychological, psychoanalytical, and neo-analytical practices in favor of Pavlovian neurophysiological reflexology adopted from Soviet psychology (Schultz-Hencke 1950; Gross 1996, 48–49). Initially, the future role of psychotherapy and psychoanalysis was still publicly debated.[10] However, Pavlov contended that all behavior is regulated by the brain and needs to be explained in physiological terms. The alignment of scientific views and research in the GDR with Soviet paradigms (Pavlovization) during the 1950s and early 1960s led to a continued emphasis on biological concepts within the academic fields of psychiatry (Eghigian 2005, 186–188). New somatic and psycho-pharmacological therapies in psychiatric hospitals further promoted this trend. Locally, marginal efforts of social psychiatric reformist forces existed, yet they were not implemented nation-wide (Steinberg 2016). Showing that the relationship between stimulus and reaction depends on the intactness of the cerebral cortex tissue, Soviet psychiatry, and Pavlov's theses in particular, excluded any immaterial, mental element in the formation or treatment of psychic processes. In the Soviet Union, and the GDR psychoanalysis was driven "underground" and persisted disguised in new terminology and was practiced in a group-oriented approach (Etkind 1997; Antic 2016; Leuenberger 2001).

Introduced around 1950, one year after the founding of the East German state, Pavlov's radical behaviorism enabled orthodox Marxists to trace back any still occurring psychic illnesses to either remnants of the old class order or defects caused in the brain. Although orthodox Marxism contended that being (*Sein*) determines consciousness (*Bewusstsein*) and that the abolition of class conflict would subsequently lead to the removal of psychic conflicts, psychic illness was defined as an internal physiological problem that therefore needed to be resolved not from outside but rather from within the body and the mind (Maaz 1990, 195). From the 1950s onward, the public effort to promote health among the East German population was increasingly defined by the Communist Party (SED). As the psychiatric care system was aligned with the organizational structure of work brigades and systematic planning in the economic sphere (Drechsler), little room existed within this collective, future-driven society for remembering the aftereffects of psychological traumas related to the Second World War.

CODA: REFRACTED MEMORY AND THE MEDICAL HUMANITIES

The connections between the private and public worlds, individual and community shaping collective experience in the aftermath of the war, need to be restored through a historical investigation of posttraumatic stress and related psychological disorders that remained unrecognized in postwar Germany after 1945. Since the 1960s, this oversight has contributed to a narrow moral assessment of Germans' failure in the early postwar years to deal with the crimes and atrocities they had inflicted on others. In recent decades, the historical dissociation from psychological harm after 1945 has shifted toward the other extreme, a public proliferation of memories related to the traumas the Germans themselves experienced during the war.

In this essay, I have shown that opening new archives and discursive realms—including medical records, narrative case files, psychiatric studies, or eyewitness accounts by those involved in the reorganization of the professional and academic field in the second half of the twentieth century—can compel us to unlearn established understandings of the early postwar era as an all-pervasive "sphere of resilience and amnesia." While conventionally academic clinicians or trained historians have written the history of psychiatry, I argue that literary and cultural scholars attuned to the emerging Medical and Health Humanities can interlink the history of medicine, including its scientific registers and claims to objectivity, with cultural debates about the unsettled memory regarding such multi-layered historical violence. In other words, while medical histories can be infused with attention to historical and narrative contingency, revealing their constructed nature, cultural histories in the narrower sense and their literary and cinematic imaginaries benefit from being situated within larger, heterogenous fields of knowledge productions.

Moreover, what becomes visible at the intersection of public memory and the postwar history of psychiatry is the urgent need to create discursive spaces that can render the unaccounted-for traumatic experience of patients in East German/Soviet psychiatric care as well as the recollections by families of victims of Nazi psychiatry. Films such as *Verwahrt und Vergessen?—Psychiatrie in der DDR* (Shut Away and Forgotten? Psychiatry in the GDR) (2022) by Ulli Wendelmann and Claudia Grüner signal this need for a shift in memory debates toward more locally scaled and regional histories. Lastly, tracing the entwined trajectories of the fields of psychiatry, psychoanalysis, and psychotherapy in the twentieth century across the rupture of 1945 also inevitably brings into focus how therapists and professional medical disciplines reconstructed their pasts in the changed discursive contexts of post-1989 after East European state socialism collapsed and Germany unified (Leuenberger 2002; Leuenberger 2006). While Dagmar Herzog's 2017 study *Cold War Freud* is brilliantly argued, thoroughly researched, and transnational in scope, it curiously confines the history of Eastern Europe and the Soviet Union to one extensive footnote (Herzog 2017, 217n17). At the same time, a slew of exciting new scholarship has emerged in recent years that challenges any totalizing understanding of regime-conforming healthcare under socialism, revealing transnational and intra-German (East/West) contacts in social medicine and psychiatry in the later twentieth century. What needs to be further explored are the incongruities between official Sovietized history and alternative therapeutic practices or psychoanalysis "in the cracks" of Eastern Europe. Reconsidering transnational and intra-German (East/West) contacts in the fields of social medicine and psychiatry during the Cold War era, Eastern and Central Europe need to be linked up with the broader historiography of twentieth-century psychiatry (Marks and Savelli 2015; Solomon 2018). In addition, the varying effects of turning to Soviet psychiatry and Pavlov's theses in Eastern European countries in the 1950s have to come into view.

Regarding Germany's collective memories of the Second World War and its aftermath, the hope would be that the dialectics between processes of numbing and reliving these traumatic events begin to articulate a story that accounts for both the multiple psychological impacts of war violence and mass death on the German population itself and their historical role as implicated subjects—as perpetrators, supporters, and bystanders. While the memory of the Holocaust is duly, of course, front and center of Germany's recent public memory, palpably absent to this day is a reflexive mnemonic field where the force of inter- and transgenerational trauma that cuts across familial spaces in the twentieth/twenty-first century, can be registered. Indeed, a rich body of literary works is devoted to these issues. However, viable public spheres of mourning are still needed, where the grievability of lost (non-Jewish) German lives can be contemplated. It appears that the specters of (post)war suffering either hover intangibly, in perpetual search of spaces able to memorialize loss and grief, or they periodically accrue meanings of unrealized pasts, producing an excess of representation. What may future memorial landscapes look like that possibly refract those multiple pasts?

NOTES

1. The International Psychoanalytic Association, which held its first post-Second World War meeting in Zurich in 1949, underscored the need to steer clear of the influence of sociological factors on the mind. Psychoanalysts in the USA, in Western and Central Europe and in Latin America would heed this call, "whether out of personal predilection or institutional pressures, or some combination of the two" (Herzog 2017, 4). It was only the "grotesque debacle" fought out through the 1950s and 1960s over financial compensation for mental health damages

experienced by Jewish survivors that became a catalyst for changing the science of trauma and for introducing Post-Traumatic Stress Disorder (PTSD) into the *Diagnostic and Statistical Manual of Mental Disorders* in 1980 (Herzog 2017, 90).

2. For a critique of Foucault's emphasis on the contingency of mental illness, see Luhrmann (2000, 17).
3. "Aktion T-4" was a campaign of mass murder by involuntary euthanasia in Nazi Germany. The term was used in postwar trials against doctors involved in the killing. The name T-4 is an abbreviation of Tiergartenstrasse 4, the street address of the Chancellery department set up in 1940, from which the program was coordinated. In October 1939 (backdated to September 1939), Hitler signed an order that permitted the beginning of the killing of the disabled (Herzog 2018, 56–58). Between 1939 and August of 1941, some 70,000 patients of psychiatric institutions were killed. Altogether circa 160,000 patients were put to death either by gas, lethal application of drugs, or intentional starvation (in the Reich). In occupied Poland thousands of patients were shot; for all the territories occupied by German forces, there were at least 250,000 to 300,000 victims (Roelcke 2008, 229). Immediately following the war, the atrocities of Nazi psychiatry were addressed in a few publications by authors who were affected by measures of persecution. Associated with the first postwar trials, these publications quickly disappeared from public attention until the mid-1960s [in the West] (Roelcke 2008, 230).
4. In this article, I replicate the diagnostic vocabulary deployed by the medical profession at the time, even if this terminology is outdated today and risks reproducing forms of exclusion. My aim is to critically historicize psychiatric discourse as the object of analysis.
5. In the Soviet Occupation Zone, the thirty-five institutions with a bed capacity of 30,000 only held about 6,000 remaining patients, all elderly, completely neglected, and starved (Lindenberg 1949, 4); see also Roggenbau. Unless otherwise noted all translations are mine.
6. In the Soviet Occupation Zone in 1947 the number of occupied beds had more than doubled since 1945 (from 6,000 to 13, 938), and the number of the mentally ill treated in mental institutions had also significantly increased from 1946 (20,111) to 1947 (40,056) (Lindenberg 1949, 4).
7. Sabine Hanrath stresses the continuity regarding the *Anstaltspsychatrie* (institutional psychiatry) in both the GDR and FRG from 1945 until the late 1960s. She also contends, despite different debates over theory, both postwar societies eventually succeeded in developing expanded social welfare and fostering open debate over medical issues, particularly the rights of the mentally disabled (Hanrath 2003). See also Coché (2017).
8. It should be noted, however, that the Second World War is rarely addressed directly in these studies. The brain-injured served as broader category, including those who suffered from epilepsy, experienced work injury and accidents. The language deployed in Lindenberg's medical report reveals how war violence is contained by and seeps into the psychiatric discourse: First traces of war violence can only be found in war-related language, such as "verschüttet, Schädelbruch" ["buried, skull fracture"], "stumpfe Gewalt, Projektil, Granatsplitter" ["blunt impact, projectile, grenade splinter"], "Kriegsverletzungen durch Schädelschüsse" ["war injuries through skull shots"] (Lindenberg, 1947a, 226); later a reference is given by the author to his own study of 10,000 brain-injured in the First World War of which fifty suffered from "traumatic epilepsy" (characterized by spontaneous fainting or severe temper tantrums) (Lindenberg, 1947a, 227); and finally, by the end of the study, a statistics is provided: In 1947, the total number of registered brain-injured in Berlin was 3158. This included war-damaged from WW I (26%) and from WW 2 (68%), the rest was injured in accidents or otherwise (Lindenberg, 1947a, 228).
9. DEFA (Deutsche Film Aktiengesellschaft), the film company, was founded in 1946 in the Soviet Occupation Zone. See Staudte (1946), Lamprecht (1946), Klaren (1948).

10. In 1950, the weekly cultural-political paper *Der Sonntag* published Ernst Sommer's novel on Franz Mesmer (1734–1815), entitled *Nacht und Tag* [Night and Day], as serial novel. The paper juxtaposed the publication with articles by Alexander Mette about the history and future role of psychotherapy and psychoanalysis. Mette stated: "[...] certainly not of little relevance will be the fact that under conditions of a socialist society the formation of neurosis will be significantly less than in a society based on class order. Apparently, we will no longer have to face the necessity to resort to the practices of analytic psychotherapy" (Mette 1950, 13). See also Mette (1951).

WORKS CITED

Antic, Ana. 2016. *Therapeutic Fascism: Experiencing the Violence of the Nazi Order*. Oxford: Oxford University Press.

Becher, Johannes R. 1947. *Deutsches Bekenntnis*. Berlin: Aufbau.

Besold, F. 1949. "Die Wirkungsmechanismen psychoanalytischer Therapie." *Psychiatrie, Neurologie, Medizinische Psychologie* 1, no. 12: 374–376.

Beyer, Alfred. 1946. "Ein Jahr Deutsche Zentralverwaltung des Gesundheitswesens. *Deutsches Gesundheitswesen* 1, no. 21: 641–645.

Biess, Frank. 2009. *Homecomings: Returning POWs and the Legacies of Defeat in Postwar Germany*. Princeton: Princeton University Press.

Bock, Gisela. 1986. *Zwangssterilisation im Nationalsozialismus: Studien zur Rassenpolitik und Frauenpolitik*. Opladen: Westdeutscher Verlag.

Bonhoeffer, Karl. 1947. "Vergleichende psychopathologische Erfahrungen aus den beiden Weltkriegen." *Der Nervenarzt* 18, no. 1: 1–4.

Busemann, Adolf. 1947. "Psychologische Untersuchungen an Hirnverletzten." *Der Nervenarzt* 18, no. 8: 337–349.

Busemann, Adolf. 1948. "Psychologische Untersuchungen an Hirnverletzten." *Der Nervenarzt* 19, no. 3/4: 120–129.

Coché, Stefanie. 2017. *Psychiatrie und Gesellschaft: Psychiatrische Einweisungspraxis im "Dritten Reich" in der DDR und der Bundesrepublik 1941–1963*. Göttingen: Vandenhoeck & Ruprecht.

Cocks, Geoffrey. 1990. "The Professionalization of Psychotherapy in Germany." In *German Professions 1800-1950*, edited by Geoffrey Cocks and Konrad Jarausch, 308–328. Oxford: Oxford University Press.

Cocks, Geoffrey. 1994. "Repressing, Remembering, Working Through: German Psychiatry, Psychotherapy, Psychoanalysis, and the 'Missed Resistance' in the Third Reich." In *Resistance Against the Third Reich 1933–1990*, edited by Michael Geyer and John Boyer, 312–325. Chicago: University of Chicago Press.

Cocks, Geoffrey. 1997. *Psychotherapy in the Third Reich: The Göring Institute*. New Brunswick/ London: Transaction Publishers.

Cohen, Deborah. 2001. *The War Come Home: Disabled Veterans in Britain and Germany, 1914–1939*. Oakland: University of California Press.

Derbolowsky, Dr. and W. Lindenberg. 1949. "Wissenschaftliche Tagung der Psychiater und Neurologen in der SBZ, veranstaltet von der Zentralverwaltung für Gesundheitswesen, Berlin 27.–29. Mai, 1948." *PNMP* 1, no. 1/2: 53–60.

Drechsler, Erich. 1951. "Pläne zur Förderung der Volksgesundheit." *PNMP* 3, no. 8: 247–250.

Eghigian, Greg. 2005. "Care and Control in a Communist State: The Place of Politics in East German Psychiatry." In *Psychiatric Cultures Compared: Psychiatry and Mental Health Care in the Twentieth Century: Comparisons and Approaches*, edited by Hugh Freeman, 183–199. Amsterdam: Amsterdam University Press.

Etkind, Alexander. 1997. *Eros of the Impossible: The History of Psychoanalysis in Russia*. Boulder: Westview Press.
Foucault, Michel. 1954. *Mental Illness and Psychology*. Berkeley: University of California Press.
Freud, Sigmund. 1961. *Beyond the Pleasure Principle*. Edited by James Strachey. New York/London: W.W. Norton & Company.
Friedländer, Henry. 1995. *The Origins of Nazi Genocide: From Euthanasia to Final Solution*. Chapel Hill: University of North Carolina Press.
Friedrich, Jörg. 2002. *Der Brand: Deutschland im Bombenkrieg 1940–1945*. Munich: Prophyläen.
Geyer, Michael. 1997. "The Place of the Second World War in German Memory and History." *New German Critique* 71 (Spring–Summer): 5–40.
Goltermann, Svenja. 2001. "Im Wahn der Gewalt: Massentod, Opferdiskurs und Psychiatrie 1945–1956." In *Nachkrieg in Deutschland*, edited by Klaus Naumann, 344–363. Hamburg: Hamburger Edition.
Goltermann, Svenja. 2014. *War in Their Mind: German War Veterans and Their Experience of Violence in the Second World War*. Translated by Philip Schmitz. Ann Arbor: University of Michigan Press.
Gross, Friedrich-Rudolf. 1996. *Jenseits des Limes: 40 Jahre Psychiater in der DDR*. Bonn: Psychiatrie Verlag.
Hacking, Ian. 1996. "Memory Science, Memory Politics." In *Tense Past: Cultural Essays in Trauma and Memory*, edited by Paul Antze and Michael Lambek, 67–87. London: Routledge.
Hanrath, Sabine. 2003. "Strukturkrise und Reformbeginn: Die Anstaltspsychiatrie in der DDR und der Bundesrepublik bis zu den 60er Jahren." In *Psychatriereform als Gesellschaftsreform: Die Hypothek des Nationalsozialismus und der Aufbruch der sechziger Jahre*, edited by Franz W. Kersting, 31–61. Paderborn: Ferdinand Schöningh.
Henssge, E. 1949. "Reaktive psychische Erkrankungen der Nachkriegszeit." *PNMP* 1, no. 5: 133–137.
Herman, Judith. 1997. *Trauma and Recovery: The Aftermath of Violence–from Domestic Abuse to Political Terror*. New York: Basic Books.
Herzog, Dagmar. 2017. *Cold War Freud: Psychoanalysis in an Age of Catastrophes*. Cambridge: Cambridge University Press.
Herzog, Dagmar. 2018. *Unlearning Eugenics: Sexuality, Reproduction, and Disability in Post-Nazi Europe*. Madison: University of Wisconsin Press.
Kapczynski, Jennifer M. 2008. *The German Patient: Crisis and Recovery in Postwar Culture*. Ann Arbor: University of Michigan Press.
Kardiner, A. and H. Spiegel. 1947. *War, Stress, and Neurotic Illness*. New York: Hoeber.
Kemper, Werner. 1949. "Aufgaben, Grenzen und Möglichkeiten der Psychotherapie," (Lecture given at the Conference of Psychiatrists and Neurologists of the Soviet Occupation Zone [November 22 and 23, 1946], held in the offices of the German Central Administration for Healthcare, on the topic of "Organizing Care and Therapy for Psychopaths and Those Suffering from Mental Illness.") (Referat gehalten auf der Arbeitsbesprechung der Psychiater und Neurologen der Sowjetischen Besatzungszone im Hause der deutschen Zentralverwaltung zum Thema: Organisation der Geisteskranken - und Psychopathen-Fürsorge und ihre Therapie, 22. und 23. 11. 1946). *PNMP* 1, no. 1/2: 47–53.
Klaren, Georg. 1948. Dir. *Wozzeck*.
Konitzer, P. 1946. "Die Aufgaben der Deutschen Zentralverwaltung für das Gesundheitswesen in der Sowjetischen Besatzungszone." *DGW* 1, no. 1/2: 4–6.
Kristeva, Julia. 1989. *Black Sun: Depression and Melancholia*. New York: Columbia University Press.
Kröber, E. 1946. "Der praktische Arzt und die Beurteilung der Kriegsschäden des Nervensystems." *DGW* 1, no. 12: 347–352.
Kröber, E. 1948. "Die nervösen Beschwerden und ihre Behandlung." *DGW* 3, no. 9: 277–280.
Küchenhoff, Joachim and Peter Warsitz. 1991. "Psychiatrie und Psychoanalyse nach den Weltkriegen: Wiederholen oder Durcharbeiten?" In *Hard War/Soft War: Krieg und Medien 1914 bis 1945*, edited by Martin Stingelin, Wolfgang Scherer, 47–80. Munich: Wilhelm Fink Verlag.

Lamprecht, Wolfgang. Dir. 1946. *Somewhere in Berlin* (Irgendwo in Berlin).
Lerner, Paul. 2009. *Hysterical Men: War, Psychiatry and The Politics of Trauma in Germany, 1890–1930*. Ithaca, NY: Cornell University Press.
Leuenberger, Christine. 2001. "Socialist Psychotherapy and Its Dissidents." *Journal of the History of the Behavioral Sciences* 37, no. 3 (Summer): 261–273.
Leuenberger, Christine. 2002. "The End of Socialism and the Reinvention of the Self: A Study of the East German Psychotherapeutic Community in Transition." *Theory and Society* 31, no. 2 (April): 255–280.
Leuenberger, Christine. 2006. "Constructions of the Berlin Wall: How Material Culture Is Used in Psychological Theory." *Social Problems* 53, no. 1: 18–37.
Lewin, Bruno. 1949. "Neurologisch-psychiatrische Untersuchungen und Beobachtungen an deutschen Kriegsgefangenen in Ägypten 1941–47." *PNMP* 1, no. 8: 230–236.
Leys, Ruth. 2000. *Trauma: A Genealogy*. Chicago: University of Chicago Press.
Lindenberg, W. 1947a. "Fehlbeurteilung Hirnverletzter." *DGW* 2, no. 7: 225–228.
Lindenberg, W. 1947b. "Invalidität und Körperbeschädigung." *DGW* 2, no. 14: 447–450.
Lindenberg, W. 1948. "Ärztliche und soziale Betreuung des Hirnverletzten." *DGW* 3, no. 5: 145–147.
Lindenberg, W. 1949. "Die psychiatrische Versorgung in der Sowjetischen Besatzungszone seit 1945." *Psychiatrie, Neurologie, Medizinische Psychologie* 1, no. 1/2: 3–7.
Luhrmann, T. M. 2000. *Of Two Minds: An Anthropologist Looks at American* Psychiatry. New York: Vintage Books.
Maaz, Hans-Joachim. 1990. *Gefühlsstau: ein Psychogramm der DDR*. Berlin: Argon.
Marks, Sarah and Mat Savelli, eds. 2015. *Psychiatry in Communist Eastern Europe*. London: Palgrave Macmillan.
Mette, Alexander. 1950. "Hat die Psychotherapie eine Zukunft." *Sonntag*, Dec. 24.
Mette, Alexander. 1951. "Umschau." *PNMP* 3, no. 1: 93–95.
Micale, Mark S. 2008. *Hysterical Men: The Hidden History of Male Nervous Illness*. Cambridge: Cambridge University Press.
Micale, Mark and Paul Lerner, eds. 2001. *Traumatic Pasts: History, Psychiatry, and Trauma in the Modern Age, 1870–1930*. Cambridge: Cambridge University Press.
Mitscherlich, Alexander and Margarete Mitscherlich. 1967. *Die Unfähigkeit zu Trauern: Grundlagen kollektiven Verhaltens*. Munich: Piper & Co.
Mitscherlich, Alexander and Margarete Mitscherlich. 1975. *The Inability to Mourn: Principles of Collective Behavior*. Translated by Beverly R. Paczek. 1967. Reprint, New York: Grove Press.
Möller, Robert. 2001. *War Stories: The Search for a Usable Past in the Federal Republic of Germany*. Berkeley: University of California Press.
Müller-Hegemann, Dietfried. 1973. *Die Berliner Mauerkrankheit: Zur Soziogenese psychischer Störungen*. Herford: Nicolaische Verlagsbuchhandlung KG.
Naimark, Norman. 1995. *The Russians in Germany: A History of the Soviet Occupation Zone*. Cambridge, MA: Harvard University Press.
Nobbe, Dr. 1948. "Diagnose und Therapie der Geisteskrankheiten in der allgemeinen Praxis." *DGW* 3, no. 1: 15–19.
Parkinson, Anna M. 2015. *An Emotional State: The Politics of Emotion in Postwar West German Culture*. Ann Arbor: University of Michigan Press.
Pinkert, Anke. 2008. *Film and Memory in East Germany*. Bloomington: Indiana University Press.
Radetzky, R. v. 1946. "Ein Jahr Gesundheitspolitik." *DGW* 1, no. 17: 497–499.
Reinisch, Jessica. 2013. *The Perils of Peace: The Public Health Crisis in Occupied Germany*. Oxford: Oxford University Press.
Roelcke, Volker. 2008. "Trauma or Responsibility? Memories and Historiographies of Nazi Psychiatry in Postwar Germany." In *Trauma & Memory: Reading, Healing, and Making Law*, edited by Austin Sarat, 225–242. Stanford: Stanford University Press.

Roggenbau, Heinrich Christel. 1949. "Über die Krankenbewegung an der Berliner Universitäts-Nervenklinik in den Jahren 1933–1945. *PNMP* 1, no. 1/2: 129–132.
Schagen, Udo. 1999. "Gesundheitspolitik im Nachkriegsdeutschland." In *Das Gesundheitswesen der DDR-Eine historische Bilanz für zukünftige Gesundheitspolitik*, edited by Anita Rausch, Lothar Rohland, and Horst Spaar, 163–169. Berlin: Eigenverlag.
Schmitz, Willi. 1949. "Kriegsgefangenschaft und Heimkehr in ihren Beziehungen zu psychischen Krankheitsbildern." *Der Nervenarzt* 20, no. 7: 303–311.
Schulte, Walter. 1948. "Psychogene organ-neurologischer Krankheiten." *Der Nervenarzt* 19, no. 3/4: 129–135.
Schulte, Walter. 1953. "Cerebrale Defektsyndrome nach schwerer Hungerdystropie und Möglichkeiten ihrer Kompensierung mit einem Blick auf Heimkehrerdepressionen und forensische Komplikationen." *Der Nervenarzt* 24, no. 10: 415–420.
Schultz-Hencke, H. 1946. "Arzt und Psychotherapie." *DGW* 1, no. 9: 247–252.
Schultz-Hencke, H. 1949. "Der heutige Stand der 'grossen Psychotherapie.'" *PNMP* 1, no. 8: 246–248.
Schultz-Hencke, H. 1950. "Offener Brief an den Verfasser des Aufsatzes 'Psychotherapie in der modernen Gesellschaft D. Müller-Hegemann.'" *PNMP* 2, no. 1: 84–89.
Schwarz, Hans. 1950. "Psychisches Trauma und Neurologie." *PNMP* 2, no. 10: 289–300.
Sebald, W. G. 1999. *Luftkrieg und Literatur*. Munich: Hanser Verlag.
Sebald, W. G. *On the Natural History of Destruction*. 2003. Translated by Anthea Bell. New York: Random House.
Seidel, Ralf and Wolfgang Franz Werner. *Psychiatrie im Abgrund: Spurensuche und Standortbestimmung nach den NS-Psychiatrie-Verbrechen*. 1991. Cologne: Rheinland-Verlag.
Shephard, Ben. 2001. *A War of Nerves: Soldiers and Psychiatrists in the Twentieth Century*. Cambridge: Harvard University Press.
Solomon, Susan Gross. 2018. "East European Public Health and the Cold War: In Search of Circulation." *Revue d'études comparatives Est-Ouest* 1: 7–43.
Staudte, Wolfgang. Dir. 1946. *Murderers Among Us* (Die Mörder sind unter uns).
Steinberg, H. 2016. "25 Years after Re-Unification of Germany: An Overview on Eastern German Psychiatry. Part 1: Post-War Era, Pavlovization, Psychopharmacological Era and Social Psychiatric Reform Movement." *Fortschritte der Neurologie-Psychiatrie* 84, no. 8 (April): 196–210.
Ulrich, Bernd. 1992. "Nerven und Krieg: Skizzierung einer Beziehung." In *Geschichte und Psychologie: Annäherungsversuche*, edited by Bedrich Loewenstein, 163–192. Pfaffenweiler: Centaurus Verlagsgesellschaft.
Vischer, Adolf. 1918. *Die Stacheldrahtkrankeit: Beiträge zur Psychologie des Kriegsgefangenen*. Zurich: Rascher Verlag.
Weisse, Klaus and Matthias Uhle. 1990. "Entwicklungsformen und derzeitige Wirkungsbedingungen der Psychiatrie in der DDR." In *Psychiatrie im Wandel: Erfahrungen und Perspektiven in Ost und West*, edited by Achim Thom and Erich Wulff, 440–462. Bonn: Psychiatrie Verlag.
Wendelmann, Ulli and Claudia Grüner. Dir. 2022. *Verwahrt und Vergessen? – Psychiatrie in der DDR*. Co-produced with RBB.
"Wer ist der Angeklagte? Gedanken bei der Rückkehr von Kriegsgefangenen." 1950. *Sonntag* Jan. 8.

PART VII

Animals and the Environment

CHAPTER TWENTY-THREE

The Animals among Humankind: Fables of Reason in Johann August Unzer's Medical Weekly *Der Arzt*

BRIAN MCINNIS

Johann August Unzer's Enlightenment weekly *Der Arzt: eine medicinische Wochenschrift* (1759–64, The Doctor: A Medical Weekly)[1] attracted broad readership by combining science writing with entertainment for lay readers/listeners, educated elites, and medical professionals. Unzer was born in 1727 in Halle as the son of a hatmaker. In 1737, he entered the Latin School at the local Pietist Glaucha Institutes, now known as the Francke Foundations. He attended Halle's new Prussian university, the Fredericiana, and studied medicine with Friedrich Hoffmann student Johann Gottlob Krüger. Building on Krüger's work, Unzer challenged local philosopher Georg Friedrich Meier and argued for the influence of the physical body on the emotions. Unzer earned his doctorate in medicine in 1748 with the publication of a dissertation on sneezing. In 1750, he moved to Hamburg and shortly thereafter to Altona to open his private medical practice. Unzer trained his skills in writing about science with articles in the *Hamburgisches Magazin* from 1750 to 1752. He further honed his literary tone editing and publishing the weekly magazines *Gesellschaftliche Erzählungen für die Liebhaber der Naturlehre, der Haushaltungs-Wissenschaft, der Arzney-Kunst und der Sitten* (1753–54, Societal Review for the Lovers of the Natural Sciences, Homemaking Sciences, Medicine, and Morals) and *Der physikalische und ökonomische Patriot. Oder Bemerkungen und Nachrichten aus der Naturhistorie, der allgemeinen Haushaltungskunst und der Handlungswissenschaft*

(1756–58, The Physical and Economic Patriot. Or Comments and Reports from Natural History, General Homemaking, and Economic Sciences).

With the weekly magazine *Der Arzt,* Unzer both disseminated medical knowledge and entertained his audience. Almost all articles come from Unzer's pen, though several summarize or translate existing work. The journal features topics such as diagnosing illness, fever, pox, other diseases, emotions, exercise, healthy lifestyle, food and drink recommendations, tobacco, alcohol, coffee, perception, imagination, bloodletting, digestion, hypochondria, frostbite, supposed reader letters, several stories, and critiques of the medical profession. In this article, I argue that Unzer deploys the popular Enlightenment form of the fable to respond to social conditions shaped by an outbreak of an epizootic, a disease widespread in an animal population, and to a perceived imbalance in political power. Non-human animals play a central role in this text. I therefore employ aspects of Cultural and Literary Animal Studies (CLAS) to open this text to meanings beyond its stated moral that focuses more traditionally on the human sphere. My paper begins with a summary of the fable, a brief overview of one version of CLAS that is particularly productive for the analysis of Unzer's fable, and a summary review of its interface with Enlightenment poetics. I then read the fable parallel with historical documents to develop an interpretation that explores the relations of the non-animal humans, humans, and their environment. I argue that Unzer knowingly morphs the form for his own ends, choosing prose and extending the length to meet his periodical medium and his message. The text questions the political status quo by encouraging humans to reflect on their political power, suggesting the possibility of non-human political agency, and satirizing the political failings of aristocrats.

Unzer's fable "Erzählung, wie sich die Thiere einstmals der Vernunft zu ihrer Wohlfahrt bedient haben" (Story of How the Animals Once Used Reason for Their Benefit, Issue 192, 1762) deviates from the prevailing verse fable model of popular authors such as La Fontaine, Hagedorn, Gleim, and Gellert to follow Lessing's recommendation to craft fables in prose (Lessing 1997). This tale also departs from Lessing's call for brevity with a length that extends to more than twenty-eight hundred words (Lessing 1997). Set in Greece and Italy, it portrays humans and animals lodging complaints with Jupiter about a deadly cattle epidemic ("Viehseuche") and thereby focuses on community responses to the pestilence rather than describing the contagion's symptoms, causes, transmission, or mortality. The protests confound the patriarch. He initially wishes to reassert authority with his thunderbolts, but refocuses on prevention of additional animal annihilation. After consulting with his wife, he reluctantly gives animals reason so that they may evaluate their situation to promote survival. Yet with added faculties of reason, they develop subsequent complaints that once again overwhelm Jupiter. He then sends Minerva to open the philosophical schools in Greece to promote thinking and wisdom, and the Greeks become the "Lehrmeister der Nationen und der Nachtwelt" (teachers of nations and posterity). The fable closes with an appeal to humans to use reason to pursue their health and welfare. No published interpretation of this fable is known. Research on *Der Arzt* has focused on hypochondria (Bilger), on the weekly's contexts, contents, contributions to the history of ideas, on reception (Reiber), and on aging (Wesselmann). In the following, I extend a social-historical interpretation through a Cultural and Literary Animal Studies reading.

The interactions between gods, humans, and non-human animals invite an Animal Studies reading of Unzer's fable. In shaping my reading, I refer primarily to the work of Roland Borgards, Stephanie Waldow, and Sebastian Schönbeck. Borgards defines one version of Cultural Literary Animal Studies as constellations of texts, concepts, and practices through which researchers negotiate knowledge about animals and related concepts (Borgards 2016, 234). This theoretical lens operates in four ways: first, it contextualizes definitions and practices; second, it historicizes texts, primarily with cultural knowledge preceding and contemporaneous to a given text; and, third, it analyzes how literary texts represent, observe, and reflect knowledge about animals and their environments in order to identify the structures of knowledge, to evaluate its historical change, and to make visible the limits of specified knowledge. Finally, CLAS evaluates how the literary and aesthetic modes shape politics and materiality (Borgards 2016, 226, 228–231). The proposed interplay between creating context, integrating history, and evaluating politics expands the interpretation of a fable beyond a singularly allegorical reading.

Stephanie Waldow's essay "Von schlauen Füchsen und sprechenden Pferden. Die Fabel als 'animots'" (On Clever Foxes and Talking Horses. The Fable as "Animots") offers important arguments for the re-evaluation of fables and for the contributions of Enlightenment poetic theory to human relations with non-human animals. In Unzer's fable, humans and animals share a common spoken language. Waldow argues that language is the space in which the relationship between animal and human occurs (Waldow 2015, 141). She suggests that the unique lesson of the fable may be to acknowledge Giorgio Agamben's claim in *The Open: Man and Animal*, that the human must acknowledge his non-humanness in order to be human (142). Waldow's essay surveys Enlightenment contributions to the differentialist versus assimilationist debate about the proximity of humans to animals that will be addressed later. In his book *Die Fabeltiere der Aufklärung: Naturgeschichte und Poetik von Gottsched bis Lessing* (The Animals in Fables of the Enlightenment: Natural History and Poetics from Gottsched to Lessing), Sebastian Schönbeck foregrounds analysis of the differentialist vs. assimilationist positions, of anthropocentrism, of animal characteristics and abilities, including speech and reason, and of a fable's moral in the poetics of Gottsched, Breitinger, and Lessing, and in the natural history of Linneus and Buffon. Waldow and Schönbeck's work enable contextualized assessment of the similarity/dissimilarity of animal/human relations, anthropocentrism, and the representable characteristics of animals in the fable for my reading of Unzer.

Unzer establishes a tone for the fable in part through his use of epigraphs. The magazine *Der Arzt* frequently quotes literary and scientific authors, mirroring the assumed shared references between Unzer as author and editor, and his readers. In this issue, the author cites modern polymath Albrecht von Haller and Roman author Virgil, spanning the interests of Enlightenment readers and encouraging them to educate themselves. As the first of two quotations, Unzer cites Haller's poem "Gedanken über Vernunft, Aberglauben und Unglauben" (Thoughts on Reason, Superstition, and Scepticism) when he underscores the importance of reason from one of the final stanzas:

> Vernunft kann, wie der Mond, ein Trost der dunklen Zeiten,
> Uns durch die braune Nacht mit halben Schimmer leiten. (Haller 36, v. 359–360)

> [Reason can, like the moon, a solace in dark times,
> Guide us with a partial shimmer through dusk's light.]

This is perhaps a typical Enlightenment credo of faith in reason to lead society through the dim metaphorical night of eighteenth-century existence. Indeed, reason plays an outsize role in the fable as a source of friction between Jupiter and the animals. Reason shines, but here with only a partial-strength glimmer. This sentence stands on its own and conveys hope in the efficacy of reason as a guide through a difficult time. What shapes this epigraph and the initial tone of the fable is what is left out. Unzer purposely excludes the subsequent two lines from Haller's poem:

> Der Wahrheit Morgen-roth zeigt erst die wahre Welt,
> Wann Gottes Sonnen-Licht durch unsre Dämmrung fällt.
>
> (Haller 36, v. 361–362)

> [The dawn of truth first shows the real world
> When God's sunlight falls through our twilight.]

In Haller's poem, the light of God's truth far outshines that of humans and fully illuminates their existence, overpowering the mere shimmer of their reason. By excluding God's reason in this excerpt, Unzer lets humans play a greater role in the represented world, even if their contributions do not compare to those of the divine. The Virgil epigraph echoes Haller's sentiment that humans struggle amid the moon's pale shine. In this narrative and throughout his magazine, Unzer crafts a largely secular world that relies on human reason, human creation, and human science.

A traditional interpretation of this fable might claim that possessing power increases and reinforces one's blindness to the needs of society. It might highlight the unity of animals and humans in their dismay at livestock deaths, and their objection to Jupiter's inaction to halt the losses (Unzer 1762, 8: 145), despite his role as a unifier of the community (Stapleton 1986b, 126). They jeer at Jupiter and protest that "Er schuf die Thiere, um nur etwas zu vernichten zu haben" (8: 145). (He created the animals only to have something to destroy.) This rebuke sets off a series of psychological reactions as Jupiter cannot endure the animal and human critiques and lamentations. His immediate impulse is to grab his thunderbolts to forcefully shake the animals into submission: "Diese Reden verdrossen ihn und der Mächtige griff nach seinen Donnern" (8: 145) (These discourses annoyed him and the powerful [god] seized his thunderbolts.) He rebukes the animals for their ego, but suffers under his own. The narrator casts the sky god as uninformed about and uninterested in the causes of the animal deaths: "[…] Jupiter hatte zwar die Thiere erschaffen […] ohne die geringste Einsicht von ihrem Mechanismo zu haben. Niemand wußte weniger, woran die Thiere starben, und niemand hatte sich weniger darum bekümmert als Jupiter. Gleichwohl war das Wehklagen nicht länger auszustehen" (8: 145–146). (Indeed, Jupiter had created the animals […] without having the slightest understanding of their being. No one knew less from what the animals perished and no one had occupied himself less [with this issue] than Jupiter. Nonetheless, the lamentations became intolerable.)

He is the disengaged and ignorant pater familias who turns to his wife, Juno, to assess the conflict. She suggests that the difference between humans and animals exists because the animals lack the understanding to preserve their own health and persuades him to grant animals reason to provide for their well-being and self-preservation:

> Hast du ihnen wohl die geringste Einsicht zu ihrer Wohlfahrt und Erhaltung gegeben? Warum entzogest du ihnen in einer so wichtigen Sache die Vernunft und das Nachdenken? Du hattest es ja wohl recht darauf angefangen, sie zu vernichten? Wie sollen die armen Thiere ihren Untergang verhüten, da sie weder wissen, was ihnen schade, oder nütze, noch wie es anzufangen sey, um ihre Fehler wieder gut zu machen? Gieb ihnen also nur den Gebrauch des Verstandes, so werden sie bald selbst die Mittel erfinden, sich von ihrem Untergang zu erretten.
>
> (8: 146)

> [Have you given them even the smallest insight into their well-being and self-preservation? Why did you withdraw reason and reflection in such an important matter? You had likely began it to destroy them? How should the poor animals avoid their destruction when they neither know what harms or helps them, nor how they might begin to make amends for their mistakes? Just provide them the use of the understanding and they will soon create the means to rescue themselves from their demise.]

Though Jupiter derides the complaints of humans and animals, he listens to this rebuke by his wife.

A traditional reading might highlight how application of reason leads to personal knowledge and social responsibility, while circumvention of reason leads to psychological self-challenges such as self-doubt and ineffective leadership. Jupiter grants the animals reason as an act of divine spiritual animation, as encompassed in the Greek *pneuma*: "Alsobald schnob Jupiter einen gelinden Wind aus seinen Nasenlöchern unter die Thiere, und so war es geschehen. Die Vernunft wandelte ihnen an, wie ein kleines Fieber. Sie hielten sich gar nicht dabey auf, daß sie vernünftig dächten; noch weniger bewunderten sie es" (8: 146). (At once, Jupiter exhaled a light breeze from his nostrils among the animals and it was done. Reason came over them like a slight fever. They didn't stop to notice that they thought rationally, even less did they admire it.) Gradually, the animals progress through stages of self-awareness and thought as they first say "Ich bin, und ich denke" (I think and I am), then aver "Wir sind, darum denken wir" (We are, therefore we think), then echo Descartes's *cogito* with "Wir denken, darum sind wir" (We think, therefore we are). When they recognize the other in the moment of stating "Du bist" (You are), they discover new worlds encompassed in intersubjectivity (8: 147). One could understand the rational evolution of the animal characters thought processes through Descartes and Fontenelle to Leibniz as an awakening of the individual. One could question Jupiter's impulsiveness, tendency to violence, and reticence to hear critique as evidence of underdeveloped leadership.

A traditional interpretation might view the constellation of animals, gods, and humans as an allegory of the human sphere. The humans exhibit the faculty of reason and appear briefly at the story's beginning and again at its close. The animals represent an active and empowered cross section of people who apply reason to redefine their role in the social system and reconsider their daily life choices. The animals comprise another group of people, the masses, who learn from the exercise of reason how to voice their opinion to the political elites. As head of the Etruscan pantheon and head figure in Unzer's fable, Jupiter represents an aristocrat, possibly a king, who in a narcissistic fashion ignores the needs of the people. He derides the masses' use of reason to promote their self-preservation, to propose changes to their lives, and to question the existing order. In the case of the cattle, this means complaining about the "crudities" of a diet based on raw grass and about how to maintain health without shelter from [inclement] weather: "Wie ist es möglich, sagte der Sprecher in der Versammlung, daß wir gesund bleiben können, da wir das rohe Gras fressen, wie es aus der Erde hervor wächst, und sogar unter freyem Himmel schlafen?" (Unzer 1762, 8: 149). (How is it possible, said the speaker in the assembly, that we can remain healthy when we eat the raw grass as it grows out of the ground and even sleep in the open air?) Such complaints could easily be human concerns, and their organization with a speaker before an assembly mimics human democratic government like the one in Great Britain. Complaints voiced by animals yet understandable to humans promote an allegorical interpretation of the animal characters as merely people. At the same time, Minerva clarifies that humans who do not use reason as society expects, for example, to preserve one's health or to tame one's desires, are mere animals (8: 155).

What would it mean to reconsider this animal-human divide? Unzer's tale participates in Enlightenment debates about the fable and the continuity between animals and humans as shaped by Johann Christoph Gottsched, Johann Jakob Breitinger, and Christian Fürchtegott Gellert. Key differences include the extent to which animals use reason and human speech. Sebastian Schönbeck outlines how Gottsched's *Versuch einer critischen Dichkunst* (1730, 1st ed.) requires that authors represent animals as they exist in nature, deploy the literary animals to educate readers, and avoid depicting the animals as wondrous, unnatural, or chimerical (Gottsched 1730, 161; Schönbeck 2020, 42–43). Humans differ from animals in their human speech and use of reason. In the fable, the fantastic subgenre features irrational animals or inanimate objects that speak and act as if they were human (Gottsched 1730, 126; Schönbeck 2020, 47). Gottsched thus follows the Cartesian differentialist position in separating humankind from animals based on the capabilities of human speech and reason (Schönbeck 2020, 36, 48, 56–62). Over time, Gottsched alters his positions, conceding in the third edition that poets are allowed free rein to create talking plants and animals (Gottsched 1742, 207). In the fourth edition, he mandates rules for the Aesopian fable that such talking non-humans should build character and motivate plot through their recognized species characteristics, i.e. that a fox is sly (Gottsched 1751, 447; Schönbeck 2020, 63). Despite these expanded allowances for the use of talking non-humans in the fable, educating humans remains his focus and he maintains a differentiation of humans and other beings (Schönbeck 2020, 64).

Gellert and Breitinger present more assimilationist arguments for the relation between non-human animals and humankind than Gottsched, and Unzer develops a similarly assimilationist perspective. Gellert draws on experience to note that animals act according to specific reasons and possess a language of facial expressions, cries, and body language through which they communicate their perceptions (Gellert 1994, 15, 17). The fable author provides animals with a higher degree of understanding and the capability to speak in a humanly comprehensible language (17). Though this acknowledges some differences between human and non-human animals, they are smaller than Gottsched's and the fable author works to more closely connect human and non-human animals.

Breitinger also argues for a similarity between human and non-human animals based in daily experience, language use, and poetics. In most cases, humans live in a relationship with various animals like they live among persons who speak different languages (Breitinger 1740, 202). As Gellert notes, the human-animal interaction is advanced such that they almost talk to each other. Their understanding goes both ways: animals understand some human language, and they use a natural language to communicate their thoughts "almost as well" as people from another nation (203). One must only develop human language in animals for them to be comparable to humans (202). Moreover, animals engage humans with an appearance of reason (202). Breitinger seems to grant space for animal understanding, even if it does not manifest as abstract reason.

The close proximity of animals and humans in daily life provides an impetus to represent an interdependence between them in the fable. Like Gottsched, Breitinger seeks a precedent for animal-human interaction and draws on Biblical fables, idiomatic language, allegories, and symbols (Breitinger 1740, 200–201). The representation of humans and non-human animals together in the fable derives in part from Breitinger's psychological definition:

> Die Fabel ist ... ein lehrreiches Wunderbares. Diesselbe ist erfunden worden, moralische Lehren und Erinnerungen auf eine verdeckte und angenehmergetzende Weise in die Gemüther der Menschen einzuspielen, und diesen sonst trockenen und bitteren Wahrheiten, durch die künstliche Verkleidung in eine reizende Maske, einen so gewissen Eingang in das menschliche Herz zu verschaffen, dass es sich nicht erwehren kann, ihren heilsamen Nachdruck zu fühlen.
>
> (166)

> [The fable is an instructive marvelous [work]. It was created to instill moral teachings and memories into the minds of humans in a hidden and enjoyably amusing manner, and to provide these otherwise dry and bitter truths, through the artistic disguise of an alluring mask, with such a certain entrance into the human heart that it cannot resist feeling their healing power.]

The combination of an "instructive marvelous" echoes the Horatian call that literature should enlighten and entertain. Yet the inclusion of the marvelous (*Wunderbares*) also specifies reception to the extent that the text's moral beliefs and memories should secretly enter the reader's heart. Its effect is pervasive: they will not be able to resist feeling its healing power. Moreover, moral lessons, remembrances, and punishments are the only means for humans to achieve peace and happiness. In this sense, he grants moral literature a dietetic and medical function (Breitinger 1740, 167). Thus, Breitinger imagines Aesopian fables achieve a secretive and certain moral transformation of readers, in part by deploying speaking and reasoning animal characters and through use of the marvelous. A desire for the new led to the inclusion of gods or even talking and thinking non-living beings (184–185). Ultimately, Breitinger opines that the fable opens a new world: that of our interdependence with animals and non-living beings: "Nun führet uns die Fabel [...] in eine neue Welt, sie eröffnet uns das Commercium mit den Thieren und leblosen Geschöpfen selbst, sie ist ihr Dolmetsch gegen uns" (185–6) (Now the fable leads us [...] into a new world, it opens up for us the interaction with animals and non-living beings, it is their translator for us).

Unzer's fable similarly masks its moral and sparks reader interest through this fantastical story of gods and reasoning animals talking with humans. The text promotes assimilation of animals and humans in episodes that illustrate animal speech and reflection or show the similarity of human and animal reason. In the opening scene, animals and humans speak and complain together to Jupiter about the pandemic deaths and his unwillingness to halt its scourge. Later, Juno aims to reduce Jupiter's impatience with the reproachful reflecting animals by noting a common development in the human and animal application of reason to life. She observes that each plays with reason because of its initial novelty. She continues that humans only become useful to the world when they transition from thinking "I think, therefore I am" to asking "why do I exist?" and noting that animals will also progress in a similar manner (8: 148). The animals approximate human social forms in their organization in assemblies with representative speakers. Animals ask why sickness and death must exist, much like humans question the existence of evil in Leibniz's *Theodicy* (8: 148). Jupiter acknowledges similar uses of reason shared by humans and animals and laments that they do not evaluate their own actions, but hold him accountable for their sickness and weaknesses (8: 152). Jupiter views the humans and animals equally, and he vows to revoke their reason equally (8: 153). Humans and animals protest deaths together, they challenge species-typical behaviors together, and they are each threatened with a loss of reason.

Though the narration of the fable as a whole represents a position of assimilation between humans and non-human animals, Jupiter's daughter Minerva increases the differentiation between humans and animals at the conclusion when she argues that while animals may survive without reason, humans need reason to survive (Unzer 1762, 8: 154). This argument is more anthropocentric because it deems reason superfluous to animals, but necessary for humans. Similarly anthropocentric, Minerva argues that humans appear in Jove's image. Some humans use reason well when they honor Jupiter and acknowledge his work or study other human beings to teach the laws of virtue and of nature (8: 154). She effectively separates humans and animals through a dichotomy of instinctual drives and reason that strongly reduces animal perception and thought: "Gleichwie die Vernunft mit zu seiner [dem Menschen] ersten Anlage gehöret, so ersetzet sie auch bey ihm den Mangel der starken sinnlichen Triebe, wodurch du die Thiere regierest; und wenn sie sich derselben nicht immer zu ihrem wahren Besten bedienen, so ist dasselbe mit den Trieben nicht anders beschaffen" (8: 154). (Just as reason belongs to his [the human being's] primary faculties, it also replaces for him the weakness of the strong sensual drives through which you cannot control the animals; and although they do not always use it [reason] to their greatest benefit, it is no different with the drives.) Minerva travels to Greece and teaches use of reason and pursuit of well-being through the philosophical schools (8: 155). Jupiter and Minerva thus act to further differentiate animals and humans based on the pursuit or avoidance of well being.

The seeming equality of humans and non-human animals at the beginning of the fable prompts political ramifications. In the beginning, the animals and humans are equally incensed at the livestock plague. Both protest to no effect and then ridicule Jupiter for his creation of life and pernicious destruction through the epizootic. From the first paragraph of this fable, the non-human animals protest the seemingly senseless destruction of animal life. Once they receive the *pneuma* from Jupiter and begin to develop their own reason, they question Jupiter as the seat of power regarding the means of their survival. In protesting the epizootic and lodging complaints to Jupiter, the animals question the singularity of human reason and political action. From the cattle to the donkeys, from the birds of prey to the bees, the animals demonstrate growing self-knowledge and join human beings as political subjects. The animals implore gods and humans to pay greater heed to animal needs as part of a more inclusive set of actionable concerns.

The non-human animals question why they must submit to Jupiter's inattention and lack of knowledge. They are subjects as rational beings who make decisions, but are also subordinated to Jupiter's whims. Juno and Minerva provide Jupiter with a kind of cultural translation about the needs of the animals and humans. Juno implores him to give animals reason for their welfare and self-preservation so that the animals may correct their missteps (Unzer 1762, 8: 146). Minerva chides him for considering rescinding humanity's reason and trains humans in thinking while accepting the loss of reason among animals (8: 153–155).

The fable's depiction of Jupiter, Juno, and Minerva implies the necessity to reconsider extant social structures. The local political model relies on hereditary patriarchy, with Jupiter making final decisions. He is much more effective as a governmental leader because he solicits and accepts some suggestions from his wife and daughter. The fable models limited reform of government, but changes only begin from within the aristocratic pantheon. Though the animals theoretically have a space to share their concerns, as noted earlier, Jupiter easily becomes overwhelmed by their demands and in frustration complains about their requests. His wife and daughter are the ones who moderate his impatience and his inclination to immediate punishment, destruction, revocation of rights, and disregard of human and animal interests. Juno and Minerva help ensure that animals and humans do not succumb to the disease so that he has a populace to govern.

The fabric of this fable includes interwoven strands of local knowledge about animals that reveal how animal sickness hampered movement and challenged sectors of the agricultural economy, how animals play a role in representation of political systems and structures of power, and how the animals challenge prevailing theological and philosophical positions about whether only humans have souls. The conceit of the epizootic seems like a chance decision, yet the author creates a situation that approximates historical realities. Cattle plagues were a recurring problem in the German lands and Europe during the eighteenth century, with three strong waves hitting parts of the continent from 1711 to 1717, most of Europe from 1744 to 1757, and again parts of Europe from 1769 to 1786 (Hünniger 2011, 9).

The second wave of pestilence likely informed Unzer's choice of a cattle plague and its representation. This surge from 1744 to 1757 subsided only five years prior to the fable's publication in 1762, and readers would have remembered animal suffering and governmental restrictions on human and animal movement. In Unzer's tale, there is significant yet unelaborated animal suffering due to mortality. Pestilence could also be devastating for humans. Mary Lindemann notes that the plague asserted its virulence among humans and animals in almost every generation from 1350 to 1721. There were limited subsequent waves, but its lethality (60 percent for bubonic plague, nearly 100 percent for lung-based pneumonic plague) always evoked fear (Lindemann 2010, 56–58). Yet Dominick Hünniger concludes that when writers marked an infectious wave as a cattle epidemic, the academic authors knew it only affected cattle, even though they did not know why it could not transfer to humans (2011, 99). Even if sick animals seemingly posed no health threat to humans, infested cattle also meant significant financial and nutritional losses.

Unzer's nondescript and limited dramatization of the cattle epizootic may reflect uncertainty about the cross-species transferability and about the diverse and sometimes conflicting analyses of symptoms, causes, and transmission of the cattle epidemic. This doubt arose in part from a lack of specialists in veterinary medicine. Universities only began to address the shortage with the Europe-wide founding of numerous schools of veterinary medicine in the 1760s (Hünniger 2011, 67). Many authors publishing on the eighteenth-century cattle epidemics were human physicians and lacked the knowledge of animal illness that herders and butchers had (Hünniger 2011, 68). They struggled with the realization that cattle did not communicate initial symptoms, but only when the disease was in full force (Hünniger 2011, 69).

Halle doctor Friedrich Hoffmann summarized symptoms of the first eighteenth-century epizootic that remained valid for the second wave. He wrote in 1716 that few trained scientists and physicians pursued research and treatment of animal epidemics due to a lack of interest and prestige (3–4). Hoffmann catalogued symptoms of the cattle infection that included chills and fever, hair standing on end, hanging of the head, sleepiness, loss of appetite, glassy and teary eyes, thick mucus dripping from the nose, constipation, diarrhea, etc., yet Hünniger notes that the long lists of symptoms were common in other sicknesses (Hoffmann 1716, 7; Hünniger 2011, 73–74). Hoffmann hypothesized that the epidemic was an airborne disease and might be caused by delayed burial of human corpses after battles or related to an insect infestation (grasshoppers and inchworms) (Hoffmann 1716, 7). Others linked the disease to stomach worms, and analyses allowed for diverse local causes (Hünniger 2011, 80). Though humans were not subject to its infection, they and other animals such as dogs, cats, goats, and sheep could carry the contagion and infect other cattle (Hoffmann 1716, 8). Unzer excludes the specifics of the pandemic disease, but represents social responses to it.

Unzer's depiction of a cattle pandemic revisited a local problem. Beginning in the 1750's, Braunschweig-Lüneburg to the west and south of Hamburg and the duchies of Mecklenburg-Schwerin and Mecklenburg-Strelitz to its east experienced significant epizootic events. In August 1755, Duke Christian Ludewig of Mecklenburg tightened the existing restrictions on cattle markets by extending closures from infected areas to the entire principality. In addition, the duke ordered a cessation of livestock trading from infected or adjacent areas. Further, the administration required the residents, servants, and "Schutzverwandte" (protected persons) to avoid infected zones, thereby restricting human movement (Ludewig 1755, 2r). These historical realities relegate real world animals to a subservient role in relation to humans because of the animals' functions to transport, to labor for, and in some cases, to feed humans.

The literary animals in Unzer's story challenge the subservient animal role by communicating with people in human language and by petitioning Jupiter for changes to their housing and their diet. One purpose of their protest may be to question the habitual, pseudo-fixed notion of existing animal habits and animal husbandry. For example, the cattle protest always eating raw grass and lack of protection from weather that may cause colds. The comparative anatomist Buffon's *Natural History* describes grass as a diet particularly appropriate for cattle with their four stomachs and the related ability to digest large volumes of material (Buffon 1807, 5: 211, 229–230). However, oxen and cattle working the fields require more nutrition and he recommends hay or straw with bran or oats, or grass with small quantities of ash, elm, or oak leaves. Alfalfa and other legume plants such as sainfoin and lupin, turnips, and boiled barley are particularly nutritious and the cattle will not overeat them (5: 223, 233–234). Farmers also frequently fatten oxen and cattle for slaughter with supplementary bran, grain, and again turnips (5: 213). Johann Bernhard von Fischer in his *Liefländisches Landwirthschaftsbuch* confirms grass as a first choice of feed followed by straw from barley, rye, and oats (Fischer 1753, 165). To fatten calves, he recommends a combination of wheat with beer or milk (171). With regard to shelter, Fischer and Buffon underscore the necessity of warm, close stalls for survival in winter, particularly for calves, though Fischer notes that not all farmers can provide weatherproof protection for their herd (Fischer 1753, 169; Buffon 1807, 5: 223). The complaints by Unzer's cattle would seem to request a richer, tastier, more nutritious and robust diet than the normal grass. Their requests that press Jupiter for additional protection in winter echo the documented insufficient practices for protecting animals in harsh weather conditions. The reader of this fable can readily imagine that the cattle's and other animals' concerns about the quality of food and shelter would be survival concerns of animals newly provided with and proficient in reason. In an allegorical reading, subsistence concerns would have been front of mind for a majority of the rural population in Mecklenburg subject to serfdom.

The protests of the literary animals against the arrogance of Jupiter also echo dissatisfaction of knights and farmers toward the dukes of Mecklenburg-Schwerin. In the immediate contemporary history, this could have been prompted by Duke Christian Ludewig's closure of all livestock markets in 1755, which would have temporarily restricted the ability of farmers and landowners to sell animals and reduced their income (Ludewig 1755, 1r). In November 1760, his successor Duke Friedrich ordered checkpoints established surrounding animal plague zones with workers funded by the affected districts to prevent transport of potentially infected livestock or animal products (Friedrich 1760, 2v–3r). These restrictions would have likely reawakened anger over the forceful attempts of Carl Leopold (1649–1747), duke from 1713 until 1728, to fund a standing army through taxes and thereby rid the principality of foreign troops (Heitz 1991, 304–305). Carl Leopold fought with the knights and church over his attempts to establish more wide-ranging absolutism, and further disadvantaged the farmers and citizens of small towns who supported him (304–305). He aggravated the grievances most members of other classes had toward the Mecklenburg dukes. His opposition to the Holy Roman Emperor's politics of compromise prompted the emperor to replace him as duke. Within Unzer's fable, Jupiter's tendency to initially disregard the animal concerns would have seemed familiar to the aggrieved knights, clergy, and citizens of Mecklenburg-Schwerin and interested observers from nearby Hamburg, the duchy of Hannover, or Brandenburg-Preußen. Like Carl Leopold, Jupiter initially works to minimize the political participation of the animals under his control.

Finally, in using reason, the literary animals participate in the scientific, theological, and philosophical debates about humans' uniqueness because they possess a soul and the potential loss of human preeminence if animals also have souls. The contemplation of animals who reason as animals with souls comprises one of the potentially most inflammatory ramifications of this fable. Günter Frank notes that the theories in the German Enlightenment as to whether animals have souls fell on a spectrum of positions: (1) animals do not have a soul (Descartes); (2) the rationality of humans and animals results from an interdependence of sensual stimuli and sensual responses (Hobbes); (3) animals have a soul, but it is not eternal and they do not have the same self-consciousness of humans (Christian Thomasius); (4) animals have a soul different in kind from a human soul (Leibniz), (5) humans and animals each have a soul, but humans uniquely have an ability to formulate concepts and to use language (Christian Wolff); (6) animals have a soul similar to humans (Ribov, Schneider) (Frank 2001, 253–261). The animals in Unzer's story specifically develop concepts and use language, surpassing the divide presupposed by Wolff. The fable tellingly narrates the development of an animal consciousness that transitions from perception to practice of comparison, judgment, and argument, to Descartes's self-awareness and self-definition in thinking, to a recognition of others thinking in a community of thought, to a recognition of others as other, and to the discovery of incredible variety in the world of others (Unzer 1762, 8: 147). The animals illustrate a reinvention of the self through the practice of reason.

The cattle, donkeys, and other domesticated and wild animals in the fable with souls also affirm contemporary connections in the natural sciences between the nerves, sensibility, and animal souls. Stephanie Eichberg argues that Albrecht von Haller's experimental studies of pain in animals rested on an assumption that the visible signs of animal unrest were prompted by similar mental states as in humans (2009, 286). Human perception of pain relied upon reflection of a given perception (287). The experimental study prompted the question of how strong of an analogy could be made between the structure and function of the human brain and the animal brain. Haller's work indicated that this difference was small (288). In granting animals reason and demonstrating their anthropomorphized applications of reason, Unzer was in a sense following the trend of experimental biology, yet reaching beyond its proofs. The fable was a literary, not a scientific work, yet it challenged prevailing assumptions about the existence of an animal soul.

Unzer's fable is more than mere entertainment. By adopting an assimilationist position regarding animals and humans, Unzer supports the arguments of Gellert and Breitinger on the animal-human relationship over the position of Gottsched. Like Breitinger, Unzer's representation of the marvelous aspires to an interdependence of non-human and human actors through an engaging format. The depicted relationship is also one of equality. From this position, the animals implicitly question the assumed uniqueness of human reason and the singularity of human political action to establish themselves as political subjects. The fable alludes to the necessity of political change from an imagined setting of a despotic ruler that may have seemed all too familiar to the readership in Hamburg and surrounding kingdoms.

Unzer's idea of reasoning animals ultimately challenged prevailing Cartesian, Thomasian, and Wolffian positions, buoyed by the assumptions of an animal soul in the experiments on pain by Albrecht von Haller.

Unzer's fable reveals some problematic social reactions to disease. Zoonotic diseases such as the plague challenged government officials to develop a public health policy by necessitating quarantines. The infections likely prompted some uncertain responses among the populace as families and animal herders struggled to ascertain whether a given disease could infect humans. Local authors played a key role in communicating a disease's threat, symptoms, and potential treatments. As a practicing physician, Unzer would have experienced the illnesses circulating among his patients in Hamburg Altona and read about pathogens from across the German lands and Europe. The Cultural and Literary Animal Studies approach recovers concepts that significantly expand traditional readings with additional cultural and historical insights. This approach enables an illumination of conflicts such as the differentiation versus assimilation of animals and humans that makes the fable more relevant today, for example, in light of ongoing research into the complexities of animal language and emotions.

The literary form "fable" invites a literal reading focused on the nature of human and non-human relationships, the question of whether disease is zoonotic, and social responses to change while informing more reflective readings. This fable supports allegorical readings that critique political leadership, open the possibility to social reform, and implicitly challenge conservative religious positions on the animal-human divide. The focus on animal fortunes promises to entertain a broad reading or listening audience. Unzer included other essays in *Der Arzt* on fever or smallpox, but by occasionally deploying a literary genre, he broadened his audience and could engage more people in the pursuit of health. Doctor-writers such as Unzer contributed significantly to the dissemination of health knowledge, the deployment of creatively rational thought, and thereby to the project of Enlightenment.

NOTE

1. All translations are mine, unless otherwise noted.

WORKS CITED

Borgards, Roland. 2016. "Tiere und Literatur." In *Tiere: Kulturwissenschaftliches Handbuch*, edited by Roland Borgards, 225–244. Stuttgart: Metzler.

Breitinger, Johann Jakob. 1740. *Critische Dichtkunst Worinnen die Poetische Mahlerey in Absicht auf die Erfindung im Grunde untersuchet und mit Beyspielen aus den berühmtesten Alten und Neuern erläutert wird*, Zürich/Leipzig: Orell, Gleditsch.

Buffon, Georges Louis Leclerc de. 1807. *Buffon's Natural History. Volume 5*, edited by James Smith Barr. London.

Eichberg, Stephanie. 2009. "Constituting the Human via the Animal in Eighteenth-Century Experimental Neurophysiology: Albrecht von Haller's Sensibility Trials." *Medizinhistorisches Journal* 44, no. 3-4: 274–295.

Fischer, Johann Bernhard von. 1753. *Liefländisches Landwirthschaftsbuch*, Halle im Magdeburgischen: Gebauer.
Frank, Günter. 2001. "Seele oder Maschine? Der Streit um die Tierseele in der deutschen Aufklärung." In *Die Seele der Tiere*, edited by Friedrich Niewöhner and Jean-Loup Seban, 249–266. Wiesbaden: Harrassowitz.
Friedrich, Herzog zu Mecklenburg. 12 November 1760. *Edict wegen der Vieh=Seuche und der gegen Verschleppung derselben anzuordnenden Postirungen*. Schwerin: Bärensprung.
Gellert, Christian Fürchtegott. 1994. "Von denen Fabeln und deren Verfassern." In *Gesammelte Schriften V. Poetologische und Moralische Abhandlungen. Autobiographisches*, edited by Jung, Werner, John F. Reynolds, and Bernd Witte, 1–99. Berlin/New York: De Gruyter.
Gottsched, Johann Christoph. 1730. *Versuch einer critischen Dichtkunst*. Leipzig: Breitkopf. 1st ed.
Gottsched, Johann Christoph. 1742. *Versuch einer critischen Dichtkunst*. Leipzig: Breitkopf. 3rd ed.
Gottsched, Johann Christoph. 1751. *Versuch einer critischen Dichtkunst*. Leipzig: Breitkopf. 4th ed.
Haller, Albrecht von. 1965. "Gedanken über Vernunft, Aberglauben und Unglauben." In *Die Alpen und andere Gedichte*, edited by Adalbert Elschenbroich, 23–38. Stuttgart: Reclam.
Heitz, Gerhard. 1991. *Kaiser, König, Kardinal: Deutsche Fürsten 1500–1800*, edited by Rolf Straubel and Ulman Weiss, 303–310. Leipzig: Urania.
Hoffmann, Friedrich. 1716. *Heilsame Vorschläge wie der graßirenden Seuche unter dem Horn-Vieh vorzubauen und was vor Mittel dazu dienlich: Auf Gutbefinden des Collegii Sanitatis zu Halle herausgegeben*. Halle: Renger.
Hünniger, Dominik. 2011. *Die Viehseuche von 1744–52: Deutungen und Herrschaftspraxis in Krisenzeiten*, Neumünster: Wachtholz.
Lessing, Gotthold Ephraim. 1997. "Abhandlungen zur Fabel." *Werke und Briefe in zwölf Bänden*, edited by Günter E. Grimm, vol. 4, 345–411. Frankfurt: Deutscher Klassiker Verlag.
Lindemann, Mary. 2010. *Medicine and Society in Early Modern Europe*. Cambridge: Cambridge University Press.
Littlewood, R. Joy. 2006. *A Commentary on Ovid's Fasti: Book 6*. Oxford: Oxford University Press.
Ludewig, Christian, Herzog zu Mecklenburg. 1755. *Herzoglich-Mecklenburgisches Patent wegen der einzustellenden Horn-Vieh-Märkte und sonstiger Verfügung gegen die Vieh-Seuche*. Schwerin: Bärensprung.
Schönbeck, Sebastian. 2020. *Die Fabeltiere der Aufklärung: Naturgeschichte und Poetik von Gottsched bis Lessing*. Stuttgart: Metzler.
Schönbeck, Sebastian. 2019. "Return to the Fable: Rethinking a Genre Neglected in Animal Studies and Ecocriticism." In *Texts, Animals, Environments: Zoopoetics and Ecopoetics*, edited by Frederike Mittelhoff, Sebastian Schönbeck, Roland Borgards, and Catrin Gersdorf, 111–125. Freiburg im Breisgau, Berlin, Wien: Rombach.
Stapleton, Michael. 1986a. "Juno." In *The Illustrated Dictionary of Greek and Roman Mythology*, 126. New York: Bedrick.
Stapleton, Michael. 1986b. "Jupiter." In *The Illustrated Dictionary of Greek and Roman Mythology*, 126–128. New York: Bedrick.
Unzer, Johann August. 1762. "Erzählung, wie sich die Thiere einstmals der Vernunft zu ihrer Wohlfahrt bedient haben." In *Der Arzt: eine medicinische Wochenschrift* 8: 145–155. Hamburg: G.C. Grunds Erben.
Virgil. 1983. *The Aeneid*. Translated by Robert Fitzgerald. New York: Random House.
Waldow, Stephanie. 2015. "Von schlauen Füchsen und sprechenden Pferden. Die Fabel als 'animots.'" In *Von armen Schweinen und bunten Vögeln: Tierethik im kulturgeschichtlichen Kontext*, edited by Stephanie Waldow, 141–155. Paderborn: Fink.

CHAPTER TWENTY-FOUR

Dangerous Bodies: Witches in German Fairy Tales and the Literary Imagination

NICOLE THESZ

In the Grimms' tales, witches feature widely as malevolent females, usually older, and sometimes disabled, women who seek to thwart human happiness and usurp the place or resources of humans. They stand—from society's perspective—for "fear," as Ronald Hutton eponymously contends. And certainly, women in particular had much to fear from being considered a witch. Heinz Rölleke points out, for example, that the Grimms' main contributor, the impoverished Dorothea Viehmann, made no mention of witches in her tales, possibly to avoid any association with this persecuted figure in the social and literary imagination (Rölleke 2010, 229). Indeed, witches fare miserably in the Grimms' tales, being burned, barreled, and otherwise tortured to death.[1] I will argue, however, that folk and fairy tales to varying extents allow for a dual perspective that mirrors social sensibilities as well as hinting at the supposed witch's personal struggles.

The witch in "Hänsel und Gretel" ("Hansel and Gretel," KHM 15) of the Grimms' *Kinder- und Hausmärchen* (*Children's and Household Tales*) is not only sneaky and insatiable, luring the siblings into her cannibalistic realm, but she is also elderly, lacking in physical strength, and near-sighted.[2] The antagonist of "Jorinde und Joringel" ("Jorinda and Joringel," KHM 69) turns brides into birds, perhaps out of a pathological envy of the girls' romantic potential. A similar motive is seen in "Rapunzel" (KHM 12), where the sorceress jealously guards her "adoptive" daughter, fearing her loss as much as envying the attractiveness of the younger female.[3] However, not all fairy-tale witches are deprived of sexuality or fertility. Some double as hyper-protective mothers who seek to procure advantageous marriages for their biological daughters, e.g., "Brüderchen und Schwesterchen" ("Little Brother and Little Sister," KHM 11), suggesting an overlap with the evil stepmother type, while the stepmother in "Schneewittchen" ("Snow White," KHM 53) is driven to pursue her witchcraft and annihilate her competitor out of furious envy. Yet these witches may also, as Barbara Gobrecht contends, serve to convey the human vulnerability to temptation and greed (Gobrecht 2010, 118, 120). Strikingly, the above-mentioned fairy-tale witches are seldom linked, implicitly or explicitly, to evil forces outside of themselves. Their acts are evil, unnatural, and supernatural, but these appear to be inherent behaviors or born of personal vendettas. In addition to discussing fairy tales, this article also explores a literary reworking of the notion of witchcraft, Wilhelm Meinhold's novel *Maria Schweidler, die Bernsteinhexe* (*The Amber Witch*, 1843). Like the earlier fairy tales, this novel presents a notion of witchcraft that diverges from historical accounts in that the narrator alternately dispels and affirms superstitions, indicating Meinhold's perception of a society almost—but not quite—ready to abandon beliefs about supernatural evils in its midst.[4]

Traditional suspicions of witchcraft were directed at members of society who had supposedly formed a pact with the devil (cf. Thurston, Hutton), a notion that undergirds the intense fears fueling witch hunts.[5] In contrast, tales interrogate the emotional factors associated with the witch characters, whose status in the literary imagination ranges from not-quite human to non-humans mimicking human appearance and behaviors to take advantage of human victims. The emotional dimension of the humanoid role, which can include witches, fairies, nixies, and various temptresses, is especially true for female characters, who are frequently marked by supernatural beauty, dangerous or transgressive sexuality, social isolation, or creativity.[6] These literary witches at times point toward "functional" explanations of beliefs in and hunts of "witches,"[7] though scholars are hesitant to attribute witch hunts to fundamental belief patterns, given the high regional and historical variability in eruptions of these persecutions (Thurston 2007, 13–14; Hutton 2017, 14).[8]

In literary scenarios, female temptresses helped to express deviant behavior on the part of men (e.g., in Ludwig Tieck's *Der Runenberg*, 1804), while the thoughts of lascivious relations with the devil could also help to demonize sexual freedoms that were not conducive to orderly family and social structures. The depicted proximity of female creativity, hysteria, and transgression to the witch type in tales served to warn women against neglecting so-called feminine duties, thus also discouraging competition from female artists or a reworking of creative and social standards based on women's writing or art (cf. Treder). Rather than acknowledging the long history of fears of witches at the margins of civilization, Bruno Bettelheim famously interpreted the witch as a projection of children's oral desires on the mother figure (1989, 159). At the same time, social marginalization of both men and women—the elderly, the disabled, the eccentric—and its association with witches could help to attribute blame to the individuals, rather than the societies that cast them out, while it would be easier to attack the marginalized than the well-connected. Yet such functional explanations, though not completely invalid, are too tidy to completely reflect historical and psychological realities. Altogether, they may be more useful in understanding fictional scenarios than in the anthropological interpretation of fieldwork on beliefs and behaviors with respect to perceived threats from witchcraft.

The intimate link between the supposed witches and the envisioned evil beings who inspire and direct them is weakened in storytelling as compared to the popular beliefs that fueled witch persecutions. James M. McGlathery examines the role of witch-like female figures in tales in which they use their powers in service of love, as seen, e.g., in "Die Gänsehirtin am Brunnen" ("The Goose-Girl at the Well," KHM 179), where the elderly witch tricks a prince into coming to her home and falling in love with a princess who was temporarily bewitched, albeit for her own protection (McGlathery 1991, 115). Such encounters have led me to emphasize the affinity that witches have for human fates and emotions (Thesz 2021, 99). I revisit this interpretation here with respect to the emphasis on female witches' bodies in literary depictions—portrayals that counter the historical emphasis on witches as destructive devil's associates, according to beliefs ranging from antiquity to the early modern period (and today).[9]

As Joseph Pentangelo suggests, unexplained illnesses such as epilepsy at times led to accusations of bewitchment, as patients blamed neighbors for sudden and frightening afflictions (2021, 65–67). Yet "witchcraft" was not always interpreted as a selfish or harmful pursuit. Witches or hags in folktale can, for example, be characterized as "an older woman knowledgeable in occult or magic arts" (McGlathery 1991, 113). This perspective would suggest not vicious intent, but rather a body of professional knowledge. Indeed, this focus is found with respect to occult figures as related to a variety of medical practitioners over the course of history. Altogether, the witch character and related figures (e.g., the "Kräuterhexe," *herbalist witch*, in German culture or the "cunning folk" of British tradition) are relevant in providing a historical and philosophical link in the chain of development of medicine from individuals that could be considered to be spiritual figures, shamans, herbal practitioners, or providers of gynecological care, etc. In these figures—both literary as well as historical—humanity begins to envision its control over biological fate.

The interest in biological existence—its natural mysteries and vulnerability—extends to fairy-tale depictions of witches. Not only is their power of vital interest, but their own embodiment seems to be at stake in lore about humanoid females. What are their experiences, parameters, desires, and vulnerabilities? The literary—and historical—focus on the bodies of witches (as opposed to the vague or absent description of most women in fairy tale, as seen in the stereotypical and unspecific beauty of maidens) is evident in "Hansel and Gretel," in which siblings are abandoned, encounter a witch, escape by burning her, and are reunited with their father. The Grimm tale was actually less an established folktale than a work inspired by a number of mainly literary and literary-inspired sources, such as Giambattista Basile's "Ninnillo and Nennella" (1634), Charles Perrault's "Le petit Poucet" (1697), and Marie d'Aulnoy's "Finette Cendron" (1697).[10] Although the Grimms' intent "was to collect variants, not to invent them," their middle and upper-middle class sources such as the Wild and Hassenpflug sisters were in fact responding to what they perceived as the Grimms' aesthetic expectations for engaging narratives (Blécourt 2008, 43–4). Thus, source studies of tales such as "Hansel and Gretel" or "Snow White" indicate that the "folk beliefs" contained in the Grimms' tales concerning witches were highly influenced by French, Italian, and other literary tales and their stock characters. In turn, Grimms' tales became influential in shaping popular ideas about female identity, and thus also about the experience of female bodies.

With respect to "Hansel and Gretel," the brothers increased their focus on the witch's body and health from edition to edition. Their attention to detail suggests a complex vision of this character type in German culture and the Grimms' specific imagination.[11] In the first publication in 1812, the children's attacker is already "eine kleine steinalte Frau" ("a little woman, as old as the hills") who hides her viciousness behind a "feine Stimme" ("gentle voice") ("Hänsel and Gretel," 2016, n.p.; Ashliman 2002, online, n.p.). Yet Wilhelm Grimm (or storytellers consulted after the initial telling by Dortchen Wild) inserted further intimations of a vulnerable physical body, giving evidence of the mixture of fascination, fear, and revulsion with respect to female agents in tales. The witch is, in 1812, still somewhat pitiable due to her small size, and this appearance contrasts with her supernatural forces, which perhaps explains the Grimms' choice to remove the adjective "klein" in following editions.[12] Moreover, she is either extremely near- and far-sighted or has some other condition that prevents her from recognizing that Hansel is poking a stick, rather than his well-fed finger, out of his cage (her bad eyesight is merely implied in 1812). This depiction inserts grotesque humor and thereby prevents the audience from sentimentalizing the pathetic victimhood of the child, but also levels the playing-field between young and old, human and supernatural creature. Dehumanizing the antagonist, the Grimms (from the 1850 edition onwards) frame the statement about visual impairment as one about the entire "species" of witches[13]: "[d]ie Hexen haben rote Augen und können nicht weit sehen, aber sie haben eine feine Witterung, wie die Tiere, und merken's wenn Menschen heran kommen [sic]" (Grimm 2017, 101; "Witches have red eyes and cannot see very far, but they have a sense of smell like animals and know when humans are approaching," Ashliman 2002, online).[14] By adding this characteristic detail, the Grimms "fleshed out" the antagonist, who in her appetite for human flesh resembles the ogres and ogresses found in French tales, i.e., d'Aulnoy's "Finette Cendron" and Perrault's "Le petit Poucet" that feature abandoned and endangered children.

Across regions and times, witches have been thought to be either humans who choose to practice evil or supernatural beings; the latter view seems to predominate in the Grimms' tales. Fairy-tale witches have the distinct advantage (over many other supernatural characters) of appearing to be human (in part due to powers of transformation), and thus tricking their victims. The particular witch in "Hansel and Gretel" is disadvantaged through age, size, ability, and indeed does not use magic much (except perhaps to construct her edible cottage). Yet her realm is tainted by her evil, in the Grimms' depiction, who added after 1812 the term "Hexenwald" or *witches' forest* to the description of the woods in order to emphasize the tale's Manichean struggle.[15] Moreover, the witch is disparaged as the narrator attributes to her an animal's sense of smell. This reference to her uncanny ability to straddle different states of being or species experiences, I would argue, creates a sense of distrust that accentuates her activity in trapping and dissimulating in service of her cannibalistic urges. However, this detail can also be understood as the privilege of the humanoid witch (and her species) to enjoy superhuman senses, which implies a human marveling at her enhanced faculties. To the witch, in this description, a facet of the world opens up that is closed to humans—the witch is more attuned to nature and surroundings, and this is not only the mark of a predator, but also provides her with a sense of transcendence and power as compared to her human counterparts. Ultimately, this detail becomes suggestive of a more positive or curious approach to witches on the part of storytellers, who definitely feared but also secretly admired them in various literary depictions.

Nevertheless, one editorial change on the part of the Grimms does point toward the overlap of documented folk beliefs and this literary depiction. While Wilhelm Grimm tended to enhance, sanitize, and add Christian references to tales in the course of editions, he in fact toned down religious connotations in the context of "Hansel and Gretel." In both 1812 and later versions, Gretel pleads to God when the witch announces her plan to eat Hansel, plump or not. Yet, in later editions, Grimm deleted the idea that God warns Gretel by communicating the witch's evil plan to the girl[16]; instead she herself interprets the situation ("[a]ber Gretel merkte was sie im Sinn hatte" [Grimm 2017, 103]; "[b]ut Gretel saw what she had in mind," Ashliman 2002, online, n.p.) and then comes up with the famous trick to ask for a demonstration of how to enter the oven. While the pious Grimms credited God's help in such stories as "The Robber Bridegroom" (KHM 40), where the heroine's escape from a band of criminal cannibals is due to luck in 1812, and then to divine assistance in later versions,[17] they removed this vital human-divine connection in "Hansel and Gretel." Is this discrepancy rooted in storytelling logic or in the context of the witch narrative? Given the fact that the Grimms in other tales sacrificed logic to propriety (see Rapunzel's slip-up about her pregnancy) and generally enhanced Christian elements (e.g., "The Robber Bridegroom" and "Godfather Death" [KHM 44]), it is possible that they sought here to distance Christianity from any dealings with a witch. Even though the witch's thoughts were certainly knowable to God—in the story's logic—it may be that the volatile situation was, to their minds, best limited to the human and humanoid sphere. In fact, Gretel's power at this moment—over the witch and over her brother—makes her a formidable character, and it is indeed somewhat unusual for female human characters to pass judgment, punish others, or to wield existential power. Having been a victim in the woods—and nearly of burning—Gretel herself is implicated in some of the isolation, ruthlessness, trickery, and power that the witch has embodied in this tale (and in others) up to this point.

The Grimms' "Snow White" contains a similarly prominent female figure in the popular imagination: the heroine's stepmother (in 1812, the biological mother), who is also a witch and uses magic to poison her (step)daughter. Much like "Hansel and Gretel," this tale emphasizes the female antagonist's body—in fact, more so than the body of the youthful love interest. In contrast to the witch in "Hansel and Gretel," Snow White's jealous parent is described as very beautiful (though aging) and evidently consumed by her desire for beauty, attention, and implicitly the sexual attentions of men. From the standpoint of a feminist, symbolic interpretation, Sandra Gilbert and Susan Gubar envision the queen as a quintessentially active heroine: "a plotter, a plot-maker, a schemer, a witch, an artist, an impersonator, a woman of almost endless creative energy" (Gilbert and Gubar 1979, 38). Her evil intentions are obvious in the Grimms' fairy-tale context. Perhaps more importantly, the image of deviant femininity in this tale is also linked to a description of bodily functions: when the stepmother first recognizes the young Snow White's beauty, her heart reacts with panic and revulsion: "wenn sie Sneewittchen erblickte, kehrte sich ihr das Herz im Leibe herum, so hasste sie das Mädchen" (Grimm 2017, 258; "whenever she looked at Snow-White her heart turned over inside her body, so great was her hatred for the girl" [Ashliman 2005, online, n.p.]). While this might simply be the description of a deeply jealous, but otherwise "normal" second wife, the Grimms' embellishments add to the sense of a non-human force gaining hold of or revealing itself in the antagonist. Snow White's stepmother is marked by a metaphorical "Unkraut in ihrem Herzen" (Grimm 2017, 258; "weed in her heart" [Ashliman 2005, n.p., online]), which could be construed as simply flowery speech, were it not for the narrative segue into the queen's demand for organs from her stepdaughter—lungs and liver—that would be proof of the latter's death and perhaps even a mode of incorporating her youth and vitality. As such, the stepmother embodies a number of beliefs surrounding witches: the focus on beauty, the antisocial hatred, the emphasis on her body, and the intended consumption of the victim (aligning, for example, with reports of witches killing and eating young children [Hutton 2017, 69]).

Interestingly, the queen's first attack on her stepdaughter proceeds without magic, featuring disguise and attempted strangling. Nevertheless, the narrative is quite explicit about the queen's focus on physical experiences.[18] When the mirror reveals the truth about Snow White's survival, the queen's body expresses and reinforces her murderous rage: "[es] lief ihr alles Blut zum Herzen" (Grimm 2017, 262; "all her blood ran to her heart" [Ashliman 2005, online, n.p.]). This physical reaction precipitates the second attempt and the eruption of her true identity as she fashions the poisoned comb with the "Hexenkünsten, die sie verstand" (Grimm 2017, 262; "art of witchcraft" [Ashliman 2005, online])—the reference to which now confirms earlier suspicions on the part of the audience. Strikingly, however, the Grimms' 1812 version still described this encounter as free of magic—the queen simply finds a new disguise and uses a poisoned comb.[19] Ultimately, the apple episode, which is the queen's third attempt in Grimm (and the only one in the 1937 Disney version)—concocted in "eine[r] ganz verborgene[n] einsame[n] Kammer" (Grimm 2017, 263; "her most secret room" [Ashliman 2005, online])—provides an evocative image of hidden witchcraft, at least when associated with the mention of magic, as in the post-1819 editions.[20] Not only is this reference to a secret room a symbolic representation of the queen's accessing of her true identity as a presumably not-quite-human witch—a fact she has kept hidden in her attempt to occupy the privileged spot as a legitimate, human queen—but also a nod to historical fears about occult work in the service of evil. Given the lack of reference to witchcraft in the "Snow White" version of 1812 and 1819, the plot may there be read as a representation of criminal behavior[21]; ultimately, however, Wilhelm Grimm clearly chose in later editions to enhance this tale through a frisson of terror through more explicit allusions to magic.

Perhaps most important for the reception of witches in the nineteenth-century imagination is the extent to which the narrative's plot is driven by the queen's strong, uncontrollable bodily presence, lust, and passion—Snow White's cool composure is the Apollo to the queen's Dionysian abandon. Yet, as in "Hansel and Gretel," there is a hint that the heroine herself is—though innocent—inherently prone to being transformed by the sheer token of her female identity. Much as Anne Sexton in "Snow White and the Seven Dwarfs" (1971) imagines the princess herself, in the end, turning to the mirror in self-obsession (Sexton 1981, 229), the Grimms' heroine is dehumanized in her stepmother's eyes as an "Ausbund von Schönheit" (Grimm 2017, 263; "specimen of beauty" [Ashliman 2005, online, n.p.]), then as a corpse, and finally as an onlooker to the stepmother's horrible death. She may or may not turn to fits of envy later in life (as Sexton imagines it), but she is not merciful, much like the kingdom into which she has married; jointly, the ruler and the former victim enact a public display of capital punishment. That the use of burning-hot iron shoes is reminiscent of witch persecutions, in which hot iron was said to bring about repentance (Hutton 2018, 32), not only indicates that the authorities have pegged the stepmother as a witch, but also suggests that interrogation, trial, and execution have been conveniently and cruelly conflated at the wedding ceremony. The public destruction of her body serves both to gain revenge and to reinforce the (male) ruler's power. However, taking into account the overall picture—including the 1812 and 1819 versions and the related Basile tale "The Young Slave" (1634), all free of explicit witchcraft—the non-violent apprehension of the queen speaks to her powerlessness: her deeds can be deemed those of a jealous murderess, but not of a supernaturally gifted being.

The witch as a classic hindrance to romantic relationships reappears in "Jorinda and Joringel," in which the antagonist transforms young girls into birds and holds suitors captive by petrifying them in her garden. Aside from hints at "sexual envy" and her role as "villainess" in the romantic tale, the witch may be part of a longer tradition of assigning emotional concerns to the female realm, while the elderly woman is by necessity a comic, rather than romantic figure (McGlathery 1991, 128–129). As in other Grimms' tales, the description of the antagonist, an "Erzzauberin" (Grimm 2017, 347) or master witch, provides a mixture of Gothic horror, stereotypes, shape-shifting,[22] and impressions of ill health. Not only does this "alte Frau" (Grimm 2017, 347; "old woman," my translation) transform into a cat or owl (cf. beliefs about owls and witches in a number of cultures) during the daytime, but her human shape at night is that of an elderly, repulsive hag.[23] The tale's introduction simply mentions the old woman's status as a witch with two animal alter egos. Interestingly, the nuances of her horrible appearance and brutality are not tangible until the young couple actually encounters her, disoriented in her castle's proximity and presumably lured into the witch's trap. At this moment, they have become separated as Jorinda is transformed, mid-song, into a nightingale. Only as night falls and the witch's animal form wanes does she appear in the space of the narrative: "die Eule flog in einen Strauch, und gleich darauf kam eine alte krume Frau aus diesem hervor, gelb und mager: große rote Augen, krumme Nase, die mit der Spitze ans Kinn reichte" (Grimm 2017, 348–349; "the owl flew into a bush, and out of it appeared a stooped old woman, yellow and skinny, great red eyes, and a crooked nose that bent down to her chin," my translation). While the first impression of Hansel and Gretel's captor is somewhat positive—we have not yet witnessed her cruelty—the witch in "Jorinda and Joringel" has already harmed the couple when we meet her. Her reputation precedes the story's unfolding; thus, less focus is placed on the witch's experience and possible motivations for her actions. Her grotesque appearance, frailty, and possible illness (seen in the red eyes, albeit without mention of visual impairment) are cast as species markers, rather than disabilities, and her layered identity—as cat, human, and owl—marks her as a predator and a hunter of humans who not only imprisons young maidens but also preys upon and eats birds and other animals of the woods. She is voracious and cruel, and her appetites are as uncontrolled as those of the antagonists in "Hansel and Gretel" or "Snow White." However, the witch's defeat in "Jorinda and Joringel" is, as in "Hansel and Gretel," laughably easy: a touch with the magical red flower renders her powerless and thus irrelevant; her fate is unspoken, and she fades into the background. This denouement renders crystal-clear the truth of her situation: she is an elderly woman completely helpless in the face of the superior strength of others. It is frailty, and not power, that marks the classic fairy-tale witch's biological existence and emotional state. That jealousy drives the hag's actions is indicated in her last-ditch, rather pathetic attempt (as "die Alte," Grimm 2017, 350; "the old one," my translation) to flee with Jorinda's cage when Joringel appears armed with the red flower—symbolic of passion, aggression, and youth. Both physical frailty and greed ultimately align these witches with the human condition and the fear of obsolescence. However, the literary witches' vulnerabilities are partially covered up by means of superhuman powers that serve to make them projection screens for human anger and resentment. The failure, time and again, to win the objects of their desire makes witches convenient antagonists, for they allow the human audience to vicariously triumph over adversity but also to despise the unattractive and pathological other. Unlike the historical fears that led people to believe evil had been wrought by a member of their community, the emotional and cognitive function of these fairy-tale witches lies in mediating feelings of spite, weakness, projection, and catharsis.

As the Grimms explored dramatic and cathartic witch representations, the question of evil, and its apprehension, received a more cerebral treatment in Wilhelm Meinhold's *Maria Schweidler, die Bernsteinhexe* (1843; *The Amber Witch*). The short novel juxtaposes a melodramatic account of a witch trial with a skeptical perspective offered in the frame narrative. The narrator contends that he found a seventeenth-century manuscript recording a witch trial in his church on the island of Usedom. In fact, however, the story of the priest's daughter, Maria, who is accused of witchcraft after being framed by an actual witch, was only supposedly based on a historical case in which a pastor's daughter was burned at the stake in the early seventeenth century (Burns 2011, 627–631; Vredeveld 2014, 200–202). Meinhold creates a narrative in which early modern violence is ultimately tamed by enlightened individuals and possible supernatural intervention, inserting fairy-tale hues by having the young victim saved in the last moment by her educated aristocratic suitor.

The frame narrative's seemingly authentic account takes readers to an early-seventeenth-century Europe marked by warfare and rampant superstitions at the cusp of new, scientific paradigms. The core tale's narrator, the accused teenager's father, pastor Abraham Schweidler, believes in his daughter's innocence but does not in fact reject the existence of witches. His description (in historicized dialect) of the mean-spirited neighbor, Lise Kolken, supports folk beliefs of a constant battle between good and evil, and his observations (and personal animosity) appear to offer near-conclusive evidence of Lise's pact with the devil or a demon (though he, too, relies on hearsay; Meinhold 2014, 54). Moreover, the pastor hears reports of a conversation between Lise and the district Sheriff (who supports the accusations against Maria because he hopes to coerce her into a relationship with him) in which Lise demands payment for supposed bewitchments she has strategically placed on residents and animals of her village in order to frame the young girl (Meinhold 2014, 85–86). In fact, the pastor believes until the end in Lise's supernatural dealings, and the events of the core narrative bear this out—complicating Meinhold's overall Enlightenment message. Only certain individuals (above all, Maria's suitor, Rüdiger von Nienkerken[24]) in this early-modern society have moved beyond superstition, and Meinhold's frame narrative, including footnotes deriding folk beliefs (e.g., Meinhold 2014, 64, 71, 77, 82), are designed to criticize the witch trials of early modern Europe, all the while letting the core story stand as a quasi-Gothic and sometimes sentimental story of persecution and victimhood of an innocent girl by both patriarchal structures and a vengeful female witch.

Although Meinhold does not refer specifically to the fairy-tale genre, the inclusion of witchcraft, the conflict between maiden and witch, and the last-minute saving by the "prince" (in this case, a *Junker* or nobleman) indicate connections to traditional tales. At the same time, Meinhold provides insights into the social dynamics in a rural area marked by the ravages of war and capricious authorities. This case study of a witch trial develops an unlikely heroine, whose high level of education (she is fluent in Latin) and intelligence (seen in the cutting logic and wit in her statements at the trial) add to impeccable integrity (construed here as bedrock faith). Given the stylized and sentimental rewriting of what would have been horrific realities, Meinhold touches upon instruments of torture but focuses on the maiden's integrity and beauty. Her imagined and actual body is relevant as a victim of hunger (after raids to the village), repository of innocence (her father's perspective), lust (the *Amtshauptmann* or Sheriff, wardens, and others), desire (the *Junker*), fallenness (the prosecutors and villagers), and beauty, as recognized even by the prosecutors, who on the one hand show her deference and on the other hand believe her appearance to be all the more proof that the devil would put great effort into pursuing her. Although the narrative does not offer many specifics (except red cheeks and long hair), Maria's beauty is prominent in the tale and stands in metonymically for her body in most scenarios. Notable exceptions would be hints at her physical experience and enjoyment (she bathes nude in the sea and is shown throughout desiring the Junker), a kiss on the mouth by the Swedish king Gustav Adolf (which indicates her willingness to use her beauty for a moment of political recognition), as well as reports of her meeting with the Junker in the woods as he is disguised in a wolf's pelt. Moreover, a brief description early in the novel of the Sheriff's sadistic killing of a wolf with instruments of torture is explicitly used to presage Maria's fate, allowing Meinhold to spare too much mention of the maiden's body (Meinhold 2014, 45).

The trial's climax takes place in the torture chamber, as the audience and her father (as the narrator of the core story) are introduced to the intended sequence of torture techniques; the warden's sadistic pleasure at describing each instrument and its effects serves to condemn earlier historical practices (perhaps Meinhold's political aim) as well as to increase the audience's investment in the heroine's fate. Yet images of physical pain, blood, and death will be reserved in the narrative for the antagonist and presumed witch Lise Kolken and the mention of a previous victim of witch hunts, whose blood is still visible on the instruments and the martyring robes (Meinhold 2014, 101, 103); the latter's body thus stands in for Maria's potential trajectory much as the wolf's did. In contrast, Meinhold mentions Maria's youth and beauty in general terms, while focusing mainly on her face and hands as chaste representatives of her innocent body—similar to the vague description of fairy-tale heroines. Thus, as he prepares us to imagine her body in various horrible situations (seen in the Gothic horror of the warden's explanations of the methods he plans to use on Maria; Meinhold 2014, 101–103), he seeks to maintain polite boundaries. An exception to this sparing of physical detail is found at the trial in the baring of Maria's chest to exhibit a mole that an accuser contends was the mark of the devil (Meinhold 2014, 91–92). The father's problematic marveling at his child's white skin (which reminds him of his deceased wife's appearance[25]) at this public display may suggest Meinhold's aim to criticize society's physical and political power over her body. At the same time, this comment might simply serve to sentimentally express the protagonist's innocence.

The heroine's steadfastness in view of suffering is ultimately not broken by physical pain; as she is fitted with the thumbscrews, it is the father's outcry at the judge's command "Schraubet!" (Meinhold 2014, 105; Screw! 2005, 64) that interrupts the process, causing Maria to "confess" to witchcraft and to an allegiance to the devil in order to spare her father the terrible spectacle of torture. Thus, Meinhold instrumentalizes fantasies about the heroine's beautiful body being assaulted by the prosecutors, but suspends these Gothic (and realistic) images in the hypothetical realm so as not to subvert the sanitized, sentimental plot line. (Similarly, she is repeatedly in danger of being raped by soldiers and prison wardens, but is miraculously spared, as a narrative means to preserve the image of absolute innocence in both senses of the word.) The maiden's body first serves to elicit suspense, compassion, admiration, and horror, but is ultimately saved and becomes the object of the Junker's renewed romantic attentions. As an idealized object of both victimhood and infatuation, the protagonist's body thus resembles that of fairy-tale heroines, while her near-martyrdom as a suspected witch illuminates the sexualization and feminization of witches in the early modern German imagination.[26]

Despite its overall critical treatment of superstition and patriarchal force, Meinhold's narrative also problematically cements the stereotype of elderly women as witches in the figure of Lise Kolken, who is described as spiteful, stingy, as associating with an evil spirit or demon, and being called a witch by the narrator throughout, even before Lise apparently frames Maria and bewitches villagers and their livestock. In fact, Meinhold repeatedly evokes Lise's physical traits, which he explicitly links to traditional beliefs. For example, he leitmotivically refers to her as "gluderäugig" and having red eyes; the old-fashioned term "gluder(n)" (passim) could refer to squinting, crossed eyes, and eyes darting about.[27] Moreover, Lise is described passim as an old witch, "alte Hexe" (2014, 45), skinny and sallow; she is consistently hard-hearted, demanding, and greedy. When crossed, she mumbles threats under her breath. Since she later confesses and dies in a mysterious fashion amid circumstantial evidence (her husband's strange, violent death and anti-religious behavior after a life of piety; a witness having heard her discuss payment for witchcraft; her presence when animals and humans suffer of mysterious ailments), the narrative leaves little space for following the enlightened hero—the Junker von Nienkerken—in seeking rational explanations for events (such as the Sheriff dying because his horse slips on a bridge greased by a vengeful man). In contrast, the father (and narrator), Schweidler, never abandons his supernatural reading of Kolken's role in his daughter's torment. Although Lise's hard-hearted behavior could have simply derived from suffering and hunger and her attempt to instigate a witch trial might be an act of non-magical revenge, Schweidler's overall likable portrayal prevents the narrative from questioning his perspective and thus moving beyond Schweidler's fairy-tale type-casting of marginalized women as witches.

Ultimately, the comparison of a number of Grimms' tales and Meinhold's novel indicates that Hutton's assessment of the feminization and sexualization of witchcraft in the early modern period, and in particular in the German context, holds true in literary depictions. These narratives arise from the overlap between related physical imaginaries: the female body, the "body" of nature (associated with the feminine), the lust of the devil for the female body (and vice versa), the lacking rationality of women, and the model of "fallen" matter all center on obsessions with the female body. Moreover, Maria Schweidler's portrayal suggests that witchcraft in literature serves both to imagine victimhood and to legitimize societal preoccupations with desire, the physical experience, and transgression. Much as in fairy tales, Maria's isolation is both a romantic plight and the projection of human fears of being outcast, which can result in a death sentence. At the same time, the witch figure is—as Bettelheim hinted (albeit with misleading claims about gender roles) regarding "Hansel and Gretel"—a projection of fears of starvation, of depravity, of loss of community (much as Lise will demand rations but never agrees to share hers), and of affliction.[28] In contradistinction to Christian beliefs of the sacred body that represents and gives life, the witch's body (after "marrying" the devil) is life-draining, faith-sapping, and dangerous precisely in its supposed perversion of female submissiveness, receptivity, and role as preserver of human life.

NOTES

1. See, for example, the witch in "Die zwei Brüder" ("The Two Brothers," KHM 60) (who is burned), in "Die weiße und die schwarze Braut" ("The White Bride and the Black Bride," KHM 135) (killed in a barrel studded with nails), or the stepmother-witch in "Sneewittchen" ("Snow White," KHM 53), who is forced into hot iron slippers.
2. Unless otherwise specified, the Grimms' tales are cited from the 1857 edition of the *Kinder- und Hausmärchen* edited by Heinz Rölleke (Grimm, Reclam, 2017).
3. As I have argued elsewhere, this tale type shows the flexibility of the warden character, who is an ogress (Basile), fairy (de la Force and Schulz as well as Grimm 1812) or witch (Grimm 1857) in narratives that otherwise agree on the essentials of the plot (Thesz 2021, 100). The source study by Bolte and Polívka focuses less on the supernatural wardens than on the promise of children before their birth, often in exchange for satisfying cravings (or compensating for theft) (Bolte and Polívka 1994, 97–99).
4. In the preface, Meinhold claimed to have based this text on a manuscript he found that detailed a seventeenth-century witch trial of the daughter of his predecessor, Abraham Schweidler. As B. Burns and Harry Vredeveld explain, Meinhold had set out to dupe leading philologists and theologians who claimed to be able to ascertain the authenticity of biblical texts; although Meinhold contended that his hoax had been successful, doubts had begun to arise and, as Vredeveld writes, forced Meinhold to publicly discuss his novel's false claims (B. Burns 2011, 627–631; Vredeveld 2014, 200–202).
5. In addition, politically motivated accusations arose in some regions (cf. Thurston 2007, 13, 110; Hutton 2017, 51).

6. Ruth Bottigheimer has observed that the Grimms' tales emphasize both the social and physical isolation of female characters; she draws attention to the proximity of this marginalization and the persecution of fairy-tale women as witches (Bottigheimer 1987, 101–105).
7. The "functional" explanation of witch persecutions focuses on probable roles such accusations played in a given society, e.g., allowing groups to scapegoat individuals and thus helping to relieve social tensions.
8. It is striking that the "species lore" of European tale traditions differs considerably from the focus of historical and anthropological studies of folk beliefs concerning individuals or groups in league with the devil, spirits, or demons; moreover, throughout history and cultures, accusations of witchcraft have been made again men, women, and children, whereas literary witches are usually female (cf. Thurston 2007; Hutton 2017; and Millar 2021, 693).
9. It must be noted that folk tales inconsistently judge magic; even when the supernatural is employed beneficently by elderly wielders of magic (e.g., in "The Goose-Girl at the Well"), they are still frequently deemed witches, whereas girls (e.g., Cinderella characters) appropriating the supernatural are not.
10. See a wide range of sibling tale variants listed by Johannes Bolte and Georg Polívka. For example, the means and circumstances of escape may include the burning (killing) of the witch (ogre/ogress) or her/their child/children or the witch's pursuit of the children and bursting after she attempts to drink up the body of water they cross (Bolte and Polívka 1994, 115–126).
11. The female witch has become emblematic for German folktale, perhaps even more so than the wicked stepmother figure. As Bottigheimer writes, twentieth-century critics such as Bettelheim ignore cultural specifics by drawing simplistic psychoanalytical conclusions about the significance of witches as projection screens for children's fears (Bottigheimer 1989, 296–298).
12. In 1857, she is simply "eine steinalte Frau" (Grimm 2017, 101).
13. https://de.wikisource.org/wiki/H%C3%A4nsel_und_Grethel_(1850).
14. As Heinz Rölleke points out, the Grimms' later versions of "Hansel and Gretel" draw substantially on August Stöber's "Das Eierkuchenhäuslein" (1842) (Rölleke 1983, 16–19). For example, the comment that the witch did not see that Hansel was presenting a little bone instead of his finger seems to derive from Stöber (Stöber 1842, 107); however, the claim about witches' eyesight and red eyes does not appear in Stöber's tale, and thus is taken from another source or from Wilhelm Grimm's own imagination.
15. See https://de.wikisource.org/wiki/H%C3%A4nsel_und_Gretel_(1812) and Grimm 2017, 103. The *Hexenwald* first appears in 1843: https://de.wikisource.org/wiki/H%C3%A4nsel_und_Grethel_(1843).
16. The connection to God is removed beginning in the fourth edition of the *Children's and Household Tales* (https://de.wikisource.org/wiki/H%C3%A4nsel_und_Grethel_(1840)). The idea of God presenting insights is still present in 1812, 1819, and 1837: "Gott aber gab es Gretel ein und sie sagte: 'ich weiß nicht, wie ich das anfangen soll, zeigs mirs erst, setz dich drauf, ich will dich hineinschieben'" (https://de.wikisource.org/wiki/H%C3%A4nsel_und_Gretel_(1812)); "However, God let Gretel know this, so she said, 'I don't know how to do that. First show me. You sit on the board, and I will push you inside'" (Ashliman, comparison 1812/57, 2002).
17. For both versions of "The Robber Bridegroom," see: https://sites.pitt.edu/~dash/grimm040.html.
18. In contrast to the written tale, the 1937 Disney version *Snow White and the Seven Dwarfs* more vividly depicts the queen's witchcraft, showing her physical transformation into, as opposed to simply disguise as, an old peddler woman. Cinematically, Disney and his team explore the transgressive excitement with regard to this larger-than-life figure, who dominates the screen through drama, color, expressiveness, and her insecurities.

19. "Darnach sann sie den ganzen Tag und die Nacht, wie sie es doch noch fangen wollte, und machte einen giftigen Kamm, verkleidete sich in eine ganz andere Gestalt, und ging wieder hinaus" (https://de.wikisource.org/wiki/Sneewittchen_(Schneewei%C3%9Fchen)_(1812)); "Then for an entire day and a night she planned how she might catch her. She made a poisoned comb, disguised herself differently, and went out again" (https://sites.pitt.edu/~dash/type0709.html#snowwhite).
20. The first mention of "Hexenkünsten" is in the 1937 edition: https://de.wikisource.org/wiki/Sneewittchen_(1837).
21. To be fair, potion-making could already signify witchcraft.
22. The Mesopotamians and Greeks had imagined various female supernatural demons that attacked young brides as well as preyed upon men, a complex that is relevant for the witch's attack on Jorinda and Joringel; Romans believed specifically in owls or similar flying creatures, the murderous *strix* or *striges* (singular and plural), though the association between witches and owls was shared by various cultures spanning South and North America (Hutton 2017, 67, 69–70).
23. However, in Hutton's survey of anthropological studies, the witches were usually thought to be humanoid in the daytime, and owls or other flying creatures at night (2017, 67).
24. A name that alludes, perhaps, to the idea of a "new," more enlightened Church.
25. "Ach Gott, sie war geradeso weiß auf ihrem Leibe wie meine Selige" (Meinhold 2014, 91; "Well-a-day, her body was just as white as my departed wife's," Meinhold 2005, 56).
26. Hutton perhaps too summarily relies on Jacob Grimm's statements in *Deutsche Mythologie* regarding this feminization, given that there are German literary depictions of male witches as well (cf. Hutton 2017, 72).
27. For example, the judge repeats beliefs that the narrator has already voiced regarding "typical" appearances of witches, which Lise matches perfectly (including her odd, bleating voice): "Denn er hätte schon öfters in Erfahrung gezogen, daß alle alte [sic] Weiber, so rote Gluderaugen und eine finnige Kehle hätten, auch Hexen wären" (Meinhold 2014, 82; "for that he had often been told that all old women who had red squinting eyes and sharp voices were witches," Meinhold 2005, 42). Kolken's stereotypical characterization is repeated throughout the novel without any hint of irony. See also the Grimms' *Deutsches Wörterbuch* entry for "gludern," which provides a wide range of usages, including "glotzen," "einen finstern Blick haben," "schielen," "heimlich nach etwas sehen" (https:// dwds.de/wb/dwb/gludern). An online source on Northern Germany describes "gludern" as "böse ansehen, wütend ansehen, schielen" (https://www.niederdeutsche-literatur.de/dwn/dwn_he.php?W_ID=21781; accessed August 12, 2022).
28. See Bettelheim (1989, 159–166).

WORKS CITED

Bettelheim, Bruno. 1989. *The Uses of Enchantment: The Meaning and Importance of Fairy Tales*. New York: Vintage.

De Blécourt, Willem. 2018. "Contested Knowledge: A Historical Anthropologist's Approach to European Witchcraft." In *Cultures of Witchcraft in Europe from the Middle Ages to the Present: Essays in Honor of Willem de Blécourt*, edited by Jonathan Barry, Owen Davies, and Cornelie Usborne, 1–22. Cham: Palgrave Macmillan.

De Blécourt, Willem. 2008. "On the Origin of *Hänsel and Gretel*: An Exerscise [sic] in the History of Fairy-Tales." *Fabula* 49, no. 1–2: 30–46.

Bolte, Johannes and Georg Polívka. 1994. *Anmerkungen zu den Kinder- und Hausmärchen der Brüder Grimm: Jacob Grimm und Wilhelm Grimm. Werke*, edited by Ludwig Erich Schmitt. Sect. 5. Vol. 2. Hildesheim: Olms-Weidmann.
Bottigheimer, Ruth. 1989. "Bettelheims Hexe: Die fragwürdige Beziehung zwischen Märchen und Psychoanalyse." *Psychotherapie, Psychosomatik, Medizinische Psychologie* 39, no. 8: 294–299.
Bottigheimer, Ruth. 1987. *Grimms' Bad Girls and Bold Boys: The Moral and Social Vision of the Tales*. New Haven: Yale University Press.
Burns, B. 2011. "Truth, Fiction, and Deception in Meinhold's Maria Schweidler, die *Bernsteinhexe*." *Neophilologus* 95: 627–638.
Gilbert, Sandra M. and Susan Gubar. 1979. *The Madwoman in the Attic: The Woman Writer and the Nineteenth-Century Literary Imagination*. New Haven: Yale University Press.
Gobrecht, Barbara. 2010. "Hexen, Zauberinnen und weise Frauen in europäischen Zaubermärchen." In *Abenteuer am Abgrund – Außenseiter im Märchen: Forschungsbeiträge aus der Welt der Märchen*, edited by Harlinda Lox and Renate Vogt, 116–135. Krummwisch: Königsfurt-Urania.
Grimm, Jacob and Wilhelm. 2016. "Hänsel und Gretel." https://de.wikisource.org/wiki/H%C3%A4nsel_und_Gretel_(1812). Accessed 28 May 2022.
Grimm, Jacob and Wilhelm. 2002. "Hansel and Gretel" (a comparison table of the 1812 and 1857 editions), edited by D. L. Ashliman. https://sites.pitt.edu/~dash/grimm015a.html. Accessed 28 May 2022.
Grimm, Jacob and Wilhelm. 2017. *Kinder- und Hausmärchen*, edited by Heinz Rölleke. Stuttgart: Reclam.
Grimm, Jacob and Wilhelm. 2005. "Little Snow White," edited by D. L. Ashliman. https://sites.pitt.edu/~dash/grimm053.html. Accessed 10 June 2022.
Grimm, Jacob and Wilhelm. "Little Snow White," 1812 edition, edited by D. L. Ashliman. https://sites.pitt.edu/~dash/type0709.html#snowwhite. Accessed 25 July 2022.
Grimm, Jacob. 2002. "The Robber Bridegroom," translated by D. L. Ashliman. https://sites.pitt.edu/~dash/grimm040.html. Accessed 10 June 2022.
Grimm, Jacob and Wilhelm. "Sneewittchen." 1812 edition. https://de.wikisource.org/wiki/Sneewittchen_(Schneewei%C3%9Fchen)_(1812). Accessed 8 Nov. 2022.
Hutton, Ronald. 2018. "Witches and Cunning Folk in British Literature 1800–1940." *Preternature* 7, no. 1: 27–49.
Hutton, Ronald. 2017. *The Witch: A History of Fear, From Ancient Times to the Present*. New Haven, CT: Yale University Press.
McGlathery, James M. 1991. *Fairy Tale Romance: The Grimms, Basile, and Perrault*. Urbana: University of Illinois Press.
Meinhold, Wilhelm. 2005. *The Amber Witch*. Translated by Lady Duff Gordon. *ProjectGutenberg*.
Meinhold, Wilhelm. 2014. *Maria Schweidler, die Bernsteinhexe*. Berlin: elv.
Millar, Charlotte-Rose. 2021. "Diabolical Men: Reintegrating Male Witches into English Witchcraft." *The Seventeenth Century* 36, no. 5: 693–713.
Pentangelo, Joseph. 2021. "Burning Feathers: A Hint of Hysteria in a Connecticut Witchcraft Case." *Folklore* 132, no. 1: 59–71.
Rölleke, Heinz. 1983. "August Stöbers Einfluss auf die *Kinder- und Hausmärchen* der Brüder Grimm: Zur Textgenese der KHM 5 und 15." *Fabula* 24, no. 1–2: 11–20.
Rölleke, Heinz. 2010. "Außenseiter in den *Kinder- und Hausmärchen* der Brüder Grimm." In *Abenteuer am Abgrund – Außenseiter im Märchen: Forschungsbeiträge aus der Welt der Märchen*, edited by Harlinda Lox and Renate Vogt, 224–248. Krummwisch: Königsfurt-Urania.
Sexton, Anne. 1981. "Snow White and the Seven Dwarfs." In *The Complete Poems*. Foreword by Maxine Kumin, 224–229. Boston: Houghton Mifflin.
Stöber, August. 1842. "Das Eierkuchenhäuslein." *Elsässisches Volksbüchlein: Kinder- und Volksliedchen, Spiele, Sprüche und Märchen*, 102–109. Straßburg: G. L. Schuler.

Thesz, Nicole. 2021. "Humans and Non-Humans: Uncanny Encounters in the Grimms' Tales." In *A Cultural History of Fairy Tales*. 6 vols, edited by Anne E. Duggan. *A Cultural History of Fairy Tales in the Long Nineteenth Century*. Vol. 5, edited by Naomi Wood, 83–103. London: Bloomsbury.

Thurston, Robert. 2007. *The Witch Hunts: A History of the Witch Persecutions in Europe and North America*. Harlow: Pearson.

Tieck, Ludwig. 1992. "Der Runenberg." *Der blonde Eckbert. Der Runenberg. Die Elfen*. Stuttgart: Reclam.

Treder, Ute. 1984. *Von der Hexe zur Hysterikerin: Zur Verfestigungsgeschichte des "Ewig Weiblichen."* Bonn: Bouvier.

Vredeveld, Harry. 2014. "Pia fraus: Anachronisms, Fake Latin, and Stolen Colors in Wilhelm Meinhold's *Maria Schweidler, Die Bernsteinhexe*." *Monatshefte* 106, no. 2: 200–212.

CHAPTER TWENTY-FIVE

"Vollkommene Organismen:" The Beginnings of a Literary Imagination of the Microbiome

DAVINA HÖLL

THE MICROBIOME AND ITS CHALLENGES FOR THE NATURAL SCIENCES AND THE HUMANITIES

For centuries, microbes have been a source of fascination and horror. As invisible life forms that cannot be seen with the naked eye, they have challenged our understanding of the world and our place in it. The perception of the minutiae transgressing material, epistemological, as well as aesthetical borderlines and thus questioning the notion of humanness itself often found its equivalent in picturing the microbe as a monstrous threat (Höll 2021b), which had to be fended off or combated against. The declaration of a metaphorical and virtual war against microbes (Lederberg 2000; Gradmann 2007, 334–337; Berger 2009, 186; Hänseler 2009, 109) led to the implementation of strict anti-microbial practices, which can be described as a form of "antibiotic thanatopolitics" according to Penelope Ironstone (2018, 331). This involved the widespread use of antibiotics and disinfectants in the years following the Second World War (D'Abramo and Neumeyer 2020, 326). As a result, the approach to the microbial "Other" has been decidedly necropolitical (Mbembe and Corcoran 2019) and was just recently revived by the pandemic experience of Covid-19 (Höll and Bossert, forthcoming 2024). Driven by

Parts of the research for this paper were funded by the Deutsche Forschungsgemeinschaft (DFG, German Research Foundation) under Germany's Excellence Strategy—EXC 2124–390838134 at Eberhard Karls University Tübingen.

fears of a perceived end of the antibacterial era (Landecker 2016), a veritable paradigm shift in conceptualizing human-microbe relationships has emerged in scientific and popular discourses in recent years (Bapteste et al. 2021).

Microbiome research has revealed the manifold intricacies of the relationships between humans and microbes, with about 40–100 trillion microorganisms living on and in our bodies and constituting the human microbiome. The microbiome is linked to all human body organs, and the hope is that its biomedical study holds the key to combating many of our time's most significant health challenges (Hanage 2014, 247f). Numerous research studies focus on infectious diseases and the challenges of current and future epidemics and pandemics; other studies suggest links between the composition of the human microbiome and various physical and mental illnesses. The highly diverse accesses to the microbiome impressively show that the way microorganisms interact in and with the human body has a significant influence on the development of a variety of physical—not only infectious—diseases, such as diabetes (Al Ishaq et al. 2023), allergies (Zubeldia-Varela et al. 2022), or asthma (Aldriwesh et al. 2023). However, microbiome research does not focus on physical diseases alone. The disposition for mental illnesses, such as depression and anxiety disorders, also seems closely related to the microbiome (Mitrea et al. 2022). As the influence of microorganisms and microbiomes on the development of diseases is becoming increasingly evident, it is also becoming more and more apparent that they are indispensable for becoming healthy and maintaining health—and not only for human life. Just as humans contain and depend on microbiomes, so do all other life forms—such as animals or plants—as well as all habitats of these life forms, such as soil, air, or water bodies.

Assessing microbes' impact on other living things is a complex endeavor. First and foremost, the decidedly holistic perspective offered by the microbiome concept fundamentally challenges the prevailing antagonism between humans and microbes. Microbes are no longer seen only as a pathogenic threat but as essential to almost all life forms on Earth. Recent scientific research clearly shows that the categorization of microbes into "good" and "bad" can no longer be sustained (Beck 2021) since, for example, pathogenicity is not an ontological status of microbes but depends, among other things, on the bodies they encounter and their condition (Casadevall and Pirofski 2014; Greenhough et al. 2018). Dichotomous ways of thinking are outdated and must be overcome to enable innovative and forward-looking research that goes beyond targeting microbes as causative agents of disease and death, a mindset that is also reflected at the level of language (Höll and Bossert, 2022a, 106–108). Speaking about microbe-human relationships in terms of "invasion" is a long handed-down topos (Hänseler 2009, 119). Conceptualizing and speaking about microbes as threatening invaders by using war metaphors reinforces a distinct antagonistic conception of microorganisms, especially in infectious diseases and epidemic or pandemic events. Moreover, as Priscilla Wald has shown, talking about "viral invaders" and "germ warfare" links the politics of anti-microbial warfare to the macrobial politics of war (Wald 2008, 164). This fatal conflation of microbic and macrobic rhetoric became apparent again during the Covid-19 pandemic (Höll 2021c, 194) when, as early as March 2020, French president Emmanuel Macron, in his address to the nation, declared "Nous sommes en guerre" ["We are at war"], and US "wartime" President Donald Trump denoted SARS-CoV-2 as the

"China virus," also exhibiting the distinct xenophobic dimension of military metaphors in the context of pandemics (Craig 2020, 3).

Science and society are becoming increasingly aware that "we have never been individuals" (Gilbert, Sapp, and Tauber 2012) but "contain multitudes" (Yong 2017) that connect us with our interior and exterior human and nonhuman environments. Microbiome research also challenges our concepts of the (human) self and its autonomy (Rees et al. 2018; Ironstone 2018), drawing attention to humanities fields such as philosophy, ethics, literature studies, and the arts (cf. Greenough et al. 2020; Höll and Bossert 2022b) by emphasizing the need to (re-)consider the role of microbes in our understanding of the world and our place in it. These challenges of conceptualizing both the human and nonhuman life worlds and their interrelations have led to inspiring theories and visions of cross-species futures (Braidotti, 2013; Haraway, 2008, 2016; Helmreich, 2014; Kirksey, 2014). These approaches highlight the interconnectedness of all life on Earth, proclaiming a series of "turns." Donna Haraway, for instance, emphasizes the "multispecies" nature of humans (Haraway 2008), thus providing one key starting point for the "species turn in anthropology" (Kirksey and Helmreich 2010, 546). Rosi Braidotti (2013, 60) calls for a "post-anthropocentric turn" in the humanities, opening perspectives about the microbial world. And while Stefan Herbrechter observed a "microbial turn," stressing that "[h]uman entanglement with the microbial is thus another attack on human or humanist narcissism, hubris and human exceptionalism" (Herbrechter 2018, 355–356), Jamie Lorimer announces a "probiotic turn," promoting "human interventions that use life to manage life, working with biological and geomorphic processes to deliver forms of human, environmental, and even planetary health" (Lorimer 2020, 2).

MISSING MICROBIOMES: A LITERARY HISTORY OF THE MICROBIOME YET TO COME

The interface of art and science has always been a space for innovative, even transgressive, thinking. Art and literature can act as sensitive indicators of social and scientific changes. Microbes are a potent symbol for the entanglements of terrestrial and even extra-terrestrial living beings, as "[t]he most likely type of life to be encountered on any planetary body beyond Earth, if we find it at all, will be microscopic" (Cockell 2016, 167). Even before their discovery by the Dutch cloth merchant Antonie van Leeuwenhoek (1632–1723), there were various philosophical, theoretical, and proto-scientific attempts to fathom the infinitely small. Very early, art and literature, with their seismographic power, explored the fascination and fear that enshrouded the potential of a microworld beyond the spheres of human perception, as one of the earliest artistic depictions of microbes—the colored engraving created by the London caricaturist William Heath (1794/5–1840) in 1828, impressively shows. The picture bears the title "Monster Soup" (Heath 1828) and became an icon of what I call the *microgothic* (Höll 2021b, 25). By downscaling "the fear, anxiety, and dread that often pervades the relationships of humans with the nonhuman world" (Keetley and Sivils 1) to the microbial level, the microgothic imagines and describes microbes as invisible monstrous hazards "from a nonhuman outside that imperils the human inside" (Höll 2021b, 24). William Heath's caricature thus features a Victorian Lady holding a tea cup containing London drinking water swarming with "all monstrous, all prodigious things, [...] hydras, and gorgans, and chimeras dire" (Heath 1828) about to enter her body. The etching is not only remarkable in terms of microbial aesthetics but also regarding its quasi-prophetic power. Even though the frightful, until then rather fantastic assumption that tiny monstrous microorganisms inhabiting London's drinking water supply—the River Thames—could threaten the well-being of the metropolis' population had been discussed before, it became a scientific fact only at the end of the century. During the next two hundred years, the microgothic imagination and aesthetic were revisited and revived numerous times in such different genres as Mark Twain's novel fragment *Three Thousand Years Among the Microbes* (1905) or BioArtist Anna Dumitriu's discussion of the "Bacterial Sublime" (2012). Consequently, literary history is (literally)[1] populated by a wide diversity of microorganisms constituting a veritable literary microbiome, although literary studies are still rather unconscious of it. When microbes become an issue of literary studies, it often is in the context of discussing the aesthetic and epistemological challenges of the advances of microscopy (cf. Forsberg 2021; Košenina 2001; Lightman 2010; Nicolson 1976; Siebenpfeiffer 2017) or within the discourses of infection and infectious disease (cf. Outka 2020; Wald 2008; Strowick 2009; Briese 2003; Otis 1999), culminating in a decidedly *microgothic* imagination of the microcosm and its interconnectedness with human life (Höll 2021b).

Recently Martina King has provided a comprehensive *Literaturgeschichte des Mikrobiellen* focusing on the "golden age of microbiology" between 1880 and 1920, the only monograph-length study of the microbial in literary history so far. In her study, she traces two key concepts of the bacteriological discourse around 1900: The microbe as a "kollektives Wissenssymbol" ["collective symbol of knowledge"] that becomes a focus of modern diversity ["Projektionsfigur moderner Diversität") and the core narrative of the "Mikrobenjagd" ["microbe hunt"] based on the imperative to "find the microbe and kill it" that provides "Spannung, Orientierung und kollektive Identitätsstiftung" ["tension, orientation, and collective identity formation"] (King 2021, 554). However, King's readings of a wide range of turn-of-the-century texts also imply the paradigm shift of microbiomic narration. Without even once mentioning the technical term of the microbiome itself,[2] King provides the seeds for a (pre-)history of the literary microbiome (511–518). She shows that already around 1900, people realized that "[d]er Mensch ist keine Reinkultur, sondern ein unberechenbar komplexes System" ["[t]he human being is not a pure culture, but an unpredictably complex system"] (273). This revelation, King argues following Silvia Berger (252), meant "Komplexitätszuwachs und Ausdifferenzierung" ["increased complexity and differentiation"], (273) inducing "parasitologisch-ökologische Vorstellungen" ["parasitological-ecological conceptions"] that perceived the body as "offenes System ohne stabile Grenzen, das dauerhaft fremde Organismen einlässt und beherbergt" ["open system without stable boundaries that permanently admits and harbors alien organisms"] (512). King concludes that in this line of reasoning, man and microbe exist and interact in "bewegliche[n] Gleichgewichtszustände[n]" ["mobile states of equilibrium"] in which the human body becomes both an "autonomer Organismus" ["autonomous organism"] and a "heteronomer Container für ein Gewimmel von unsichtbaren Untermietern [...] für ein

Leben im Leben" ["heteronomous container for a bustling crowd of invisible subtenants [...] for a life within a life"] (512). Although these early ecological conceptions are not identical to today's understanding of the microbiome, they show that alternative discourses on human microbe relationships existed alongside the dominant medical discourse of infection from early on. Today, with the recognition of microbiomes as interconnected systems within and on living organisms and, by some, as living organisms themselves, it is unsurprising that the primary metaphor used to understand the complexities of human-microbe relationships is the one of ecology (e.g., Bapteste et al. 2021). As Nicolae Morar and Brendan Bohannan show, besides conceptualizing the microbiome as an "organ," "immune system," "superorganism," or "holobiont," the most common and comprehensive way of understanding the purported paradigm shift in human-microbe interaction is through an "ecosystem view" (162).

While the concept of modern microbial ecology emerged in the 1950s (Konopka 2009, 92), as did, interestingly, the first mention of the term "microbiome," the idea of conceptualizing microbial realms as miniature versions of macro ecosystems can be traced back to the nineteenth century (Grote 2022). The current definition of the term "microbiome" in the Oxford English Dictionary (OED) is a fusion of two terms: "micro," denoting something very small, and "biome," describing the plant and animal communities within a significant climate or habitat. The term "microbiome" is defined in two ways by the OED. First, the microbiome refers to "the population of microorganisms inhabiting a particular environment, such as the body, which form a microbial community or ecosystem" ("microbiome," 2020). Second, the microbiome is described as "the collective genomes of all microorganisms inhabiting a specific environment, particularly the body" ("microbiome," 2020). Despite the significant difference between referring to a population or collective genomes, both definitions are semantically rooted in ecology ("microbiome," 2020). Nobel Laureate and pioneer of microbiome research, Joshua Lederberg, already demanded to actively replace "the war metaphor with an ecological one" in 2000 (Lederberg 2000). In the center of the "ecosystem view" of the microbiome is the notion of transcorporeal (Alaimo 2010) entanglement reflected in shared environments of human and nonhuman life forms, perpetual processes of exchange, as well as physiological co-dependencies that ultimately change the conception of what (human) life is (Rees et al. 2018).

While the microbiome has been studied in various academic disciplines recently, this ecological perspective on microbes has received little attention in literary studies.[3] Even in science fiction, a genre at the forefront of dealing with emerging technologies, scientific advances, and novel knowledge, the microbiome "is not yet as prominent a theme [...] as genetic engineering or cloning" (Vint 2020, 113). To address this lacuna, my paper wants to begin at the beginnings of microbiome imagination by analyzing one of the founding texts of modern microbiology, Christian Gottfried Ehrenberg's *Die Infusionsthierchen als vollkommene Organismen: Ein Blick in das tiefere organische Leben der Natur* (1838). Although it is not a work of fiction *per se*, some of its core convictions were perceived as such by his contemporaries and have initiated the gradual oblivion of the once-famous scientist (Grote 2022, 4). However, from today's perspective, against the backdrop of the multiple crises of the Anthropocene, they seem to gain new momentum. Ehrenberg's visions of universal, sentient, and sociable micro life that either benefits or threatens human life are a reminder of the deep connection between science and imagination.

BEGINNING AT THE BEGINNINGS: CHRISTIAN GOTTFRIED EHRENBERG'S *DIE INFUSIONSTHIERCHEN ALS VOLLKOMMENE ORGANISMEN* (1838) AND THE EARLY MICROBIOME IMAGINATION

Christian Gottfried Ehrenberg (1795–1876) was a German zoologist and microscopist regarded as the most important forefather of modern microbiology. As an outstanding scholar, he was a member of the Royal Prussian Academy of Sciences, the Royal Society of London, the Russian Academy of Sciences, and the American Academy of Arts and Sciences. In 1877, Ehrenberg was posthumously awarded the first Leeuwenhoek medal. He was extraordinarily productive and exceptionally well-connected with the international scientific community of his time. He was in frequent correspondence with Charles Darwin (1809–82) and Thomas Henry Huxley (1825–95) and traveled the world, joining Alexander von Humboldt (1769–1859) on his Siberian expedition (Grote 2022, 2). In 1838, he published his influential work *Die Infusionsthierchen als vollkommene Organismen*. The text, the title of which translates as "The Infusoria as perfect organisms" (Grote 2022), presented the collected findings of his exploration of the microcosmic *terra incognita* that rendered him a "Humboldt in miniature" (Grote 2022, 2). He pursued the claim of pure empiricism and scientific exactness in exploring and describing the microcosm. He thus resolutely opposed the "höchst wunderbaren, alle philosophischen Ansichten vom Leben und der Entstehung der Organismen" ["most wonderful, philosophical views of life and the origin of organisms"] (Ehrenberg 1838, VI) as speculations of contemporary natural philosophy (Grote 2022, 5; Geus 1987, 231ff.). Instead, he states:

> Es ist unter Anderm die stille und ernste Aufgabe einer langen Reihe von Jahren meines Lebens gewesen, diese vor allen so merkwürdigen, riesenhaft grossen, aber in das Dunkel der Kleinheit verhüllten, Naturverhältnisse näher und immer näher zu betrachten und zu prüfen, das Fabelhafte von dem Wirklichen zu sondern und das Wirkliche in eine systematische leicht fassliche Uebersicht zu bringen.
>
> [Among other things, it has been the quiet and solemn task of a long series of years of my life to consider and examine ever more closely these natural relationships, which are above all so strange and so gigantic, but are veiled in the darkness of smallness; to separate the fabulous from the actual and to bring the actual into a systematic, easily comprehensible account.]
>
> (Ehrenberg 1838, VI)

Ehrenberg's contemporaries praised his microscopic endeavors (Geus 1987, 237, 241) as skillful and meticulous. However, he did not always live up to this praise, as some of his "findings" were marked by "erheblich[er][…] Phantasie" ["considerable imagination"] (Geus 1987, 240). While many of his often ground-breaking observations and conclusions could be reproduced and thus proven later, other "findings" fell into the realm of imagination. Based on the conviction that the infusoria as "perfect organisms" were as complexly organized and had the same main organs as their macrobic counterparts, Ehrenberg was convinced that he could prove that microbes have complex digestive and reproductive organs, just like highly developed life forms. Proving the existence of these organs was of such importance to Ehrenberg that he even featured his discovery in the study's dedication to the Prussian crown prince Friedrich Wilhelm (1795–1861), emphasizing that "das Kleinste [...] mit den verschiedensten thätigen Organen so wundervoll und unbegreiflich ausgestattet ist, dass es sich ganz gleichmässig und gleichwürdig in die Reihen der grösseren Lebensformen stellt" ["the smallest [...] is so wonderfully and incredibly equipped with the most diverse active organs that it places itself quite evenly and equally in the ranks of the larger life forms"] (Ehrenberg 1838, n.p.). Within the study, Ehrenberg devoted specific sections to the genealogies of knowledge regarding the existence of digestive (Ehrenberg 1838, 519f.) and reproductive organs (Ehrenberg 1838, 382f.) of infusoria, putting himself at the top of these epistemic histories.

Although Ehrenberg would later be proven wrong, particularly with respect to these crucial aspects, he based his misconception on the conviction that "unimposing, apparently simple organisms represented a part of Nature not inferior to animals." In doing so, he ultimately "rehabilitated creatures largely marginalized by natural history" (Grote 2022, 3). He starts the introduction of his pioneering study with the passionate statement that,

> In den reinsten Gewässern und auch in den trüben, stark sauren und salzigen Flüssigkeiten der verschiedensten Erdzonen, in Quellen, Flüssen, Seen und Meeren, oft auch in den inneren Feuchtigkeiten der lebenden Pflanzen und Thierkörper, selbst zahlreich im Körper des lebenden Menschen, ja wahrscheinlich auch periodisch getragen im Wasserdunst und Staube der ganzen Atmosphäre der Erde, giebt es eine den gewöhnlichen Sinnen des Menschen unbemerkbare, Welt sehr kleiner lebender organischer Wesen [...].
>
> [In the purest waters, just as in the turbid, strongly acidic, and salty liquids of the most diverse earth zones, in springs, rivers, lakes, and seas, often also in the inner dampness of living plants and animal bodies, even in the body of the living human being, probably periodically also carried in the steam and dust of the entire atmosphere of the Earth, there exists a world of very small living organic beings unnoticeable to the ordinary senses of man [...].]
>
> (Ehrenberg 1838, V)

This very first sentence of his book is a bold move since the ontological status of microbes was still highly disputed at the time. Ehrenberg stresses the sheer ubiquity of the minutiae populating every part of the Earth's surfaces, life forms, waters, and even the air, and he assigns them a specific place in the world of the living. In the tradition of Leeuwenhoek's "animalcules," he calls them "Thierchen" ["little animals"]. In the following, Ehrenberg acknowledges that these invisible micro creatures have given great cause for speculation since their discovery. They have often been portrayed "unter der Feder leicht bewegter und phantastischer Schriftsteller"[4] ["under the pen of lightly moved and fantastic writers"] as "monströse Geisterwelt, voll [...] theils grauenhafter, theils wunderlich verzerrter, nicht recht lebender und nicht recht lebloser Formen" ["monstrous spirit world, full of partly gruesome, partly whimsically distorted, not quite living and not quite lifeless forms"] (Ehrenberg 1838, V). In doing so, he gives an account of the widely popular perception of the microbial realm as a distinct microgothic sphere. As an integral part of popular discourse, contemporary imagery, and literary imagination, the microgothic also fuelled early forms of the phenomenon that Martina King, adapting Nancy Tomes (2002), termed "microbe entertainment" (King 502).

Additionally, Ehrenberg openly attacks views contrary to his own convictions on the form and function of microbes by ridiculing them. He depreciates his colleagues as "phantastische[r] Schriftsteller" and thus places their work more near speculative fiction than natural science trying to secure his own position in emerging microbiology. However, it was not only "das Mystisch-Wundervolle, Abentheuerliche und Sonderbare der Formen und ihrer Kleinheit" ["the mystical-wonderful, the oddness and strangeness of their forms and their smallness"] (Ehrenberg 1838, I) that fascinated Ehrenberg. Microbes' "physiologischen höchst wunderbaren Eigentümlichkeiten" ["most wonderful physiological peculiarities"] (V) made them "notwhendig" ["necessarily"] (V) and should therefore attract "das Interesse aller nachdenkenden Menschen" ["the interest of all contemplating people"] (I). Since "[a]lle Freunde des Wissens, und selbst die gelehrtesten und tiefsten Forscher von Leibnitz und Boerhave" ["[a]ll friends of knowledge, and even the most learned and profound researchers of Leibnitz and Boerhave"] were inevitably drawn to the microcosm, according to Ehrenberg, a plethora of attributes were assigned to its inhabitants—most of them erroneously (VI).

In the following, Ehrenberg provides an overview of the history of microbiology from ancient times to the early nineteenth century, before the concept of microbiology as a scientific discipline existed as such (cf. Grote 2022). He stresses that the interest in microorganisms was mainly centered in the medical field. In doing so, Ehrenberg traces what he perceived as an international history of scientific misconceptions of the microscopic world. To remedy this circumstance, he created a catalog of the now "begründeten" and "besonders merkürdigen Eigenschaften und Verhältnisse der Infusorien" ["well-founded" and "particularly peculiar properties and conditions of infusoria"] (Ehrenberg 1838, XIII). This extensive list contains thirty scientific "facts." Concerning the idea of an early microbiomic imagination, Ehrenberg's assumptions can compete with today's most progressive approaches to the microbial realm. The most crucial of his findings and elaborations later in his study in this regard are that microorganisms are ubiquitous and make up "die grössten numerischen bekannten Verhältnisse des selbstständigen Lebens; [...] die Hauptzahl, vielleicht die Hauptmasse der thierisch belebten Organismen auf der Erde," that "alle Infusorien sind organisirte, zum grossen Theil, wahrscheinlich alle, hoch organisirte Thiere" ["the largest numerical known proportions of independent life; [...] the largest number, perhaps the largest mass, of animate animal organisms on the earth"], having complex digestive and reproductive organs. Moreover, Ehrenberg was deeply convinced that they have a distinct "Gesellschaftstrieb" ["social drive"] (20) and possess "Geistesfähigkeiten" ["mental abilities"] (XIV), which ultimately make them "Bürger einer unserm Urtheile fern liegenden grossen Welt" ["citizens of a great world far removed from our judgment"], who share "den Genuss einer empfindungsreichen Existenz, so stolz wir uns auch geberden mögen" ["the enjoyment of sentient existence, however proud we may behave"] (Ehrenberg 1838, 60–70).

The perspective of the microcosmos that Ehrenberg develops in his monumental study is exceptionally far- and short-sighted, taking, on the one hand, a proto-ecological perspective on the microcosm but, on the other, denying "the existence of living microbial pathogens" (Grote 2022, 1). His contemporary American colleague Thomas Henry Huxley (1825–95) describes his observations as "wonderful monuments of intense and unremitting labor, but at least as wonderful illustrations of what zoological and physiological reasoning should *not* be" (Huxley 1851, 436; cf. Williams and Huxley 1998). With this ambiguity, Ehrenberg's work is an extraordinary example of the complex twists and turns of knowledge-making, and the role imagination, creative boldness, and unpopular and marginalized ideas play within these processes. It became Ehrenberg's misfortune, "mehr als andere vor ihm gesehen, das Gesehene aber falsch gedeutet zu haben" ["having seen more than others before him, but having misinterpreted what he saw"] (Geuss 1987, 245). He was among the first to fathom microorganisms' far-reaching impact on Earth's living and non-living matter. However, because of his urge to show the perfection of these "vollkommene Organismen" ["perfect organisms"] and to assign them their rightful place in the hierarchy of life, he not only endowed them with non-existent organs and corresponding abilities but also entirely dismissed their pathogenic potential as "unbewiesene Behauptung und Aberglaube" ["unproven assertion and superstition"] (Ehrenberg 1838, XIII):

> Die unsichtbaren Infusorien schaden zuweilen und allein, wie es scheint, durch Tödten der Fische in Teichen, durch Verschlammen des klaren Wassers, durch Sumpfgeruch und durch Schreck abergläubischer Menschen. Dass sie die Sumpffieber, Pest und andere Krankheiten bedingen, ist unwahrscheinlich und nie glaubwürdig nachgewiesen.
>
> [The invisible infusoria sometimes only do harm, it seems, by killing fish in ponds, muddying clear water, smelly swamps, and frightening superstitious people. That they cause swamp fever, plague, and other diseases is unlikely and has never been credibly proven.]
>
> (XIII)

Ehrenberg's rejection of microbes' possible pathogenicity—as they might only harm as a side-effect of environmental changes they induce and become lethal only, if at all, "durch Schreck abergläubischer Menschen"—might seem incomprehensible to us today. Back in the early beginnings of modern microbiology, however, it was a stance not uncommon. However, history took a different path; it took another half century before the pathogenicity of microbes would become a proven fact. The following two hundred years witnessed the advent of modern bacteriology and medical microbiology centered on microbes as harbourers of the most deadly diseases, such as smallpox, cholera, tuberculosis, influenza, Ebola, HIV, and recently, Covid-19. This focus led to the "war on microbes" of an anti-bacteriological era (Landecker 2016), with a distinct "thanatopolitical" (Ironstone 2018) or "micronecropolitical" (Sütterlin, 2023) agenda.

Ehrenberg wanted to exclude the medical discourse from the discourse on microorganisms and, by doing so, excluded himself from the discipline he helped to found (cf. Grote 2022). At the time, he created a counternarrative that earned him mostly ridicule. However, from today's standpoint, he prefigured a concept of the world of microbes that stresses all living beings' interconnectedness and perpetual circulatory processes at the core of current microbiology (Grote 2022, 6), especially concerning the concept of the *microbiome*. With that, Ehrenberg's zealous opus magnum *Infusionsthierchen*—in which he did nothing less than catalog and describe all known microbial life forms, including several of those he had discovered himself—became a pioneering work. Despite its refusal to recognize the pathogenic potential of the "vollkommene Thierchen," it paved the way for modern microbiology and, at the same time, can be read as a kind of science fiction gaining momentum almost two hundred years after its publication. A (close) reading of Ehrenberg's controversial work shows that microbial thinking outside the medical framework can be traced back at least to the nineteenth century and since then "has been highlighted as an elemental, creative biological force" (D'Abramo 2020). As the antibiotic era seems to be ending, it is all the more important to look for alternative conceptions of human microbe coexistence or "microontologies" (Hird 2009). Ehrenberg's thinking of microbial ecology and the microbiome *avant la lettre* has shown that non-antagonistic ways of perceiving the omnipresence of invisible, micro life have existed all along. Returning to the beginnings of this microbiomic thinking might spark novel approaches to life in an entangled world. With its curious reception history, which oscillates between admiration, contempt, and mockery, Ehrenberg's passionate and empathetic devotion to the world of the microcosm that he developed in his *Infusionsthierchen als vollkommene Organismen* is also an appeal to look for forgotten, ridiculed, or marginalized thoughts, ideas, and imaginations past and present to bring them (back) into "das helle Licht der wissenschaftlichen Erkenntnis" ["the bright light of scientific knowledge"] (Ehrenberg VIII).

CONCLUSION: READING MICROBIAL NARRATIVES AGAINST THE GRAIN

Through the power of imagination, speculation, and thought experiments, especially regarding an epistemological object that still puzzles science and society, we can explore the unknown and attempt the "wondrous but next to impossible" (Hird 2009, 20) and create intellectual spaces that embrace the possibility of (momentary) failure. Ehrenberg rejected the role of microbes in causing disease and was wrong. The knowledge about microorganisms' potential pathogenicity and the development of means to answer it—namely disinfectants and anti-microbials—changed human history forever. Unarguably, at least for a time, it made human life less vulnerable and longer lasting. However, with the sword of Damocles of the "silent pandemic of antibiotic resistance" (UK Government) hanging over us, thinking about the microbial world in terms of controlling and eradication has literally come to a dead end. Already in 2000, Joshua Lederberg, regarding the fight against microbes, declared that it will always be "our wits versus their genes" (286), a veritable battle of the microbial David against the human Goliath. As we become increasingly aware of the highly complex entanglements of the macro- and microcosms that constitute our life world, we have to renounce the "war against microbes" for good and explore new ways of thinking human-nonhuman-microbial entanglements, also by venturing into non-anthropocentric perspectives. Ehrenberg's marveling at "vollkommene Organismen" is a reminder of the power of (scientific) imagination in all its complexity and, sometimes, untimeliness. For him, microbes were "eine[r] der würdigsten Gegenstände des Nachdenkens und der wissenschaflichen Forschung" ["one of the worthiest objects of reflection and scientific research"] (1838, V), even though he did not believe in any direct impact these tiny beings had on human well- or ill-being. He did not perceive them as "die kleinsten [...] Feinde der Menschheit" ["the smallest enemies of humankind"] (Gradmann 2007, 330) and also mostly refrained from anthropomorphizing them. Valuing microbes for themselves and imagining a coexistence beyond anthropocentrism—paradoxically, maybe for humankind's own good—seems to be one of the most significant challenges of our time.

Current microbiome research is shifting paradigms concerning how we perceive humanity's place within the order of things. The analysis of Ehrenberg's pro-microbial counternarrative has demonstrated that going back might be a fruitful step toward looking ahead. Reading microbial narratives such as Ehrenberg's—fictional, factual, or in-between—against the grain to excavate forgotten, suppressed, ridiculed, or marginalized approaches of human microbe relationships that, through acknowledgment and critical discussion, may stimulate visions of imaging the microbiome beyond the infection paradigm and human hubris.

NOTES

1. See Calhoun's (2020) fascinating article about the microbiomes of books and the more-than-human, multi-species co-production of literature. Also see the intriguing work of Nicole Karafyllis.
2. Instead, King focuses on the concept of symbioses (352), which is deeply linked to that of the microbiome (cf. Gilbert, Sapp and Tauber 2012).
3. Notable exceptions are Vint (2020, 2021); Herbrechter (2018); Magnone (2016); Weed (2019); Sütterlin (2023).
4. I would like to thank Mathias Grote for pointing out that with the term "Schriftsteller," Ehrenberg seems to refer to rival scientists—as authors of scientific works—rather than actual writers of (phantastic) fiction.

WORKS CITED

Alaimo, Stacy. 2010. *Bodily Natures: Science, Environment, and the Material Self*. Bloomington: Indiana University Press.

Aldriwesh, Marwh G., Abrar M. Al-Mutairi, Azzah S. Alharbi, Hassan Y. Aljohani, Nabeel A. Alzahrani, Reham Ajina, and Abdullah M. Alanazi. 2023. "Paediatric Asthma and the Microbiome: A Systematic Review." *Microorganisms* 11, no. 4: 939. https://doi.org/10.3390/microorganisms11040939.

AL-Ishaq, Raghad Khalid, Samson Mathews Samuel, and Dietrich Büsselberg. 2023. "The Influence of Gut Microbial Species on Diabetes Mellitus." *International Journal of Molecular Sciences* 24, no. 9: 8118. doi:10.3390/ijms24098118.

Bapteste, Eric, Philippe Gérard, Catherine Larose, Manuel Blouin, Fabrice Not, Liliane Campos, Géraldine Aïdan, et al. 2021. "The Epistemic Revolution Induced by Microbiome Studies: An Interdisciplinary View." *Biology* 10, no. 7: 651. doi:10.3390/biology10070651.

Braidotti, Rosi. 2013. *The Posthuman*. Cambridge: Polity Press.

Beck, A. 2021. "Microbiomes as Companion Species: An Exploration of Dis- and Re-entanglements with the Microbial Self." *Social and Cultural Geography* 22, no. 3: 357–375. https://doi.org/10.1080/14649365.2019.1593490

Berger, Silvia. 2009. *Bakterien in Krieg und Frieden: Eine Geschichte der medizinischen Bakteriologie in Deutschland 1890–1933*. Göttingen: Wallstein.

Briese, Olaf. 2003. *Angst in den Zeiten der Cholera: Über kulturelle Ursprünge des Bakteriums. Seuchen-Cordon I*. Berlin: De Gruyter.

Calhoun, Joshua. 2020. "Book Microbiomes." In *The Unfinished Book*, edited by Alexandra Gillespie and Deidre Lynch, 460–473. Oxford: Oxford University Press. https://doi.org/10.1093/oxfordhb/9780198830801.013.32.

Casadevall, Arturo, and Liise-anne Pirofski. 2014. "Microbiology: Ditch the Term Pathogen." *Nature* 516, no. 7530: 165–166. doi:10.1038/516165a.

"Christian Gottfried Ehrenberg." 2023. American Academy of Arts & Science. Accessed March 15, 2023. https://www.amacad.org/person/christian-gottfried-ehrenberg

Cockell, Charles S. 2016. "The Ethical Status of Microbial Life on Earth and Elsewhere: In Defence of Intrinsic Value." In *The Ethics of Space Exploration*, edited by James S. J. Schwartz and Tony Milligan, 167–179. Cham: Springer International Publishing. https://doi.org/10.1007/978-3-319-39827-3_12.

Craig, David. 2020. "Pandemic and Its Metaphors: Sontag Revisited in the COVID-19 Era." *European Journal of Cultural Studies* 23, no. 6: 1025–1032. https://doi.org/10.1177/1367549420938403.

D'Abramo, Flavio and Sybille Neumeyer. 2020. "A Historical and Political Epistemology of Microbes." *Centaurus* 62, no. 2: 321–330. https://doi.org/10.1111/1600-0498.12300.

Dumitriu, Anna. 2012. *The Bacterial Sublime*. https://annadumitriu.co.uk/portfolio/the-bacterial-sublime/.

Ehrenberg, Christian G. 1838. *Die Infusionsthierchen als vollkommene Organismen: ein Blick in das tiefere organische Leben der Natur: nebst einem Atlas von vierundsechszig colorirten Kupfertafeln, gezeichnet vom Verfasser*. Leipzig: Voss.

Forsberg, Laura. 2021. *Worlds Beyond: Miniatures and Victorian Fiction*. New Haven: Yale University Press.

Geus, Armin. 1987. "Christian Gottfried Ehrenberg und 'Die Infusionsthierchen als vollkommene Organismen – ein Blick in das tiefere organische Leben der Natur' (1838)." *Medizinhistorisches Journal* 22, no. 2–3: 228–245.

Gilbert, Scott F., Jan Sapp, and Alfred I. Tauber. 2012. "A Symbiotic View of Life: We Have Never Been Individuals." *The Quarterly Review of Biology* 87, no. 4: 325–341. https://doi.org/10.1086/668166.

Gradmann, Christoph. 2007."Unsichtbare Feinde: Bakteriologie und politische Sprache im deutschen Kaiserreich." In *Bakteriologie und Moderne: Studien zur Biopolitik desUnsichtbaren 1870–1920*, edited by Philipp Sarasin, Silvia Berger, Marianne Hänseler, and Myriam Spörri, 327–374. Frankfurt am Main: Suhrkamp.

Greenhough, Beth, Andrew Dwyer, Richard Grenyer, Timothy Hodgetts, Carmen McLeod, and Jamie Lorimer. 2018. "Unsettling Antibiosis: How Might Interdisciplinary Researchers Generate a Feeling for the Microbiome and to What Effect?" *Palgrave Communications* 4, no. 1: 149. doi:10.1057/s41599-018-0196-3.

Greenhough, Beth, Cressida Jervis Read, Jamie Lorimer, Javier Lezaun, Carmen McLeod, Amber Benezra, Sally Bloomfield, et al. 2020. "Setting the Agenda for Social Science Research on the Human Microbiome." *Palgrave Communications* 6, no. 1: 18. https://doi.org/10.1057/s41599-020-0388-5.

Grote, Mathias. 2022. "Microbes before Microbiology: Christian Gottfried Ehrenberg and Berlin's Infusoria." *Endeavour* 46, no. 1–2: 100815. https://doi.org/10.1016/j.endeavour.2022.100815.

Hanage, William P. 2014. "Microbiology: Microbiome Science Needs a Healthy Dose of Scepticism." *Nature* 512, no. 7514: 247–248. doi: 10.1038/512247a.

Hänseler, Marianne. 2009. *Metaphern unter dem Mikroskop: die epistemische Rolle von Metaphorik in den Wissenschaften und in Robert Kochs Bakteriologie*. Zürich: Chronos.

Haraway, Donna. 2008. *When Species Meet*. Minneapolis: University of Minnesota Press

Haraway, Donna Jeanne. 2016. *Staying with the Trouble: Making Kin in the Chthulucene*. Durham: Duke University Press.

Heath, William. 1828. *Monster Soup*. Coloured etching. https://wellcomecollection.org/works/qqcx38hr

Heise, Ursula K. 2020. "Multispecies Futures and Study of Culture." In *Futures of the Study of Culture*, edited by Doris Bachmann-Medick, Jens Kugele, and Ansgar Nünning, 274–287. Berlin/Boston: De Gruyter.

Helmreich, Stefan. 2014. "Homo Microbis: The human microbiome, figural, literal, political." *Threshold* 42: 52–59. https://doi.org/10.1162/thld_a_00076.

Herbrechter, Stefan. 2018. "Microbes." In *The Edinburgh Companion to Animal Studies*, edited by Lynn Turner, Undine Sellbach, and Ron Broglio, 354–366. Edinburgh: Edinburgh University Press. https://doi.org/10.1515/9781474418423-026.

Hird, Myra J. 2009. *The Origins of Sociable Life: Evolution after Science Studies*. Basingstoke: Palgrave Macmillan.

Höll, Davina. 2019. "'Der Tod Ist Hundertfach in Jedem Mundvoll Luft, Den Wir Einatmen': Unheimliche Grenzgänge Zwischen Mensch und Umwelt. 'Ecogothic' in Ricarda Huchs ‚Erinnerungen von Ludolf Ursleu dem Jüngeren.'" *Studia Germanica Gedanensia* 40 (December): 218–226. https://doi.org/10.26881/sgg.2019.40.18.

Höll, Davina. 2021a. *Das Gespenst der Pandemie: Politik und Poetik der Cholera in der Literatur des 19. Jahrhunderts*. Stuttgart-Bad Cannstatt: frommann-holzboog.

Höll, Davina. 2021b. "Microgothic: Microbial Aesthetics of Haunted Nature." In *Haunted Nature*, edited by Sladja Blazan, 21–42. Cham: Palgrave Macmillan. https://doi.org/10.1007/978-3-030-81869-2_2.

Höll, Davina. 2021c. "Zu Einer Ethik Der Ästhetik in Pandemischen Zeiten." *Zeitschrift Für Praktische Philosophie* 8, no. 1: 181–208. https://doi.org/10.22613/zfpp/8.1.8.

Höll, Davina and Leonie N. Bossert. 2022a. "'What Would a Microbe Say?:' Paving the Way to Multispecies Communication." In *Multiple Knowledges: Learning from/with Other Beings. Multiples Wissen: Lernen von/mit anderen Entitäten*, edited by Pawel Piszczatowski, Joanna Godlewicz-Adamiec, Piotr Kociumbas, and Justyna Włodarczyk, 103–118. Göttingen: V&R unipress. https://doi.org/10.14220/9783737013826.103.

Höll, Davina and Leonie N. Bossert. 2022b. "Introducing the Microbiome: Interdisciplinary Perspectives." *Endeavour* 46, no. 1–2: 100817. https://doi.org/10.1016/j.endeavour.2022.100817.

Höll, Davina and Leonie N. Bossert. 2024. "Narrating the Uncanny Triad: Imagining Microbe, Animal, and Human Entanglements within the Planetary Health Humanities." In *Planetary Health Humanities and Pandemics*, edited by Heike Härting and Heather Meek. London: Routledge.

Huxley, Thomas Henry. 1851. "Zoological notes and observations made on board H.M.S. Rattlesnake during the years 1846–50." *Annals and Magazine of Natural History* 8, no. 48: 433–442.

Ironstone, Penelope. 2018. "Me, My Self, and the Multitude: Microbiopolitics of the Human Microbiome." *European Journal of Social Theory* 22, no. 3: 325–341. https://doi.org/10.1177/1368431018811330.

Käser, Rudolf. 2013. "Living with Rats and Mosquitoes: Different Paradigms of Cohabitation with Parasites in a German Narrative of Contagion around 1930." In *Contagionism and Contagious Diseases*, edited by Thomas Rütten and Martina King, 185–208. Berlin/Boston: De Gruyter. https://doi.org/10.1515/9783110306118.185.

Karafyllis, Nicole Christine, Jörg Overmann, and Ulrich Johannes Schneider, eds. 2021. *Die kontaminierte Bibliothek: Mikroben in der Buchkultur*. Leipzig: Leipziger Universitätsverlag.

Keetley, Dawn and Matthew Wynn Sivils. 2017. "Introduction." In *Ecogothic in Nineteenth-Century American Literature*, edited by Dawn Keetley and Matthew Wynn Sivils, 1–20. New York: Routledge.

King, Martina. 2013. "Anarchist and Aphrodite: On the Literary History of Germs." In *Contagionism and Contagious Diseases: Medicine and Literature 1880–1933*, edited by Thomas Rütten and Martina King, 101–130. Berlin/Boston: De Gruyter.

King, Martina. 2021. *Das Mikrobielle in der Literatur und Kultur der Moderne: Zur Wissensgeschichte eines ephemeren Gegenstands (1880–1930)*. Berlin/Boston: De Gruyter.

Kirksey, Eben. 2014. *The Multispecies Salon*. Durham: Duke University Press.

Kirksey, Eben and Stefan Helmreich. 2010. "The Emergence of Multispecies Ethnography." *Cultural Anthropology* 25, no. 4: 545–576.

Konopka, Allan. 2009. "Ecology, Microbial." In *Encyclopedia of Microbiology*, edited by M. Schaechter, 91–106. Amsterdam: Elsevier. https://doi.org/10.1016/B978-012373944-5.00002-X.

Košenina, Alexander. 2001. "Schönheit Im Detail Oder im Ganzen? Mikroskop und Guckkasten als Werkzeuge und Metaphern der Poesie." In "*Das Schöne Soll Sein." Aisthesis in der deutschen Literatur: Festschrift Für Wolfgang F. Bende*, edited by Peter Heßelmann, 101–127. Bielefeld: Aisthesis.

Landecker, Hannah. 2016. "Antibiotic Resistance and the Biology of History." *Body and Society* 22, no. 4: 19–52. https://doi.org/10.1177/1357034X14561341

Lederberg, Joshua. 2000. "Infectious History." *Science* 288, no. 5464: 287–293. https://www.science.org/doi/10.1126/science.288.5464.287

Lightman, Bernard. 2010. "The Microscopic World." *Victorian Review* 36, no. 2: 46–49. https://doi.org/10.1353/vcr.2010.0006.

Lorimer, Jamie. 2020. *The Probiotic Planet: Using Life to Manage Life*. Minneapolis: University of Minnesota Press.

Magnone, Sophia Booth. 2016. "Microbial Zoopoetics in Octavia Butler's Clay's Ark." *Humanimalia: A Journal of Human-Animal Interface Studies* 7, no. 2: 109–130.

Mbembe, Achille and Steve Corcoran. 2019. *Necropolitics: Theory in Forms*. Durham: Duke University Press.

"microbiome," n. (2020). *OED Online*. Oxford: Oxford University Press. www.oed.com/view/Entry/365863. Accessed March 13, 2023.

Mitrea, Laura, Silvia-Amalia Nemeş, Katalin Szabo, Bernadette-Emőke Teleky, and Dan-Cristian Vodnar. 2022. "Guts Imbalance Imbalances the Brain: A Review of Gut Microbiota Association With Neurological and Psychiatric Disorders." *Frontiers in Medicine* 9 (March): 813204. https://doi.org/10.3389/fmed.2022.813204.

Morar, Nicolae and Brendan J. M. Bohannan. 2019. "The Conceptual Ecology of the Human Microbiome." *The Quarterly Review of Biology* 94, no. 2: 149–175. https://doi.org/10.1086/703582.

Nicolson, Marjorie Hope. 1976. *Science and Imagination*. Hamden: Archon Books.

Otis, Laura. 1999. *Membranes: Metaphors of Invasion in Nineteenth-Century Literature, Science, and Politics*. Baltimore/London: Johns Hopkins University Press.

Outka, Elizabeth. 2020. *Viral Modernism: The Influenza Pandemic and Interwar Literature*. New York: Columbia University Press.

Ratcliff, Marc. 2009. *The Quest for the Invisible: Microscopy in the Enlightenment*. Farnham: Ashgate Pub.

Rees, Tobias, Thomas Bosch, and Angela E. Douglas. 2018. "How the Microbiome Challenges Our Concept of Self." *PLOS Biology* 16, no. 2: 1–7. https://doi.org/10.1371/journal.pbio.2005358.

Siebenpfeiffer, Hania. 2017. "Die Kunst des Minutiösen: Mikroskopie, Mikrografie und Mikropoetik bei Barthold Heinrich Brockes und Robert Hooke." In *Medienphilologie: Konturen Eines Paradigmas*, edited by Friedrich Balke and Rupert Gaderer, 240–268. Göttingen: Wallstein.

Slovic, Scott, Swarnalatha Rangarajan, and Vidya Sarveswaran, eds. 2022. *The Bloomsbury Handbook to the Medical-Environmental Humanities*. London: Bloomsbury.

Strowick, Elisabeth. 2009. *Sprechende Körper, Poetik der Ansteckung: Performativa in Literatur und Rhetorik*. München: Fink.

Sütterlin, Nicole A. 2023. "The Art of Living Well with Worms: Interspecies Relationships in Olga Flor's Posthuman Novel *Ich in Gelb* (2015)." *Gegenwartsliteratur: A German Studies Yearbook* 22.

Tomes, Nancy. 2002. "Epidemic Entertainments. Disease and Popular Culture in Early-Twentieth Century America." *American Literary History* 14, no. 4: 626–652.

Twain, Mark. 1968. "Three Thousand Years Among the Microbes." In *Mark Twain's Which Was the Dream? And Other Symbolic Writings of the Later Years*, edited by John Sutton Tuckey and Walter Blair, 433–533. California: University of California Press.

Vint, Sherryl. 2020. "Microbial Life and Posthuman Ethics from the Children Star to the Highest Frontier." In *Posthuman Biopolitics*, edited by Bruce Clarke, 111–132. Cham: Springer International Publishing. https://doi.org/10.1007/978-3-030-36486-1_6.

Vint, Sherryl. 2021. *Science Fiction*. Cambridge: The MIT Press.

UK Government. Department of Health and Social Care. *The Silent Pandemic of Anti-microbial Resistance*. https://www.gov.uk/government/speeches/the-silent-pandemic-of-antimicrobial-resistance. Accessed March 16, 2023.

Wald, Priscilla. 2008. *Contagious: Cultures, Carriers, and the Outbreak Narrative*. Durham: Duke University Press.

Weed, Kym. 2019. "Microbial Perspectives: Mark Twain's Imaginative Experiment in Ethics." *Literature and Medicine* 37 (1): 219–240. doi:10.1353/lm.2019.0008.

Williams, David M. and Robert Huxley. 1998. "Christian Gottfried Ehrenberg (1795–1876): The Man and His Legacy." *The Linnean* 1: 1–88.

Yong, Ed. 2017. *I Contain Multitudes: The Microbes Within Us and a Grander View of Life*. London: Vintage.

Zubeldia-Varela, E., TC Barker-Tejeda, D. Obeso, A. Villaseñor, D. Barber, and M. Pérez-Gordo. 2022. "Microbiome and Allergy: New Insights and Perspectives." *Journal of Investigational Allergology and Clinical Immunology* 32, no. 5: 327–344. https://doi.org/10.18176/jiaci.0852.

INDEX

www.ingramcontent.com/pod-product-compliance
Ingram Content Group UK Ltd.
Pitfield, Milton Keynes, MK11 3LW, UK
UKHW050950290926
15470UKWH00005B/1743

9 781350 296183